INTRODUCTION TO
HEALTH SERVICES

0-8273-5010-4

90000

9 780827 350106

For D. and N. Williams
and J., C., J. C., and N. Torrens

INTRODUCTION TO HEALTH SERVICES

FOURTH EDITION

Edited by

Stephen J. Williams, Sc.D.

Professor of Public Health
Head, Division of Health Services Administration
Graduate School of Public Health
San Diego State University
San Diego, California

Paul R. Torrens, M.D., M.P.H.

Professor of Health Services Administration
School of Public Health
University of California, Los Angeles
Los Angeles, California

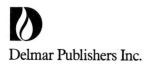

Delmar Publishers Inc.

NOTICE TO THE READER

Publisher and author do not warrant or guarantee any of the products described herein or perform any independent analysis in connection with any of the product information contained herein. Publisher and author do not assume, and expressly disclaim, any obligation to obtain and include information other than that provided to them by the manufacturer.

The reader is expressly warned to consider and adopt all safety precautions that might be indicated by the activities described herein and to avoid all potential hazards. By following the instructions contained herein, the reader willingly assumes all risks in connection with such instructions.

The publisher and author make no representations or warranties of any kind, including but not limited to, the warranties of fitness for particular purpose or merchantability, nor are any such representations implied with respect to the material set forth herein, and the publisher and author take no responsibility with respect to such material. The publisher and author shall not be liable for any special, consequential, or exemplary damages resulting, in whole or in part, from the readers' use of, or reliance upon, this material.

Delmar Staff
Senior Administrative Editor: Bill Burgower
Associate Editor: Elisabeth F. Williams
Project Editor: Mary Beth Ray
Senior Production Supervisor: Larry Main

For information, address Delmar Publishers Inc.
3 Columbia Circle, Box 15-015
Albany, New York 12212

Printed in the United States of America
Published simultaneously in Canada
By Nelson Canada
A Division of The Thomson Corporation

4 5 6 7 8 9 10   99 98 97 96 95 94

Library of Congress Cataloging-in-Publication Data
Introduction to health services/edited by Stephen J. Williams, Paul
   R. Torrens.—4th ed.
      p. cm.
   Includes index.
   ISBN 0-8273-5010-4 (textbook)
      1. Medical care—United States.   2. Health services
administration—United States.   I. Williams, Stephen J. (Stephen
Joseph), 1948–   II. Torrens, Paul R. (Paul Roger), 1934–
   [DNLM: 1. Health Services—United States.   W 84 AA1 I9]
RA395.A3I495   1993
362.1′0973—dc20
DNLM/DLC
for Library of Congress   92–18592
                                                    CIP

Introduction to the Series

This Series in Health Services is now in its second decade of providing top quality teaching materials to the health administration/public health field. Each year has witnessed further strengthening of the market position of each of the principal books in the Series, also reflecting the continued excellence of the products. Each author, book editor, and contributor to the Series has helped build what is widely recognized as the top textbook and issues collection of books available in this field today.

But we have achieved only a beginning. Everyone involved in the Series is committed to further expansion of the scope, technical excellence, and usability of the Series. Our goal is to do more for you, the reader. We will add new books in important areas, seek out more excellent authors, and increase the physical attributes of the book to make them easier for you to use.

We thank everyone, the authors and users in particular, who have made this Series so successful and so widely used. And we promise that this second decade will be dedicated to further expansion of the Series, and to enhancement of the books it contains to provide still greater value to you, our constituency.

Stephen J. Williams
Series Editor

Delmar Series in Health Services Administration
__ Stephen J. Williams, Sc.D., Series Editor

Introduction to Health Services, fourth edition
   Stephen J. Williams and Paul R. Torrens, Editors

Health Care Economics, fourth edition
   Paul J. Feldstein

Health Care Management: A Text in Organization Theory and Behavior, second edition
   Stephen M. Shortell and Arnold D. Kaluzny, Editors

Ambulatory Care, Management, second edition
   Austin Ross, Stephen J. Williams, and Eldon L. Schafer, Editors

Health Politics and Policy, second edition
   Theodor J. Litman and Leonard S. Robins, Editors

Strategic Management of Human Resources in Health Services Organizations
   Myron D. Fottler, S. Robert Hernandez, and Charles L. Joiner, Editors

SUPPLEMENTAL READER:
Contemporary Issues in Health Services
   Stephen J. Williams

Contributors

Lu Ann Aday, Ph.D.
Professor of Behavioral Sciences
School of Public Health
The University of Texas Health Science Center
Houston, Texas

A. E. Benjamin, Jr., Ph.D.
Professor in Residence and Associate Director
Institute for Health and Aging
School of Nursing
University of California, San Francisco
San Franciso, California

William L. Dowling, Ph.D.
Clinical Professor of Health Services
School of Public Health and Community Medicine
University of Washington
Vice-President, Planning and Policy Development
Sisters of Providence Corporation
Seattle, Washington

Connie J. Evashwick, Sc.D.
President
CEA—Consulting & Evaluation Associates
Los Angeles, California

Claudia L. Haglund, M.H.A.
Director, Corporate Planning
Sisters of Providence Corporation
Seattle, Washington

Alma L. Koch, Ph.D.
Associate Professor of Public Health
Graduate Program in Health Services Administration
Graduate School of Public Health
San Diego State University
San Diego, California

Philip R. Lee, M.D.
Professor of Social Medicine
Director, Institute for Health Policy Studies
University of California, San Francisco
San Francisco, California

Bryan R. Luce, Ph.D.
Senior Research Scientist
Director, Medical Technology Assessment Program
Batelle Human Affairs Research Centers
Washington, D.C.

Lawrence A. May, M.D., F.A.C.P.
Assistant Professor of Medicine
University of California, Los Angeles
Los Angeles, California

Stephen S. Mick, Ph.D.
Associate Professor
Department of Health Services Management and Policy
School of Public Health
The University of Michigan
Ann Arbor, Michigan

Ira Moscovice, Ph.D.
Professor and Associate Director
Institute for Health Services Research
University of Minnesota
Minneapolis, Minnesota

Mary Richardson, Ph.D.
Assistant Professor & Director, Graduate Program in Health Services Administration
Department of Health Services
University of Washington
Seattle, Washington

William Shonick, Ph.D.
Professor
Division of Health Services
School of Public Health
University of California, Los Angeles
Los Angeles, California

Paul R. Torrens, M.D., M.P.H.
Professor of Health Services Administration
School of Public Health
University of California, Los Angeles
Los Angeles, California

Gary S. Whitted, Ph.D., M.S.
Division Vice President
Managed Care and Employee Benefit Operations
Travelers Insurance Companies
Hartford, Connecticut

Stephen J. Williams, Sc.D.
Professor of Public Health
Head, Division of Health Services Administration
Graduate Program in Health Services Administration
Graduate School of Public Health
San Diego State University
San Diego, California

Contents

Foreword

Dramatic changes have occurred in our nation's health care system since the first edition of this book appeared in 1980. Yet the challenges and opportunities to provide the best possible health care for all of our citizens remain much as they were more than a decade ago. Ultimately, we still have a long way to go to ensure that the great promise of our health care system becomes reality for everyone.

We live in an exciting time in health care and medicine. We have reached frontiers in science that promise greater rewards in preventing, detecting, and curing disease than we could ever have imagined. We must make sure that this great knowledge is transformed into medical practice and provided to our citizens; that is the primary goal of the nation's health care system. As providers, administrators, and policy makers, that should be our goal as well.

Introduction to Health Services has, since its inception, served to inform and educate its audience about the health care system in an objective, analytical, and thoughtful manner. By bringing together some of the nation's most knowledgeable and articulate observers of the health care system, and by carefully crafting a logical, well-planned framework, the editors have designed a highly effective and informative work.

Everyone involved in health care has a duty to understand how the system functions and an obligation to participate in our search for better approaches. This book can be an integral component of the reader's search for such understanding.

It is also a personal pleasure, as a contributor to earlier editions of the book, including the first edition, to note the continued success of *Introduction to Health Services*. The editors have indeed served their readers well.

William C. Richardson, Ph.D.
President, The Johns Hopkins University
Baltimore, Maryland

Preface

For over 50 years our nation has faced a crisis in health care. We have struggled with the fundamental goals of providing cost-effective, high-quality care to all Americans. Yet politically, economically, and socially acceptable answers to these problems have continued to elude us.

The debate has continued and intensified since the last edition of this book was published. The nature of the system continues to evolve, but dramatic changes still may be needed. The objective of this book remains the same as in earlier editions: to educate the reader about the organization, structure, and operation of the nation's health care system in such a manner as to help him or her serve more effectively as provider, manager, decision maker, and analyst.

The fundamental structure of the book has been retained from previous editions. The book begins with an overview (in Part One) of the nation's health care system, as presented in Chapter 1. The overview provides an opportunity to set the stage for the chapters that follow as well as to present a coherent and relatively comprehensive perspective on the nation's health care system; each of the system's components is dissected and discussed individually in subsequent chapters. While the bulk of the book presents detailed analyses of each component of the system, it is always important to remember the larger contexts and interrelationships within which each of these components functions.

Part Two discusses the causes and characteristics of health services utilization in the United States. The nature of disease and illness is discussed in Chapter 2, particularly in the context of the principal categories of illness that lead to the use of health care services. Chapter 3 presents a comprehensive and integrated examination of the characteristics of utilization of services in the United States with particular emphasis on the variables that are associated with utilization.

Part Three presents detailed discussions of individual provider settings within which health care is offered to patients. The first chapter in this section, Chapter 4, discusses the history and current functions of public health services. Public health services remain our principal line of defense against disease and illness in society. Although public health services account for a relatively small fraction of health care expenditures, their importance far outweighs our spending in this area. In addition, the history and role of public health services in the United States is of immense importance in helping us address such societal issues as the priorities that we should assign to health care versus other activities in our economy, the obligations of government to protect the population collectively, and the responsibilities for ensuring access to care for individuals who lack services.

Chapter 5 focuses on the provision of ambulatory health care services. The increasing importance of ambulatory care in facilitating the integration of care is a key theme of this chapter and parallels the increasing focus of the book on the competitive marketplace, systems of care, and the financing of health care services.

Chapter 6 discusses the role of the hospital as well as the internal structure and operation of these important institutions. The hospital, too, has changed dramatically over the past few years as reflected by the changing content of this chapter. Hospitals have increasingly sought a more competitive posture for themselves individually and collectively, have aligned themselves with other organizations, and have battled for market share to ensure their long-term viability. The hospital is also changing in response to technological developments, changes in the role and power of the physician, and other developments. And, of course, as discussed throughout the book, dramatic changes in the way hospitals are paid, by both the private and public sectors, are forcing equally dramatic responses by all institutional providers of care.

Both long-term care and mental health services are undergoing change; the rate of change in these two areas is probably accelerating at a somewhat slower pace than is the case for the hospital or ambulatory care. Nevertheless, very significant changes have occurred since the last edition of the book in both long-term care and mental health services. The focus in Chapter 7 on the continuum of care is particularly germane to the increasing integration of providers in organized systems of care. Chapter 8 is an up-to-date and comprehensive discussion of the history and current status of mental health services in the United States. Change in this area has been more evolutionary than revolutionary, but the challenges for our society continue to grow.

Part Four deals with the nonfinancial resources needed to provide health care services. One of the most important of these resources is the technology used by physicians and other providers in identifying and combating illness. Technology is integral to the health care system since the nature of the technology often determines how care is provided, affects the structure of the institutions that provide care, and influences financing mechanisms. Advancements in technology and their critical evaluation can lead to lower morbidity and mortality and increased rationalization of resources. These key issues are discussed in detail in Chapter 9.

The second major area of resources used in the provision of health care is people. The health care system is one of the largest employers in the United States and as such is key to the economic well-being of the nation. In addition, of course, the increasingly specialized personnel required today make possible the provision of sophisticated, high-quality care. Trends and issues regarding health care personnel are discussed in detail in Chapter 10.

Part Five addresses financial resources: sources of funds, uses of funds, reimbursement mechanisms, incentives, insurance approaches, and related topics. This part begins with Chapter 11, which primarily focuses on reimbursement and financing mechanisms. Two new chapters have been added to the book to substantially expand this content section. Chapter 12 comprehensively addresses the insurance industry, employee benefits, and insurance plans. Chapter 13 discusses managed care plans, programs, and policy issues.

Part Six (Chapter 14) has been revised to discuss more concisely and directly measurement of system outcomes: quality of care, regulation and planning, and evaluation of services. Part Seven addresses, in Chapter 15, national health policy formation and execution. To conclude the book, Chapter 16 reviews our options for the future and possible directions for achieving national health care goals.

The nation has undergone many years of significant and wide-ranging changes in health care. Most Americans would probably like a health care system that is somewhat apolitical and more focused on meeting the health care needs of the American population. The reality, of course, is that politics are integral to all decision making. As a result, understanding the political process, and its implications, is critical to any realistic appraisal of where our health care system has been and where it is headed in the future. Thus Chapters 15 and 16 serve a very important function in helping the reader to evaluate the shifting political winds and the implications for the nation's health care system.

Chapter 16 also pulls together a number of key integrating concepts discussed throughout the book. But this chapter only sets the stage for the reader's further integration of knowledge and personal assessments of the health care system and thoughts about his or her role in that system.

It is important for readers to think through their value systems and personal ethical perspectives in reading this book. Health care cannot be divorced from individual and societal opinions and biases. Understanding one's personal perspectives is the key to forming assessments about where the health care system has been and the directions that are appropriate for the future.

As a nation, we have made dramatic changes in how we provide health care services. The rate of change itself may change in the future; but the fact remains that we will likely continue to modify the delivery system, attempt new approaches, discontinue old approaches, and make other judgments that will significantly affect how health care is provided, whom services are provided to, and how the bill is paid. Everyone—providers, payers, and consumers alike—has a key and active role in the health care system. The better everyone understands his or her role and the system itself, the better prepared all Americans will be to develop the best possible system.

As in the previous edition, a multidisciplinary approach is used. Empirical research is presented and summarized. The comments of colleagues, readers, and students have been integrated into the book.

Many people assisted in the preparation of the manuscript, reviewing drafts prepared for this edition, and in putting together the final manuscript itself. We are grateful to all who helped.

The goal of this book, to reiterate, is to provide information and a useful perspective from which readers can analyze what they do as a part of providing or consuming services. It is hoped that whatever this book can contribute to each individual's understanding of the system and its complex interactions will lead to a more rational, fair, and equitable system for all Americans.

Stephen J. Williams
Paul R. Torrens

PART ONE

Overview of the Health Services System

Chapter 1

Historical Evolution and Overview of Health Services in the United States

Paul R. Torrens

This chapter introduces the development, background, concepts, and issues of health care in the United States. The first section presents the historical evolution and development of health services in this country; the second section describes the current organization of services. Combined, these sections set the stage for the detailed analyses of the latter chapters in the book.

Historical Evolution of Health Services in the United States

The modern American health care system has had three important periods of development and has now entered a fourth. The first period began in the mid–nineteenth century (1850) when the first large hospitals, such as Bellevue Hospital in New York City and Massachusetts General Hospital in Boston, began to flourish. The development of hospitals symbolized the *institutionalization of health care* for the first time in this country. Before this time, health care in the United States was a loose collection of individual services functioning independently and without much relation to each other or to anything else. By today's standards, the first hospitals were not very remarkable, but they did provide the first visible institutions around which health care services could be organized.

The second important historical period began around the turn of the century (1900) with the *introduction of the scientific method into medicine* in this country. Before this time, medicine was not an exact science, but was instead a rather informal collection of unproved generalities and good intentions. After 1900, stimulated by the opening of the new medical school at the Johns Hopkins University in Baltimore, medicine acquired a solid scientific base that eventually transformed it from a conscientious but poorly equipped art into a detailed and clearly defined science.

With the coming of World War II, the United States underwent a major social, political, and technological upheaval whose effect was so marked that it ended the second and signaled the beginning of the third period of health care development.

3

The scientific advances continued unabated, but now they were paralleled by a *growing interest in the social and organizational structure of health care*. During this time, attention was first directed toward the financing of health care, with the resultant formation of health insurance plans such as Blue Cross and Blue Shield. This was also the time of increasing concentration of power in the federal government, as witnessed by the Hill-Burton Act (Hospital Survey and Construction Act), by the huge research budgets of the National Institutes of Health (NIH), and, more recently, by the passage of Medicare. Finally, during this period the principle of health care as a right, not a privilege, was widely discussed and generally accepted.

Since the early 1980s, the health care system in this country has moved into the fourth phase of its development, an era of *limited resources, restriction of growth, and reorganization of the methods of financing and delivering care*. Before this period, it had been presumed that the health care system would always be encouraged to grow and expand, both in size and in complexity, and that there would always be sufficient resources to support that expansion. Now it seems that the limits of our resources are being approached and that the health care system is being forced to consider options or alternatives to unrestricted growth and expansion.

Indeed, recent reimbursement policies introduced by Medicare and by employer-controlled insurance systems have caused a decrease in the numbers of inpatient days provided by hospitals each year and a reduction in the operating size of many hospitals. In the same vein, expert observers have suggested that the United States is rapidly approaching a major surplus of physicians and have advised that the numbers of new physicians being produced each year be greatly reduced. On all sides, there are pressures for smaller size, pressures to use less, and pressures to reduce expenditures in health care.

At the same time, the 1990s are witnessing the appearance of many new organizational models in health care. The idea of the health maintenance organization is spreading throughout the country, assuming widely different formats in different locations and situations. A variety of new enterprises have appeared to provide special services to patients and families at home. New intermediary organizations are appearing to provide reviews of quality of patient care and utilization of services. The term "joint venture" has become an accepted part of our health care language, now used to describe new forms of partnership activities between hospitals and physicians, hospitals and insurance companies, and hospitals with other hospitals. Virtually no health care organizational model has been left untouched by recent trends and changes.

Predominant Health Problems

Since the dawn of recorded history, human beings have repeatedly suffered the sudden and devastating appearance of epidemics of infectious disease. Plague, cholera, typhoid, smallpox, influenza, yellow fever, and a host of other diseases raged almost at will, creating havoc wherever they struck.

During the period 1850–1900 in this country, these epidemics of acute infectious diseases were the most critical health problem for the majority of Americans. Of particular importance were those diseases related to impure food, contaminated water supply, inadequate sewage disposal, and the generally poor condition of urban housing. During this time, for example, a cholera epidemic occurred throughout the country, resulting in an official death toll of 5071 in New York City alone and an unofficial toll several times higher. During this same period, yellow fever killed 9,000 in New Orleans in 1853, 2,500 in 1854 and 1855, and another 5,000 in 1858. Abraham Lincoln regularly sent his family away from the White House during the summer months to escape the "fevers," probably malaria, that swept through Washington.

By 1900, the epidemics of acute infectious disease had been brought under control due to improving environmental conditions. In the latter years of the nineteenth century, cities had begun to

TABLE 1-1. Death Rates for Leading Causes of Death, 1900 and 1990; United States

1900		1990	
Causes of Death	*Crude Death Rate per 100,000 Population per year*	*Causes of Death*	*Crude Death Rate per 100,000 Population per year*
All causes	1,719.0	All causes	848.4
Pneumonia and influenza	202.2	Diseases of the heart	288.1
Tuberculosis	194.4	Malignant neoplasms	196.4
Diarrhea, enteritis, and ulceration of the intestine	142.7	Cerebrovascular accidents	55.2
Diseases of the heart	137.4	Accidents	36.3
Senility, ill-defined or unknown	117.5	Chronic obstructive pulmonary diseases	35.8
Intracranial lesions of vascular origin	109.6	Pneumonia and influenza	29.8
Nephritis	88.6	Diabetes mellitus	18.9
All accidents	72.3	Suicide	14.3
Cancer and other malignant tumors	64.0	Chronic liver disease and cirrhosis	11.4
Diphtheria	40.3	Homicide	9.8

SOURCES: *Vital Statistics of the United States.* (1972). Washington, DC: U.S. National Center for Health Statistics. *Monthly Vital Statistics Report.* (September 27, 1990). U.S. National Center for Health Statistics, vol. 39, no. 6.

develop systems for water purification, for sanitary disposal of sewage, for safeguarding the quality of milk and food, and for monitoring the quality of urban housing. Health departments had begun to grow in numbers and in strength, and had begun to apply the methods of case finding and quarantine with satisfying results. Indeed, by 1900, as table 1-1 shows, those epidemics that had plagued humanity for centuries were now eliminated as major causes of death in the United States.

After 1900 the predominant health problems that attracted the attention of the health services system were those acute events, either infectious or traumatic, that affected individuals one by one. The pendulum had swung away from epidemics of acute infections that affected large numbers of people toward conditions of a personal nature that require individualized treatment. As table 1-1 shows, pneumonia and tuberculosis were the primary causes of death in 1900, with heart disease, nephritis, and accidents close behind.

Relieved from the burden of epidemic illnesses, the newly developed medical sciences turned their attention to better surgical techniques, the discovery of new sera for the treatment of pneumonia, and the development of new tests for more accurate and rapid diagnoses. Hospitals began to grow rapidly, medical schools flourished, and there was a general air of excitement that suggested the world was on the brink of significant advances in the treatment of individual illnesses.

Significant advances *were* being made. In Baltimore and Boston, the students of William Halsted, the pioneer surgeon at Johns Hopkins Hospital, began to operate on patients whose disease had previously been beyond the ability of surgeons. Advances in obstetrics now made it safer for women to have babies, and for the first time women did not approach childbirth with the fear of dying in delivery. Research work by two physicians, Banting and Best, in the laboratories of the University of Toronto led to the discovery of insulin in 1922, and for the first time diabetes could be effectively treated. Other research by Whipple, Minot, and Murphy on the causes of pernicious anemia led to successful medical treatments for that condition and further spurred the rush to find new treatments for other age-old conditions.

There were new discoveries on all fronts, each of which contributed some new advances in medical treatment. In 1928, however, in a cluttered laboratory at St. Mary's Hospital in London, a Scottish researcher, Alexander Fleming, produced the first of several discoveries that were to lead to the treatment of patients with penicillin for the first time in 1941. This discovery absolutely revolutionized medical care and totally changed the patterns of disease that threatened humanity. Within a few years after the treatment of the first patients with penicillin, antibiotics became readily available, and acute illnesses that had previously caused serious illness and possible death now meant nothing more than the discomfort of an injection and a few days of disability. Many older people experienced the incredible effects of the antibiotic era. When they had contracted pneumonia as children, their families had admitted them to hospitals and despaired for their lives; now, as older adults, they were told they had "a little pneumonia," given an injection of penicillin, and treated at home.

With the arrival of the antibiotic era in the 1940s and the subsequent conquest of acute infectious disease, the predominant problems of Americans became chronic illnesses. Since acute infections were no longer snuffing out the lives of children, people were living longer and beginning to manifest long-term chronic diseases such as heart disease, cancer, and stroke. As shown in table 1-1, these three conditions alone now account for two-thirds of all deaths. A similar review of the causes of disability would show arthritis, blindness, arteriosclerosis, and other chronic diseases to be the predominant causes of morbidity and limitation of function.

The rather sudden appearance of acquired immune deficiency syndrome (AIDS) in almost epidemic proportion in the early 1980s has further highlighted the changing pattern of disease. AIDS is apparently initiated by a viral infection that triggers extensive damage to an individual's immune system, leading to susceptibility to other infections and various forms of cancer. This combination of viral disease, immune system defects, and cancer as manifest in AIDS is probably only the first of many such new combinations of disease causation we must face. Chronic illness will certainly continue to be the predominant health problem of the American people in the future. Increasingly important will be chronic illness related to genetic makeup, personal lifestyles, and environmental hazards. Evidence is accumulating that suggests that many of the important chronic illnesses are related to how we live our personal lives, what hazards we subject ourselves to, and what dangers we allow our environment to impose on us. As we move into the 1990s, it is clear that chronic illnesses, particularly those related to genetic, environmental, and lifestyle causes, will be increasingly important.

The predominance of chronic illness as the major threat to health in the future raises a number of issues relevant to health professionals. First, as May points out in Chapter 2, the entire method of defining a chronic illness and determining its prevalence must be reexamined to obtain a more accurate picture of the situation. At the present time, a chronic disease is identified or documented on the basis of the first appearance of symptoms or on positive laboratory test results. In most cases, however, it is known that the disease process started long before the appearance of symptoms. In a practical sense, this forces one to ask: when should a chronic disease be considered to be present? The implications of the answer to this question for the planning and financing of health services could be enormous.

Chronic illnesses also have two important characteristics that directly affect both prevention and treatment. First, as was pointed out earlier, they often begin early in life, long before overt symptoms appear, the exact starting date for a chronic disease is never known. For example, many studies of apparently healthy young people who were victims of automobile accidents or other sudden death show that large percentages have already begun to develop early signs of chronic illness, detectable by pathological examination but not yet by clinical tests. Second, once a chronic illness is present, it remains with the patient forever. The *disease* is not cured by medical treatment; rather, its more prominent *symptoms* or external manifestations are treated.

Unfortunately, although the pattern of predominant illnesses has changed from epidemics of acute infections in the 1850s, to individual acute conditions in the 1900s, to chronic illnesses generally in the 1950s, and to special chronic illnesses in the 1980s, thinking about prevention and treatment has only recently begun to change. Acute infections very conveniently have a clear-cut beginning, middle, and end; as a result, they are amenable to one-shot solutions. If there is an epidemic caused by contamination of the water supply, the construction of a sewage treatment facility will eliminate it completely. If there is a threat of poliomyelitis infection, the ingestion of polio vaccine once or twice will permanently protect a population.

With chronic illnesses, however, prevention and treatment cannot be a one-shot affair, even though this is still how our health care system approaches them. Arteriosclerotic heart disease, for example, begins early in life and is probably affected by diet, cigarette smoking, stress, obesity, and several other factors that are directly related to personal habits and life-style. Prevention of these conditions cannot be accomplished by giving a person a single lecture on the evils of high-cholesterol food or the dangers of heavy cigarette consumption. Rather, prevention must be long-term, continuous, and aimed at bringing about major changes in an individual's knowledge of disease, personal values, and behavior patterns. Unfortunately, that understanding has been a long time in coming, but now seems to be taking hold quite strongly. The death

rate from heart disease has been dropping each year for the last 15 years, a result that is generally attributed to more aggressive early treatment and to major improvements in the prevention of some of the important causative factors.

Optimal treatment for long-term, continuous illness requires a system of health care that is, in itself, long-term and continuous. Unfortunately, the organization of our health services is still modeled on the disease patterns that were predominant in the 1900–1945 period and concentrates on individual episodes of illness as if they were separate and distinct entities. As a result, the health care system is primarily short-term and discontinuous in nature, and it treats chronic illness as if it were merely a series of separate acute episodes. This trend is further reinforced by the current method of financing of health services, with its great emphasis on paying for individual services rendered rather than on the long-term, continuous nature of the underlying disease process.

It should be noted that efforts are beginning to be made to develop longer-term and more continuous systems of financing and organizing patient care. There have been serious discussions regarding the development of a system of long-term care insurance and several long-term care insurance products have been introduced for early trial. Persons eligible for Medicare, the federally sponsored health insurance for those over 65 years of age, are being encouraged to join health maintenance organizations (HMOs). State and local governments are encouraging the creation of new case-management programs to improve the coordination of health and welfare services for the elderly.

It is entirely possible (and, indeed, probable) that the predominant disease patterns will be changing again in the future, creating an entirely different set of conditions that may require an entirely different array of services and interventions. It will be important for future generations of health professionals to watch for changes in predominant disease patterns to ensure a health care system that is genuinely pertinent and responsive to the problems of the day.

Technology Available to the American People

During the various developmental periods of the American health care system, what technology was available to handle the diseases that affected the American people? What tools were available to heal workers to conquer these conditions?

In the period 1850–1900, only a very rudimentary technology was available for the treatment of disease. The scientific base of medicine was still very narrow, and the number of effective medical treatments was very limited. Indeed, a great deal of energy and effort was expended on treatment, but whether a patient recovered from an illness usually depended more on the patient and the disease rather than the treatment.

Physicians during this period of time were poorly trained. They usually obtained their skills by serving apprenticeships with physicians already in practice and then taking short courses at unsophisticated medical colleges. What physicians had to offer was usually contained in their black bags, which they took with them wherever they went. They spent a good deal of time in patients' homes and almost no time at all in hospitals. In general, their practice was little different from that of their predecessors for centuries before them.

Nurses during the period 1850–1900 were not much better trained. Generally they were members of religious groups who volunteered to work in the few hospitals that existed, or they were poor, desperate, discarded women who frequented these institutions anyway and were pressed into service. Their work was nonscientific in the extreme and consisted simply of assisting patients with their usual bodily functions in any way possible. Not until the first training program for nurses was organized at Bellevue Hospital in the 1860s was there any formal preparation for this important role anywhere in the country.

As for hospitals themselves, they were merely places of shelter and repose for the sick poor who could not be cared for at home. Anyone who could stay at home usually did so, since hospitals had little to offer that would not be obtained at home if one had the money. Indeed, the hospitals of those days were often a direct threat to the lives of patients, since they were dirty, crowded, and disease-ridden. Infectious diseases frequently spread rapidly among hospitalized patients, and during the typhus epidemics of 1852 in New York City, for example, the highest mortality for the disease was among the patients and staff of the hospitals themselves.

After 1900 conditions began to change, spurred on by the new discoveries that were emerging from the research laboratories in this country and in Europe. In 1912, for example, a Polish chemist, Casimir Funk, published a paper, "The Etiology of Deficiency Diseases," in which he described "vitamines" and opened a whole new field of disease conditions to treatment. In 1908, James MacKenzie, in London, published his famous book *Diseases of the Heart,* and patients throughout the world were the beneficiaries. In countless medical schools and hospitals throughout this country and Europe, major scientific advances were achieved, each of which contributed to easier and safer diagnosis and treatment of acutely ill patients.

The medical schools led the way in many of these advances as a result of some basic reforms that took place in the early 1900s. Before this time, a large number of small, poorly staffed, free standing medical colleges existed throughout the country, 14 in Chicago alone in 1910 and 10 each in Missouri and Tennessee. In 1910, Abraham Flexner undertook a study of medical education for the Carnegie Foundation for the Advancement of Teaching and in his report, *Medical Education in the United States and Canada,* recommended that medical education in this country undergo radical reform. In particular, he strongly urged that the training of physicians be made a university function and that it be based on a firm scientific foundation. On the basis of Flexner's recommendations and the support of the Rockefeller Foundation, many of the small unaffiliated schools began to close and many of the remaining ones became part of universities, with the important result that physicians began to be trained as scientists as well as practitioners.

Gradually, physicians began to have more effective tools with which to work, and the range of their capabilities expanded rapidly. They still continued to spend the majority of their time in their offices or in patients' homes, but they now also began to look to the hospital for the care of their more severely ill patients. A small but gradually increasing number of physicians began to specialize in a particular area of medicine; however, by 1940, more than 80 percent were still in general practice.

Hospitals in the 1900s began to play an increasingly important role in health care. As more technology developed, it tended to be concentrated in hospitals, with the result that patients and physicians began going to hospitals for the technology to be found there. St. Luke's Hospital in New York City, for example, was 50 years old in 1906 when it opened its first private patient pavilion. Before that time, there had been no reason for private patients to go to a hospital, because they could usually get the same type of care in their homes. Now, however, hospitals began to offer services and skills that were not available anywhere else.

Although the period 1900–1940 was one of rapid growth in scientific technology, it was nothing compared to what happened with the advent of World War II. With the start of the war, this country mounted a massive effort to organize the best talents available for the care of the wounded and for the solution of the health care problems generated by the war. For the first time, relatively large efforts in research were begun under the direction of the federal government, and the results were impressive. The development of antibiotics accelerated rapidly, new surgical techniques for the treatment of trauma and burns were discovered, and new approaches to the transportation of the sick and wounded were developed. The range and breadth of problems that were subjected to organized investigation was remarkable, opening the way for an even more greatly expanded research

effort after the war ended. In 1950, the size of the research commitment begun during World War II had risen to $73 million per year, $35 million of which was distributed through the National Institutes of Health (NIH). By 1974, this expenditure had risen to an annual research budget of $2.5 billion, with $1.6 billion coming from a now greatly expanded NIH.

After World War II, hospitals were no longer the same. Previously, they had been places for the care of patients, with great emphasis being placed on the caring function. Now they became extensions of research laboratories, placed where medical science was practiced and where curing was the order of the day. New procedures, new equipment, and new techniques all flourished to such a degree that the hospitals were now captured by their technology. The technology itself was the motivating force for hospitals, and most major decisions were based on that technology.

The operation of these newly complex institutions called for waves of new workers, each more specialized and more highly skilled than the last. Before the war there had been approximately 20 major categories of health workers; by the 1970s there were hundreds. With the increasing specialization of services and skills, there was also an increasing interdependence of health workers on each other and an increasing reliance on the health care systems to integrate the work of so many separate groups.

Physicians were seriously affected by these trends. With the explosive growth of scientific knowledge after World War II, it was impossible for one physician to know everything, and so the trend toward specialization in a particular subarea of medicine had a strong impetus. Before the war, approximately 80 percent of physicians had been general practitioners and 20 percent specialists. In the years after the war, these percentages were reversed. In their training and practice, physicians focused increasingly on the scientific aspects of diagnosis and treatment, and as a result spent more time in hospitals and less time in patients' homes. The hospital became the emotional center of the physician's life, since it was here that the most important, most challenging and most interesting aspects of training or treatment occurred.

These trends affected nursing and the other health professionals to only a slightly lesser degree. The training of nurses and other health professionals became increasingly more scientific, more specialized, and more lengthy during the years after World War II. The desire to be recognized as competent in a particular area led to the proliferation of professional groups and to formal accreditation on the basis of scientific training and ability. It also led to university-based training programs in all of the health professions.

Today the technology available to the American health care system has advanced to an incredible degree. Organ transplantation, gene therapies for various conditions, laser beam surgical techniques . . . are all accepted as merely the expected developments of the technological age. The merging of technologies from fields other than medicine, such as the development of computerized axial tomographic systems and magnetic resonance imaging systems, has further added to the immense range of technology available to the health care system. However, this explosion of technology in recent years has not been without its problems. Indeed, the technology itself has *caused* a rather serious set of problems with which future generations of health care professionals must grapple.

One interesting problem introduced by technology is evaluation of the various new discoveries and techniques. Much new (and even some old) technology is adopted without appropriate evaluation of how effective it really is, and even more important, how much more effective it might be than already existing technology. Only limited examination of the cost implications of new technology is usually done before that technology is widely distributed throughout the health care system. Although it has not been customary to evaluate the effectiveness and the cost of technology in the past, economic pressures on the health care system in the future will certainly demand more care-

ful evaluation and scrutiny of technology before it is put into place for regular use.

Possibly a more important problem of medical technology is its impact on the form and configuration of the health care system and on the values and patterns of practice of the professionals in that system. In many ways, the American health services system has been captured by its technology and has been subtly and seductively shaped by its demands. Decisions regarding the design of programs and institutions, the training of personnel, and the distribution of services have been governed by technological considerations that loom larger every year.

A still more profound effect of technology is its ability to insinuate itself into the values of not just the system but also of the people who work in the system. The student entering a health profession rapidly learns that academic success and, later, professional success, comes from mastery of the scientific technology. Increasingly, the student views excellence as being reached through technical achievements and gives decreasing importance to the more personal, nontechnical aspects of disease. By the time the student becomes a fully accepted member of the profession, a value system has been established that views illness as a series of technical problems to be solved by the application of specific technical solutions. This value system is then reinforced in practice by the expectations of the public and by the requirements of the regulators, both of whom have come to view quality in terms of technical excellence. The result frequently is professional performance that is excellent in technical terms and rather poor in human terms.

A quite different problem of technology arises not from its excessiveness but rather from its inequitable distribution to society. There is more technology available than can be provided equitably to all people due to limits on funding, and large portions of society do not benefit as much as they should from technological advances. Marked differences exist, for example, in mortality and morbidity measures for white and nonwhite segments of society, possibly indicating an unequal access to modern health care technology. The answer obviously is to improve the health services system to ensure adequate distribution of available resources.

In summary, virtually no technology was available to treat disease before the 1900s. Technology began to appear and grow rapidly after the turn of the century. World War II fostered an incredible surge of research endeavors, with the result that the health care system began to be overwhelmed by the range and diversity of available technology. By the 1990s, the American health care system had been captured by its technology, and the challenge was to regain mastery over the giant that had been created.

Social Organization for the Use of Technology

How has our society organized to use the technology available to it? What has been the predominant view of the role of society in health care? During the period 1850–1900, no organized program was available for the use of whatever technology existed. Public services were rudimentary and were concentrated on a very narrow range of problems. There were hospitals in a few areas, but they were generally started by religious or charitable groups for the care of those who were obviously and publicly impoverished. The predominant ethic of the time was that people should care for themselves and be self-sufficient. If they become dependent, they should take advantage of and be grateful for the various charities established for these purposes.

This philosophy of rugged individualism and relative lack of large-scale social organization for health care predominated in this country until the 1930s, when the Great Depression struck with full force. At that time, economic forces beyond the comprehension of most Americans struck down many people, destroying their lives and leaving them destitute. The traditional belief in being totally and personally responsible for all aspects of one's life was badly shaken by the events of the Depression.

With the arrival of Franklin Roosevelt in the White House, the New Deal was launched and a wide array of social programs appeared, all aimed at repairing the damage of the Depression. The importance of the New Deal in terms of American social thought cannot be underestimated since, for the first time, American society created large-scale national programs to assist those who could not assist themselves.

In health care, governmental activity was still minimal, limited to a few specific areas of grant-in-aid programs to states to improve certain public health services such as infectious disease control and maternal and child health. Although the services were limited and aimed primarily at the poor, this small start did signify an assumption of responsibility by the national government for health care, at least for those who could not care for themselves.

The next major change in social organization and social thinking came with the arrival of World War II. As part of the mobilization effort, millions of men and women entered military service and in return received a wide array of health services simply by virtue of that service. The significance was twofold: (1) the services themselves were provided without charge by salaried physicians working for the government; and (2) they were provided as a right of those in the service and were clearly not charity for people who could no longer take care of themselves, as previous governmental efforts had been.

Not only did World War II accustom the country to large-scale health care programs provided by the society to its members, it also encouraged the growth of the health insurance industry. During the war, a freeze was imposed on wages and salaries so that very little collective bargaining for increases in salary could occur. However, considerable activity did occur in the development of pensions, disability programs, and health insurance plans, with the result that the health insurance industry began to flourish. This industry provided the American public with a new form of social organization—the "third party," or fiscal intermediary. Before the development of health insurance, the public had no form of social organization to protect it from a sudden onslaught of medical bills. With the arrival of this new phenomenon, health insurance, the American public began to gain experience in the cooperative effort of pooling many individual contributions for a common group objective—protection from financial disaster.

The period immediately after World War II witnessed the slow, tentative growth of the "Blue" plans, Blue Cross and Blue Shield, nonprofit community-based health care plans that insured against hospital and medical costs. With the success and growth of Blue Cross and Blue Shield, commercial insurance companies also entered the field, offering health insurance plans to employers and industry as part of their life/health/retirement/disability packages. With the rapid advances made by Blue Cross/Blue Shield and the commercial insurance carriers, the percentage of Americans covered by some form of health insurance rose from less than 20 percent before World War II to more than 70 percent by the early 1960s.

In the early 1960s, a major battle was fought and won by those advocating a greater societal role in the organization of health services. The battle involved the creation of government-sponsored health insurance plans for people over the age of 65 and resulted in the passage of legislation that created Medicare. Although Medicare itself was directed primarily to the needs of the country's elderly, its impact was soon felt throughout the entire health care system. The creation of the Medicare program had two immediate major social implications. First, Medicare provided financing for health care for all persons over the age of 65 simply on the basis of age; need was not a factor. The American society, in effect, determined that there were certain things the society should do for all of its members, regardless of individual need, since society could ensure equity. The second

major effect of Medicare was the assumption by the federal government of the responsibility for planning, financing, and monitoring a significant portion of the health care services in this country. The society not only wanted social insurance programs for health care, but also wanted the federal government to assume a central role in operating these programs.

A further significant change in the social organization of health care in this country occurred in the mid–1960s with the development of the Neighborhood Health Centers program of the U.S. Office of Economic Opportunity. In the War on Poverty, a number of health programs were funded for underserved areas of the country, each of which was required to have significant participation of consumers, often through governing boards and committees. This involvement of consumers was a substantial change from the past and soon became standard policy in new governmental programs. This philosophy was vigorously put forward in the National Health Planning and Resources Development Act of 1974, which required a majority of consumers on all local health planning boards. Although the health planning effort in this country has recenlty been dismantled to a large degree, the involvement of consumer advocates in health policy matters continues and will clearly be an increasingly important aspect of the U.S. health care system in the future.

It is interesting to note that, although consumer participation in local, state, and national health policy has decreased as a result of the demise of the health planning network, its decrease has been more than compensated for by the growth of employer and industrial involvement in health affairs. The growth of employer health care coalitions, and the more active involvement of various large employer purchasers of health insurance in matters of health policy, have created a new consumer advocacy force that promises to become an important part of the U.S. health care system in the future.

In the late 1970s and early 1980s, the health care system of this country, as noted previously, entered the fourth phase of its development, an era of *resource limitation, restriction of growth, and reorganization of systems of financing and of providing health care.* With the federal Medicare program experiencing increases in expenditures of 20 percent or more per year, interest has shifted toward a reduction of benefits, greater cost sharing by the elderly themselves, and a limitation on reimbursements to providers of service. Energies have now become focused less on the development of new services or the expansion of coverage and more on the control of costs through limitations and reductions. Indeed, recent changes in the manner in which Medicare reimburses hospitals ("Diagnosis-Related Groups") have been designed to encourage hospitals and doctors to provide less in the way of services and to sharply curtail or limit the number of services provided. In turn, this has led to a gradual shrinkage in the actual supply of staffed and operating hospital beds in the United States within the last few years.

These developments, to be discussed in detail in later chapters that deal with health care financing, planning, policy, and regulation, have also served to reinforce the increasingly powerful central role played by the federal government in the direction of health services. The federal government now not only controls a significant amount of the financial support for health care (approximately one-third of the total health care expenditures from all sources) but also, by using these massive resources in a unified and centralized manner, is able to set many of the rules by which, health care, governmentally funded or not, is provided. The health care system of this country, although by no means federally operated, certainly is federally dominated.

This country entered the twentieth century with the social philosophy that people should care for themselves or be satisfied with charity. In midcentury, it adopted the philosophy that society should care for those who, through no fault of their own, could no longer take care of themselves. Finally, toward the end of the century, it had moved to a philosophy that society, operating through the national government, should assume responsibility for solving certain large-scale problems of life for all of its members, even if some individual members can solve these problems for themselves. In very recent years, the country has begun to realize that some of the programs that it proposed earlier to solve one set of problems (for example, the development of a Medicare health insurance plan to protect the elderly from the economic effects of illness) have, in turn, created new problems (such as the rising cost of health care for everybody).

Summary of Historical Trends

The past 125 years of history have witnessed major changes in the American health care scene (table 1-2). The predominant health problems of our people have changed from epidemics of acute infections to a different kind of "epidemic," chronic illness. The range of technology available has mushroomed from about none in 1850 to a condition of such abundance now that the health care system has been virtually overwhelmed and captured by the technology it has created. Society's social values have changed from a *laissez-faire* approach in the 1850s that depended on individual initiative or organized private charity to one that now assumes the central role of the federal government in the organizing and financing of health care in the United States by means of various health insurance and regulatory mechanisms.

Overview of Health Services in the United States

When visitors from abroad, particularly those engaged in health services in their own country, come to the United States, they frequently want to know about the American health care system and how it works. They are usually puzzled by the answer they get:

There isn't any *single* "American health care system." There are many separate subsystems serving different populations in different ways. Sometimes they overlap; sometimes they are entirely separate from one another.

TABLE 1-2. Major Trends in the Development of Health Care in the United States, 1850 to Present

Trends	1850–1900	1900 to World War II	World War II to Present	Future
Predominant health problems of the American people	Epidemics of acute infections	Acute events, trauma, or infections affecting individuals, not groups	Chronic diseases such as heart disease, cancer, stroke	Chronic diseases, particularly emotional and behaviorally related conditions
Technology available to handle predominant health problems	Virtually none	Beginning and rapid growth of basic medical sciences and technology	Explosive growth of medical science; technology captures the health care system	Continued growth and expansion of technology, with attempts to repersonalize the technology
Social organization for the use of technology	None; individuals left to their own resources or charity	Beginning societal and govermental efforts to care for those who could not care for themselves	Health care as a right; governmental responsibility to organize and monitor health care for everyone	Greater centralization of responsibility and control in federal government; greater use of organized systems of health insurance and financing to shape and control developments within the health care system

SOURCE: Torrens PR: *The American Health Care System: Issues and Problems.* St. Louis, Mosby, 1978.

Sometimes they are supported with public funds, and at other times they depend solely on private funds. Sometimes several different subsystems use the same facilities and personnel; at other times, they use facilities and personnel that are entirely separate and distinct.

It should not be surprising that there is a multiplicity of health care systems (or subsystems) in the United States, given the historical development of health services in this country. In the earliest days, health care was entirely a private matter, and people were expected to take care of themselves by obtaining services of private physicians and nurses when needed, purchasing medications from drugstores and chemist shops, and paying for all these services personally. For those persons who could not take care of themselves, charitable institutions were established as voluntary, nonprofit corporations to provide charity health care. These

groups usually centered their efforts on hospitals and were usually located in the larger towns and cities of this country.

In the early twentieth century, a new element was added with the development of the city/county hospitals. These hospitals were established by local governments to care for the poor in their area who could not get care either by their own efforts or from the voluntary nonprofit charity hospitals. These public facilities were generally large, acute care, general hospitals, with busy clinics and emergency rooms and with close connections to local government ambulance services, police departments, and other community services. At the same time, state governments were developing mental hospitals. The cities had previously been responsible for the care of lunatics and the insane, but after the turn of the century, state governments began to assume this burden. Every state soon had at least one mental hospital where the emotionally disturbed were offered what little care was available.

With the explosive growth in the size of the federal government and in the numbers of persons in the armed forces during World War II, a separate system of care developed for active-duty military personnel and their dependents, retired military personnel, and veterans. These were almost entirely self-contained systems, employing salaried physicians and nurses, working entirely in military or veterans hospitals directly operated by the federal government.

As the cost of health care began to increase rapidly after World War II, the United States experienced a rather sudden and somewhat bewildering development of a wide variety of health insurance plans. The first to be operated were community-based nonprofit Blue Cross and Blue Shield plans, developed by hospital and physician associations to spread the cost of health care more widely among the population. These were followed by labor union health and welfare trust funds, established as a consequence of benefit negotiations for union members. At the same time, the private, for-profit commercial insurance companies expanded their efforts on behalf of both individuals and large groups of employees. Finally, several large government-sponsored and publicly supervised health insurance plans evolved, such as Medicare and Medicaid, the latter to aid the medically indigent.

Private medical practitioners, voluntary nonprofit hospitals, city and state government hospitals, military and veteran hospitals, and health insurance plans with a variety of forms and origins all developed in the United States at the same time, separately, and for specific purposes. The resulting picture has been described as having a rich diversity of opportunities and approaches for meeting the health care needs of a population that has in itself a rich diversity of people and situations. It has also been described as chaotic, uncoordinated, overlapping, unplanned, and wasteful of precious personal and financial resources. The reality probably lies somewhere in between.

If there is no single, easily described American health care system, at least some of the subsystems that compose the larger entity can be identified. Although an endless set of variations is possible, it seems appropriate to examine four models or subsystems of health care in the United States, each of which serves a different group. By looking at the components, the system as a whole may be better understood. These systems serve (1) regularly employed, middle-income families with continuous programs of health insurance coverage: (2) poor, unemployed (or underemployed) families without continuous health insurance coverage; (3) active-duty military personnel and their dependents; and (4) veterans of U.S. military service. For each of these systems, the manner in which basic elements of health care are provided is reviewed.

Employed, Insured, Middle-Income America (Private Practice, Fee-for-Service)

It is appropriate for two reasons to consider the system of health care used by the typically employed, insured, middle-income individual or family. First, this system is frequently described as *the* American health care system (all others, therefore, immediately becoming somehow secondary to it); second, this system is frequently said to include the best medical care available in the United States and perhaps anywhere in the world.

The most striking feature of the employed, insured, middle-income system of care is the absence of any *formal* system. Each family puts together an *informal* set of services and facilities to meet its own needs. The system, therefore, has no formal structure or organization and is different for each individual or family. Indeed, each family's system may vary widely according to the particular situation in which it is used. The only constant feature of this system is the family itself, all other aspects are transient, changeable, and widely varied.

Two other characteristics are also immediately noteworthy. First, the service aspects of the system focus on and are coordinated by physicians in private practice. Second, the system is financed by personal, nongovernmental funds, whether paid directly by consumers or through private health insurance plans. As the system is described, it will become readily apparent that these two features are not only important descriptively; they have been important in shaping the system in its present form.

Public health and preventive medicine services for the employed, insured, middle-income system are provided by two different sources. Those services designed to protect large numbers of people, such as water purification, sewage disposal, and air pollution control, are provided by local or state governmental agencies. Frequently, these agencies are called *public health departments.* They usually provide their services to the entire population of a region, with no distinction between rich and poor, simple or sophisticated, interested or disinterested. Indeed, these mass public health services are common to all the systems of health care to be discussed. Those public health and preventive medicine services that are aimed at individuals, such as well-baby examinations, cervical cancer smears, vaccinations, and family planning, are provided by individual physicians in private practice. If a middle-income family desires a vaccination in preparation for a foreign trip or wants the blood cholesterol level of its members checked, the family physician is consulted and provides the service. If it is time for the new baby to have its first series of vaccinations, the family pediatrician is usually the one who provides them.

Ambulatory patient services, both simple and complex, are also obtained from private physicians. Many families use a physician who specializes in family practice, while others use an array of specialist physicians such as pediatricians, internists, obstetrician/gynecologists, and psychiatrists who provide both primary care and specialty services. When special laboratory tests are ordered, X-ray films required, or drugs and medications prescribed, private commercial for-profit laboratories or community pharmacies are used. Many of these services, from individual preventive medicine services to complex specialist treatments, are financed by individuals through out-of-pocket payment, since most health insurance plans do not provide complete coverage for these needs. When the middle-income family begins to use institutional services, such as hospital care, the source of payment shifts almost completely from the individual to third-party health insurance plans.

Inpatient hospital services are usually provided to the employed, insured, middle-income family by a local community hospital that is usually voluntary and nonprofit. The specific hospital to be used is determined by the institution in which the family physician has medical staff privileges. Generally, the smaller, less specialized, more local hospitals will be used for simple problems, whereas the larger, more specialized, perhaps more distant hospitals will be used for more complicated problems. Many of these larger hospitals have active physician training programs, conduct research, and may have significant charity or teaching wards. The employed, insured, middle-income family obtains its long-term care from a variety of sources, depending on the service required. Some long-term care is provided in hospitals and, as such, is merely an extension of the complex inpatient care the patient has already received. This practice was more common in the past, but utilization review procedures have increased the pressure on hospitals to reduce the length of time people are hospitalized. More commonly, long-term care is obtained at home through the assistance of a visiting nurse or voluntary nonprofit community-based nursing service. If institutional long-term care is needed, it is probably obtained in a nursing home or a skilled nursing facility, usually a small (50–100 patients) institution, operated privately, for profit, by a single proprietor or small group of investors. Recently, there has been a general increase in size (100 + patients per facility) and a trend toward absorption of individual facilities into larger multifacility proprietary chains. The employed, insured, middle-income family usually pays for its long-term care with its own funds, since most health insurance plans provide relatively limited coverage for long-term care.

When employed, insured, middle-income families require care for emotional problems, they will again use a variety of mostly private services. However, as the illness becomes more serious, families may, for the first time, rely on government-sponsored service. When emotional problems first begin to appear in the employed, insured, middle-income family, the patient will probably turn to the family physician, who may provide simple supportive services such as tranquilizers, informal counseling, and perhaps referral for psychological testing. The physician may even arrange for the patient to be hospitalized in a general hospital for a rest, for "nervous exhaustion," or for some other non-psychiatric diagnosis. If the emotional problems become more severe, the family physician may refer the patient to a private psychiatrist, or to a community mental health center that most likely will be a voluntary nonprofit agency or under the sponsorship of one (such as a voluntary nonprofit hospital). If hospitalization is required, the psychiatrist or the community mental health center is likely to use the psychiatric section of the local voluntary nonprofit hospital if it seems that the stay in a hospital will be a short one. If the hospitalization promises to be a long one, the psychiatrist may use a psychiatric hospital, usually a private, nongovernmental community facility.

In those cases in which very extended institutional care is required for an emotional problem and the patient's financial resources are relatively limited, the middle-income family may request hospitalization in the state mental hospital. This event usually represents the first use of government health programs by the middle-income family, and as such it frequently comes as a considerable shock to patient and family alike.

In summary, the employed, insured, middle-income family's system of health care is an informal, unstructured collection of individual services put together by the patient and the private physician to meet the needs of the moment. The individual services themselves have little formalized interrelationship, and the only thread of continuity is provided by the family's physician or by the family

itself. In general, all the services are provided by nongovernmental sources and are paid for by private funds, either directly out-of-pocket or by privately financed health insurance plans.

For all of its apparent looseness and lack of structure, the employed, insured, middle-income family's system of health care allows for a considerable amount of decision and control by the patient, more than that of the other systems to be discussed. The patient is free to choose the physician, the health insurance plan, and frequently even the hospital. If additional care is required, the patient can seek out and use (sometimes overuse) that care to the limit of the financial resources available. If the patient does not like the particular care being provided, dissatisfaction can be expressed in a more effective manner; the patient can seek care elsewhere from another provider. Even with the newer managed care approach to health insurance, which attempts to influence people to obtain care from lower-cost physicians and hospitals, the influences are indirect and economic in nature (i.e., a discount for using the lower-cost providers) and certainly not coercive or directive (i.e., mandating that a person can use only certain providers in order to be insured at all).

On the other hand, the employed, insured, middle-income family's system of care is a poorly coordinated, unplanned collection of services that frequently have little formal integration with one another. It can be very wasteful of resources and usually has no central control or monitor to determine whether it is accomplishing what it should. Each individual service may be of very high quality, but there may be little evidence of any "linking" taking place to ensure that each service complements the others as effectively as possible.

One special subset of the middle-income model now involves millions of patients in this country. When people reach age 65, they are automatically eligible for Medicare, the federally sponsored and supervised health insurance plan for the elderly. A patient covered by Medicare benefits can utilize the same system of care as the middle-income family, including private practice physicians and voluntary nongovernment hospitals. The main difference now is that the bills are paid by a federal government health insurance plan, rather than the usual private plan in which the typical middle-income family is enrolled. The physicians are the same and the hospitals are the same; only the health insurance plan is different.

Many employed, insured, middle-income families no longer receive their various health services in piecemeal fashion, one at a time, from various independent practitioners who have no formal relationship to one another. Now, instead, many people belong to health maintenance organizations (HMOs) that contract to provide an organized package of health services in an integrated and intentionally coordinated program. These HMOs usually do not provide much in the way of long-term care but do provide just about everything else to some degree. It should be noted that, whereas in the past, HMO membership was usually made up of people under the age of 65, recent changes in the Medicare program have created incentives for people over the age of 65 to join HMOs as well as incentives for HMOs to enroll them. As a result, elderly people are now joining HMOs in the same fashion as younger people have in the past.

Unemployed, Uninsured, Inner City, Minority America (Local Government Health Care)

A second major system of health care in the United States serves those people who are not regularly employed, don't have continuous health insurance coverage, and often are minority group members living in the inner city. While the specific details may vary from city to city, the general outline is well known in all major cities of the country. If it was important to study the system of health care for the employed, insured, middle-income population because it represented the *best* health care possible in this country, it is equally important to study the care of the poor, unemployed, and uninsured, since it frequently represents the *worst*.

The most striking feature of the health care system of the poor, inner-city resident is exactly

the same as that characterizing the middle-income family system: there is no *formal* system. Instead, just as in the middle-income system, each individual or family must put together an *informal* set of services, from whatever source possible, to meet the health care needs of the moment. There is one significant difference, however: The poor do not have the resources to choose where and how they will obtain their health services. Instead, they must take what is offered to them and try to put together a system from whatever they are told they can have.

There are two important characteristics of the system. First, the great majority of services are provided by local government agencies such as the city or county hospital and the local health department. Second, the patients have no real continuity of service with any single provider, such as an employed, insured, middle-income family might have with a family physician. The poor family is faced with an endless stream of health care professionals who treat one specific episode of an illness and then are replaced by someone else for the next episode. While the middle-income system of health care can establish at least some thread of continuity by the ongoing presence of a family physician, the poor family cannot.

The poor obtain their mass public health and preventive medicine services, including a pure water supply, sanitary sewage disposal, and protection of milk and food, from the same local government health departments and health agencies that serve the middle-income system. In contrast to the middle-income system, however, the poor also get their individual public health and preventive medicine services from the local health department. When a poor family's newborn baby needs its vaccinations, that family goes to the district health center of the health department, not to a private physician. When a low-income woman needs a Papanicolaou smear for cervical cancer testing or when a teenager from a low-income family needs a blood test for syphilis, it is most likely that the local government health department will give the test.

To obtain ambulatory patient services, the poor

family cannot rely on the constant presence of a family physician for advice and routine treatment. Instead, they must turn to neighbors, the local pharmacist, the health department's public health nurse, or the emergency room of the city or county hospital. It has often been said that the city or county hospital's emergency room is the family physician for the poor, and the facts generally support this contention: When the poor need ambulatory patient care, it is quite likely that the first place they will turn is the city or county hospital emergency room.

The emergency room also serves the poor as the point of entry to the rest of the health care system. The poor obtain many of their ambulatory services in the outpatient clinics of the city and county hospitals. To gain admission to these clinics, they must frequently first go to the emergency room and be referred to the appropriate clinic. Once out of the emergency room, they may be cared for in two or three specialty clinics, each of which may handle one particular set of problems but none of which will take responsibility for coordinating all the care the patient is receiving.

When the poor need inpatient hospital services, whether simple or complicated, they again usually turn to the city or county hospital to obtain them. Admission to the inpatient services of these hospitals is usually obtained through the emergency room or the outpatient clinics, thereby forcing the poor family to use these ambulatory patient services if they wish later admission to the inpatient services. The poor may also turn to the emergency room, the outpatient clinics, and the inpatient ward or teaching services of the larger voluntary nonprofit community hospitals. Since these hospitals are frequently teaching hospitals for the training of physicians, they often maintain special free or lower-priced wards. It is to these wards that the poor are usually admitted. Since the care in the teaching hospitals is generally as good as or better than any that might be obtained at the local city or county hospitals, many poor are willing to become teaching cases in the voluntary nonprofit hospitals in exchange for better care in better surroundings.

By and large, however, city and county hospitals carry the largest burden of inpatient care for the poor.

If the long-term care situation of middle-income people is generally inadequate, the long-term care of the poor can only be described as terrible. In contrast to the system of care for the middle-income families, most of the long-term care of the poor is provided in the wards of the city and county hospitals, although not by intent or plan. The poor simply remain in hospitals longer because their social and physical conditions are more complicated and because the hospital staffs are reluctant to discharge them until they have some assurance that continuing care will be available after discharge. Since this status is often uncertain, poor patients are likely to be kept longer in the hospital so that they can complete as much of their convalescence as possible before discharge. Most of the long term care of the poor is provided in the same types of nursing homes or skilled nursing facilities that are used by the middle-income—either the smaller (50–100 patients) facilities, operated for profit by a single proprietor, or the larger (100+ patients) facilities operated by a proprietary chain. One major difference between the systems used by the poor and the middle-income is the quality of the facility used. The middle-income generally have access to better-equipped and better-staffed nursing homes, while the poor are admitted to less expensive, less well-equipped facilities. Another important difference between the middle-income and the poor is that employed, insured, middle-income patients are more likely to pay for their own care in these institutions, while the poor have their care paid by welfare, Medicaid, or other public funds.

It is interesting to note that the system of health care for the employed, insured, middle-income utilizes entirely private, nongovernmental facilities until long-term care for mental illness is required; at that point, a governmental facility, the state mental hospital, is used. By contrast, the system of health care for the poor is composed almost entirely of public, government-sponsored services until long-term care is required. This care is usually provided in private, profit-making facilities, the first such use of private facilities by the poor.

The convergence of the poor and the middle-income systems of care in the private profit-making nursing homes is important, since it represents an important feature of our multiple subsystems of health care. In many cases, several systems of health care that are otherwise separate and distinct will merge in their common use of personnel, equipment, and facilities. The emergency rooms of the city or county and voluntary nonprofit teaching hospitals, for example, will serve as the source of emergency medical care for the middle-income family that cannot reach its own family physician. They will also serve as the family physician for the poor family that has none of its own. The private, for-profit nursing home will serve as the source of long-term care for the middle-income family, and may provide the same function for the poor. The radiology department of the voluntary nonprofit teaching hospital will provide X rays for the middle-income patient whose care is supervised by the private family physician, as well as for the poor patient whose care is supervised by a hospital staff physician in training. This does not mean that there is any real, functional integration of the separate systems of care because of their use of the same facility or personnel. Rather, the model is more like that of a busy harbor in which a variety of ships will berth side by side for a short period of time before going their separate ways for separate purposes.

In their use of services for emotional illnesses, the poor return once again to an almost totally public, local government system. Initial signs of emotional difficulties are haphazardly treated in the emergency rooms and outpatient clinics of the city or county hospital. From here, patients may be referred to the crowded inpatient psychiatric wards of these same hospitals, but are just as likely to be referred to community mental health centers operated by local governmental or voluntary nonprofit community agencies. When long-term care in an institution is required, the poor are sent to the psychiatric wards of the city or county hospital, and from there to the large state governmental mental hospitals, frequently many miles away.

In the past, health services for the poor were usually free, at least to the patients. The local health department, the city or county hospital or the state mental hospital generally did not charge for its services, regardless of the patient's ability to pay. In the last few years, both local health departments and city and county hospitals have been forced to initiate a system of charges for services that were previously free. They have done this to recapture third-party payments to which the poor patient might be eligible, and patients who are unable to pay are still ordinarily provided the services they need. The imposition of these charges for previously free health services has probably changed the perception of these programs by the poor, but it is still too early to determine the implications of these changes.

As with the employed, insured, middle-income system, there is a subset of the health care system for the poor that requires special comment. Certain persons who are poor enough by virtue of extremely low income or resources may qualify for Medicaid, the federal-state cooperative health insurance plan for the indigent. Under Medicaid people whose income and resources are below a level established by the individual states can use a state government-sponsored health insurance program to purchase health care in the private, middle-income marketplace. The purpose of this program is to move the poor out of their usual local government health care system and into the supposedly better private practice health care system of the middle-income. Unfortunately, the ability of Medicaid to move the poor into a better system of care had been limited by the reluctance of private physicians and private hospitals to assume responsibility for many Medicaid patients. This reluctance has been based on what has been seen as a low rate of reimbursement by Medicaid for services provided, an often cumbersome system of paperwork and prior authorizations in order to provide care and a frequently irrational system of retroactive denials of payment for services already provided.

Medicaid has succeeded to a degree in helping poor patients move from local government hospitals into voluntary nonprofit teaching hospitals, but its greatest effect has probably been in moving poor patients into private, profit-making nursing homes and skilled nursing facilities. In some states, for example, more than 60 percent of all patient bills in private nursing homes are now paid by the Medicaid program, providing some indication of the importance of this program to the provision of long-term care. And for all its problems, the Medicaid program has allowed certain aspects of the employed, insured, middle-income system of health care to be shared with the poor, inner-city minority system of health care—a blending, merging, or sharing of resources and services that is characteristic of the American health care system and that makes it so difficult to evaluate any one subsystem cleanly and separately.

Unfortunately, with the recent tendency to cut back on the Medicaid program at both the national and state levels, this movement of poor patients into the middle-income system may abate considerably and may even be reversed. As less and less Medicaid money becomes available to purchase care in the middle-income system for poorer patients, they may increasingly have to fall back once again on the resources of the city and county public hospital, as in the past.

A second subset of the system of care for the poor and uninsured is that system that exists for poor people who turn 65. Immediately on reaching age 65, they are eligible for Medicare and ostensibly should be able to take their new insurance coverage and move into the private, middle-income system of care. Unfortunately, this movement from public to private provider systems by poor people who become 65 years of age is limited by the deductible and coinsurance features of Medicare. Under Medicare everyone (poor included) is expected to spend several hundred dollars for health care first, before Medicare begins to pay bills. Even when this deductible requirement is met, the el-

derly person is also required to pay the first $500 or so for each hospitalization, in addition to the previously mentioned deductible. The level of available cash to pay these deductibles and coinsurance limits the ability of many poor people to take full advantage of the benefits of Medicare when they become eligible at age 65.

In summary, the system of health care for the poor is as unstructured and informal as that for the employed, insured, middle-income, but the poor have to depend upon whatever services the local government offers them. The services are usually provided free of charge or at low cost, but the patient has relatively little opportunity to express a choice and exercise options. Poor patients often cannot move to another set of services if they dislike the one first offered, since those first offered are usually the only services available.

Like the system of health care for the middle-income, the system for the poor is poorly coordinated internally and almost completely unplanned and unmonitored. It is certainly as wasteful of resources as the middle-income system, but because it is a low-cost, poorly financed system, the exact amount of waste is difficult to document. At the same time, the great virtue of the health care system for the poor—its openness and accessibility to all people at all times for all conditions (albeit with considerable delays)—is difficult to evaluate adequately as well.

Certainly, the most important issue for the system of care that presently serves the poor is whether it will be able to survive much longer without a new source of financial support. As more and more city and county governments find themselves in deep financial difficulties, as more and more states and local areas pass laws limiting the amount of tax revenue a local (or even a state) government can raise, the financial situation of local government units becomes increasingly shaky; so too does the financial situation of the public health and hospital services they provide. The key issue in the survival of the system that provides care for the poor is financial, and the prospects are increasingly bleak.

Military Medical Care System

A person joining one of the uniformed branches of the American military sacrifices many aspects of civilian life that nonmilitary personnel take for granted. At the same time, however, this person receives a variety of fringe benefits that those outside the military do not enjoy. One of the most important of these fringe benefits is a well-organized system of high quality health care provided at no direct cost to the recipient. Certain features of this military medical care system (the general term used to include the separate systems of the U.S. Army, Navy, and Air Force) deserve comment. First, the system is all-inclusive and omnipresent. The military medical system has the responsibility of protecting the health of all active-duty military personnel everywhere and of providing them with all the services they may eventually need for any service-connected problem. The military medical system goes where active-duty military personnel go, and assumes a responsibility for total care that is unique among American health care systems.

The second important characteristic of the military medical care system is that it goes into effect immediately whether the active-duty soldier or sailor wants it or not. No initiative or action is required by the individual to start the system; indeed, the system frequently provides certain types of health services, such as routine vaccinations or shots, that the soldier or sailor would really wish not to have. The individual has little choice regarding who will provide the treatment or where, but at the same time, the services are always there if needed, without the need to search them out. If a physician's services are needed, they are obtained; if hospitalization is required, it is arranged; if emergency transportation is necessary, it is carried out. There is little that the individual can do to influence how medical care is provided, but at the same time, there is never any worry about its availability.

The third important characteristic of the military health care system is its great emphasis on keeping personnel well, preventing illness or injury, and finding health problems early while they are still amenable to treatment. Great stress is placed on preventive measures such as vaccination, regular physical examinations and testing, and educational efforts toward prevention of accidents and contagious diseases. In an approach that is unique among the health care systems of this country, the military medical system provides health care and not just sickness care.

In the military medical system, the same mass public health and preventive medicine services that are provided to a locality or a community by a local government health department or health agency may also be provided to the active-duty military personnel. However, whenever the personnel are actually within the boundaries of a military reservation or post, an additional set of mass public health and preventive medicine servicers may be provided by the military itself. Sanitary disposal of sewage, protection of food and milk, purification of the water supply, and prevention of vehicular or job-related accidents may be provided for by a local government agency, but each military installation will usually have a second separate system of its own, staffed by its own public health and safety officers. Individual public health and preventive medicine services are also provided by the military medical system according to a well-organized, regularly scheduled routine of yearly examinations, surveys of patient records, vaccinations, and other measures. The persons providing the specific preventive service (for example, a routine tetanus shot) are usually medical corpsmen or other nonphysician personnel; however, their work is carried out according to carefully developed guidelines and will be monitored by well-trained supervisory medical personnel.

Routine ambulatory care is usually provided to most active duty military personnel by the same medics who provide the individual preventive services. These services are usually provided at the dispensary, sick bay, first aid station, or similar unit that is very close to the military personnel's actual place of work. These ambulatory services may also be provided by physicians or nurses at the same locations, but this is less likely. More complicated ambulatory patient care services are usually provided by physicians, frequently specialists, working at the same dispensary or medical station as the medics or, more likely, in a clinic or outpatient department of a larger facility such as a military hospital. Patients are usually referred by medics or physicians who have first cared for the patients for simpler problems; laboratory tests, X-ray examinations, and medications are obtained at the same military facility to which the patient is referred.

The simplest hospital services are provided using short-stay beds at base dispensaries, in sick bays aboard ship, or at small base hospitals on various military installations around the world. Usually the range of services that can be offered at these installations is limited, and referral to larger institutions is routinely carried out if a more complex problem is suspected. More complicated hospital services are provided to active-duty military personnel in regional hospitals that possess a wide variety of specialized services and facilities. Frequently, these hospitals also have large teaching and training programs, where the atmosphere and the quality of care are similar to what might be expected at a university hospital or a large community teaching hospital.

The military medical system does not pretend to offer the same extensive range of long-term care services that it provides for more acute short-term problems. The military medical system does provide care for potentially long-range problems in military hospitals, as long as there is some reasonable expectation that the patient will someday be able to return to full active duty. Whenever it is determined, however, that the problem is genuinely long-term in nature and that complete return to active duty is not possible, the patient is given a medical discharge from the service and long-term care will be provided through the Veterans Administration (VA) facilities.

If military personnel develop emotional difficulties, care is most likely to be provided initially by the medical corpsperson and then by a physician assigned to that military unit. These personnel will provide short-term nonpsychiatric support and

counseling, and possibly prescribe certain medications, such as tranquilizers. For more severe problems, the patient is referred to the psychiatric services of larger military hospitals where the severity of the problem will be determined. If the problem is short-term and is not believed to affect the patient's work seriously, an attempt may be made to provide the short-term treatment at the military hospital itself, first on an inpatient and later on an outpatient basis. More likely, if there is a significant psychiatric diagnosis, the patient will be given a medical discharge, with follow-up care to be provided through the psychiatric services of the VA hospitals.

In general, the military medical system is closely organized and highly integrated. A single patient record is used, and the complete record moves from one health care service to another with the patient. Once the need for health care is identified, the system itself arranges for the patient to receive the required care and usually even provides transportation to the services. The patient does not have to search out the necessary service or determine how to use it. This service is provided at no cost to the patient, requires little effort by the patient to initiate it, and generally involves a high-quality product. The system is centrally planned, uses nonmedical and nonnursing personnel to the utmost, and is entirely self-sufficient and self-contained. The services are provided by salaried employees in facilities that are wholly owned and operated by the system itself. The system is not generally available to persons who are not active-duty military personnel or their dependents, although in cases of emergency or pressing local need, they can be. Generally, the patient has little choice regarding the manner in which services will be delivered, but this drawback is counterbalanced by the assurance that high-quality services will be available when needed.

Dependents and families of active-duty military personnel are served by a special subsystem of military medicine that combines the services of the middle-class middle-income system and the active-duty military system. The dependents and families of active-duty military personnel are covered by an extensive health insurance plan, the Civilian Health and Medical Program of the Uniformed Services (CHAMPUS), provided, financed, and supervised by the military. This health insurance plan allows dependents and families of active-duty personnel to purchase medical care from private practitioners, from health maintenance organizations, and from local community nonmilitary hospitals when similar services cannot be provided at a military installation within a reasonable distance. The dependents and families of active-duty military personnel can also use the same military services that the active-duty personnel use, provided space and resources are available and military authorities determine that this procedure is appropriate. The resulting subsystem of care for military dependents and families generally allows them to participate to some degree in two separate systems of care: the middle-class, middle-income private practice system and the military medical system. Their participation in either is generally not as clearly focused or as active as it would be for someone firmly planted in either system exclusively, but it still provides them with two viable options for obtaining care.

Veterans Administration Health Care System

Parallel to the system of care for active duty military personnel is another system operated within the continental United States for retired, disabled, and otherwise deserving veterans of previous U.S. military service. Although the VA system is in many respects larger than the system of care for active-duty military personnel, it is not nearly as complete, well integrated, or extensive. At the present time, the VA system focuses largely on hospital care, mental health services, and long-term care. It operates 171 hospitals throughout the country that provide most VA care. In recent years, the VA has increasingly provided outpatient services and now maintains more than 200 outpatient clinics; however, the majority of VA health care is still focused on the hospitals.

A second important characterisitic of the VA system is the great preponderance of male patients with multiple-system problems. By and large, the patients using the VA health care system are older, inactive men in whom the occurrence of multiple and chronic physical and emotional illnesses is much higher than in the general population.

A third important feature of the VA system is its existence as only one part of a much larger system of social services and benefits for veterans. Many of the people eligible to use the VA health care system are also receiving other kinds of financial benefits as well; indeed, access to the VA health care system is sometimes directly dependent on eligibility for financial benefits of various kinds. These include educational assistance grants, disability compensation, and home loans. Since health care is only one of many VA programs, a great variety of social services interact with and compete for available resources.

A further feature of the VA health care system is its unique relationship with organized consumer groups. Since the VA is organized to provide care exclusively for veterans, and since many of those veterans are members of local and national veterans' clubs and associations, the VA health care system is constantly in direct communication with groups representing the interests of veterans. In a manner that is unparalleled in any other health care system in this country, the interests of the veterans are constantly conveyed to individual VA hospitals, to the VA administrative body in Washington D.C., and to the U.S. Congress. In no other health care system in this country does organized consumer interest play such a constant, important, and influential role.

Since the VA system is primarily a hospital system, there are few attempts to provide general public health services or routine ambulatory care services. Veterans usually obtain these services from some other system of care, either the middle-income system or the local government system that serves the urban poor. The VA does provide the more complicated ambulatory services, usually through its hospital outpatient clinics. This care is in preparation for possible hospital admission or as follow-up after hospitalization. Many veterans who require these services obtain them from other systems of care and come to the VA system only after a condition is apparent and hospitalization is required. Admission to VA hospitals can be gained through the ambulatory patient care services operated by the VA itself, by direct referrals from physicians in private practice, or by referrals from hospitals in the community. The services in VA hospitals are provided by salaried, full-time medical and nursing personnel; as in the military medical system, most of the VA hospitals are self-contained, relatively self-sufficient units that require little outside support or staff.

The VA health care system provides a tremendous quantity of long-term care for both physical and emotional illnesses. Indeed, the VA is probably the largest single provider of long-term care in the country, if not the world. In addition to providing considerable long-term care in the acute, short-term care hospitals, the VA also operates a number of domicilaries and nursing homes and pays for care in local community nursing homes and skilled nursing facilities. As of early 1982, 18 VA hospitals also offered hospice or hospice-like care to their patients who were dying of cancer.

The VA system of care is difficult to describe fully for two important reasons. First, it is a system that does not attempt to provide a complete range of services, but instead concentrates on acute hospital services and on long-term care for physical and emotional problems. Second, eligibility for entry into the system is somewhat unclear and sometimes open to variable local interpretation. The system is designed to serve veterans with service-connected disabilities, but offers services to other veterans if they cannot obtain adequate care elsewhere and if adequate VA resources are available. In practice, the actual eligibility requirements and patient mix vary substantially from one VA hospital to the next.

If the system of health care for active duty military personnel focuses on preventive, ambulatory, and acute inpatient care, the VA system of care stresses long-term, chronic inpatient care for both physical and emotional problems. Whereas the military medical system offers a complete, well-integrated, well-coordinated package of health care services, the services that the VA offers are primarily hospital-related. In contrast to the military medical system, which actively seeks out and offers services to patients as part of their work environment, the VA provides its services to patients only when they come forward to seek them. If they do not seek out the care, the VA system does not actively pursue them. Despite these reservations about the VA as a complete system of health care, it should be stressed that the VA serves as the primary source of inpatient hospital care for hundreds of thousands of veterans each year and is a potential source of inpatient care for millions more. As such, it is the largest single provider of health care services in this country and must be considered an integral, important component of the American health care scene, both now and in the future.

Health Services: A Summary of Perspectives

In reviewing each of these four major systems of health care for Americans—the system for employed, insured, middle-income families who use the private sector services; the local government system for the urban poor; the military medical system for active-duty military and their dependents; the VA system for veterans—it becomes apparent that there are a number of additional systems that could have been included as well. Other systems of health care include the one used by rural farming families and the Indian Health Service operated for Native Americans by the federal government. There are also many possible variations within the four systems discussed here. The purpose, however, is not to be exhaustive in describing the systems themselves but rather to point out that there are multiple systems providing services to different populations with different needs. No one system predominates in terms of persons served or benefits provided. Indeed, the purpose here is to point out that there is no one single American health care system but rather a mosaic of subsystems, each with its own characteristics and moving in its own direction.

Is it bad to have so many separate subsystems? Why is it even worth pointing out the obvious fact that many such systems exist? Several pressing reasons exist for reviewing this country's compartmentalized organization of health care. The first and most important reason is quite simple: To improve health service to everyone in the country, an understanding of the component parts of the present health care structure is essential. Without a fundamental understanding of the separate component parts, it is impossible to understand the whole structure. Without an understanding of the interaction among the component parts, one cannot design really appropriate and effective interventions and changes.

The second reason for considering the various separate systems of health care in this country is the vigorous competition for scarce resources of money, people, and facilities. Although the four systems described are separate from one another, they all compete for the same resources since they are all dependent on the same economy and the same supplies of health personnel and skills.

Whenever there is vigorous competition for resources, two things frequently happen. First, the stronger, more vigorous, more aggressive, or better connected competitors obtain the larger portion of the resources, whether or not this outcome is justified by their needs. In practice, this has meant that the middle-income/private practice system, the military medical system, and the VA system have all done relatively well, while the local government health care system for the poor has always been severely underfinanced and understaffed, a situation that seems to be getting progressively worse.

Second, intense competition for resources frequently results in wasteful duplication and ineffective use of resources. For example, in the same region, a city or county hospital, a private teaching hospital, a military hospital, and a VA hospital may all be operating exactly the same kind of expensive service, although only one facility might be needed and where undoubtedly one large integrated service would provide more efficient use of resources than four smaller ones. Because each institution is part of a separate system, serves a different population, and approaches the resource pool through a different channel, no really purposeful planning or controlled allocation of resources is possible. In the past, this situation might have been acceptable because the resources seemed endless, but in these days of very limited resources, this is no longer acceptable.

In addition to this economic inefficiency, there are other reasons for looking with a critical eye at multiple systems of care, reasons that are related to quality and accessibility of services. Unfortunately, not all of these subsystems of care serve people in the same way with the same results. There is great inequality among the various systems of health care, with the result that different people receive different levels of care simply by accident of birth or membership in a special group. Since all the separate systems of health care in this country ultimately depend on public funds for their continued existence, it is imperative that the inequalities among them be removed as rapidly as possible. This does not necessarily mean eliminating the various separate subsystems of care, but rather requires that all the systems rise to a common high level and equitably share responsibilities and resources.

In recent years, there have been various approaches to the problem of reorganizing these separate subsystems of care so that they function together in a more integrated and effective fashion. Although these proposals have often been limited to specific aspects, such as financing or quality of care, their overall purpose has generally been to move the various pieces of the American health care system into a better and more efficient relationship with each other. These approaches are interesting not only in themselves but also as examples of approaches that will be used to change the American health care system in the future. The specific scenarios may change, but the types of approaches will continue to be proposed, just as they have been in the past.

Two proposals can be mentioned briefly, not because they are unimportant but rather because the possibility of their implementation is so slight that they have relatively little practical impact. The first of these might be described as a *laissez-faire,* free-market approach that implies in effect, "Leave everyone alone, stop meddling, stop regulating, and let the workings of the marketplace with its active competition eventually force the health care system to reorganize." The second approach, at the other political and social extreme, implies, "What this country needs is a single, government-controlled health care system, such as the British National Health Service, which would allow for greater centralized control and planning for all aspects of the system." Although some aspects of the marketplace approach are increasingly being applied, the free-market proposal as a total system reform has gained little general support. In the same fashion, the national health service approach has stimulated some interest but little active support. Both of these approaches as total system reforms have been viewed as politically, organizationally, and socially impractical for the United States at this time.

Another approach that has been considered has been the health planning approach. With the passage of the original Comprehensive Health Planning legislation and, more important, with the passage of the National Health Planning and Resources Development Act of 1975, it had been thought that providers, consumers, and public officials might come together and develop plans for all states and localities that would then become blueprints for a more rationally organized system of care. This hope did not turn into reality, and with the demise of the health planning system, this approach toward more rational coordination of health care services has been virtually abandoned for the time being. It seems clear that more rational allocation of resources will be increasingly impor-

tant in the future, but it is doubtful that there will be a return to anything resembling an intentionally planned and integrated health care system, controlled by a government-sponsored health planning system.

A somewhat different approach to rationalizing the American health care system focuses on the use of financing mechanisms to encourage or force increased coordination of effort throughout the system. The proponents of this approach suggest that the power to withhold financial reimbursement to providers who do not comply with efforts to improve the system would be so strong as to be irresistible. Although the argument is used most visibly by many of the proponents of a national health insurance plan, this approach has become more apparent in the way the Health Care Financing Administration (HCFA) uses Medicare funds to encourage compliance with its long-range objectives. It is also becoming increasingly obvious in the way certain employer health care coalitions are using their influence over the industrial concerns' health insurance dollars as a means of making their wishes known. Indeed, it would have to be said that the greatest forces shaping the organization and functions of the health care system today are financial, and the greatest power to affect how the system will work in the future is in the hands of the large third-party payers for health care. In the absence of any other effective mechanism to reorder and reorganize the health care system, control of the financing mechanisms is being substituted for other forms of planning or supervision.

Another possible solution, which has yet to receive considerable attention, is the public utility approach. In this approach toward a more rational health care system, all the components of the health care system, or at least the large institutional ones, would be placed under the regulatory supervision of public bodies that would have total control over licensing, financing, mode of function, packages of services to be offered, personnel development, and so forth. Both public and private components could continue to exist as they do at present under their own auspices (just as individual utilities do now, for example), but what they would be able to do and how much they would be allowed to charge would be controlled by a single regulatory agency. A strong argument for this approach is that all of these regulatory efforts are now conducted in a poorly coordinated and often conflicting fashion by multiple regulatory agencies. Having one single body would remove much of the present jungle of regulatory efforts. A strong argument *against* such a body is that immense power over the system would be given to a single superagency. Practically speaking, in the present antiregulatory political climate in this country, there is little enthusiasm for this approach.

A final approach toward rationalization of the present system might be called incremental tinkering and it is one that tacitly assumes that no major, sweeping, overall reorganization is possible. The proponents of this approach try instead to do whatever they can to increase rationality whenever an opportunity occurs anywhere in the system. A new piece of state legislation here, a new form of federal health insurance there, a new form of local cooperative planning are all added in piecemeal fashion, with no great effort to relate them to each other or to some underlying master plan. The hope in this approach is that all the individual accretions to the system will provide for a more efficient and integrated end product.

These six approaches are obviously not mutually exclusive, so it is entirely possible that someone might support several of them because they work well together. Someone interested in reorganizing the health care system through health planning might also want to institute a national health insurance program because it would provide the centralized financial leverage for mandatory health planning. In the same fashion, someone might propose a mostly *laissez-faire* approach to any intentional reorganization and also support a national health insurance plan that would allow all people to make their own choices in an open market.

In the future, all six approaches (and possibly more) will probably continue to be fostered and most likely no single approach will predominate. What certainly will continue, however, will be efforts to bring the various pieces of the subsystems and the various subsystems themselves into a more efficient and effective new relationship with one another and with the consumers who must use them. Indeed, this issue is so important and so central to all our other interests that the future of health care in this country will be shaped by the direction our society decides to follow in this regard.

PART TWO

Causes and Characteristics of Health Services Use in the United States

What conditions/types of illness do ppl seek care for?

How has this changed?

Does supply/distrib of providers have an impact?

Chapter 2

The Physiologic and Psychological Bases of Health, Disease, and Care Seeking

Lawrence A. May

In this chapter, the physiological bases of disease and the psychological characteristics of care-seeking behavior are explored. The concepts of illness and disease and the complexities surrounding the exact definitions of diseases are discussed. The orderly relationship among pathologic abnormality, physiologic alteration, and clinical manifestations of disease are presented, especially as they relate to care-seeking behavior. The influence of biologic, pharmacologic, and environmental factors on changing disease patterns is reviewed, and some of the effects of these changing disease patterns on the health services system are demonstrated as a prelude to the remaining chapters of the book.

Defining Illness and Disease

The distinction between illness and disease is essential for the understanding of care-seeking behavior. Illness is a lay experience that connotes both a physical and a social state (1). It is an individual's reaction to a biologic alteration and is defined differently by different people according to their state of mind and cultural beliefs. The term *illness,* therefore, is imprecise and represents an individual response to a set of physiologic and psychological stimuli.

By contrast, *disease* is a professional construct. It is perceived as being precise and reflecting the highest state of professional knowledge, particularly that of the physician. The definition of disease is used as the vehicle for informing the patient of the presence of pathology, as a means for deciding on a course of treatment, and as a basis for comparing the results of therapy. It becomes an essential element in the planning and organization of the health care system and in the allocation of resources within that system.

The accurate definition of disease is so important that it is crucial to recognize that considerable imprecision exists in the process of medical diagnosis. An individual physician using the best professional judgment available may diagnose a disease in a particular patient, but this definition

31

may not be shared by other physicians. Even when the definition of a particular disease is similar in different patients, the impact of the diagnosis on those patients may vary widely depending upon how the definition is applied and on the unique social and biologic characteristics of individual patients.

Attempts to link illness (the individual's perception of loss of functional capacity) with disease (the professional's definition of a pathologic process) is even more complicated. Illness may occur in the absence of real disease, and disease may be present in the absence of perceived illness. It is illness, the individual's perception of impaired function, and not disease that stimulates care-seeking behavior, making the relationship between these two concepts important to understand.

There can be difficulty in defining illness and disease, and significant cognitive dissonance between physician and patient may result. Mitral valve prolapse, a rather common abnormality of a heart valve with a prevalence of 5–10 percent of the population, has had an assortment of symptoms attributed to it. Fatigue, irritability, dizziness, and palpitations have all been suggested as symptoms of this condition. However, a study at Duke University failed to reveal any difference in symptoms in the patients with objectively conformed mitral valve prolapse from a group that had been referred for echocardiographic studies in which no mitral valve prolapse was discovered (2). Although the control group in this study was not selected randomly, it illustrates that symptoms may exist and be attributable to a medical disease that are, in fact, equally prevalent in a similar population without the disease.

This problem is further illustrated in the case of _hypertension, which physicians acknowledge as an asymptomatic condition, but one to which patients attribute a wide variety of symptoms. The generally acknowledged symptoms of headache, ringing in the ears, and nosebleeds failed to be confirmed as having any greater prevalence in those with hypertension than those without. The need for patients who perceive themselves as ill to have a disease explanation for their symptoms can pose a major

challenge to physicians; and if a medical explanation for essentially functional symptoms is provided, notable care-seeking behavior can result.

A powerful example of this has been the possible association of chronic fatigue with persistent infection with the Epstein-Barr virus (3). This was originally reported in a group of 90 patients who were evaluated for persistent fatigue by several physicians near Lake Tahoe in California (4). The media coverage of this situation created a tremendous interest on the part of patients in determining whether they might be suffering from a disease for which there is admittedly no cure, and for which such poorly defined parameters exist, that physicians cannot conclude that the disease actually exists. (A similar historical example was hypoglycemia, which produced numerous physical visits for glucose tolerance tests that are generally felt to be unnecessary; true hypoglycemia is rare and symptoms are generally absent in patients with blood sugar levels below the reported normal levels.) The search for an etiologic agent in the well-described syndrome of chronic fatigue has led investigators to consider other etiologic agents, such as herpes virus type 6. Other authors have offered enteroviruses, Borrelia, and a novel retrovirus as possible etiologic agents for chronic fatigue syndrome. The ability of science to establish specific etiology to relatively commonly described and experienced syndromes is apparently limited. (5).

The complexity of defining disease and its interaction with care-seeking behavior is well illustrated by the condition diabetes mellitus. Both the general public and the health care professional understand that diabetes results in an elevated blood sugar level, but the physiologic bases of this metabolic alteration can vary widely (6). In one person, the disease may result from impaired secretion of insulin by the pancreas, or it may be caused by a resistance to sufficient amounts of insulin in a patient who is obese. Diabetes mellitus may result from the imposition of a normal physiologic condition such as pregnancy, or it may be due to the use of exogenous drugs such as diuretics or steroids.

Aside from the varying causes of an elevated blood sugar level (referred to as *hyperglycemia*), an important issue is the amount of hyperglycemia that defines a patient as diabetic. Various criteria have been suggested to define who is diabetic, using different numerical measures of elevated blood sugar level, but these criteria do not necessarily separate those who feel healthy, nor do they define a level at which treatment is indicated (7). The myriad criteria that have been applied to diabetes at one time or another would define anywhere between 4 percent and 40 percent of the population over age 60 as having diabetes. In recognition of the fact that even objective measures of disease or health such as blood sugar determination are variable, great effort was expended to reach a consensus on what level of blood sugar elevation defines diabetes. The criteria state that the level must be consistently elevated in the fasting and postprandial states and that this level must be found on two separate occasions. The current criteria for diagnosing diabetes are a fasting blood sugar level of 140 and a blood sugar level of more than 200 measured two hours after eating on two separate occasions. The previously widely used glucose tolerance test is expensive, unnecessary, and results in an excessive number of false-positive readings sacrificing specificity in a way that is unacceptable (8).

The problem illustrated by diabetes extends to many other disease conditions that are defined by an abnormal laboratory measurement or blood test result. Hypertension is a common medical problem resulting from a variety of physiologic bases, including abnormalities in hormone production and use, improper resetting of neurologic control centers, or acquired loss of blood vessel elasticity secondary to atherosclerosis.

In view of the variety of causes of hypertension, the selection of an arbitrary number to define individuals or members of a population as having an abnormal condition is a difficult and possibly futile effort. The blood pressure reading of 140/90

has been offered as the boundary of normality, but the meaning of this reading in different persons may vary markedly. A blood pressure of 150/100 in a 72-year-old woman has quite different implications from the same reading in a 26-year-old man. An elevated blood pressure after a half hour of bed rest means something quite different from an elevated blood pressure in a person waiting anxiously for half an hour in a physician's office.

To complicate matters further, as with diabetes, there is no direct relationship between the presence of elevated blood pressure and the development of either perceived symptoms or actual pathologic damage to body organs, at least at the lower ranges of hypertension. Some people with only slight hypertension will attribute a variety of functional complaints to their "blood pressure," whereas others with dangerously elevated levels may not have any symptoms and perceive themselves as being well (9, 10).

The definition of diabetes or of hypertension is relatively straightforward when compared to diseases that cannot be numerically defined, such as rheumatoid arthritis. The definition of this disease is clinical rather than numerical and is based on the presence of four or more diagnostic characteristics determined by the American Rheumatism Association to be valid criteria for the disease. Even with the use of this symptom aggregation approach, there are still many professionals who confuse rheumatoid arthritis with degenerative joint disease and with other forms of arthritis. Further, even with this more orderly approach to the definition of this disease, the ability to measure its impact on a population is comparatively limited.

In summary, the definition of disease is a more imprecise and inexact process than is usually thought. Although it is frequently associated with apparently solid, objective measurements such as blood sugar levels or blood pressure, the implications of these values may vary widely. Finally, the relationship between illness, which is a personal observation by patients, and disease, which is a scientific judgment by professionals, needs to be understood and constantly remembered.

Disease Processes: The Physiologic Bases of Disease

The major pathophysiologic processes involved in disease production are vascular, inflammatory, neoplastic, toxic, metabolic, and degenerative. These processes give rise to disease conditions, but their expression is modified by factors in the host such as age, immunologic status, medication ingestion, concurrent disease, or psychological perceptions. The combination of the pathophysiologic processes and the different host factors creates the various patterns of disease presentation.

Vascular abnormalities may produce disease in a variety of ways in multiple-organ systems. The gradual narrowing and eventual blockage of blood vessels by the deposit of fatty materials in the walls and lumina of the vessels is a characteristic of arteriosclerotic cardiovascular disease. Vascular disease may also be produced by the more rapid occlusion of a blood vessel by an embolus, material from a distant site floating in the bloodstream. Other disease pictures may be produced by bleeding from a ruptured blood vessel in the brain or elsewhere. In some disease conditions, such as stroke, the same clinical picture may result from any one of these three causes. Whatever the initial cause, gradual occlusion, embolus, or rupture, the result is damage to brain tissue and resultant paralysis. It is usually easy to determine that a cerebrovascular accident (stroke) has occurred, but it is frequently impossible to determine whether it was caused by gradual occlusion, embolus, or rupture of a blood vessel.

Inflammation is the basis of disease in many organ systems, but the physiologic basis of that inflammation may be infectious, autoimmune, traumatic, or something else. A single inflamed joint may be due to autoimmune inflammation, the presence of uric acid crystals, or degeneration of cartilage as a consequence of age and use, or it may be due to infection with bacteria or virus. The failure to identify the specific etiologic factor can be highly destructive to the patient or at least fail to resolve the problem in the appropriate amount of time. Therefore, having defined both the type of disorder and the mechanism of inflammation, physicians must seek to identify the underlying agent in the process of inflammation.

Neoplastic disease is caused by an abnormal new growth of tissue. Benign neoplasms are abnormal growths that remain localized and do not spread to distant locations in the body. Malignant neoplasms, generally called *cancer,* by contrast, not only grow locally and invade surrounding tissues but also spread to distant sites in the body, producing metastases. Benign neoplasms may cause considerable damage by continued local growth and pressure on surrounding tissues, such as pressure on the brain from a benign growth on its surface. Malignant neoplasms, by contrast, invade the organs directly and disrupt their normal functioning by replacing normal tissue with diseased tissue. Neoplasms may occur spontaneously or may be caused by environmental, toxic, or host factors (11,12,13,14,15).

Toxic bases for disease involve the presentation to individual organs of chemical materials that are inherently damaging. These materials may originate from environmental pollutants, from the use of potentially damaging materials such as alcohol or cigarettes, or from the ingestion of medications. Alcohol, for example, is toxic to the liver under appropriate conditions, causing hepatitis, fibrosis, and eventual cirrhosis. Cobalt in beer can be toxic to heart muscle cells, bee stings may damage the glomerulus of the kidney, and asbestos may contribute to the development of lung cancer. Cigarette smoking may destroy, inflame, or alter the cells of the lung, producing emphysema, chronic bronchitis, or cancer. Digitalis, an ordinarily useful drug in the treatment of various heart conditions, in excess doses may produce toxicity and life-threatening arrhythmias. In a society with an increasing amount of environmental pollution, drug use, and industrial exposure, toxins are unfortunately becoming a more common cause of disease. The widening hole in the ozone layer is producing precipitous increases in the incidence of cutaneous malignancies (16).

Metabolic diseases are caused by chemical disorders within body cells, usually secondary to excess or deficiency of a hormone or nutrient. The excess or deficiency of a thyroid, parathyroid, or adrenal cortical hormone causes clinical disease pictures that are easily recognized by well-trained physicians. A deficiency of insulin, secreted by glands in the pancreas, gives rise to diabetes, as mentioned earlier. Deficiency of important nutrients, caused either by a scarcity of the elements in the diet or by an inability to absorb and use them, results in a wide variety of clinical pictures ranging from anemia to pellagra. The incidence of deficiency states in the developed world is still staggering, and simple supplementation with such minerals as iodine or such vitamins as vitamin A have produced dramatic improvement in health status (17).

Degeneration is the final pathophysiologic cause of disease, and may occur as a primary idiopathic disorder or secondary to another process such as aging. Physicians generally resist accepting degeneration as an explanation for disease, but there are many diseases that currently cannot be otherwise explained. For example, many people with senile dementia have a pathologic process of unexplained primary degeneration of brain cells. Degenerative joint disease is usually related to age and may be accelerated by unusual use or trauma, but it remains primarily a degenerative process with no specific vascular, metabolic, or inflammatory explanation.

It should also be clear that a particular disease can be caused or affected by a variety of pathophysiologic mechanisms. Peptic ulcer, for example, is a common disease with a multifactorial physiologic basis. The ulceration of the mucosal lining of the duodenum is caused by gastric acid, may occur in genetically predisposed people, and may be abetted by the toxic effect of drugs such as aspirin or corticosteroids that impair the protective barrier of the mucosa. After all the insights about ulcer pathogenesis, both psychologic and dietary, the real cause may emerge to be an infectious agent known as Helicobacter pylori (18). There

may be a secondary inflammation producing pain or obstruction, and the ulcer may erode a blood vessel, producing bleeding. To say that any single pathophysiologic process "causes" ulcers would be misleading.

Once the initial pathophysiologic process has given rise to a particular disease entity, its clinical manifestations are modified by a variety of host factors such as age, immunologic status, medication ingestion, concurrent disease, or psychological makeup. For example, in a healthy person with high tolerance for pain, a case of herpes zoster (shingles) may be perceived as a minor discomfort, whereas in a person with a low threshold for pain, it may become a disabling illness for which professional attention and potent analgesics are required. Under the influence of a concurrent disease or the ingestion of drugs such as steroids, which suppress the immunologic response, a usually nonpathogenic fungal infection may produce serious illness. A minor inflammation of the connective tissue such as cellulitis, for example, may become a serious, life-threatening problem in a diabetic with an impaired vascular, sensory, or immunologic status. In a genetically susceptible host, an infectious agent may precipitate an inflammatory response and antibody production leading to systemic lupus erythematosus, whereas in a genetically nonsusceptible host it may not produce any effect.

Thus, there are a variety of pathophysiologic processes that can initiate disease, but the expression of the disease itself may be modified by a variety of factors in the host. Any review of a particular disease entity, therefore, should include consideration of both aspects, so that a complete understanding of the disease can be developed.

Symptom Production and the Pathologic Process

A pathologic process may begin and exist silently for some time without producing any evidence of physiologic alteration. Although the disease is present and active, it may be undiscovered. In many chronic disease situations, it is now well known that the disease condition may be present for a considerable length of time before becoming detectable by current diagnostic procedures. Atherosclerosis, for example, has been detected at autopsy in healthy young 18-year-olds dying from accidental causes (19,20); many prostatic cancers are discovered at autopsy that were never recognized during life.

After a pathologic process has been present for a time, it may not only begin to produce physiologic alterations that can be discovered by appropriate diagnostic tests but may also begin to produce clinical symptoms that are, for the first time, recognized by the patient or the physician. There can be a significant time lag, however, between the onset of physiologic alteration and the production of symptoms, just as there was between the onset of the pathologic process and the physiologic alteration. A pathologic process may be present and discoverable by diagnostic tests long before it produces sufficient symptoms for a patient to feel its presence. Atherosclerosis and atherosclerotic vascular disease illustrate this continuum of pathologic process, physiologic alteration, and symptom production and are reviewed to provide further insight into the disease process.

Atherosclerosis is a pathologic process characterized by focal accumulation of lipids and complex carbohydrates, producing a secondary narrowing of the arteries. The process affects arterial vessels of the body in the cerebral, coronary, peripheral, and abdominal circulations and is now the leading cause of death in the United States.

As mentioned previously, atherosclerosis without physiologic alteration has been documented in 18-year-olds. At this stage, it is a subclinical or presymptomatic process and can be identified only by direct examination of the blood vessels.

Coronary artery disease is a specific manifestation of atherosclerosis in the arteries that provide blood to the heart muscle. As it becomes progressively more serious, it interferes with arterial capability for providing sufficient oxygen to meet the heart muscle's metabolic demands. As the reduc-

tion in oxygen supply worsens, ischemia of the heart muscle may occur. With still further progression, any increased demand on the cardiac muscle, as in any kind of exertion, may produce angina pectoris, or chest pain, the cardinal symptom of coronary artery disease.

Long before the angina is present, coronary artery disease may be identified by an abnormal electrocardiogram (EKG). If an EKG with the patient at rest does not produce evidence of disease, frequently an EKG during controlled exercise will yield the necessary evidence. In these cases, the coronary artery disease may not be sufficiently serious to produce EKG changes during normal demands on the heart, but the increased cardiac demands associated with exercise will provide the necessary diagnostic evidence.

These clinical changes may not evoke any symptoms, but eventually the patient may experience intermittent chest pain on exertion and seek medical care. At this time, the chances of obtaining an abnormal EKG and conforming the presence of coronary artery disease become much greater, but even at this stage a patient may have typical angina pain with an apparently normal EKG. The difficulty of defining the specific relationship between pathology and symptoms may be even greater. Both resting and exercise EKGs produce a number of false-positive and false-negative results. The absolute criterion for the definition of coronary artery disease becomes ateriography, the injection of dye to outline the coronary artery and the areas of narrowing. However, it should be understood that many people with no symptoms have demonstrable coronary artery disease, and that many others with classic anginal symptoms and characteristic EKG abnormalities have coronary arteries free of atherosclerosis (21). It has been well established in the literature that the same objective alterations in the EKG and classic symptoms may be produced by spasm rather than occlusion of the coronary arteries (22).

In patients with occlusive coronary artery disease, atherosclerosis may eventually occlude a coronary artery completely causing the heart muscles supplied by the artery to die. This clinical event is known as *myocardial infarction,* commonly called a "heart attack," and is accompanied by prolonged chest pains, nausea, sweating, shortness of breath, and weakness. However, the arterial occlusion and subsequent tissue death may occur silently and without symptoms, to be discovered by EKG at some later date.

Following the pathologic process a step further, loss of heart muscle function secondary to coronary artery disease may affect the heart's ability to maintain adequate circulation to the rest of the body and may produce a range of secondary signs and symptoms in other organs. As the heart becomes weaker, there may be progressive difficulty in breathing, swelling of the legs and feet, inability to maintain blood supply to the brain and subsequent faintness, and impairment of kidney function with reduction of urinary output. These events are sometimes labeled by the single clinical description of *heart failure.*

Atherosclerosis is a generalized disease and is usually not limited to the coronary arteries; similar events occur in the blood vessels of other organs. This process may produce primary effects in organs that are not related to the secondary effects of heart failure described above. Abdominal pain, bowel necrosis, neurologic deficits, strokes, renal failure, calf pain, and aortic aneurysms may all be produced by atherosclerotic damage to the arteries of various organs. The combination of this primary damage to the organs themselves and the secondary effects of heart failure is complicated and serious, dramatically illustrating why atherosclerosis is such a major cause of morbidity and mortality.

The Physiologic Bases of Disease

Over the years, the pattern of diseases affecting the U.S. population has changed profoundly, generally as a result of changes in the environment, in the population's demographic composition, and in medical practice. Infectious diseases as the major cause of mortality have been replaced by chronic diseases associated with aging. At the turn of the

century, infectious diseases struck the young and healthy and spread rapidly, often resulting in death. The confluence of improved sanitation, a higher standard of living, antibiotics, and vaccines reduced death and disability from infectious diseases so markedly that they are now a comparatively minor cause of death (see Chapter 1).

The treatability of syphilis, for example, has reduced its incidence and impact markedly, and cases with the secondary or tertiary manifestations of this potentially devastating disorder are now increasingly rare. Smallpox, polio, mumps, diphtheria, measles, pertussis, rubella, tetanus, typhoid, and cholera, all once highly prevalent, have now all but disappeared. Bacterial infections of childhood and infantile diarrheas of all kinds are now effectively treated with antibiotics and intravenous feedings; as a result, they do not present the threat they did at the turn of the century.

While these disease entities have been diminishing or disappearing, new disease patterns have been emerging to take their place as the most important threat to life and health. Some of these patterns have resulted from the removal of diseases in early life (e.g., childhood infections), which has allowed time for diseases in later life (e.g., atherosclerosis) to appear. Other disease patterns, however, are comparatively new, are far more prevalent than they once were, and are the result of new forces in modern life and environment.

Other disease patterns are comparatively new. Tuberculosis illustrates how a disease can come under control only to reassert itself with an influx of immigrants from areas where the disease is still endemic, and the emergence of the disease in a more virulent form among a vulnerable population such as those with the HIV virus. Tuberculosis, once the scourge of our public hospitals, is again emerging as a major public health crisis (23).

Changes in the incidence and prevalence of some cancers, for example, provide dramatic evidence of these patterns. In the early part of the century, cancer of the lung was not a major cause of death, but it began to increase in men as the rate of cigarette smoking in men increased. The incidence of lung cancer in women lagged behind that of men until recently, when it began to rise to a comparable level, probably secondary to the increase in cigarette smoking among women.

In the same vein, there has been a rise in endometrial carcinoma in women, attributed at least in part to the increased use of estrogens by postmenopausal women (24,25). Pancreatic cancer has increased in recent years and is occurring at a younger age than previously, but no clear explanation of this changed disease pattern has been proposed. The etiologic factors contributing to the increased risk of pancreatic cancer have been subject to vigorous epidemiologic debate. Coffee in its caffeinated and decaffeinated forms has been implicated, with considerable refutation of these arguments (26). Again, recent years have seen a marked rise in mesothelioma, a previously rare type of lung cancer, probably secondary to the markedly increased use of asbestos in manufacturing and construction.

In the same fashion, improvement in our medical technology has changed the patterns of disease, not just by wiping out previously existing scourges but also by creating new ones. The morbidity and mortality of common diseases such as pneumonia and wound infections have been replaced by serious infections with once nonpathogenic bacteria that are now resistant to antibiotics. Patients whose own defense mechanisms have been compromised by corticosteroids, immunosuppressive agents, and cancer chemotherapy are now susceptible to serious infections with fungi, yeast, protozoa, or bacteria that are not normally harmful (27).

A dramatic expression of a new disease pattern is illustrated by acquired immune deficiency syndrome (AIDS), a state of serious impairment in an individual's immune mechanisms, giving rise to greatly increased susceptibility to a variety of infectious and neoplastic diseases (28). The initial descriptions of a series of previously rare infections in young and otherwise healthy homosexual men gave rise to the discovery of a condition with myriad pathologic manifestations as well as profound social and economic implications (29,30).

The human immunodeficiency virus (HIV) infects individuals and in selected cases produces a profound alteration and suppression of the host's natural immunity. The entity might therefore be considered an infectious disease because there is a specific infectious agent responsible for initiating the disease process. It must, however, also be acknowledged as an immunologic entity because the virus seems to produce no signs or symptoms but rather alters the immune system. The prevalence of infection seems to be far greater than the development of clinical expression, since there is a large population who have antibodies from the infection but who have no medically defined disease and another large population who have much milder manifestations of infection in a condition termed AIDS-related complex (ARC). Among actual AIDS patients, the manifestations of the illness cover a wide clinical spectrum, including *Pneumocystis carinii* infections of the lung, *Cryptosporidium* infections of the bowel, *Cytomegalovirus* infections of the eye, and Kaposi's sarcoma of a generalized nature.

While AIDS illustrates a fascinating new disease, its impact on care-seeking behavior may be greater than anticipated and, indeed, greater than any previous disease condition. Its existence and rapid spread have markedly changed social and sexual behavior among both the homosexual and heterosexual communities. Many people are voluntarily seeking blood tests for confirmation of possible AIDS, and serious consideration is being given to the imposition of mandatory testing for AIDS in certain special situations of travel or employment. The potential for health care workers to be infected, and conversely the risk that caretakers may transmit the virus to patients, has created considerable concern and debate about testing, as well as fear among health care providers (31). The onset of an unexplained febrile illness in a sexually active person increasingly raises the fear of AIDS and stimulates a request for medical care for diseases that may be self-limited and for which no care would have previously been sought or needed. Recognition of the importance of the immune system as a critical link in the body's response to disease has increased society's awareness of possible immunity-related illnesses and has generated greater interest and greater use of health services in this regard.

A substantial percentage of hospitalizations are now attributable to drug toxicity and the secondary effects of new surgical procedures such as ileojejunal bypass for morbid obesity or the complications of kidney dialysis for chronic renal disease. A wide spectrum of diseases has been attributed to drug toxicity, but among the most interesting was an epidemic produced by a contaminated, over-the-counter L-tryptophan preparation. A new syndrome called eosinophilia-myalgia was produced by a widely used nonprescription medicine with profound social and scientific implications (32). Cardiac pacemakers prolong life but also produce a new spectrum of morbidity, as do other new prosthetic devices such as cardiac valves, artificial joints, or silicone implants. The lack of prospective studies illustrated by the breast implant controversy suggests how important it is that we monitor new technology and medical procedures from their inception. Organ transplantation has created an entirely new spectrum of biologic diseases based on intentional destruction of the body's immunologic system, its own basic protection from disease. Patients with bone marrow or renal transplants require considerable care and present diseases that are rare if they occur at all in normal, nonimmunosuppressed populations. The potential for transplanting other organs creates considerable flux in the biologic nature of disease and has frightening implications for the ability of persons to provide and pay for these services.

The increased effectiveness of medical intervention is also having a considerable effect on the patterns of disease by changing the gene controlling the incidence of certain diseases. Improvements in prenatal and high-risk obstetric care allow completion of pregnancies in diabetic women who otherwise may not have reproduced. This development may increase the prevalence of an already common disease such as diabetes. The successful introduction of vigorous physical therapy and prophylactic antibiotic use have increased the survival of patients with cystic fibrosis, and a few have successfully reproduced. The impact of the longer-term survival on the gene pool for this disease remains to be seen, but it is a good example of some of the potential hazards caused by new technology.

An additional powerful influence affecting our patterns of disease is environmental change. Motor vehicle accidents are an increasingly important cause of morbidity and mortality, and directly reflect our increasing use of the automobile for transportation. Pollution of air and water has already been suggested as at least partially causative in a number of conditions, and toxic aspects of industrial work environments have been suggested as the cause of many more. Indeed, it has been argued that as many as three-fourths of all cancers may be in part environmentally determined.

Dietary habits have also been suggested as contributing to changes in disease patterns in recent years. The most obvious result of dietary change is obesity, which is associated with hypertension, heart disease, and diabetes. Diverticulosis, hemorrhoids, appendicitis, and even cancer of the colon may be a consequence of changes in the amount of fiber in the Western diet. Epidemiologists have implicated certain foods as possible causes of atherosclerosis (33). Increased salt intake has already been indicated in certain aspects of hypertension, and increased ingestion of refined sugars has definitely been associated with increased incidence of dental caries and possibly with several other conditions.

In summary, in addition to a wide variety of causes of disease and a wide variety of responses in individual hosts, the overall pattern of disease in a society can change markedly over time. In this country, the pattern of disease has moved from one of acute infectious disease several generations ago to one of chronic disease today. Further, the pattern of disease has been influenced by our ability to wipe out certain diseases, thereby allowing others to be expressed. Finally, many aspects of modern life, such as improved medical technology and environmental pollution, have caused disease patterns that have never existed before.

Social and Cultural Influences on Disease and Behavior

It has been estimated that 70 percent to 90 percent of all self-recognized illness is not generally treated in the conventional medical care delivery system (34). Conversely, it is reported that more than half of the visits to physicians are related to patient-identified problems for which no ascertainable biologic basis can be determined. It is clear, from this finding, that seeking medical care may or may not be associated with actual pathologic processes, and that social and cultural values greatly influence the individual's decision to visit a physician (35, 36).

A large number of physician visits are for complaints in which the physiologic function is well within normal limits, but for which the patient feels that some abnormality exists. Many people seek medical attention, for example, when bowel function is basically normal and no serious pathology can be documented. For some reason, either internally generated or imposed by the prevailing culture, these patients believe that the situation is not quite right and seek medical attention. They have somehow been led to expect bowel function that is different from what they are experiencing, and a medical remedy is sought.

Symptoms of fatigue may be attributed by the patient to a nondisease such as hypoglycemia (37). Conversely, a disease with a well-defined physiologic basis may not produce care seeking, since it may not be interpreted as a disease. The teenager with acne, for example, has a problem with a well-understood physiologic basis and an obvious clinical manifestation. The potential patient, however, may interpret it as a normal consequence of adolescence that will eventually resolve and for which treatment is either ineffective or unavailable (38). Seeking care for serious conditions is often delayed because of fear, denial, incorrect knowledge, or financial concerns (39).

Disease and the perception of illness are not the only reasons people seek medical care. Normal physiologic processes frequently are the occasion for seeking care. Pregnancy or contraception are certainly not pathologic or disease processes, but they usually require professional attention. Heavy menstrual flow, missed or irregular periods, and menopause are basically normal physiologic processes, and yet medical attention is frequently sought concerning them.

An event of modern times illustrates how medicalized normal physiologic processes can become and the interaction of social factors in creating the need for medical care. The increasing rates of infertility and the frighteningly high incidence of cesarean sections are modern medical problems. Many have attributed the current rates of infertility to the frequent delay in childbearing (40). This decrease in fertility has been well documented and has created substantial medical and psychologic problems and a tremendous base for care seeking. The rate of cesarean section is sometimes linked to this phenomenon and to the complex interaction of physician fear of litigation, the presence of monitoring equipment that allows detection of abnormalities that might not have affected the outcome, and the technologic advances that allow cesarean section to be performed with less morbidity than formerly existed. It is not only the perception of illness or the presence of disease, but also the alterations in normal physiological functions and changes in medical practice influenced by social and technologic interventions, that create some of the reasons for care-seeking behavior.

Indeed, in many cases, medical care is sought because the patient is healthy and wants to remain that way. Parents bring infants and small children to the pediatrician for routine evaluations in order to ensure that the child is developing normally. Adults visit their physician periodically for an examination, a chest X-ray film, a Papanicolaou smear, prostrate-specific antigen blood test, or mammogram. Indeed, all care-seeking behavior is carried out in a framework that is intensely affected by current social, cultural, and political values, regardless of the type or severity of the pathologic process. Cultural influences frequently determine what society considers to be a medical problem, whereas economic or political realities determine whether medical care is sought. The complex interactions of people and doctors, the personal and cultural influence on disease, and the perception of symptoms have been extensively reviewed in the literature.

Zborowsky (41) studied the differences in attribution between Italian and Jewish patients. Italians were generally satisfied and ceased demanding medical care once pain relief was obtained, Jews were reluctant to take medication and continued to be concerned with the underlying cause of their discomfort rather than simply relief of pain. It can be anticipated that they would continue to seek care until they were reassured that there was no serious underlying pathology.

The deep psychologic meaning of disease was explored by Cassel (42) in an article on suffering. He argued that suffering was experienced by people. It was not a physical construct, and it was often underappreciated by practicing physicians. He illustrated his point by suggesting that pain in circumstances such as childbirth, in which it is expected, rarely produces suffering and does not call for much care seeking because of discomfort. In contrast, situations in which pain is unexplained may give rise to considerable suffering and continued care seeking. He again argues that the physician's failure to appreciate and deal with the bases of suffering may lead to a failure to reassure the patient.

The complex psychologic underpinnings of care seeking are indicated by the remarkable ability of patients to respond to placebos. Placebos, which have been effective in reducing not only subjective symptoms but also objective test results, are a testament to the importance of symbolic intervention. They argue for a complex interaction between physician and patient on both verbal and nonverbal levels and demonstrate that the encounter itself and the therapeutic relationship have meaning to the individual who seeks medical services (43). Many authors have recently argued that physicians do not fully recognize the social and cultural determinants of care seeking. An illuminating article on the couvade syndrome demonstrated failure by physicians in a prepaid practice to recognize the influence of a woman's pregnancy on the husband's medical complaints (44). In the couvade syndrome, husbands of pregnant women have symptoms such as nausea, vomiting, anorexia, pain, and bloating—feelings often experienced by their wives—while having no objective organic abnormalities. In this study, husbands of pregnant women had two times the number of physician visits, four times the number of symptoms, and two times the number of prescriptions without any increase in actual pathology during the period of their wives' pregnancy as compared to other periods. The study illustrates the myriad influences on the production of symptoms and the need to seek medical care. It has increasingly been argued that consumerism and a critical analysis of health care needs and physician limitations can give rise to a more productive physician-patient relationship (45). Health care administrators must understand the complex influences on care seeking and design systems that identify both the physical abnormalities and the cultural determinants that provide the impetus for seeking medical services.

In our society, which is often characterized by an insatiable appetite for the consumption of medical resources, a converse picture exists where appropriate care seeking is delayed. Investigators have sought to define the basis for delay in care seeking. It is widely believed that earlier diagnosis of cancer produces a better prognosis. Failure or delay in seeking care is a substantial problem. Social scientists and administrators must determine why women fail to get recommended Pap smears and mammograms, and have to consider the reluctance to have such screening procedures as flexible sigmoidoscopies to detect colon cancers. Commonly advanced reasons are time, discomfort, and finances). In addition, cancer's image as a progressive disease with modest potential benefit from existing therapies persists. Studies have revealed that many people believe the treatment of cancer is often worse than the disease. Several studies have tried to document the basis for delay in melanoma diagnosis, and note that many patients with melanomas visited the physician for reasons other than the suspicious skin lesion (47,48). The educational, psychological, racial, and financial characteristics of the population may have a profound effect on their care-seeking behavior, and consequently the ultimate efficacy of medical care.

As social and cultural values change, the understanding of what constitutes disease and the subsequent care-seeking patterns may change as well (49,50). The transference of marital adjustment and childrearing problems from the category of family problems best handled by a member of the clergy to psychologic problems best handled by a physician or psychologist is one example of this trend. The interpretation of poor school performance as a result of a medical problem has received wide attention under the general category of learning disabilities. Dyslexia, a specific process suggesting that intelligent people may have difficulty learning to read, has been considered a disease to be treated by neurologists, psychologists, optometrists, and pediatricians. The medicalization of academic underachievement is a case study worth further investigation (51,52). The recent shift toward the description of alcoholism as a disease requiring medical treatment is another. A further example is the court decision changing abortion from a criminal act to a recognized medical service. The numerous manifestations of psychological problems represent many examples of difficult-to-define illness with a substantial political and value-laden component.

In all of these examples, it should be noted that the underlying pathologic process has not changed; rather, it is the perception of these processes as disease or not that has been altered. In other circumstances, even our perception of certain conditions as illnesses does not change; instead, external social values change the way we react to them. Psychologic factors may even increase the incidence of the most common diseases (53).

For example, the increased mobility and weakened family structure of modern American life have made it more difficult to care for elderly and infirm family members at home. Smaller housing units, increased numbers of families in which both adults are employed, and a variety of other social pressures have altered the ability to handle the health problems of the elderly in the fashion of the past. Instead, society has created a new network of health institutions—nursing homes—to provide professional care for pathologic processes that previously were handled at home. The underlying pathologic processes have remained the same. It is the societal response to them that has changed (54).

The Influence of Supply

Within the total spectrum of pathologic processes that affect the health of people in this country, it is important to note that some processes receive much more interest and attention from the health care system than others. It is also important to speculate about why this occurs.

The structure and availability of health services contribute significantly to the amount and nature of the care that will be sought. Once the patient makes the initial decision to seek professional attention, much of the additional medical care results directly from the decisions of the physician (50). The physician usually decides what laboratory tests, X-ray films, treatment procedures, and hospitalizations are necessary, and in so doing shapes a particular pattern of care for each patient. In some ways, these decisions by the physician also shape the health care system itself by creating a demand

physician induced demand

for certain services. As long as the demand exists, the institutions, programs, and services will expand to fill the need.

But does the process work this way, or is the reverse true? Do pathologic processes stimulate patients to visit physicians, who, in turn, demand certain services as a result of their decisions? Or do the specialized services become available to physicians, thereby influencing the manner in which they approach disease, and do physicians then shape patients' perceptions and demands on the basis of what they know is available (55). There is some evidence to suggest that the latter is true, at least in part, and is becoming progressively more important.

Physicians generally do most of their training in hospitals and are introduced early to the use and benefits of sophisticated procedures and tests. The availability of these tests and treatments then influence the physicians' view of disease, since they now make possible the treatment of conditions that were previously beyond consideration. The surgical treatment of degenerative processes such as hip replacement for osteoarthritis, laser treatment for diabetic retinopathy, and replacement of diseased heart valves with prosthetic devices have all created many new options for the physician. They have also created new reasons for patients to seek care. *ear tubes*

Unfortunately, the development of these new approaches is not always in keeping with the real need for care among patients, as determined by the pathologic processes that threaten them. The mere fact that a particular process, such as arthritis or alcoholism, has a major impact on public health does not necessarily mean that sophisticated technology will be developed to deal with it. Instead, the more sophisticated technologies are frequently developed in areas of lesser importance, leaving more serious problems relatively less well attended. Patients' perceptions of illness and its importance are then shaped more by areas where major technology is available than by areas of perhaps greater need.

The influence of suppliers on the demand for medical care has increased in the past several years. There has been a significant increase in the offering of specialized "boutique" medical services, which may not be appreciated initially by the public but which are actively marketed and eventually widely used. The proliferation of weight control, substance abuse, eating disorder, and impotence programs are but a few examples of providers generating a perception of need and stimulating care-seeking behavior. *plastic surgery*

Eating disorder—with its hallmark diseases bulimia and anorexia—illustrates the complex interface between physiology and psychology. How does a normal behavior that results in episodic weight gain and weight loss differ from the behavior of those individuals who binge-eat and use diuretics, laxatives, and enemas as a means of accelerating weight loss? At what point does a natural interest in weight and appearance become a pathologic process in need of costly professional intervention? While physicians and psychologists may debate the definition of disease, the frequent bombardment of radio and television advertising creates the perception of illness in a certain number of individuals who would not previously label themselves as ill. While advertising may make a segment of the population aware of an advance, such as intraocular lens implants for the elderly who might have otherwise considered it unaffordable, the consistent interest in generating new sources of income by health care institutions and providers may be creating an unnatural emphasis on illness for which biologic and behavioral variation are more likely explanations.

It is unclear whether the development of pathologic processes or the availability of services to treat them creates the demand for health care. It is clear, however, that the use of medical services is the result of a unique interaction involving the pathologic processes themselves, the patient's and the physician's perceptions of them, and the availability of services to deal with them (56). Each of these elements must be considered if the use of health services is to be better understood by all concerned.

References

1. Apple, D. (1960). How laymen define illness. *Journal of Health and Human Behavior. 1.* 219–225.
2. Retchin, S. M., Fletcher, R. H., Earp, J. A., et al. (1986). Mitral valve prolapse: Disease or illness? *Archives of Internal Medicine. 146.* 1081.
3. Tobi, M., & Straus, S. E. (1985). Chronic Epstein-Barr virus disease. A workshop held by the National Institute of Pathology and Infectious Disease. *Annals of Internal Medicine. 103.* 251–254.
4. Centers for Disease Control. (1986). Chronic fatigue possibly related to Epstein-Barr virus in Nevada. *MMWR (Mortality, Morbidity Weekly Report). 35.* 350–352.
5. Buchwald, D., Cheny, P. R., & Peterson, D. L. (1992). A chronic illness characterized by fatigue, neurologic and immunologic disorders in active herpes virus type 6 infection. *Annals of Internal Medicine. 116.* 103–113.
6. Siperstein, M. D. (1975). The glucose tolerance test: A pitfall in the diagnosis of diabetes mellitus. *Advances in Internal Medicine. 20.* 297–323.
7. O'Sullivan, J. B. & Mahan, C. M. (1968). Prospective study of 352 young patients with diabetes. *New England Journal of Medicine. 278.* 1038–1041.
8. National Diabetes Group. (1979). Classification and diagnosis of diabetes mellitus and other categories of glucose intolerance. *Diabetes. 28.* 1039–1057.
9. Mabry, J. (1964). Lay concepts of etiology. *Journal of Chronic Diseases. 17.* 371–386.
10. Weiss, N. S. (1972). Relation of high blood pressure to headache, epistaxis and selected other symptoms. *New England Journal of Medicine. 287.* 631.
11. Ballard, Barbash, R., Schatzkin, A., Carter, C. L., et al. (1990). Body fat distribution in breast cancer in the Framingham study. *Journal of the National Cancer Institute. 82.* 286–290.
12. Merliss, R. R. (1971). Talc-treated rice and Japanese stomach cancer. *Science. 173.* 1141–1142.
13. Selikoff, I. J., Churg, J., & Hammond, E. C. (1964). Asbestos exposure and neoplasia. *Journal of the American Medical Association. 188.* 22–26.
14. Poskanzer, D. C., & Herbst, A. L. (1977). Epidemiology of vaginal adenosis and adenocarcinoma association with exposure to stilbestrol in utero. *Cancer. 39 (suppl).* 1892–1895.
15. Farrow, D. C. & Davis, S. (1990). Diet and the risk of pancreatic cancer in men. *American Journal of Epidemiology. 132.* 423–431.
16. Glass, A. G., & Hoover, R. N. (1989). The emerging epidemic of melanoma and squamous cell skin cancer. *Journal of the American Medical Association. 262.* 2097–2100.
17. Tonglet, R., Bourdoux, P., Minga, T., et al. (1992). Efficacy of low oral doses of iodized oil and the control of iodine deficiency in Zaire. *New England Journal of Medicine. 326.* 236–241.
18. Peterson, W. J. (1990). Peptic ulcer—an infectious disease? *Western Journal of Medicine. 152.* 167–171.
19. Enos, W. F., Beyer, J. C., & Holmes, R. H. (1958). Pathogenesis of coronary disease in American soldiers killed in Korea. *Journal of the American Medical Association. 158.* 912–914.
20. McNamara, J. J., Molot, M. A., Stremple, J. F., et al. (1971). Coronary artery disease of combat casualties in Vietnam. *Journal of the American Medical Association. 216.* 1185–1187.
21. Miranda, C. P., Lehmann, K. G., & Lachterman, B. (1991). Comparison of silent and symptomatic ischemia during exercise testing in men. *Annals of Internal Medicine. 114.* 649–656.
22. Fuster, V., Badimon, L., Badimon, J. J., et al. (1992). Mechanisms of disease: The pathogenesis of coronary artery disease in the acute coronary symptoms. *New England Journal of Medicine. Part I, 326.* 242–250. *Part II, 326.* 310–318.
23. Bloch A. B., Rieder, H. L., Kelly, G. D., et al. (1989). The epidemiology of tuberculosis in the United States. *Seminars in Respiratory Infection. 4.* 157–170.
24. Schwarz, B. E. (1981). Does estrogen cause adenocarcinoma of the endometrium? *Clinical Obstetrics and Gynecology. 24.* 243–251.
25. Voigt, L. F., Weiss, N. S., Chu, J., et al. (1991). Progestogen supplementation of exogenous estrogens and risk of endometrial cancer. *Lancet. 338.* 274–277.
26. Gordis, L. (1990). Consumption of methylxanthine-containing beverages and risk of pancreatic cancer. *Cancer Letter. 52.* 1–12.
27. Stamm, W. E. (1981). Nonsocomial infections: Etiologic changes, therapeutic challenges. *Hospital Practice. 16.* 75–88.
28. Centers for Disease Control. (1981). Kaposi's sarcoma and pneumocystis pneumonia among homosexual men—New York City and California.

MMWR (Morbidity, Mortality Weekly Report). 30. 305–308.

29. Wachtel, T., Piette, J., More, V., et al. (1992). Quality of life in persons with human immunodeficiency virus infection: Measurement by the medical outcomes study instrument. *Annals of Internal Medicine. 116.* 129–137.

30. Fauci, A. S. (1991). Immunopathogenetic mechanisms in human immunodeficiency virus (HIV infection). *Annals of Internal Medicine. 114.* 678–693.

31. Centers for Disease Control. (1991). Recommendations for preventing transmission of human immunodeficiency virus and hepatitis B virus to patients during exposure to prone invasive procedures. *MMWR (Morbidity, Mortality Weekly Report). 8.* 1–9.

32. Varga, J., Uitto, J., & Jimenez, S. A. (1992). The cause and pathogenesis of the eosinophilia-myalgia syndrome. *Annals of Internal Medicine. 116.* 140–147.

33. Turpeinen, O. (1979). Effect of cholesterol-lowering diet on mortality from coronary heart disease and other causes. *Circulation. 59.* 1–7.

34. Dingle, J. H., Badger, G. F., & Jordan, W. S. (1964). *Illness in the home: A study of 25,000 illnesses in a group of Cleveland families.* Cleveland, OH: Western Reserve University.

35. Zola, I. K. (1966). Culture and symptoms: An analysis of patients' presenting complaints. *American Sociological Review. 31.* 615–630.

36. Stoeckle, J. D., & Barsky, A. J. (1980). Uses of social science knowledge in the doctoring of primary care. In Eisenberg, L., & Kleinman, A. (Eds.). *The Revelance of Social Science for Medicine* (pp. 223–240). Hingham, MA: D. Reidel Publishing Company.

37. Meador, C. K. (1965). Art and science of nondisease. *New England Journal of Medicine. 272.* 92–95.

38. Ludwig, E. G., & Gibson, G. (1969). Self perception of sickness and the seeking of medical care. *Journal of Health and Social Behavior. 10.* 125–133.

39. Battistella, R. M. (1971). Factors associated with delay in the initiation of physicians' care among late adulthood persons. *American Journal of Public Health. 61.* 1348–1361.

40. DeCherney, A. H., & Berkowitz, G. S. (1982). Female fecundity and age. *New England Journal of Medicine. 306.* 424–426.

41. Zborowsky, M. (1952). Cultural components in responses to pain. *Journal of Social Issues. 8.* 16–30.

42. Cassell, E. J. (1982). The nature of suffering and the goals of medicine. *New England Journal of Medicine. 306.* 639–644.

43. Brody, H. (1982). The lie that heals: The ethics of giving placebos. *Annals of Internal Medicine. 97.* 112–118.

44. Lyokinji, M., & Lamb, G. S. (1982). The Couvade symptom: An epidemiologic study. *Annals of Internal Medicine. 96.* 509–511.

45. Jensen, P. S. (1981). The doctor-patient relationship: Headed for impasse or improvement? *Annals of Internal Medicine. 95.* 769–771.

46. Love, N. (1991). Why patients delay seeking care for cancer symptoms. *Postgraduate Medicine. 89.* 151–158.

47. Krige, J. E., et al. (1991). Delay in the diagnosis of cutaneous melanoma: A prospective study in 250 patients. *Cancer. 68.* 2064–2068.

48. Hennrikus, D., et al. (1991). A community study of delay in presenting with signs of melanoma to medical practitioners. *Archives of Dermatology. 127.* 356–361.

49. Parsons, T. (1958). Definitions of health and illness in the light of American values and social structure. In Jaco, E. G. (Ed.). *Patients, physicians and illness* (pp. 165–187). Glencoe, IL: Free Press of Glencoe.

50. Fuch, V. (1974). *Who shall live? Health, economics and social choice.* New York: Basic Books.

51. Shaywitz, S. E., Escobar, B. A., Shaywitz, J. M., et al. (1992). Evidence that dyslexia may represent the lower tail of a normal distribution of reading ability. *New England Journal of Medicine. 326.* 145–150.

52. Rosenberger, P. B. (1992). Dyslexia—is it a disease? *New England Journal of Medicine. 326.* 192–193.

53. Cohen, S., Tyrrell, D. A., & Smith, A. P. (1991). Psychological stresses: Susceptibility to the common cold. *New England Journal of Medicine. 325.* 606–612.

54. Somers, A. R. (1982). Long term care for the elderly and disabled: A new health priority. *New England Journal of Medicine. 307.* 221–226.

55. Stoeckle, J. D., Zola, I. K., & Davidson, G. E. (1963). On going to see the doctor, the contributions of the patient to the decision to seek medical aid: A selective review. *Journal of Chronic Diseases. 16.* 975–989.

56. Rosenstock, I. M. (1966). Why people use health services. *Milbank Memorial Fund Quarterly. 44 (Part 2).* 94–127.

Chapter 3

Indicators and Predictors of Health Services Utilization

Lu Ann Aday

[handwritten margin notes:]
Rel betw. access + utilization
what factors ult. deter. who receives care?
what role do beliefs play?
trends in site (utiliz. by)
popul. char. that influence care seeking
why?

insur., mg. care, regular source of care
impact on utiliz

The utilization of health services is concerned with who does and does not receive medical care and why; and, for those who do, how much and what types of care they consume. Utilization data may be obtained from surveys asking people about their health care; from files of practicing physicians; or from hospital or other institutional record sources.

From the point of view of health policy, planning, program administration and evaluation, and knowing who did not receive care and why are equally as or more important than describing the actual utilization patterns for those who do.

Health policy analysts and program evaluators, for example, want to know the impact of health policies or programs or changes in these over time (e.g., Medicaid, Medicare) on whether the people most directly targeted by the programs are actually served and/or use services at higher or lower rates as a result. Health planners are concerned with identifying areas of greatest need or highest potential demand in the target communities for new health care delivery organizations. Health care program administrators want to know the share of the health care market captured by their facility and whether special programs they may have developed are having the desired impact on changing patterns of care (e.g., seeing women earlier in their pregnancy, reducing inpatient utilization). Physicians and nurses are concerned with patients who delay obtaining care in response to serious symptoms and with those who fail to comply with prescribed medical regimens. Social workers, discharge planners, and case managers need to take into account social and psychological, as well as physiological, factors in formulating appropriate patient care plans. All of these issues are informed by understanding approaches to conceptualizing, measuring, and predicting health services utilization behavior.

The discussion that follows reviews 1) ways in which the utilization of health services has been conceptualized and measured, 2) major analytic models that have been developed to explain health care-seeking behavior, 3) selected empirical findings on utilization, and 4) current policy issues that can benefit from studies of health care utilization.

Conceptualization and Measurement of Health Services Utilization

Utilization may be characterized in a number of different ways. Four principal dimensions of the concept are, however, reflected in most empirical indicators of utilization: type, purpose, site, and time interval of use.

The *type* of utilization refers principally to the category of service rendered—physician, dental or other practitioners' services, hospital or long-term care admissions, prescriptions, medical equipment, and so on. The *purpose* refers to the reason care was sought: for health maintenance in the absence of symptoms (primary prevention), for the diagnosis or treatment of illness in the interest of returning to a previous state of well-being (secondary prevention), or rehabilitation or maintenance in the case of a long-term health problem (tertiary prevention). Another reason for rendering care is the maintenance or custodial care of medically fragile or dependent adults or children, in which the personal, as well as medical care, needs of the patient are met. The *site* or organizational unit refers to the place services were received. It might be in an inpatient setting (e.g., short-term-stay hospital, mental institution, nursing home) or ambulatory setting (e.g., hospital outpatient department or emergency room, physician's office, health maintenance organization [HMO], public health clinic, community health center, freestanding emergency center), or the patient's home. The *time interval* refers to measures of 1) contact, based on whether the service was received during a particular time period (e.g., proportion seeing a physician within the last year); 2) volume, the total units of service received during that period (e.g., mean number of visits in a year for those seeing a physician); or 3) episodic patterns, based on the patterns of providers, referrals, and continuity of care for a given occurrence or episode of illness.

These dimensions are not mutually exclusive. A single utilization indicator may, in fact, be descriptive of a number of different dimensions. The "proportion seeing a physician in the year for a particular symptom" reflects, for example, the type, purpose, and time interval of utilization. It is important to understand, however, that different indicators may well reflect different stages of or reasons for seeking care. In choosing a relevant utilization indicator, it is important to consider the precise dimension(s) one is interested in examining and what measures best operationalize it. Further, the process of selecting the appropriate models and variables for predicting or explaining utilization should be guided by their relevance to the particular dimension(s) of utilization being considered.

Analytic Models of Health Services Utilization

Over the past 25 years there has been considerable interest in integrating the multiplicity of factors found to be associated with health services utilization into conceptual models to guide the conduct of research for understanding who uses health care services, who does not, and why. The development of these models is of interest from both more theoretical and applied points of view. They contribute to an understanding of health care behavior in a broad sense by clarifying how it might be influenced by social, psychological, economic, institutional, and other factors. They also provide guidance for practical health policy decisions about what might be changed to facilitate individuals' or groups' receiving care when they need it.

There has been a considerable interest expressed in recent years with developing a systems approach to understanding utilization behavior that would integrate the range of institutional and individual factors associated with decisions to seek care. This systems perspective is represented to a considerable extent by the Behavioral Model of Health Services Utilization introduced by Ronald Andersen in 1968 and expanded by Andersen, Aday, and their colleagues to have broad applicability for measuring access to medical care

(1,2,3,4,5,6,7). The discussion that follows describes the Andersen and Aday framework and the contributions and limitations of this and other major conceptual models in understanding health care utilization behavior.

Behavioral Model of Health Services Utilization

The expanded Behavioral Model of Health Services Utilization is portrayed in figure 3-1 and the principal indicators used to operationalize various aspects of the model appear in table 3-1.

Utilization, particularly as it might indicate the population's or a subgroup's access to medical care, is often evaluated in a political context. For example, major health care financing (e.g., Medicare and Medicaid) and organizational programs (e.g., community health center, preferred provider arrangements) have been concerned with improving target groups' ability to obtain care when it is needed. It is the effect of health policy on altering the utilization of and access to medical care that health policy makers and administrators often wish to evaluate. Thus it may well be appropriate to view health policy as the starting point for consideration of utilization behavior.

The delivery system component of the model refers to those arrangements for the potential rendering of care to consumers. It includes both their availability (volume and distribution of services) and organization (mechanisms for entry and movement through the system). These characteristics are aggregate, structural properties. The community, or a particular delivery organization, is the unit of analysis, rather than the individual.

The characteristics of the population at risk are the predisposing, enabling, and need components in Andersen's original Behavioral Model of Health Services Utilization (5).

Predisposing variables include those that describe the propensity of individuals to use services—including basic demographic characteristics (e.g., age, sex, family size), social structural variables (e.g., race and ethnicity, education, employment status, and occupation), and beliefs (e.g.,

general beliefs and attitudes about the value of health services', and/or of physicians' knowledge of disease). For example, age is highly correlated with the need for care. Variables such as ethnicity, education, and occupation suggest the importance of life-style and environmental influences on individuals' decisions to seek care. People who believe strongly in the value of health care or physicians might be more likely to seek care than those who do not have these beliefs.

The enabling component describes the means individuals have available to them for the use of services. Both resources specific to individuals and their families (income, insurance coverage) and attributes of the community or region in which an individual lives are included here. Place of residence—for example, whether one lives in a rural or urban area—may indicate geographic proximity to a source of care as well as local attitudes about health care.

Need refers to health status or illness, which is the most immediate and important cause of health service use. The need for care may be perceived by the individual and reflected in reported symptoms or disability days, for example, or evaluated by the provider in terms of the actual diagnosis or severity of presenting complaints.

Those characteristics that are biological or social givens, such as one's age, sex, race, or place of residence are termed immutable. Health policy cannot directly alter these attributes, but they are defining of target groups of interest. The more manipulable beliefs and enabling variables, such as insurance coverage, are characteristics that health policy seeks to change in order to affect these groups' access to care. They are "mutable" to or alterable by health policy.

This model has been applied to evaluate whether services are fairly or equitably distributed. To the extent that differences in utilization are explained primarily by medical need variables and demographic correlates of need (e.g., age, sex), the distribution of services is said to be equitable. If other factors (e.g., insurance coverage, income) are the most important predictors of who gets care, then an inequitable system is said to exist (8,9).

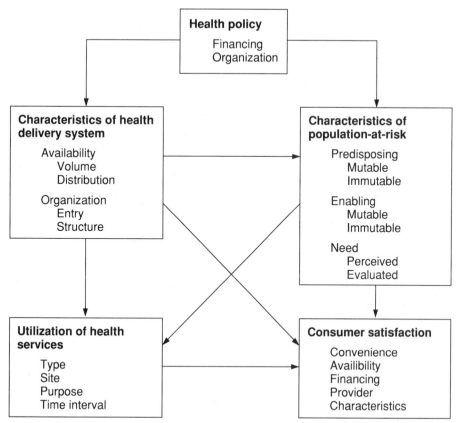

Figure 3-1. The expanded behavioral model. (SOURCE: Aday, L. A., Andersen, R., & Fleming, G. V. *Health Care in the U.S.: Equitable for Whom?* Copyright © 1980 by Sage Publications, Inc. Reprinted by permission of Sage Publications, Inc.)

A particular challenge for health services research in the context of the equity, effectiveness, *and* efficiency objectives is the development of indicators of the domains of need (including risks or conditions) for which medical care could make a difference. The service requirements to meet those needs would then become the primary policy focus of the equity objective.

In the expanded Behavioral Model, applied to measuring the concept of access, the principal outcomes of interest were objective measures of health services utilization, as well as subjective assessments by consumers of their recent utilization experiences.

A number of criticisms have been offered of this framework. Wolinsky (10) and Becker and Maiman (11), have, for example, argued that because of

the range of variables and differing levels of analysis included, it is difficult to gather data to test the complete model. Mechanic (12) notes that the major multivariate studies of health services utilization applying this and other comprehensive models of utilization behavior have failed to confirm the importance of certain psychosocial and organizational factors borne out in other studies. He offers a number of explanations for these results: 1) the measures of perceived *need* used actually incorporate concepts of psychological distress as well but are not interpreted as such, 2) the use of aggregate system-level resource availability indicators for large areas does not adequately capture the experience of individuals in their local communities, and 3) the large-scale multivariate studies fail to adequately model patient decision

TABLE 3-1. Operational Indicators of the Expanded Behavioral Model

I. Characteristics of health delivery system
  A. Availability
    1. Volume
      a. Personnel
        i. Number of primary care physicians
        ii. Number of specialists
      b. Facilities
        i. Number of hospitals
        ii. Number of hospital beds
    2. Distribution
      a. Number of personnel per 1,000 population
      b. Number of facilities per 1,000 population
  B. Organization
    1. Entry
      a. Convenience of regular source of care
        i. Availability of services at night, on weekends, and in emergencies, house calls
        ii. Mode of transportation
        iii. Travel time
        iv. Appointment system and waiting time
        v. Office waiting time
        vi. Time physician spends with the patient (on average)
      b. Sources of medical care used by those with no regular source
        i. Reasons for not having a regular source
        ii. Places that people without a regular source did or will go to for care
    2. Structure
      a. Type of regular source of care
        i. Location of provider
        ii. Type of provider
        iii. Types of paramedical provider
        iv. Specialty of attending physician
      b. Type and extent of third-party coverage
        i. Type of health plans
        ii. Extent of coverage
        iii. Out-of-pocket cost of care
II. Characteristics of population at risk
  A. Predisposing
    1. Mutable
      a. General health care beliefs and attitudes
      b. Knowledge of health care information
    2. Immutable
      a. Age
      b. Sex
      c. Family size
      d. Race and ethnicity
      e. Education
      f. Employment status
  B. Enabling
    1. Mutable

      a. Family income
      b. Type and convenience of regular source of care[a]
      c. Type and extent of third-party coverage[a]
    2. Immutable
      a. Residence
      b. Region
      c. Length of time in community
  C. Need
    1. Perceived
      a. Health status
      b. Episode of illness
      c. Symptoms of illness
      d. Disability days
    2. Evaluated
      a. Physician severity ratings of condition
      b. Physician severity ratings for symptoms

III. Utilization of health services
  A. Type
    1. Physician
    2. Dentist
    3. Hospital
    4. Long-term care
  B. Site
    1. Location of nonhospital visits with physician in the year
    2. Location of visits to a physician in connection with illness episode
  C. Purpose
    1. Prevention
      a. General preventive exam
      b. Diagnostic procedures
    2. Illness-related
      a. Response to symptoms experienced in the year
      b. Use in response to disability
    3. Custodial
      a. Nursing home stays reported in connection with illness episode
      b. Other long-term stays
  D. Time interval
    1. Contact
      a. Percent seeing provider in the year
      b. Percent hospitalized in the year
    2. Volume
      a. Mean visits in the year
      b. Mean admissions and hospital days in the year
    3. Continuity
      a. Profile of care in response to illness episodes
      b. Summary indexes of continuity of care
IV. Consumer satisfaction
  A. On most recent visit to usual source of care
  B. With medical care in general

[a] A fuller description of these indicators is provided under the entry and structure heading for the characteristics of the health delivery system.

making about the care-seeking process. He argues that in bringing the literature on larger-scale quantitative studies and smaller-scale qualitative approaches together, it is important "to recognize that what are characterized as 'illness' variables in the multivariate studies are more appropriately seen as illness-behavior measures incorporating various learned inclinations, and life events as well as physical illness" (12).

In the discussion that follows other efforts to develop comprehensive systems models of health services utilization, as well as those that focus more directly on modeling the processes for decision making surrounding illness that Mechanic describes, are reviewed.

Other Comprehensive Models of Health Services Utilization

In a comprehensive review of the literature on health services utilization in the early 1970s, McKinlay (13) identified six major approaches to characterizing the predictors of health services utilization: 1) demographic, 2) social structural, 3) social psychological, 4) economic, 5) organizational, and 6) systems (see table 3-2). They may be identified principally by the types of predictors they emphasize.

Many of these indicators are ones that appear in the Behavioral Model described earlier. Of particular interest is how the systems approach facilitates the specification of the causal linkages between variables and their direct and indirect impact on the ultimate utilization outcomes of interest. Anderson (14), for example, concludes, "What is sorely needed is careful, theoretically based attempts to explicate causal structures that incorporate major features of all [the] approaches. The social systems approach appears to provide a valuable framework in which such research can be undertaken.

A number of studies have been carried out in recent years attempting to specify and test the causal relationships implied in the Behavioral Model directly (15,16,17,18,19,20,21,22,23). Others attempt to model a somewhat different set of rela-

TABLE 3-2. Six Approaches to Characterizing the Predictors of Health Services Utilization

Model	Predictors
Demographic	Age, sex, marital status, family size, residence
Social structural	Social class, ethnicity, education, occupation
Social psychological	Health beliefs, values, attitudes, norms, culture
Economic	Family income, insurance coverage, price of services, provider/population ratios
Organizational	Organization of physicians' practices, referral patterns, use of ancillaries, regular source of care
Systems	All or most of the above considered in the context of set of interrelationships

tionships in specifying the operation of the health care system (24,25,26). The relative impact of selected indicators considered separately and in the context of analyses controlling for other factors is summarized in the discussion of empirical findings on utilization later in this chapter.

What is important to underline here is that various factors may account for who ultimately obtains care; considerable progress has been made in measuring and specifying the relationships among these different factors, and the systems perspective provides an integrative framework for considering many of these factors and their interrelationships. However, more focused studies are required to adequately model the causal relationships and internal processes associated with individual patients' decisions to seek care. The discussion that follows reviews a number of these efforts. (It draws heavily from review articles by Becker and Maiman [11], Becker et al. [27], and Janz and Becker [28].)

Models of Patient Decision Making

Suchman

The dimension of utilization that is the focus of Suchman's framework for stages of decision making about seeking medical care is an episode of illness. In Suchman's paradigm, the sequence of seeking medical care for illness is divided into five stages: 1) the experience of the symptom, 2) assumption of the sick role, 3) medical care contact, 4) dependent-patient role, and 5) recovery or rehabilitation. At each stage, the patient makes certain decisions and engages in particular types of health care behavior (29,30).

At the first stage, one perceives that something is wrong, based on the physical sensation of pain or discomfort; this is followed by a cognitive interpretation of the symptom's importance given its impact on one's functioning and finally by an emotional reaction of fear or anxiety. During this stage the patient may use nonprescribed home remedies to deal with the symptoms. Theoretically one would then move to the next stage of response and assume the sick role, although one could also deny having the illness or delay beginning to act like someone who is ill.

At the point of assuming the sick role, however, one would begin to relinquish one's usual roles and obligations, such as stay in bed or not go to work and request provisional validation for the sick role from family members or friends that constitute one's lay referral system. One may continue to use home remedies, based on their advice as well.

In the next stage, help is sought from a professional medical provider to provide legitimation of the sick role and negotiate the proper treatment for the condition. As in the previous two stages, the individual may not accept the recommended therapies and might shop around for another professional opinion.

In the dependent-patient role stage, the individual accepts professional judgment and undergoes the recommended treatment. This stage is seen as necessary to restore the patient to good health. A variety of factors, including the quality of the physician–patient relationship itself might, however, interfere with patient compliance with the recommended regimens.

In the final stage of recovery and rehabilitation, the patient is called on to relinquish the sick role and resume normal activities. Some people may refuse to give up the sick role at this point, however, and become chronic malingerers.

Suchman then proceeds to pose a theoretical explanation for the impact that social structure and associated medical orientations might have on the patient's progression through these stages. A group with more parochial or traditional, in contrast to more cosmopolitan, affiliations and a popular, rather than more scientific, orientation toward medical care would, he suggests, be more likely to delay in recognizing the seriousness of the symptoms initially, linger longer in the stage in which one uses home remedies and seeks support from family and friends, be suspicious of medical providers and maybe shop around more, fail to adhere to prescribed regimens, and relinquish the sick role as soon as possible (31).

Suchman's model is an interesting conceptual framework for the various stages many patients might go through in responding to illness. There has not, however, been strong empirical support for Suchman's formulation of the impact of the social structure and medical orientation on these stages of care seeking (33, 34).

Kosa and Robertson

Kosa and Robertson (35) have formulated another model for explaining decisions to seek medical care in the context of an episode of illness. Whereas Suchman's model tended to offer more sociological or social structural explanations for why individuals might respond differently at different stages of the illness episode, Kosa and Robertson's explanation is more psychological in focus. Behavior is motivated by the individual's psychological need to reduce the anxiety aroused by the threat of illness. Anxiety might be of two kinds: "floating anxiety" (generalized anxiety that is not directly connected with the illness episode) and "specific anxiety" (the psychological response to physical discomfort proportionate to the seriousness of the symptoms experienced).

The Kosa–Robertson formulation is a process model as well with stages organized around the episode of illness. The principal components include 1) an assessment of a disturbance in usual functioning, 2) anxiety arousal based on a perception of the symptoms, 3) the application of one's medical knowledge to address the problem, and 4) the performance of activities to alleviate the anxiety. Activities may be one of two kinds: "therapeutic interventions" that are directed at the removal of a particular health problem and its concomitant anxiety, or "gratificatory interventions" aimed at relieving the anxiety of satisfying other needs without addressing the underlying health problem directly. The model does not deny the importance of external social factors, however. Each stage of the process is influenced by these psychological dynamics as well as the culture and social groups of which one is a part (e.g., family) or with which they come in contact (e.g., professional medical providers). There has, however, not been substantial empirical verification of the Kosa–Robertson framework.

Mechanic

Mechanic is concerned more generally with the variety of factors that influence individuals' experiences of symptoms in seeking care for illness-related reasons. It is not a process model in the context of an illness episode as are the Suchman and Kosa–Robertson formulations. It addresses, however, a variety of social and psychological factors that influence patients' perceptions of the need to seek medical care. These include the following:

1) visibility, recognizability, or perceptual salience of deviant signs and symptoms; 2) the extent to which symptoms are percieved as serious (that is, the person's estimate of the present and future probabilities of danger); 3) the extent to which symptoms disrupt family, work, and other social activities; 4) the frequency of the

appearance of deviant signs or symptoms, their persistence, or their frequency or recurrence; 5) the tolerance thresholds of those who are exposed to and evaluate the deviant signs and symptoms; 6) available information, knowledge, and cultural assumptions and understandings of the evaluator; 7) basic needs that lead to denial; 8) needs competing with illness responses; 9) competing possible interpretations that can be assigned to the symptoms once they are recognized; and 10) availability of treatment resources, physical proximity, and psychological and monetary costs of taking action (included are not only physical distance and costs of time, money, and effort, but also such costs as stigma, social distance, and feelings of humiliation) [36].

These variables are identified as influencing "help seeking" from the point of view of the patient. They may or may not be associated with the need for care as defined by the provider, however. Further, Mechanic distinguishes "other-defined" from "self-defined" illnesses. The former differs from the latter in that the definition of illness originates with others in the environment, and the sick individual may resist this labeling and have to be brought into treatment involuntarily. It is, therefore, applicable to mental illness as well as situations when dependent children or adults may resist required medical treatment (37).

Health Belief Model

One of the more social psychological-oriented models for explaining decisions to seek medical care that has been subject to considerable empirical testing as well is the Health Belief Model (HBM). As originally conceived, it was applied to understanding preventive care (health behavior) but has subsequently been applied to explaining care seeking in response to illness (illness behavior) and those activities required for recovery from illness (sick role behavior) (11,27,28,38,39,40,41,42). In the HBM (see figure 3-2), a variety of diverse demographic, sociopsychological, and structural factors may influence behavior. They are, however, believed to work through their effects on the individual's subjective perceptions and motivations (beliefs), rather than functioning as direct causes of the behavior themselves.

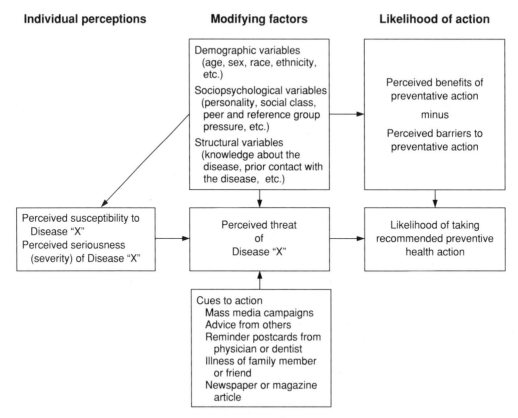

Figure 3-2. The health belief model. (SOURCE: Rosenstock, I. M. (1974). Historical origins of the health belief model. *Health Educ Monograh. 2.* 344. Adapted from Becker M. H., Drachman, R. H., Kirscht, J. P., et al. (1974). A new approach to explaining sick role behavior in low income populations. *American Journal of Public Health. 64.* 205–216. Reprinted by permission.)

The basic perceptual components of the model are as follows:

1. The individual's subjective state of readiness to take action, which is determined by both the individual's perceived likelihood of "susceptibility" to the particular illness and perceptions of the probable "severity" of the consequences (organic and/or social) of contracting the disease.
2. The individual's evaluation of the advocated health behavior in terms of its feasibility and efficaciousness (i.e., subjective estimate of the action's potential "benefits" in reducing susceptibility and/or severity), weighed against perceptions of physical, financial, and other costs ("barriers") involved in the proposed action.
3. A "cue to action" must occur to trigger the appropriate health behavior, coming from either internal (e.g. symptoms) or external (e.g., interpersonal inter-

actions, mass media, media communications) sources (11).

There is a large body of empirical evidence testing the applicability of the HBM to explaining preventive, illness-related, and sick-role (especially compliance) behavior. "Perceived barriers" appeared to be an important predictor across all of the types of behavior examined. In most of the studies perceived susceptibility to illness was associated with engaging in a variety of preventive behaviors, such as having a Papanicolaou (Pap) test, influenza vaccination, preventive dental visit, and screening for Tay-Sachs disease. The other components of the model were less strongly or consistently associated.

In prediction of illness behavior (in response to perceived symptoms), the perceived benefits of seeking care appear to be associated, while the results for the impact of perceived susceptibility are less clear and consistent across studies of this type of behavior.

The HBM has been applied to studying compliance, in particular in the context of sick-role behavior. The studies in general bear out that perceived susceptibility, severity, and benefits are associated with compliance in taking prescribed medications. Findings are more mixed regarding the impact of aspects of the model in predicting compliance with other types of prescribed regimens (27,28,29).

Many of the studies testing the HBM do not include all of the components of the framework, nor do they adequately empirically model the implied causal relationships among the variables. Less than half of the studies are prospective in design in that attitudes are measured prior to the behaviors they are supposed to predict. The issue of whether the attitudes are a cause or a consequence of behavior has, therefore, not been adequately resolved (11,27,28,39).

These and the other models discussed that deal with patient decision making concerning medical care differ in the type (lay or professional contact), purpose (preventive or illness-related), or time interval unit (contact or episode) of use being considered and the components of the decision-making process itself. They do, however, in contrast to the systems models described earlier, attempt to clarify the social psychological processes in which the individual patient engages when deciding to seek medical care. The systems framework, which begins with issues in the organization and financing of care, represents a macro perspective; and the patient decision-oriented frameworks concerned with the psychosocial dynamics that underlie decisions to seek medical care present a more micro perspective in understanding health care utilization behavior. Depending on one's perspective, both approaches are useful. From a macro public policy perspective, identifying the likely effects of changes in financing and major organizational forms for delivering care are necessary. At the same time, it is important to recognize that the way in which consumers in local communities will react to such changes will also depend on a number of micro-level social psychological factors. As David Mechanic points out, perhaps these efforts should be viewed as different but complementary ways of illuminating and understanding utilization behavior.

The traditional medical sociology literature on physician utilization would be enriched by examining psychosocial processes within an economic context that takes into account enabling variables such as access to care, the availability of providers, and scope of insurance coverage. Examining the role of cultural and social-psychological processes within the constraining influences of economic and organizational factors will result in better theory and, it is to be hoped, more adequate prediction [12].

In the section that follows, major empirical findings on the array of predictors of health services utilization are summarized separately and, when available, their effects controlling for other factors reported are discussed as well.

Selected Empirical Findings on Health Services Utilization

This summary of selected empirical findings on health services utilization will 1) review national data on the principal types of health care services—physician, dentist, hospital, and long-term care—and, when available, report data on the other major dimensions of health services utilization (purpose, site, and time interval) as they relate to these indicators; and 2) summarize the importance of a variety of predictors of health services utilization for each of these indicators, based on a review of empirical studies of their relationships to the respective use measures. These summaries draw upon a number of excellent bibliographies and reviews of health services utilization in recent years (2,14,43,44,45,46,47,48,49,50,51) as well as major national surveys of health care utilization and access (3,4,52,53,54,55,56,57). It should be noted that comparisons over time or between studies may well be affected by methodologic differences or changes in question wording across studies.

Findings: Selected Indicators of Health Services Utilization

Physician Utilization

The proportion of the population that had seen a physician at least once during the year remained relatively stable from 1958 to 1963, prior to the introduction of Medicaid and Medicare. However, it did increase slightly from 1963 (65 percent) to 1970 (68 percent), and then substantially to around three-fourths of the population in 1976 (76 percent) (3). This proportion has remained relatively stable over the last decade at around 75–77 percent (56,57,58).

The average number of visits to a physician has also remained relatively stable at around five (e.g., 4.9 in 1971 and 5.3 in 1989) over the past 20 years (56,57,58). There have, however, been substantial changes in the sites or organizational settings in which patients see physicians. In the early part of the century (1928–1931), it is estimated that 40 percent of all physician visits occurred in the home. By 1971, this proportion had dropped to less than 2 percent. During this same period, office visits increased from 50 to 70 percent of all visits (59). By 1989, the proportion seeing a physician in the office was around 60 percent, but the percent of visits to hospital outpatient clinics or emergency rooms was approximately 13, similar to the proportion of patient contacts with providers handled over the phone (around 12 percent) (57).

Around half of the U.S. population reported having a general physical exam in 1963, 1970, and 1976. However, during this period, the most frequently cited reason for having the physical tended to shift from concern about symptoms of illness to preventive care in the absence of illness per se

(3,53). The percent of women seeing a physician during the first trimester of their pregnancy has also increased substantially from 68 percent in 1970 to 76 percent in 1983, but has remained relatively stable over the past decade (56,57). From 1970 to 1976 the proportion of children one to four years of age immunized for measles and rubella increased (from 57.2 percent to 65.9 percent, from 37.2 percent to 61.7 percent, respectively), but declined in 1985 (to 60.8 percent and 58.9, respectively). There were, however, dramatic declines from 1970 to 1985 in the proportion of children having diphtheria-tetanus-pertussis (DTP) and polio vaccination (76.1 to 64.9 percent and from 65.9 to 55.3 percent, respectively) (57). The proportion of adults having selected preventive procedures (e.g., blood pressure test or Pap smear and breast examination for women) has also increased since the early 1970s. The proportion of adults reporting that they had a blood pressure check during that year, for example, increased from approximately 62 percent in 1974 to 74 percent in 1985. Corresponding changes for Pap smear and breast examination were from 54 to 63 percent, and from 56 to 68 percent, in 1973 and 1985, respectively (60,61). In the face of these increases questions have been raised about the appropriate intervals and efficacy in detecting or preventing illness of these various screening procedures relative to their cost (4).

Dentist Utilization

The percent of the U.S. population having seen a dentist during the year increased from 42.7 percent in 1964 to 50.4 percent in 1981 and 56.3 percent in 1986. The proportion of the U.S. population that had never seen a dentist also declined during this period (from 15.5 percent in 1964 to 11.0 percent in 1981 and 10.4 percent in 1986). The average number of visits for those seeing a dentist increased slightly over this same period—from 1.6 to 1964, to 1.7 in 1968 and 2.0 in 1986 (57).

The proportion of dental visits for preventive

reasons (e.g., cleaning and fluoride treatment) did increase substantially from 1964 (25 percent) to 1974 (63 percent). The rate of seeing a dentist to obtain fillings or inlays remained around 25 percent during this period, while the proportion receiving other restorative procedures, such as extractions and dentures, declined from 18 percent to 12 percent from 1964 to 1974 (62). Data from the 1986 National Health Interview Survey showed the main reasons for the last visit in the last two years for people two years of age or older to be as follows: examination or cleaning (42 percent), symptoms (24 percent), follow up on condition (11 percent), and some other reason (1 percent) (63).

Over the last 20 years, there have been major changes in how both physician and dental assistants handle preventive (e.g., examination and prophylaxis) procedures especially. In addition, an increasing number of dentists are practicing in partnerships or corporate-funded settings (64).

Hospital Utilization

In general, the proportion of the population hospitalized has declined since the early 1970s. During 1971–1972 13 percent of the U.S. population had been hospitalized (65). In 1976 the rate was 11 percent (3). It dropped to 10 percent in 1978 and to around 8 percent in 1989 (4,58,66).

The total number of hospital discharges per 1,000 population similarly tended to increase steadily until the mid–1970s, at which point it began to level off and then declined from the early 1980 on. The total days of care have declined as well since the mid-1970s, as has the average length of stay in the hospital (57,58,67,68). (Data in table 3-3 on hospital discharges and lengths of stay are based on the National Health Interview Survey [NHIS] of the civilian noninstitutionalized population of the United States. Estimates from this source will differ from those obtained directly from hospitals in the National Hospital Discharge Survey. They do, however, confirm the trends reflected in the NHIS data.)

According to the National Hospital Discharge

Survey, the numbers of operations per 1,000 males for cardiac catherizations and coronary bypass more than doubled from 1980 to 1989 (from 2.2 to 5.1 and from 1.0 to 2.3, respectively). There were increases in the rates of cesarean sections for females (from 4.8 to 6.6), but declines in inpatient operations for diagnostic dilation and curettage of the uterus (from 7.3 to 1.0) and hysterectomies (from 5.2 to 3.9). In 1989 both men and women were increasingly likely to have certain diagnostic and nonsurgical procedures while hospitalized (e.g., computerized axial tomographic [CAT] scan, diagnostic ultrasound) than had been the case in 1980, when these diagnostic procedures were relatively new (57).

There has been an increasing interest in outpatient surgery for certain conditions in recent years. Also, as mentioned previously, hospital outpatient departments and emergency rooms have come to be important sources of ambulatory physician care. The growth of freestanding emergency centers represents one effort to serve those individuals who tend to use hospital emergency rooms especially on an intermittent basis for nonurgent primary care (69).

Long-Term Care

Long-term care encompasses principally the utilization of nursing and personal care homes and mental health facilities.

The number of residents in nursing and related care homes increased from approximately 759,000 in 1969 to 1.5 million in 1985. The demand for nursing home care is expected to increase as the proportion of the population 65 and over increases and lives longer (56,57,70,71).

The rates of inpatient utilization of mental health facilities has declined substantially in recent years, reflecting efforts to deinstitutionalize this population. The rates of outpatient and day treatment mental health facilities use, on the other hand, increased substantially from the late 1960s (1969) to the late 1980s (1988): from 575.9 per 100,000 civilian population to 1234.5 and from 27.8 to 125.7, respectively. There have been particularly substantial declines in the rates of inpatient utilization of state and county mental hospitals over the past 20 years (56,57).

Findings: Selected Predictors of Health Services Utilization

In the discussion that follows, the importance of a number of variables that are considered most often in describing or explaining how utilization differs for different groups are summarized. The major types of utilization emphasized in this summary will be those just reviewed (physician, dentist, hospital, and long-term care utilization). The predictors are, in general, grouped according to the categories of the Behavioral Model of Health Services Utilization. To the extent possible, data available on the importance of the respective variables, controlling for other associated factors, are presented.

Characteristics of the Population: Predisposing Variables

Age. Age is significantly associated with all the different types of health services utilization, primarily because it is an important indicator of age-associated morbidity.

In general, the relationship between age and physician contacts and visits is curvilinear (see table 3-3). Young children and older people are more apt to contact a physician and average more visits, reflecting their age-related need for medical services. Very young children (under six) and older adults (55 and over) are also more likely to report having a general physical simply because it was "time to get a checkup" (3). A larger proportion of older adult visits are to the physician's office, compared to younger adults or especially very young children, for whom rates of telephone contact with physicians for medical advice are much higher (56,57).

The relationship between age and dentist office visits is the opposite of that observed for physician office visits. The youngest and oldest are least likely to see a dentist and average fewer visits overall (see table 3-3). Children, however, are more likely to visit a dentist for preventive reasons (examinations and cleaning) than are adults. Restorative visits for fillings and dentures tend to increase up to age 40 and then decline in the older years (62, unpublished NCHS data).

Excluding hospitalizations for delivery, the rates of admissions, discharge, and length of stay for adults tend to increase with age (see table 3-3). The rates for specific types of operations, and diagnostic and other nonsurgical procedures also vary considerably by age (56,57).

The vast majority of nursing home residents are elderly. The rate for those 65 and over is, in fact, highest for the oldest old (85 or older) (see table 3-3). Rates of institutionalization in inpatient psychiatric facilities tend to be highest for middle-aged adults (25–44 years of age) and lowest for children (under 18) (57).

Sex. Women use more health services than do men in general, which is to some extent (but not totally) a function of their obstetrics-related care.

Women are more likely to see physicians than are men and have at least one more visit on average (see Table 3-3). Findings on the relationship of sex to the use of preventive services are not consistent. In some instances, women appear to be more likely to have certain preventive procedures than do men, but in other cases, there are no sex differentials. There is substantial evidence, however, that men are less likely to see a physician in response to symptoms of illness than are women (49,50). Further, a larger proportion of men's visits are to hospital outpatient departments or emergency rooms. Women, on the other hand, are more likely to contact the physician by phone for medical advice (56,57). Overall, women are more likely to have seen a dentist and average more visits then men (see table 3-3).

Women are also much more apt to be hospitalized (see table 3-3). When admissions for obstetrical reasons are excluded, the difference diminished, however. In 1989, the National Center for

TABLE 3-3. Utilization Indicators for Selected Subgroups: United States

Selected Subgroups	Physician[a] Percent Visiting in Year	Physician[a] Mean Visits	Dentist[b] Percent Visiting in Year	Dentist[b] Mean Visits	Hospital[c] Discharges per 1,000 Population	Hospital[c] Average Length of Stay	Nursing Home[d] Residents per 1,000 Population
Total	77.7%	5.3	56.3%	2.0	92.6	7.0	46.2
Age (years)							
Under 15	82.6	4.6	53.8	1.7	44.1	5.8	—
<5	93.3	6.7	19.5	0.4	76.6	6.6	—
5–14	76.8	3.5	71.7	2.3	26.7	4.6	—
15–44	72.8	4.6	61.6	2.0	67.0	5.5	—
45–64	76.5	6.1	55.9	2.2	130.5	7.2	—
>65	86.7	8.9	42.6	2.1	265.6	8.9	—
65–74	85.1	8.2	47.3	2.4	236.7	8.5	12.5
>75	89.1	9.9	35.1	1.6	311.0	9.4	—
75–84	—	—	—	—	—	—	57.7
>85	—	—	—	—	—	—	220.3
Sex							
Male	73.0	4.8	54.1	1.8	95.0	7.3	29.0
Female	82.2	5.9	58.5	2.1	91.2	6.8	57.9
Race							
White	78.2	5.5	58.4	2.1	92.0	6.9	47.7
Black	77.0	4.9	42.6	1.3	105.2	7.6	35.0
Family income							
>$14,000	76.2	6.3	41.0	1.3	131.3	7.7	—
$14,000–$24,999	76.4	5.2	42.7	1.3	91.2	6.6	—
$25,000–$34,999	77.7	5.5	49.3	1.6	93.0	6.8	—
$35,000–$49,999	79.2	5.2	59.0	2.2	75.0	6.4	—
$50,000 or more	81.9	6.0	71.8	2.7	72.1	6.9	—
Geographic region							
Northeast	80.6	5.3	60.9	2.2	80.2	7.4	—
Midwest	78.7	5.4	60.0	2.0	98.4	7.0	—
South	76.3	5.3	49.5	1.6	106.5	6.8	—
West	76.4	5.5	59.1	2.2	75.7	7.0	—
Location of residence							
Within MSA	78.2	5.4	57.8	2.0	89.0	7.3	—
Outside MSA	76.1	5.2	51.8	1.7	105.1	6.1	—

[a] 1989 data (age-adjusted) in tables 67 and 68 in ref. 57.

[b] 1986 data (age-adjusted) in table 71 in ref. 57. Income categories differ as follows: <$10,000; $10,000–14,999; $15,000–19,999; $20,000–34,999; >$35,000.

[c] 1989 data (age-adjusted) in table 72 in ref. 57.

[d] 1986 data in table 80 in ref. 57.

SOURCE: National Center for Health Statistics. (1991). *Health, United States, 1990* (DHHS Publication No. [PHS] 91-1232). Washington, DC: U.S. Government Printing Office.

what's important?

Health Statistics Hospital Discharge Survey reported discharge rates of 105.3 per 1000 for men and 144.5 per 1000 for women, including deliveries. Excluding deliveries, the rate for women was around 111 per 1000. Men, on the other hand, average longer lengths of stay in the hospital. The rates in 1989 were 7.0 days for men and 6.1 for women, including deliveries. The average length of stay for women for deliveries was 2.9. In general, rates of inpatient surgery are higher for women than men (67,68).

The number of women in nursing and personal care homes is almost three times that of men (see table 3-3) (57,69). There are, in particular, many more of the oldest old (85 and older) among female residents of nursing homes. The admission rates to state and county mental hospitals for males (176.6 in 1986) are almost twice that of females (98.1). Men are also likely to have slightly higher rates of admission to private psychiatric hospitals (92.1 vs. 81.5), while the opposite is the case for nonfederal general hospitals (335.5 vs. 327.6) for inpatient psychiatric treatment (56,57).

Race. Whites are more likely to use certain services than are nonwhites, although the differences have narrowed considerably in recent years.

In 1989 78.2 percent of whites had seen a physician during the year, compared to 77.0 percent of blacks (see table 3-3). This represents a substantial narrowing of the differences between whites and blacks over the last 20 years. For example, in 1964, the rates for whites and blacks were 67.3 and 57.0 percent, respectively. On the other hand, the gap in the average number of visits has widened since the early 1980s. In 1983 the rates for whites and blacks were 5.1 and 4.8, respectively (56,57). In 1989 the average number of visits for whites who saw a physician was 5.5, compared to 4.9 for blacks—a differential more comparable to that almost 20 years earlier in 1971— 5.0 and 4.4, respectively (56,57,58). National survey data show that blacks may be as likely to have certain preventive procedures (blood pressure checks) or more likely to have others (Pap smears

or, to some extent, breast examinations for women) than are whites (4,7,72). Smaller proportions of black women (61.1 percent in 1988), compared to white women (79.4 percent), see a physician during the first trimester of pregnancy. This disparity has shown no signs of narrowing during the past decade (56,57). There is also evidence that blacks have lower rates of use relative to their experienced need for care (measured by disability days and reported symptoms) than do whites (3,7). Blacks are much more likely to receive care in hospital outpatient departments and emergency rooms than are whites, whereas whites more often visit or telephone physicians (56,57).

Whites are much more likely to have contacted a dentist than blacks and to average more visits once they go (see table 3-3). Whites also have higher rates of preventive dental visits than do blacks, while blacks usually see a dentist for more serious conditions and have higher rates of visits for restorative procedures (62,63).

There is evidence that hospital discharge rates for blacks, which had been higher than the rates for whites since the late 1970s, have begun to decline to be more comparable to those for whites (56,57). The average length of stay, on hospital admission, remains higher for blacks than whites (see table 3-3). However, the number of elderly blacks in nursing homes (35.0 per 1,000 population in 1985) is lower than the number of whites (47.7) (56,57).

Ethnicity. Despite improvements in the levels of access to medical care among Hispanics, there is evidence that they continue to experience barriers to obtaining care.

National Health Interview Survey data from 1978 to 1980 showed that Mexican-Americans were least likely, compared to other all major Hispanic groups, blacks, or whites to have seen a physician during the year—33.1 percent had not seen a physician. They also averaged the smallest number of visits overall (4.3). Corresponding proportions and mean visits for other groups were as follows: Puerto Ricans (20.4 percent; 6.1), Cuban-Americans (23.3

percent; 5.8) other Hispanics (23.9 percent; 5.1), blacks (23.8 percent; 4.8) and whites (23.3 percent; 4.8) (73).

In 1978–80, among people four years of age and older, Mexican-Americans were least likely to have seen a dentist in the year (34.5 percent), compared with whites (55.8 percent), blacks (36.9 percent), or any other Hispanic groups—Puerto Ricans (45.6 percent), Cuban-Americans (45.5 percent), or other Hispanics (49.8 percent). The rates of never having seen a dentist were also highest for Mexican-Americans (17.4 percent), compared with only 2.5 percent for whites, for example (73).

NCHS data confirm that Mexican-Americans were least likely to be hospitalized and also tended to spend fewer days in the hospital than most other Hispanic or non-Hispanic groups (73).

The literature on Hispanic health care suggests that language barriers, the middle-class values and attitudes of providers, longer waiting times to see a physician, and the assignment of different doctors to patients on different visits tend to characterize many Hispanics' contact with the health care system. Further, a disproportionate number of Hispanics do not have medical insurance, which is also frequently a significant barrier to their use of traditional medical services (74).

Education. The relationship of education to utilization in general varies by the type of indicator examined. It does, however, seem to be an important predictor of preventive health care utilization.

Better-educated people are, for example, more likely to have had general physicals, immunizations, tests, and procedures for preventive purposes and (for women) to have seen a physician early in pregnancy. They are also more likely to have been to a dentist and to have more visits, once they go. The relationship between education and hospital utilization tends to mirror that for income (described below). People with less education are likely to have more hospitalizations (43,49).

Characteristics of Population: Enabling Variables

Income. In the past, people with higher incomes used more health services than those with lower incomes. Since the enactment of Medicaid and Medicare in the mid–1960s, lower-income people have come to use certain services at even higher rates than those with high incomes.

In 1964, 57.5 percent of people with family incomes of less than $10,000 (in 1983 dollars) had seen a physician during the year, compared to 73.0 percent of those with family incomes of $35,000 or more (56). The corresponding percentages some 25 years later (1989) were 76.2 and 81.9 percent, respectively. Further, whereas in the past the poor tended to report fewer visits to a physician on average than did the nonpoor, they now report more (see table 3-3). The proportion of low-income adults undergoing certain preventive procedures (e.g., blood pressure check, or Pap smear and breast examination for women) continues to be lower than for higher-income individuals (4,7,72). The rates of physician contact in general, the mean number of visits, and use both of illness-related and preventive services tend to be lower for low-income, compared to high-income, children. Although the proportion of low-income women seeking prenatal care in the first trimester of pregnancy has increased substantially over the past 30 years, the rates remain lower for low-income, compared to high-income, women. There is evidence as well that low-income people continue to see physicians at lower rates, relative to the disability days or symptoms they experience, than do high-income people (43,49). Low-income people report having fewer of their visits at physicians' offices (48.5 percent for those with less than $14,000 income in 1989) than do high-income individuals (63.4 percent for those with income of $50,000 or more). They are, however, much more likely to use hospital outpatient departments or emergency rooms (18.0 and 10.7 percent, respectively) and less likely to use the phone to consult with the physician (10.8 vs. 13.6 percent) (56,57).

The proportion of low-income persons reporting

having seen a dentist during the year remains much lower than the proportion for high-income people (see table 3-3). The proportion reporting they had not seen a dentist in 1986 was also much higher for those with incomes under $10,000 (13.4 percent), compared to those with incomes of $35,000 or more (7.1 percent) (56,57). The number of visits to a dentist also varied directly with income, with higher-income people having more and low-income people having fewer visits (see table 3-3). People with higher incomes are also more likely to present more serious problems and require restorative procedures once they visit dentists. These differences by income appear to be particularly pronounced for low-income, compared to high-income children (62,63).

The numbers of hospital admissions, total days of care, and average lengths of stay are higher for low-income people, reflecting their poorer health status and more severe medical problems (table 3-3).

Residence. Rates of utilization for most types of services tend to be lower for people who live outside major metropolitan areas, especially those who live on farms or in rural communities.

The proportion of people seeing physicians and the average number of visits reported did tend to be higher for residents of Metropolitan Statistical Areas (MSAs) compared to those who live outside these areas (see table 3-3). There is evidence as well that non-MSA residents, especially those who live on farms, are less likely to have had certain preventive procedures (e.g., blood pressure check or Pap smear and breast examination for women) (3,4). Rates of contacting a physician in response to disability days or symptoms have also tended to be lower for people who live in rural areas, relative to those who live in cities (3,4). People who live outside major metropolitan areas are also more likely to see physicians at their offices and less likely to go to hospital emergency rooms or outpatient departments than are those who live in cities (56).

The proportion of people seeing dentists and the average number of visits for those who do, tend to be higher for people who live in MSAs, compared to the rates for people who live outside MSAs (see table 3-3).

Hospital discharge rates are higher for people who live outside MSAs, although their average lengths of stay are shorter (see table 3-3). This probably reflects the propensity of physicians in less densely populated areas to hospitalize their patients so they can see more patients on a single visit to the hospital.

Characteristics of the Population: Need Variables

Need is consistently borne out to be the most important predictor of the use of health services. Need indicators may be based on patient self-perceptions of their health, as well as clinical diagnoses and evaluations by medical professionals.

Perceived Need. Patient self-reports of health status include indicators of whether they perceive their health to be excellent, good, fair, or poor; the extent to which they worry about their health; whether they had to go to bed or otherwise limit their usual activities because of illness or injury, and the particular symptoms or conditions they say they have experienced.

These measures tend to be highly correlated. People with poorer health, measured in these ways, are consistently more likely to have contacted a physician in the year, average more visits when they go, have been hospitalized, and tend to stay in the hospital longer once admitted (7,43,48,49).

Evaluated Need. Providers' and patients' evaluations of medical need may not always agree. Indicators of providers' evaluations of the patients' condition include their assessment of the actual severity of presenting symptoms or complaints and diagnoses, based on laboratory tests and clinical judgments (7,43,48,49).

The type of diagnosis or disease category affects the number of physician visits and the types of provider seen. The National Center for Health Statistics reports that chronic illness, especially hypertensive disease, arthritis and rheumatism, and other diseases of the musculoskeletal system, as well as acute conditions, such as influenza, the common cold, and infectious and parasitic diseases, tend to be the most frequently mentioned reasons for seeing a physician for illness-related diagnosis or treatment (75).

Normal delivery constituted (for women) the major reason for hospitalization. Other major diagnoses for which people were hospitalized related to malignant neoplasms, fractures, pneumonia, and cerebrovascular diseases. Most of the inpatient surgery performed is gynecologic, abdominal, and orthopedic (68).

In general, as the physician-evaluated severity of a condition increases, the use of physician services also increases, although many conditions for which physicians see patients are not deemed as particularly serious by the providers (49,76).

Characteristics of the Health Care Delivery System: Special Utilization Issues

The beginning point for the consideration of the correlates of health services utilization in the Behavioral Model (figure 3-1) is health policy as it relates to the organization and financing of medical care. There have been a number of major changes under way in how medical care is organized and financed in this country in recent years, which are apt to have a profound impact on the types and volume of services consumed as well.

The numbers and kinds of health maintenance organizations (HMOs) and other primary care alternatives are increasing. Outpatient surgery and other alternatives to traditional inpatient care are being encouraged. A variety of new preferred provider alternatives are being offered to the poor. Diagnosis-related groups (DRGs) and the resource-based relative value scale (RBRVS) under Medicare have radically altered the systems of public financing of care for the elderly. Private insurers are becoming increasingly concerned about cost

shifting and are themselves beginning to forge selective contracts with providers to contain costs. Hospitals are becoming increasingly concerned about the level of uncompensated care they provide and consumers about the increasing share of health care costs they are paying out of their own pockets.

These changes portend profound changes for the access and utilization of medical care for those groups most apt to be affected by these developments—the poor, the uninsured, those with some form of public third-party coverage, and people who have tended to use hospital outpatient services for their regular source of care.

The most immediate operational indicators for the individual patient of how care is organized and financed, and which are quite often in social surveys of individuals' health care utilization, are whether one has a regular source of medical care and insurance coverage, respectively, and if so, the type of care and coverage. These are the most immediate expressions for the individual of the health care policy-oriented organizational and financial resources potentially available to that individual to enhance access (7).

In the discussion that follows some of the major issues relating to the organization and financing of care and their probable relationship to the utilization of health care services are reviewed. We discuss the findings, in general, for the relationship of regular source of care and insurance coverage to utilization and then other special issues relevant to the changing organization and financing of services in the United States that may have significant impacts on the volume and mix of health care services consumed in this country.

Organizing of Medical Care

Regular Source of Medical Care

Having a regular source of medical care is a strong and consistent predictor of health services utilization. Extensive secondary analyses of data collected in a 1982 national survey of health care utilization and access were conducted by researchers at the Center for Health Administration Studies, The University of Chicago, using the Behavioral Model of Health Services Utilization as the conceptual basis for the analyses. A variety of predisposing, enabling, and need factors were entered in multiple-regression equations for physician, hospital, and selected preventive services utilization indicators. The results demonstrated that for the range of contact measures considered (seeing a physician, being hospitalized, having a blood pressure check, or for women having a Pap smear or breast examination during the year), people who did not have a regular medical provider were much less likely to have had the service. Further, people who regularly used hospital emergency rooms for primary medical care were much less apt than those with private physicians to have seen a physician or had selected preventive procedures (e.g., blood pressure reading or breast examination) performed during the previous year. These multivariate analyses confirm descriptive findings from a variety of sources as well that document the importance of having a regular source of care in predicting health services utilization. Once entry is gained, having a regular source of care appears to be less significant in predicting the subsequent number of visits to a physician or the length of time in the hospital (7).

There have been questions raised in the literature about the causal ordering of the regular source and utilization measures—is having a regular source of care a determinant or a result of using services? Empirically based models to examine the directionality of these relationships have confirmed that having a regular source of care does indeed have a direct and causally prior impact on the decision to seek medical care (15,77).

Prepaid Systems of Care

In recent years, there has been considerable interest in encouraging the development of prepaid capitated systems of care. These generally provide for services to be rendered by a particular set of providers to an enrolled population for a set fee per person paid in advance of delivering care.

These may take a variety of forms, including having salaried physicians working for a particular delivery organization, groups of physicians contracting with the plan to provide care to enrollees, fee-for-service physicians who contract to deliver service for a negotiated fee, or arrangements in which contracting providers serve as managers or gatekeepers for the type and amount of care that plan enrollees can receive. These alternatives are promising avenues for containing the costs of medical care through encouraging more cost-effective medical practice. (See entire issue of *Health Affairs,* vol. 5, no. 1 [Spring 1986].)

Studies conducted on HMO enrollees indicate that they receive at least as many ambulatory visits as do enrollees in conventional fee-for-service plans. There also appears to be a tendency for HMOs to encourage patient-initiated and preventive service-related visits and fewer follow-up and illness-related visits.

Utilization studies provide strong and consistent evidence that HMOs are associated with lower rates of hospitalization, compared to fee-for-service arrangements. In the vast majority of studies, HMOs had lower admission rates in particular, but there was not a clear difference in average length of stay (78,79).

Questions have been raised about whether differences observed for HMO users are a function principally of the fact that HMO enrollees are often younger and in better health and have higher incomes and more education than do fee-for-service users. In the Rand Health Insurance Study (Rand Corp., Santa Monica, CA), eligible persons were randomly assigned to various levels of coverage in either a fee-for-service or an experimental group and then compared with those who had enrolled in the HMO (Group Health Cooperative in Seattle) by choice. Admission rates and hospital days per 100 persons were equivalent for the two groups of HMO patients but about 40 percent less than in the fee-for-service group. The Rand investigators concluded that population characteristics can be ruled out as an explanation for the lower hospitalization rate at Group Health Cooperative. They also concluded that the HMO did, in fact, stimulate a less hospital-intensive style of medical practice (80).

The proliferation of these modes of practice, as well as efforts in general to encourage the use of outpatient alternatives to traditional inpatient services, are apt to have major impacts on the volume and mix of services consumed in this country.

Financing of Medical Care

Insurance Coverage

There is increasing concern that the number of people who do not have insurance coverage of any kind has risen in recent years, resulting principally from cutbacks and more restrictive eligibility criteria in the Medicaid program, as well as the loss of coverage by working people during periods of high unemployment in the early 1980s. Estimates of the uninsured vary considerably—from 31 to 36 million, depending on the source and definitions used. Being uninsured is one of the principal criteria used in defining the medically indigent in this country. Increasing concern is being expressed about individuals who cannot afford to pay because they lack such coverage and the impact that their inability to pay has on their access to needed services, as well as the financial viability of institutions or providers that continue to serve them. (See Bazzoli [81] for a review of these issues.)

In the multivariate analyses of the 1982 national survey data on access and utilization described earlier, insurance coverage was another important predictor that was considered. These analyses, holding other factors constant, demonstrated that people who did not have insurance were much less likely to have seen a physician or be admitted to the hospital, to have shorter stays once admitted, and to have had routine preventive screening procedures (e.g., blood pressure checks or, for women, a Pap smear and breast examination). These findings confirm the results of many national and local studies demonstrating a positive relationship between being insured and using health care services (7,43,48,49). There is evidence in recent years as

well that people with public insurance coverage, especially Medicaid, tend to average more ambulatory physician visits than do people with private insurance coverage. This may be due to the more discontinuous patterns of care used by the publicly insured or to the fact that ambulatory physician visits are more likely to be covered by Medicaid than is the case for most private insurance policies (7). Various universal health insurance alternatives are being considered nationally to attempt to extend coverage to the uninsured. These alternatives may serve to considerably increase the ability of the uninsured to obtain care when they need it.

Methods of Payment

There has been an increasing interest in recent years in reducing the amounts that public and private third-party payers have to pay for medical care. This has taken the form of fixed, predetermined (prospective) rates of reimbursement by service or diagnosis (e.g., DRGs) or by encouraging greater cost sharing on the part of consumers.

Empirical findings on the impact of the major prospective pricing initiative in recent years (reimbursement for hospital services under Medicare on the basis of DRGs) on hospital utilization and expenditures appear mixed. Hospital admission rates, total days of care, and average length of stay have declined since the advent of DRGs. These changes may reflect a function of secular trends under way prior to the introduction of this medical program or other changes in the organization and delivery of medical care in this country in recent years (e.g., increased emphasis on nonpatient alternatives). On the other hand, there have been concerns expressed as well about provider attempts to "game" the system by modifying the diagnosis assigned to particular cases or encouraging early discharges and frequent readmissions as necessary to obtain desired levels of reimbursement (82,83,84,85,86, 87,88,89).

The evidence regarding the impact of consumer cost sharing on the patterns and amount of health services utilization are much more consistent and convincing, however. A number of studies in both the United States and Canada document as inverse the relationship between the number of physician and hospital services consumed and the amount of consumer copayment—the more consumers had to pay out of their own pockets, the less medical care they had (90,91,92). The Rand Health Insurance Study provided the most comprehensive test of the impact of consumer cost sharing on utilization. Some 2,756 families in six sites across the country, representing 7,706 individuals, were randomly assigned to five different groups representing different levels of cost sharing: those with 1) free care; 2) 25 percent coinsurance; 3) 50 percent coinsurance; 4) 95 percent coinsurance; and 5) 95 percent coinsurance with a maximum out-of-pocket expense of $150 for an individual and $450 for a family. The results of the study demonstrated that those with no or minimal coinsurance had much higher rates of physician and hospital use, and expenditures as a whole, compared to those with higher coinsurance rates (93).

The National Medical Care Expenditures Survey has similarly documented that the financial burden of out-of-pocket outlays for medical care tends to fall hardest on those with low incomes. Medical care expenses tend to comprise a larger proportion of their total income than is the case for higher-income individuals (94). Policies that encourage greater cost sharing by consumers will then undoubtedly lower their overall use of relevant services. Questions about how equitable this impact might be relate to 1) considerations of whether the utilization of necessary or more discretionary services result and 2) what the disproportionate economic consequences for low-income families and individuals might be.

This chapter has reviewed the major conceptual and empirical approaches to determining who uses medical care and why. Health services utilization measures are important indicators for evaluating the need for and impact of both national and local health policy and program activities. Major changes are underway in this country in the organization

and financing of medical care. These changes are apt to have a substantial impact on the types and amount of health care consumed in general and for certain subgroups in particular. The concepts and correlates reviewed here can be used by health care policy makers, evaluators, and program designers to assess the impact of these changes for the U.S. population as a whole and the groups particularly vulnerable to these developments both now and in the future.

References

1. Aday, L. A., & Andersen, R. (1974). A framework for the study of access to medical care. *Health Services Research. 9.* 208–220.
2. Aday, L. A., & Andersen, R. (1975). *Development of indices of access to medical care.* Ann Arbor, MI: Health Administration Press.
3. Aday, L. A., Andersen, R., & Fleming, G. V. (1980). *Health care in the U.S.: Equitable for whom?* Beverly Hills, CA: Sage Publications.
4. Aday, L. A., Fleming, G. V., & Andersen, R. (1984). *Access to medical care in the U.S.: Who has it, who doesn't.* Chicago: Pluribus Press.
5. Andersen, R. (1968). *A behavioral model of families' use of health services* (Research Series No. 25). Chicago: Center for Health Administration Studies, The University of Chicago.
6. Andersen, R. & Newman, J. (1973). Societal and individual determinants of medical care utilization in the United States. *Milbank Memorial Fund Quarterly—Health Society. 51.* 95–124.
7. Andersen, R. Aday, L. A., Lyttle, C. S., et al. (1987). *Ambulatory care and insurance coverage in an era of constraint.* Chicago: Pluribus Press.
8. Aday, L. A., & Andersen, R. (1981). Equity of access to medical care. *Medical Care. 19 (suppl.).* 4–27.
9. Andersen, R., Kravits, J., & Anderson, O. W. (eds.) (1975). *Equity in health services: Empirical analysis in social policy.* Cambridge, MA: Ballinger.
10. Wolinsky, F. D. (1980). *The sociology of health: Principles, professions, and issues.* Boston: Little, Brown.
11. Becker, M. H., & Maiman, L. A. (1983). Models of health-related behavior. In D. Mechanic (Ed.). *Hand-*

book of health, health care, and the health profes-sions (pp. 539–568). New York: The Free Press.

12. Mechanic, D. (1979). Correlates of physician utili-zation: Why do major multivariate studies of physi-cian utilization find trivial psychosocial and organi-zational effects? *Journal of Health and Social Behavior. 20.* 387–396.

13. McKinlay, J. B. (1972). Some approaches and prob-lems in the study and use of services—an overview. *Journal of Health and Social Behavior. 13.* 115–152.

14. Anderson, J. G. (1973). Health service utilization. *Health Services Research. 8.* 184–199.

15. Andersen, R., & Aday, L. A. (1978). Access to med-ical care in the U.S.: Realized and potential. *Medical Care. 16.* 533–546.

16. Evashwick, C., Conrad, D., & Lee, F. (1982). Factors related to utilization of dental services by the elderly. *American Journal of Public Health. 72.* 1129–1135.

17. Markides, K. S., Levin, J. S., & Ray, L. A. (1985): Determinants of physician utilization among Mexi-can-Americans: A three generation study. *Medical Care. 23.* 236–246.

18. Stoller, E. P. (1982). Patterns of physician utilization by the elderly: A multivariate analysis. *Medical Care. 20.* 1080–1089.

19. Wolinsky, F. D. (1976). Health service utilization and attitudes toward health maintenance organizations: A theoretical and methodological discussion. *Jour-nal of Health and Social Behavior. 17.* 221–236.

20. Wolinsky, F. D. (1978). Effects of predisposing, enabling, and illness-morbidity characteristics on health service utilization. *Journal of Health and Social Behavior. 19.* 384–396.

21. Wolinsky, F. D. (1982). Racial differences in illness behavior. *Journal of Community Health, 8.* 87–101.

22. Wolinsky, F. D., Coe, R. M., Miller, D. K., et al. (1983). Health services utilization among the noninstitution-alized elderly. *Journal of Health and Social Be-havior. 24.* 325–336.

23. Wolinsky, F. D., Coe, R. M., Mosely, R. R. et al. (1985). Veterans' and nonveterans' use of health services: A comparative analysis. *Medical Care. 23.* 1358–1371.

24. Anderson, J. G. (1973). Causal models and social indicators: Toward the development of social sys-tems models. *American Sociological Review. 38.* 285–301.

25. Shortell, S. M., Richardson, W. C., LoGerfor, J. P., et al. (1977). The relationships among dimensions of health services in two provider systems: A causal model approach. *Journal of Health and Social Behavior. 18.* 139–159.

26. Williams, S., Shortell, S. M., LoGerfo, J. P., et al. (1978). A causal model of health services for dia-betic patients. *Medical Care. 16.* 313–326.

27. Becker, M. H., Haefner, D. P., Kasl, S. V. et al. (1977). Selected psychosocial models and correlates of in-dividual health-related behaviors. *Medical Care. 5 (suppl.).* 27–46.

28. Janz, N. K., & Becker, M. H. (1984). The Health Belief Model: A decade later. *Health Education Quarterly. 11.* 1–47.

29. Suchman, E. A. (1965). Social patterns of illness and medical care. *Journal of Health and Social Behavior. 6.* 2–16.

30. Suchman, E. A. (1965). Stages of illness and med-ical care. *Journal of Health and Social Behavior. 6.* 114–128.

31. Suchman, E. A. (1966). Health orientation and med-ical care. *American Journal of Public Health. 56.* 97–105.

32. Farge, E. J. (1978). Medical orientation among a Mexican-American population: An old and a new model reviewed. *Social Science and Medicine. 12.* 277–282.

33. Geersten, R., Klauber, M. R., Rindflesh, M., et al. (1975). A reexamination of Suchman's views on social factors in health care utilization. *Journal of Health and Social Behavior. 16.* 226–237.

34. Reeder, L. G., & Berkanovic, E. (1973). Sociological concomitants of health orientations: A partial repli-cation of Suchman. *Journal of Health and Social Behavior. 14.* 134–143.

35. Kosa, J., & Robertson, L. S. (1975). The social aspects of health and illness. In J. Kosa & I. K. Zola (Eds.). *Poverty and health: A sociological analysis* (pp. 40–79). Cambridge, MA: Harvard University Press.

36. Mechanic, D. (1978). *Medical sociology: A com-prehensive text.* New York: The Free Press.

37. Mechanic, D. (1968). *Medical sociology: A selec-tive view.* New York: The Free Press.

38. Becker, M. H. (Ed.) (1974). *The health belief model*

and personal health behavior. Thorofare, NJ: Charles B. Slack.

39. Becker, M. H., Kirscht, J. P., Haefner, D. P. et al. (1979). Patient perceptions and compliance: Recent studies of the health belief model. In R. B. Haynes, D. W. Taylor, & D. L. Sackett (Eds.). *Compliance in health care* (pp. 78–109). Baltimore, MD: John Hopkins Press.

40. Kasl, S. V., & Cobb, S. (1966). Health behavior, illness behavior, and sick role behavior. I. Health and illness behavior. *Archives of Environmental Health.* 12. 246–266.

41. Kasl, S. V., & Cobb, S. (1966). Health behavior, illness behavior, and sick role behavior. II. Sick role behavior. *Archives of Environmental Health.* 12. 531–541.

42. Rosenstock, I. (1966). Why people use health services. *Milbank Memorial Fund Quarterly.* 44. 94–127.

43. Aday, L. A., & Eichhorn, R. (1972). *The utilization of health services: Indices and correlates—a research bibliography* (DHEW Publication No. [HSM] 73-3003). Washington, DC: U.S. Government Printing Office.

44. Andersen, R., & Anderson, O. W. (1979). Trends in the use of health services. In H. E. Freeman, S. Levine, & L. Reeder (Eds.). *Handbook of medical sociology* (3rd ed.). Englewood Cliffs, NJ: Prentice-Hall.

45. Anderson, O. W., & Andersen, R. (1972). Patterns of use of health services. In H. E. Freeman, S. Levine, & L. Reeder (Eds.). *Handbook of medical sociology* (2nd ed.). Englewood Cliffs, NJ: Prentice-Hall.

46. Freeburg, L. C., Lave, J. R., Lave, L. B., et al. (1979). *Health status, medical care utilization, and outcome: An annotated bibliography of empirical studies,* vols. I–IV. (DHEW Publication No. [PHS] 80-3263). Washington, D.C.: U.S. Government Printing Office.

47. Hankin, J. & Oktay, J. S. (1979). *Mental disorder and primary medical care: An analytical review of the literature* (DHEW Publication No. [ADM] 78-661). Washington, D.C.: U.S. Government Printing Office.

48. Hulka, B. S., & Wheat, J. R. (1985). Patterns of utilization: The patient perspective. *Medical Care.* 23. 438–460.

49. Maurana, C. A., Eichhorn, R. L., & Lonnquist, L. E. (1981). *The use of health services: Indices and correlates—a research bibliography, 1981.* Rockville, MD: National Center for Health Services Research.

50. Muller, C. (1986). Muller, C. Review of twenty years of research on medical care utilization. *Health Services Research.* 21. (Part I). 129–144.

51. Zuvekas, A., Arnold, J., Bracken, B. W., et al. (1986). *Second generation project for identifying medically underserved populations.* Washington, DC: Lewin & Associates.

52. Andersen, R., & Anderson, O. W. (1967). *A decade of health services.* Chicago: University of Chicago Press.

53. Andersen, R., Lion, J., & Anderson, O. W. (1976). *Two decades of health services: Social survey trends in use and expenditure.* Cambridge, MA: Ballinger.

54. Anderson, O. W., & Feldman, J. (1956). *Family medical costs and voluntary health insurance: A nationwide survey.* New York: McGraw-Hill.

55. Anderson, O. W., Collette, P., & Feldman, J. (1963). *Changes in family medical expenditures and voluntary health insurance.* Cambridge, MA: Harvard University Press.

56. National Center for Health Statistics. (1986). *Health, United States, 1985* (DHHS Publication No. [PHS] 86-1232). Washington, DC: U.S. Government Printing Office.

57. National Center for Health Statistics. (1991). *Health, United States, 1990* (DHHS Publication No. [PHS] 91-1232). Washington, DC: U.S. Government Printing Office.

58. National Center for Health Statistics. (1990). *Current estimates for the National Interview Survey, United States, 1989,* Series 10, no. 176 (DHHS Publication No. [PHS] 90-1504. Washington, DC: U.S. Government Printing Office.

59. Donabedian, A., Axelrod, S. J., Wyszewianski, L., et al. (1986). *Medical care chartbook* (8th ed.). Ann Arbor, MI: Health Administration Press.

60. National Center for Health Statistics. (1982). *Health, United States, 1981* (DHHS Publication No. [PHS] 82-1232). Washington, DC: U.S. Government Printing Office.

61. Thornberry, O. T., Wilson, R. W., & Golden, P. (1986, September 19). Health promotion data for the 1990 objectives: Estimates from the National Health Interview Survey of health promotion and disease

prevention, United States, 1985. *Advance data from vital and health statistics,* No. 126 (DHHS Publication No. [PHS] 86-1250). Hyattsville, MD: Public Health Service.

62. U.S. Department of Health and Human Services. (1980). *A decade of dental service utilization, 1964–74* (DHHS Publication No. [HRA] 80-56). Washington, DC: U.S. Government Printing Office.

63. Aday, L. A., & Forthofer, R. (in press, 1992). A profile of black and Hispanic subgroups' access to dental care: Findings from the National Health Interview Survey. *Public Health Dentistry.*

64. Rovin, S., & Nash, J. (1982). Traditional and emerging forms of dental practice: Cost, accessibility, and quality factors. *American Journal of Public Health. 72.* 656–662.

65. National Center for Health Statistics. (1976). *Differentials in health characteristics by marital status, 1971–72.* Series 19, no. 104 (DHEW Publication No. [HRA] 76-1531). Washington, DC: U.S. Government Printing Office.

66. National Center for Health Statistics. (1979). *Current estimates for the Health Interview Survey, United States, 1978.* Series 10, no. 130 (DHEW Publication No. [PHS] 80-1551). Washington, DC: U.S. Government Printing Office.

67. National Center for Health Statistics. *Utilization of short-stay hospitals, United States, 1983.* Series 13, no. 83 (DHHS Publication No. [PHS] 85-1744). Washington, DC: U.S. Government Printing Office.

68. National Center for Health Statistics. (1991, April 4). *1989 Summary: National Hospital Discharge Survey. Advance data from vital and health statistics.* No. 199 (DHHS Publication No. [PHS] 91-1250). Washington, DC: U.S. Government Printing Office.

69. Ermann, D., & Gabel, J. (1985). The changing face of American health care: Multihospital systems, emergency centers, and surgery centers. *Medical Care. 23.* 401–420.

70. National Center for Health Statistics. (1985, September 20). An overview of the 1982 National Master Facility Interview Survey of nursing and related care homes. *Advance data from vital and health statistics.* No. 111 (DHHS Publication No. [PHS] 85-1250). Hyattsville, MD: Public Health Service.

71. Andersen, R., Aday, L. A., & Chen, M. S. (1986). Health status and health care utilization. *Health Affairs. 5.* 154–172.

72. National Center for Health Statistics. (1986). *Use of selected preventive care procedures, United States, 1982.* Series 10, no. 157 (DHHS Publication No. [PHS] 86-1585). Washington, DC: U.S. Government Printing Office.

73. National Center for Health Statistics. (1984). *Health indicators for Hispanic, black and white Americans.* Series 10, no. 148 (DHHS Publication No. [PHS] 84-1576). Washington, DC: U.S. Government Printing Office.

74. Andersen, R., Giachello, A., & Aday, L. A. (1986). Access of Hispanics to health care and cuts in service: A state-of-the-art overview. *Public Health Reporter. 10.* 238–252.

75. National Center for Health Statistics. (1983). *Physician visits: Volume and interval since last visit, United States, 1980.* Series 10, no. 144 (DHHS Publication No. [PHS] 83-1572). Washington, DC: U.S. Government Printing Office.

76. Wartman, S. A., Morlock, L. L., Malitz, F. E., et al. (1983). Impact of divergent evaluations by physicians and patients of patients' complaints. *Public Health Reporter. 98.* 141–145.

77. Kuder, J. M., & Levitz, G. S. (1985). Visits to the physician: An evaluation of the usual source effect. *Health Services Research. 20.* 579–596.

78. Luft, H. S. (1978). How do health maintenance organizations achieve their savings: Rhetoric and evidence. *New England Journal of Medicine. 298.* 1336–1343.

79. Luft, H. S. (1981). *Health maintenance organizations: Dimensions of performance.* New York: Wiley.

80. Manning, W. G., Leibowitz, A., Goldberg, G. A., et al. (1985). *A controlled trial of the effect of a prepaid group practice on the utilization of medical services.* R-3029-HHS. Santa Monica, CA: Rand Corporation.

81. Bazzoli, G. J. (1986). Health care for the indigent: Overview of critical issues. *Health Services Research. 21.* 353–393.

82. Anderson, H. J. (1985). Majority of hospitals are better off under protective pricing—surveys. *Modern Healthcare. 15.* 72–74.

83. Davis, K., Anderson, G. F., Renn, S. C., et al. (1985). Is cost containment working? *Health Affairs. 4.* 81–94.

84. Dolenc, D. A. (1985). DRGs: The counterrevolution

in financing health care. *Hastings Center Report. 15.* 19–29.

85. Iglehart, J. K. (1985). Early experience with prospective payment of hospitals. *New England Journal of Medicine. 314.* 1460–1464.

86. Newcomer, R., Wood, J., & Sankar, A. (1985). Medicare prospective payment: Anticipated effect on hospitals, other community agencies, and families. *Journal of Health Politics, Policy and Law. 10.* 275–282.

87. Simborg, D. W. (1981). DRG creep: A new hospital-acquired disease. *New England Journal of Medicine. 304.* 1602–1604.

88. Spiegel, A. D., & Kavaler, F. (1985). The debate over diagnosis-related groups. *Journal of Community Health. 10.* 81–92.

89. Wennberg, J. E., McPherson, K., Caper, P., et al. (1984). Will payment based on diagnosis-related groups control hospital costs? *New England Journal of Medicine. 311.* 295–300.

90. Beck, R. G., & Horne, J. M. (1980). Utilization of publicly insured health services in Saskatchewan before, during, and after copayment. *Medical Care. 18.* 787–806.

91. Lairson, D. & Swint, J. M. (1978). A multivariate analysis of the likelihood of volume of preventive visit demand in a prepaid group practice. *Medical Care. 16.* 730–739.

92. Scheffler, R. M. (1984). The United Mine Workers' health plan: An analysis of the cost-sharing program. *Medical Care. 22.* 247–254.

93. Newhouse, J. P., Manning, W. C., Morris, C. N., et al. (1981). Some interim results from a controlled trial of cost-sharing in health insurance. *New England Journal of Medicine. 305.* 1501–1507.

94. Rossiter, L. F., & Wilensky, G. R. (1982). Out-of-pocket expenses for personal health services. *NCHSR National Health Care Expenditures Study data preview 13* (DHHS Publication No. [PHS] 82-3332). Washington, DC: U.S. Government Printing Office.

PART THREE

Providers of Health Services

Chapter 4

Public Health Agencies and Services: The Partnership Network

William Shonick

Public health services have traditionally focused on the prevention of disease. A new capitalist society—one seeking a more comfortable life for more people with its dynamism and mobility—evolved out of the decline of the relatively stable and immobile feudalism in Europe, bringing with its new ways of living and traveling the side effects of new threats to health. Disease threatened whole communities and regions with severe illness and death.

Early public health efforts in Europe, and later in America, were directed at preventing or mitigating epidemics of acute infectious diseases such as smallpox, bubonic plague, cholera, typhoid fever, malaria, yellow fever, venereal disease, tuberculosis, and the childhood diseases of measles, mumps, scarlet fever, diphtheria, and whooping cough. (The recent status of the battles against infectious diseases is described in Last (1).

The changes in living conditions created by capitalism—rapid growth of city life, worldwide exploration and trade, and formidable technology—were accompanied by an ever-changing set of diseases as people struggled to adapt to their new environment (2,3). As each new threat to public health arose, it drew a response from some leading laypeople and professionals who tried, with varying degrees of success, to organize preventive services to mitigate or eliminate it.

During the earlier stages of capitalism, the greatest scourges were epidemics of acute, infectious, and highly lethal disease. With the advent of better public health measures and other factors, such as the development of genetic immunity in large portions of the population, these health threats were superseded in importance by chronic and debilitative diseases such as emphysema, abestosis, and other pulmonary diseases; cancer; stroke and heart disease; arthritis; and mental and emotional dysfunction associated with modern life. Throughout these changes, public health practitioners, policy makers, and researchers have attempted to learn the nature of the new threats and to organize public measures to combat them. To be fully effective, these measures had to be based on a correct assessment of what caused the disease and how it spread, which led to the development of methods to control its spread.

In most cases, some form of community organization was necessary to combat the spread of disease. Since the formation of these organizations usually involved governmental authority, the term public health arose. Thus the development of public health services had four aspects: 1) identifying the diseases that were the leading causes of death and debility; 2) learning their cause and method of transmission, 3) finding methods to prevent or control them, and 4) learning how to organize society to apply the controls effectively.

In describing the organization and development of public health services in the United States, this chapter follows the pattern suggested by the actual evolution of the public health programs described above. First, the discussion identifies the major threats to health existing during a particular period, and scientific discoveries that revealed what caused the disease, how it was transmitted, and how it could be combatted. Subsequently, the chapter shows how the understanding of the disease patterns, the state of scientific knowledge, and the current configuration of society shaped the specific form assumed by the organization of public health services in response to prevailing threats to health.

The organization of American public health agencies has involved an interplay of federal, state, and local governments and authorities. Although the form and functions of public health organizations were determined largely by the four factors listed above, the structure of the public health system was also strongly affected by the roles played by these three levels of government. Great changes in these roles have occurred over time, but the most significant one for the development of U.S. public health services was the passage of the Social Security Act of 1935. For the first time, the federal government began to play a major role in the development of state and local public health services. The following discussion of the development of public health services is therefore arranged in two major sections: through 1935 and the period after 1935.

Public Health in The Period Before 1935

Local Public Health Services

During the colonial period (1620–1781), small agricultural communities generally existed. In addition to farming, they engaged in some trade, and a few port towns, such as Boston, New York, Philadelphia, and Charleston, were beginning to develop into cities. The principal health threats were epidemics of acute infectious disease, probably resulting from a combination of unsanitary and unhealthy local conditions—unsafe water supplies, swamps, and poor sanitation in housing—and diseases brought in by the crews of ships anchored in the harbors. The port towns were the sites of some of the more serious epidemics.

Local organization to counter these epidemics consisted of voluntary boards of health set up, for the most part, on a temporary basis to meet particular threats. These ad hoc boards applied what were considered to be appropriate sanctions, namely, sanitation measures and quarantine. Quarantine was the practice of confining persons who were suspected of harboring a communicable disease to restricted quarters—a house or a ship—until there was no further evidence of the disease. All individuals who had had contact with the infected person would also be confined, except for physicians, nurses, and ministers, who were permitted to enter the house or board the ship as it lay in the harbor.

After the American Revolution, local public health services were carried on much as before. Community boards, meeting as the occasion required, used their power of quarantine to isolate infected people and their power of summons to force compliance with a sanitary code. In time, a practicing local physician occasionally came to be designated as the local public health officer. For his duties he was recompensed, always modestly and often not at all. However, the continued development of sea trade increased the frequency and severity of epidemics in the port cities. The threat was abetted by the initially slow but accelerating industrial development that further increased the size and congestion of the cities—both the ports and those further inland—in which manufacturing was developing. However, the epidemics in the port cities continued to be especially severe indicating that the most serious epidemics were imported at this time.

Yellow fever attacked these port cities in a series of epidemics, of which the Philadelphia epidemic of 1793 "was in many ways the worst calamity of its kind ever suffered by an American city" (4). It was particularly serious because Philadelphia was then the capital and cultural center of the newly independent United States and virtually the entire government deserted the city. The usual measures that were followed, quarantine and sanitation, were apparently not very effective, for more than one-tenth of the population died.

Before about 1850, local public health activities were largely reactive to the onset of epidemics. Aldermen, council members, or other local elected officials generally passed ordinances establishing house and ship quarantine and sanitation measures during epidemics. On an ongoing basis, they passed ordinances providing for street drainage, cleanliness of public markets, and waste disposal. With the development of biologic science in Europe, methods of preventing and controlling outbreaks of contagious disease became more effective. As a consequence, professional health departments arose during the years 1850–1900 with full-time officials who came to be known as *health officers* appointed to lead them.

The use of quarantine and sanitation was increasingly guided by the findings of the rapidly developing bacteriologic and pathologic sciences and new knowledge about animal and human disease carriers. The development of vaccines and antitoxins made the giving and promotion of immunizing innoculations a standard public health function. Increased knowledge about the causes and method of transmission of venereal diseases and tuberculosis led local health departments to engage in case finding and some treatment of these diseases.

As 1900 approached the increased efficiency of the immunization and venereal disease and tuberculosis prevention programs resulted in a steady decline in the importance of quarantine as a method of epidemic control. (The decline of quarantine was gradual; it continued to be used, especially on arriving ships and with patients in contagious stages of tuberculosis.) The designation of quarantine as a major functional category for local health departments was gradually replaced by including quarantine under "communicable disease control" along with the other epidemic control programs that were developed as a result of the growing fund of scientific information.

In addition to sanitation and communicable disease control, the collection and analysis of vital statistics was becoming a standard local public health activity and was steadily growing in sophistication. Like many other measures, it was an American adaptation of European and especially British public health practice. Records were kept of deaths by cause and demographic classification, and in later years, physicians were required to report the incidence of communicable diseases to the local public health authority. These data were used to monitor disease rates and to alert government authorities to the development of epidemics. They were also used to establish causes of disease in association with environmental factors.

The increasing sophistication of bacteriologic and pathologic science also created a growing appreciation of the importance of appropriate laboratory facilities to determine the communicable disease agents that were prevalent in the environment or in the population. This led to the addition of a fourth function for local public health departments—maintenance of a public health laboratory. Since most private physicians had no laboratories, a public health department laboratory that could test human tissue or fluid samples—sent by private practitioners—and water or food samples—submitted by health authorities or other citizens—became an important public health facility.

By 1925, most of the causes and methods of transmission of the leading communicable diseases that had afflicted humanity for thousands of years, producing devastating epidemics in Europe and America since 1300, had been identified. Preventive measures had been developed for most of these: water and food sanitation; identification, treatment, and perhaps isolation; immunization; and control of disease carriers (particularly the mosquito, louse, and rat). The requirements for applying these controls helped to shape the structures and operations of health departments. By the 1920s, worldwide epidemic and widespread endemic occurrences of most acute communicable diseases were more due to the failure to organize public health services for an entire population than to a lack of scientific or medical knowledge for preventing them.

With localities increasingly finding it necessary—or at least desirable—to employ full-time, professionally trained staff, the size of such staff grew, especially in large cities. Toward the end of the 1800s, a medium-sized to large community with a fairly adequate public health organization had a voluntary board of health with policy-making members appointed by the executive of the local government, and a department of public health with full-time professional staff headed by a medically trained health officer. Large departments often had other health officers in addition to the head of the agency. These other health officers headed bureaus or divisions that specialized in various aspects of public health work such as communicable disease control. The head of the agency might then be designated the commissioner of health or chief health officer. Helping the health officers were public health nurses who, in large departments, might be organized in a bureau or division of public health nursing. They aided by administering immunizations and other clinics, and by making home visits to determine the need for quarantine or to encourage immunization and perform other health education functions. Together with the local coroner, they were frequently the main collectors of vital statistics.

In a large city, sanitation functions were typically headed by civil engineers who specialized in sanitation. Working under these sanitary engineers were specially trained technicians known as *sanitarians*. Sanitary engineers framed the ordinances and planned the waterworks and waste disposal sys-

tems to ensure freedom from contamination. Those who did not actually plan sanitary construction were consulted on proposals. The sanitarians inspected places of business (especially food establishments), houses, streets, and other areas for violations of the sanitary code. They often collected food and water samples and sent them to the local or state public health department laboratory for analysis. They also reported violations of the sanitary code to the health department, where the reports were routed to the appropriate health officer or sanitary engineer. Vital statistics were assembled by trained personnel, known as registrars.

The typical bureau or division of communicable disease control operated diagnostic clinics for identifying venereal disease and tuberculosis, provided or arranged for treatment, and enforced isolation or hospitalization for identified cases. In many places, attempts were made to identify and locate people from whom the disease had been acquired ("contact tracing"). This officer also offered immunization against those diseases for which vaccines and antitoxins were available and supervised vector (disease carrier) control measures such as drainage of stagnant water to control mosquito breeding and rat and louse eradiction.

The division of public health laboratories provided diagnostic services for physicians, public health clinics, and sanitarians. Samples sent to such laboratories were tested for contagious disease organisms. Many laboratories also distributed vaccines to private physicians, although in some places this was done by the division of communicable disease control.

Smaller health departments rarely had the full complement of bureaus or divisions, each performing a major specialized function and headed by a highly trained specialist (described above). They usually operated only with sanitarians and had no sanitary engineers on staff. Instead of highly trained registrars, general clerks or nurses handled whatever vital statistics were collected; communicable disease control was most likely handled by the health officer who also headed the agency; and tissue, food, and water samples were sent to the state public health laboratory for analysis. In very small health departments, a single health officer—often a part-time, local private practitioner—handled all these functions or shared them with a single public health nurse and perhaps a clerk.

In addition to changes in local public health practice resulting largely from scientific advances, the turn of the century brought with it marked changes in local health department practice due to social developments in the U.S. population. Important demographic changes were taking place in the large cities of the East Coast and the Midwest. Immigration had been an important factor in the population of the United States throughout the 1800s (5), but particularly large waves of immigrants began arriving in New York and other cities by 1892. Immigration peaked during 1901–1910 and then subsided slowly, reaching its low point during 1931–1940. Working in factories and mills, these immigrants were predominantly poor and settled into many urban ghettos, especially in New York City.

The resulting slum conditions produced illnesses similar to those that had arisen in Great Britain during the Industrial Revolution of 1750–1850, when the cities became very unhealthy and unsafe because of massive immigration from the countryside. Reformers and volunteer organizers worked and propagandized to ameliorate the living conditions of the tightly packed slums. The health condition of the immigrants—a principal concern—focused on communicable disease and infant mortality; housing, especially sanitation; and nutrition. Volunteer agencies opened milk stations in slum areas to provide uncontaminated milk and established clinics for child care. The outpatient departments of public and some private hospitals were inundated with patients seeking primary care.

This period saw the first sign of schism in public health professional circles concerning a basic issue: the appropriateness of including personal health care in a public health department. As noted previously, until about 1900 the functions of local

public health departments had generally focused on communitywide control measures—vital statistics, sanitation, communicable disease control, and public health laboratories. Sanitation was an engineering and inspection function; quarantine called for examination at times, but was basically an administrative and police activity (the government's right to quarantine superseded even property rights); and much immunization was done by private physicians with vaccines obtained from the health department. These four functions originated in the fight against epidemics of acute infectious diseases. The great improvement in the ability of local health departments to carry on the battles stemmed from scientific advances. The daily activities largely involved numbers, statistics, chemical tests, microscopes, and site inspections. It is also true that there was some laying on of hands. Blood samples were drawn, patients examined, and X rays taken. The principal aim of these activities was to determine whether the subject was infected with a communicable disease and, if so, what had to be done to prevent the spread to the community. The activities relating to sanitation often involved no contact with other people at all and immunizations entailed minimal personal contact. The basic purpose was community protection, not concern for the patient's personal care. After all, most of these activities could be carried out from one headquarters building with perhaps a few regional centers in large cities.

Given the overwhelming problems of the slums in the big cities after 1890, many in public health were saying that the most significant new need for the immigrants was for preventive health centers in their neighborhoods, oriented to personal services. In addition, the public health departments in large cities should develop chains of neighborhood public health centers. Furthermore, it was suggested that additional preventive services of a personal nature—maternal and child health (well care only) and health education, including nutrition—should be offered at these centers. The subject remained controversial until about 1910, when the New York City Health Department implemented a system of neighborhood health centers in poor areas that offered maternal and child health care, examinations (and even some treatment) for venereal disease, and tuberculosis detection. These neighborhood-based programs, involving part-time private clinicians, rapidly gained almost unanimous acceptance in professional public health circles and maternal and child health quickly became the fifth function considered to be basic to public health services.

Although the issue of public health departments providing general personal health (i.e., general medical) services became a more serious policy issue in public health circles after 1935, the expansion of local health departments into any aspect of curative or therapeutic general medicine, as opposed to preventive services, was watched closely and nervously by local medical societies even before 1935. The local and national medical societies jealously guarded their exclusive right to give medical care, and their resistance to perceived challenges often took on a truculent tone. Their insistence on the sole right to dispense personal medical treatment was largely responsible for the restriction of public health departments to communitywide activities such as communicable disease treatment and prevention and sanitation control. If a patient was completely indigent and could not afford to pay for treatment, the organized medical profession had no objection to local or other government agencies providing treatment in clinics or via government-reimbursed physicians. But the preference was for fee-for-service reimbursement to private physicians rather than the use of salaried physicians, and for welfare department rather than public health department sponsorship. During the relatively prosperous 1920–1929 period, the operation of general medical care clinics by local health departments was occasionally tolerated by the medical profession. However, during the Depression many of these programs were effectively discontinued, and the public health profession was sharply reminded that its scope did not extend to curative care.

State Public Health Agencies Before 1935

Permanent state health departments developed later than their local counterparts, as states were being pressed to exercise their police powers under the Constitution with respect to health. The power of the state to carry out functions such as protecting the health of its citizens "is generally referred to as the state's police power . . . i.e., the power to 'enact and enforce laws to protect and promote the health, safety, morals, order, peace, comfort, and general welfare of the people' . . . and local agencies, including state and local public health departments and agencies, derive their power by delegation from the state legislature" (6). The permanently organized state health department became a familiar part of state government during the years 1870–1910 when it was becoming increasingly apparent that many health problems were wider in geographic scope than the local community. As commercial and industrial development became statewide and regional rather than local, statewide public health action became necessary. One of the principal immediate factors leading to the formation of a state public health organization often was a request "from a comparatively large number of localities which shared a common problem, or when some powerful local jurisdiction such as a large city, demanded state action" (7).

The first permanent state board of health was organized in 1869 in Massachusetts. This was not surprising since the function and structure of such a department were first formulated in that state. Lemuel Shattuck, a bookseller and a student of the work of the English public health reformer Edwin Chadwick, had been campaigning for the improvement of public health measures in Massachusetts when, in 1849, he was appointed chairman of the Massachusetts Sanitary Commission, which had been created by the governor to make a "sanitary survey" of the state. The report of this commission, issued in 1850, "has become a classic in public health literature and documents" (7), with many of its recommendations serving as guides for the subsequent organization of state and local health departments. The recommenda-tions were remarkably comprehensive. In fact, many of them are still regarded as desirable even though they still remain largely unrealized to the present day.

By 1900, 40 states had state health departments, and by 1909, the remainder had organized some form of health department. The previously cited study of public health departments by Ferrell et al. (8) found that in 1925 a total of 17 states had an organized bureau of county health work with a full-time director in charge. The highlighting of his finding indicates the importance attached by public health leaders to the promotion of local health work as a function of the state health department. The interrelationship of the state and local public health agencies remains an important aspect of the public health system to the present day.

The Ferrell study found that the proportion of funds allocated for local full-time health depart-ments provided by the states varied greatly—an-other condition that still prevails. One state met 48 percent of the total expenses for full-time county health service, and in 10 states, the state's share of county budgets ranged from 20 to 30 percent of the total. The study revealed that "the trend toward increasing the aid from the state is grow-ing." (8) Functions found to be performed or pro-moted most often by state health departments in 1925 consisted of rural or district health work: development of local health units; communicable disease control, particularly tuberculosis and ve-nereal disease; vital statistics; public health labo-ratories; sanitary engineering; child hygiene; public health nursing; public health education; and food and drug regulation and control. In many states, full-time divisions were organized in the state health department to direct some of these functions.

Because this report described the situation ex-isting before the Social Security Act of 1935 began pumping federal money into the states to expand state and local health department facilities and functions, it was used as a benchmark to measure

later progress resulting from the availability of these funds.

Federal Role in Local and State Public Health Services Before 1935

Although public health services have been directly supervised or delivered almost entirely by state and local health departments, discussion of the federal role is required, as the pattern of these services has, over the years, been influenced by federal government policy. This influence was stronger after 1935 than before, but it has been there all along. The foundations for a federal role were established in the pre-1935 period, and after 1935, large-scale federal grants-in-aid and the regula-tions accompanying them increasingly determined the direction of state and local policy. Federal policy rapidly became dominant.

An intricate and unique federal system was cre-ated in which states supervised local public health, set standards, and did only a small amount of direct service delivery; localities delivered most of the direct services, and the federal government paid for these services, setting national policy in the process. The intergovernmental relations were involved and sometimes baffling.

Under the U.S. Constitution, the protection of public health is, as a general proposition, implicitly reserved to the individual states under its policy powers, since a health function is not explicitly assigned to Congress. Whenever constitutional au-thorization was invoked to justify early federal ac-tion in public health matters, one or both of two sections of the Constitution were cited. Under the first of these sections, Congress is specifically given the power to "regulate commerce with foreign nations, and among the several states." This pro-viso was used to justify the earliest federal activities centering on control of communicable diseases at ports of entry and, somewhat later, included at-tempts to control communicable diseases in inter-state commerce. Under the second proviso, that of Article I, Section VIII, Congress is empowered to "provide for the general welfare of the United States."

This clause was the justification advanced by those who sought federal intervention in health problems in the interests of countrywide uniformity, equity, and efficiency (6).

Early federal legislation, beginning in 1796, concentrated on attempting to control the introduction into the United States of communicable diseases such as malaria, yellow fever, and cholera. To this end, various laws were passed establishing aid for quarantine procedures at major ports of entry. The 1796 law merely provided for cooperation of the federal government with states and localities in enforcing state and local laws of ship quarantine. Quarantine authority itself was still regarded by Congress as resting with the states, but opposition to this view also existed.

In 1878 the Marine Hospital Service—which had been established in 1798 to provide medical care for merchant seamen—was designated as the agency that would assist any state or community requesting services in helping to prevent the introduction of contagious or infectious diseases into this country. In 1879, a National Board of Health with a four-year term of office was voted by Congress. Its duties included having "charge of interstate and foreign quarantine" (7). Because of serious dissent among its participants and various other public health bodies, the board became effectively defunct at the end of the mandated four years and officially ceased to exist in 1893. At the end of its effective life in 1883, quarantine duties were restored to the Marine Hospital Service (7). Under an 1893 act ship quarantine became a federal function, and by 1921, all quarantine stations had been acquired and were being operated by the federal government.

Congress also passed laws regulating interstate quarantine measures, with enforcement powers delegated to the National Board of Health in 1879. These powers were strengthened and specifically given to the Marine Hospital Service in 1893. Thereafter the public health aspects of the work of the Marine Hospital Service were concerned primarily with control of communicable diseases with respect to both introduction of disease from abroad

and its spread among the states. The agency used this internal power very cautiously, and for the most part, assisted states with advice and personnel only when asked, despite the 1893 law entitling it to use enforcement.

Another aspect of the Marine Hospital Service's work in communicable disease control consisted of administering federal grants-in-aid to localities and lending personnel for demonstration projects in selected states, thereby hoping to encourage better practice. This was a relatively minor facet of its operations, however.

Despite the change of the Marine Hospital Service's name first to the U.S. Public Health and Marine Hospital Service in 1902 and finally to the U.S. Public Health Service in 1912, it continued to concentrate mainly on medical care for seamen and other stipulated eligible individuals and on foreign quarantine. Beginning in 1913, however, a gradual broadening of perspective occurred when Congress began to appropriate funds for local public health research. During the years 1914–1916, the service, in cooperation with about 16 states, conducted a series of field studies in typhoid fever control. These field investigations contained a large demonstration component, and by 1917, funds were appropriated annually by Congress for rural sanitation work by the U.S. Public Health Service. The grants had to be matched by the states receiving them, an arrangement that lasted through 1934.

Between 1915 and 1935, two other sources of federal support for state and local public health activity were grants for venereal disease control and maternal and child hygiene. Grants for venereal disease control began with the Chamberlain-Kahn Act of 1918, which allocated funds to the states according to their population. Although federal appropriations for this program eventually dwindled away and ultimately disappeared by 1926, venereal disease control laws were strengthened, and programs remained in effect in many states. Grants for maternal and child health began in 1921 with the passage of the Sheppard-Towner Act. Administration of the act was assigned to the Chil-

Fed grants to support local/state efforts

dren's Bureau, which was established in 1912 as part of the U.S. Department of Labor. The Children's Bureau had been doing research and educational work on matters pertaining to the welfare of children, and had been a leading proponent of the 1921 legislation. The act provided for allocation of appropriated money among the states by a formula. Mustard writes that "between 1922 and 1927 the Division of Maternal and Infant Hygiene carried on an aggressive and productive program" (7). In 1929 the program ended when federal funds were discontinued.

Thus the period up to 1935 witnessed development of public health both as a profession and as a form of government organization to combat epidemics of acute communicable disease. The government organization was principally local, with many of the larger cities having impressive departments and boards. The states were supervising organizations that concentrated on setting standards and monitoring local service, and encouraging the formation of local health departments where none existed. Direct local public health services were also provided via state "districts" in areas that needed services but did not have a local department. By 1934, the federal government was working with states in performing quarantine services at major ports, providing modest amounts of aid to localities, and improving sanitation services in rural areas. The federal public health agency also supervised interstate quarantine on requests.

The Growing Disparity between the Tax Base and Service Responsibilities Among Levels of Government

The chapter now turns to two aspects of the interrelationship among the three levels of American government: 1) the distribution among these levels of the responsibility for delivering services to the populace and 2) the tax resources available to them.

One would suppose, on a commonsense basis, that if a particular level of government is expected to assume responsibility for a specific function,

such as providing public health protection, national tax revenues sufficient to finance it would be made available to this level. And, indeed, at the time of the inception of the United States, the proportion of the total national tax revenues collected by each level was roughly proportional to its share of the service responsibilities. Most government services were locally delivered and the local tax on agricultural real property yielded the most revenue of any tax because most people were engaged in agricultural pursuits. This was certainly true of public health. There were no state health departments and federal government involvement in public health was minimal.

But as the center of the United States economy moved from family-owned farms to a corporate, industrial, and commercial basis, the functions of the state governments, and especially the federal government, multiplied. The principal tax base became money income and the principal source of tax revenue was the income tax. The major collector for income tax (after 1913) became the federal government, with the states a poor second and the localities last.

The need for public health services increased by leaps and bounds as society became industrialized and urbanized. But the principal burden of delivering these services remained with the localities, which now had the smallest share of the total tax revenues while the federal government with its largest share of revenues carried a much smaller share of the burden. Thus, whereas the proportion of the available tax base had shifted in favor of the federal government, responsibility for health services (and other social services) remained with the state and local governments. The problem resulting from this "cultural lag" between the development of state and local service responsibilities and their tax revenue base led to a basic restructuring of the distribution of total tax revenues by government level after 1935. This change was so important that further discussion of the factors leading to the lag that caused it is warranted.

In its early years, the federal government limited its functions primarily to conducting foreign affairs, providing for national armed forces, and regulating commerce both with foreign governments and among the states. The founding fathers clearly seemed to believe that the basic regulatory and administrative unit of government, as far as the individual citizen was concerned was the state, with the federal government handling only those problems that involved all or at least several of the states. It was thus entirely appropriate that the federal government's revenues came mostly from various excise taxes and tariffs. The principal function of the tariffs was to protect the development of the infant American industry; the fact that they also produced revenue was an added benefit.

As late as 1910, 54 percent of the population was still listed as rural and only 46 percent as urban. But by 1970, 73 percent of the population was urban. Between 1910 and 1920, the majority of the population shifted from rural to urban and remained so thereafter. During this same period, there was a basic shift from a primarily agricultural population to one engaged in commerce, industry, and services.

After the Civil War, with the increase in regulatory functions to serve the burgeoning and increasingly centralized American capitalism, and with rising military expenditures, the federal government's need for additional revenue was growing into a permanent feature of national operations. As the major source of personal income shifted markedly from agricultural production or family-owned real property to nonagricultural products and services produced with corporate money and property, the federal government sought to tap these new sources of wealth.

After an attempt in 1894 to legislate a federal income tax was struck down as unconstitutional by a five-to-four decision of the Supreme Court *(Pollack v. Farmer's Loan and Trust Co.)*, the 16th amendment to the Constitution was ratified in 1913, explicitly permitting the federal government to levy taxes. Thereafter, the federal income tax rapidly became the most important single source of tax revenue for the federal government, accounting for $26 billion out of the total $35 billion, or

75 percent of federal receipts for 1950, and $173 billion out of $201 billion, or 86 percent in 1976. Customs revenues, which accounted for 84 percent of the total revenue in 1800, 91 percent in 1850, and as much as 41 percent even as late as 1900, had shrunk to less than an insignificant 1 percent by 1950.

Equally illuminating is the change over time in the percentage of total government tax revenues collected by state and local units compared with that collected by the federal government. In 1902 64 percent of total taxes were collected by the states and localities and 36 percent by the federal government. These percentages remained relatively stable until after World War II. By 1950, the picture was almost exactly the reverse of the 1900–1940 pattern, with 69 percent of all taxes being collected by the federal government. Thus, during the immediate post-World War II years, some 65 to 70 percent of all taxes were being collected by the federal government.

The shift of the major tax base from real property to cash income resulted not only in a movement in taxable resources from the states and localities to the federal level but also, and perhaps more important, in a heavily unbalanced geographic distribution of these taxable money resources (tax base) among the states. States with industrial— including large-scale, industrially organized agriculture (agribusiness)—commercial, and financial centers had high per capita incomes; those that were predominantly rural and had few or only secondary centers of industry, commerce, and finance suffered from low per capita incomes. The available base for local taxes became more and more unevenly distributed, not only among states but also among localities within states. Furthermore, the need for health services from state and local governments was often in inverse proportion to the available tax base. Study after study of expenditures for health services of the various states in the 1920s, '30s, and '40s revealed two important facts: 1) the amount spent per capita varied greatly from state to state and 2) states with a lower per capita income spent less per capita for public health than did states with higher per capita incomes, although they were spending more relative to their total tax revenues and income than were the more affluent states. In other words, poorer states were often trying harder and doing worse in providing public health than more affluent ones.

It was clear that increasing local and state taxes could not equitably provide a level of public health services to uniformly match local needs across the nation because local taxable income was generally in inverse proportion to such needs. Further, although the tax base now favored the federal government, the states' responsibility for providing public health and other services remained heavily weighted at the local level. A solution to the problem boiled down to a choice between two alternatives or some combination of them: either 1) the responsibility for many public health and other services could be directly transferred to the federal government by legislative, constitutional, or judicial action, or 2) the states could keep their responsibilities but receive money back from federal tax revenues to finance them. Federal revenues would thus be shared with the states and localities, but program control could remain largely in state and local hands. Revenue sharing did occur eventually, but with it came a shift in responsibility and program control of the public health (and other) fields to the federal government. This change corroborated the well-established maxim, "control follows the dollar."

After 1935, the principal mechanism used to correct the disparity between tax base and service responsibilities was the grant-in-aid, under which the federal government shared its tax revenues with the states and localities. Different schemes for distributing these grants among the states have been used. Some formulas are better for achieving a particular set of goals and other formulas are more suitable for other goals. We will now consider various mechanisms and their respective objectives in supplying grants-in-aid to various levels of government. Subsequent sections discuss how federal health grants actually operated with respect to state and local public health work after 1935.

Redistribution of Tax Revenues Among Different Levels of Government

Two basic methods have been used to allocate federal grant money among states and their localities—the formula grant and the project grant. Formula grants are distributed among the states according to a formula established by law. The basis for distribution may be equal allocation, variable allocation, or a combination of the two. Under the infrequently used equal allocation, an equal fixed amount is allocated to each state. Under variable allocation, certain characteristics of each state determine the percentage of the total national appropriation it receives. This type of grant allocation was the more common one for health purposes until about 1965, and it is still widely used. Its main attribute is that it permits the appropriation to be distributed in a manner that helps equalize services and tax burdens throughout the nation by adjusting the share that each state receives by the relative need of that state for the services the grant is meant to support.

The preceding discussion deals with formulas for *distributing* money among the states. Grants to states also often carry stipulations about how the money may be *spent*. Formula grants have been further identified as either general purpose (block grants) or earmarked (categorical grants), depending on the restrictions imposed. Block grants for public health departments may be used for broadly defined purposes such as improving and expanding local health department services. On the other hand, categorical grants to a local health department may be spent only for a specific type of activity, such as cancer control. It is important to note that what may seem to be a block grant at one level of administration is viewed as a categorical grant at a higher level. For example, a general-purpose grant to a local health department is a block grant for that department, but it is categorically restricted from the point of view of the local government, which may prefer to use part of it for law enforcement.

Project grants are principally designed to carry

out a particular federal program rather than to help a local health agency accomplish its own objectives. This grant transfers money directly from the federal government to a state or local government, or to any other type of government or nongovernment organization, for carrying out a specific project previously approved by the federal granting agency. The grant award is often made to one of several competing applicants. This type of grant requires an application from a would-be recipient and is not given automatically to any government unit according to a preset formula.

The Period After 1935

Local Health Department Growth, 1936–1945

The Social Security Act of 1935 established annual grants-in-aid from the federal government to the states, some of which were to further the development of full-time local health departments. This act marked the first major entrance of the federal government into a systemic nationwide relationship with state and local governments with respect to providing support for public health department operations. Although all of the act's provisions were interrelated, and a number of them affected health services, two actions directly mandated federal support for state and local public health departments. Title V, Part 1, provided grants to the states for aiding state and local health departments to provide maternal and child health services to be administered by the U.S. Children's Bureau, which at that time was part of the U.S. Department of Labor. These were categorical grants earmarked for maternal and child health. Title VI provided grants to the states to aid the work of state and local health departments. Title VI funds were administered by the U.S. Public Health Service (USPHS) and were formula block (or general) health grants that could be spent as each public health department saw fit, within very broad limits. For both Title V and Title VI grants, the states had to match federal money dollar for dollar.

The Mountin Report

The enhanced development of these departments during the years 1936–1945 has been described by Joseph W. Mountin, a USPHS assistant surgeon general well known for his public health writing, and his associates. In a USPHS monograph (9), a substantial expansion of local and state public health department services was described.

The Mountin report indicated that the number of counties covered by full-time local health services grew from 762 in 1935 to 1,577 in 1940 and then to 1,851 in 1946, and that the proportion of the population covered in the county areas outside the cities that had their own municipal health departments grew from 37 percent in 1935 to 72 percent in 1946. (Many of the counties contained large cities with their own health departments. These departments were often more richly staffed than the county departments serving the people living outside the large cities. Therefore, all of the residents of those cities were considered to be covered by appropriate local health services. The covering of increased percentages of people by public health services was therefore seen as primarily a problem for the areas, as the cities had their own municipal health departments.) The influence of these funds on the growth of local health department staffs, again exclusive of independent metropolitan centers, was equally marked, with total full-time personnel increasing from 3,435 to 10,320—more rapidly in nonmedical than in medical personnel. This improvement was accomplished in spite of the fact that "a considerable proportion of established positions for medical personnel—and others—were vacant for war-related reasons" (9). The data also indicated that at least 60 cities with populations of 10,000 or greater were added to the list of cities with "some type of full-time official public health organization." Mountin et al. define municipal health departments as "those city health units which operate under full-time technical directions and are independent of county or district organization" (9).

Despite this progress, by 1946 approximately 30 percent of the nonmetropolitan population, and almost 20 percent of the total population, still had no access to full-time local health coverage. Furthermore, some of the expanded coverage was of questionable depth, often representing a reporting artifact resulting from a simple incorporating of additional areas by consolidating several counties into multicounty health districts without a proportionate increase in staff and other needed resources. Public health professionals and analysts insistently and increasingly stressed that extending full-time local health services coverage of at least minimally acceptable quality to the entire population was an important and perhaps overriding goal of public health. It was clear that the extent of such coverage could not be accurately measured if standards defining minimally acceptable services were not available.

The Emerson Report

Because of this expressed professional desire to define minimally acceptable local health services more clearly, growth in the number of local health departments and in the numbers of types of services offered due to federal grants was accompanied by a heightened interest in defining adequate quality or depth of service. A special committee of the American Public Health Association chaired by a well-known public health officer, Haven Emerson, worked on this question. In 1945, it issued a definitive set of standards for assessing the existence of minimally adequate public health services. The committee also estimated what resources would be needed to cover the entire population with public health services that met these standards. Standards were set for staffing, types of services to be offered, organization of both the board and the department, and other matters. Staffing standards were derived by applying presumed desirable per capita personnel numbers to population size of the designated local areas. All needed improvements were projected as required increases over the 1942 data, which served as a baseline. This information was embodied in what has come to be known as the Emerson Report (10).

The section of the report dealing with the scope of function probably had the most lasting influence. The committee defined the six basic functions (which came to be known as the "basic six" functions) of a local public health department as follows:

1. Vital statistics—recording, tabulation, interpretation, and publication of essential facts of births, deaths, and reportable diseases
2. Communicable disease control—tuberculosis, venereal disease, malaria, and hookworm
3. Sanitation—supervision of milk, water, and eating places
4. Laboratory services
5. Maternal and child hygiene, including supervision of the health of school-age children
6. Health education

Public health goals for the future were described in these terms:

"The Committee is of the opinion that a present goal should be the creation of such number and boundaries of areas of local health jurisdiction in every state in the union as will bring within the reach of every person and family the benefits of modern sanitation, personal hygiene, and the guidance and protection of trained professional and accessory personnel employed on a full-time basis at public expense, selected and retained on a merit or civil service basis, and free from disturbance by the influence of partisan politics" [10:26].

The emphasis on the merit civil service system of personnel practice as a necessary reform to curb the abuses of an earlier day is worthy of note.

Developments After the Emerson Report: The Period 1946–1965

The period 1936–1945 had been one of consolidating the position of local health departments. With the federal Title V and Title VI monies and the federally mandated matching state contributions, local public health departments became well ensconced as the basic public agencies for delivering the services required to implement the standard basic six functions. The Emerson Report provided visible evidence of the forward-looking drive and professional expertise characterizing many of the leaders of public health departments. In general, leaders of the federal government's health activities accepted the role of the local health department as delineated by leading public health executives through their activities at the American Public Health Association (APHA) and worked with local and state leaders to develop public health departments with more personnel, greater depth of program activities, and wider geographic coverage. Here and there, dissent was raised about the inadequate scope of function of these departments. It was noted that times were changing and that the basic six functions would no longer suffice to adequately protect the public's health. In particular, more attention needed to be paid to preventing and controlling chronic and degenerative diseases and to providing general medical care in public health clinics for individuals with no third-party insurance coverage for paying medical bills. These criticisms began to multiply rapidly after World War II.

Mounting problems in the large cities, the growth of private health insurance that covered only the nonpoor, and the social reformism of some federal administrations and congresses all combined to put pressure on local public health departments to deliver services that were essentially alien to the spirit of the Emerson Report. The recommendations of that report had stressed preventive services based on suppressing acute infectious disease. The nature of the new demands on the local health departments and how they were met is the subject of this section. Of course, this story also must include the roles of the states and federal government, which also grew rapidly, especially that of the federal government. These will be addressed later.

A U.S. government study (11) indicated that by 1960 some 94 percent of the population was judged to have access to the services of full-time local health departments. These numbered 1,577 and covered 2,425 of the 3,072 counties in the United States. It was clear that widespread coverage had been achieved, but the depth or quality of coverage

recommended by the Emerson Report was lacking. Other data of this 1960 study indicated that the per capita personnel level recommended by the Emerson Report had not been achieved. In the all-important categories of public health nurses and dental personnel, the staffing was far short of the recommendations; the number of dental hygienists and public health nurses per population had actually declined from 1942 levels. Indeed, the overall staff-to-population ratio was somewhat lower in 1960 than the Emerson Report baseline figures showed for 1942; yet the development of the standard local public health department had gone about as far as it was to go.

Thus there is every indication that by 1960 most of the nonmetropolitan United States had access to full-time local public health department services, and the small part that did not appeared to have little need for it. "Full-time" continued to mean having only a separate public health department address (i.e., not a private physician's office) and at least one full-time employee, even if that person was only a clerk. But further public sentiment for enriching standard public health department staffs in rural and semirural areas was not strong. The political pressures for improvement in public health services were coming from another quarter—the metropolitan areas. In those areas, defined here in similar fashion to the Census Bureau's Metropolitan Statistical Area (SMA) as consisting of a large city and its surrounding trading area, two civilizations were developing—that of the central or inner city and that of the more affluent suburbs. These two cultures, although distinct, interacted with each other, usually to the detriment of the inner-city one. Members of each culture had quite different public health needs and demands. The inner-city populations and their advocates were pressing for more and better public medical services, especially primary care. The social structure of what had been working- and middle-class areas in large cities before World War II had changed, leaving them almost bereft of private physicians. In many places, they were also demanding better protection against unsafe and unclean dwellings and streets, but the demand for medical care was the more politically prominent.

Many urban areas had long had health departments that met or exceeded the minimum standards of the Emerson Report, but the standard health department was not organized to cope with the newer inner-city needs. By long-standing tradition, provision of general medical care was alien to its leadership. Fighting for improved sanitation was part of the tradition and function of local public health departments, but the widespread deterioration of the inner cities overwhelmed their resources. Coping with the ubiquitous physical devastation of slum areas and the fiscal plight of the cities was simply too much for these departments. Even standard public health activities such as public health nurse home visits often could not be properly carried out given the increasingly unsafe neighborhoods and hostile clients. The two major requirements of the inner city for public health services—medical care and aggressive enforcement of sanitation (including safety)—found the local public health department unable to respond adequately.

The demands of suburban populations focused on other issues. Their intellectual and artistic leaders demanded broadly defined environmental control (air pollution, radiation emissions, solid waste), consumer product safety, automotive safety, and similar matters. The local public health departments existing in the newly built-up suburban areas were holdovers from those that had operated in the previous rural environments and were still functioning on a relatively modest scale, focusing on an obsolete set of problems and largely ignoring the newly growing ones. They were ill-equipped and insufficiently empowered to handle these new demands and the rapid surge of development. Further, even the most efficient and forward-looking local public health leaders faced the reality that most of the problems were being caused by large, powerful industries—automotive, petrochemical, nuclear power, and extractive. They could scarcely be controlled by a local health department, even a very well managed and up-to-date one. Only re-

gional, state, and in many cases, federal (and even international for many important problems) agencies could realistically be expected to deal with them.

The confluence of the two distinct sets of problems posed by the disparate cultures in the metropolitan areas, neither of which proved very amenable to amelioration by the work of the standard local public health department as it had developed, greatly diminished the public standing of and federal support for these departments.

Congress and the White House were being pressed to consider means of using government power more effectively to make better medical care available to everyone, especially those in the lower income brackets, and to improve the quality of the environment. The leadership of the local public health department found itself faced with a changed and seemingly intractable set of problems and rapid alterations in the composition of its clientele. Various experts and commentators were counseling different courses. Some writers and practicing professionals advised local public health departments to stick to prevention, as defined in the Emerson Report. Others called for a bold expansion into delivering primary medical care. Still others sought to define the fundamental role of the local public health department as one of areawide health planning, standard setting, and monitoring. Examples abound of the probing, questioning, and exhortation that come from all sides, reflecting confusion about the "true" role of local public health departments. (Similar questions were being raised about the role of state health departments).

Perhaps the most vivid indication of attempts within the ranks to redefine the function of public health departments is provided by the annual efforts of the APHA leadership to spell them out in official policy settlements. Over the years, official APHA positions on the scope of functions and proper organization of local public health departments continued to change in recognition of changing conditions.

There was a sharp decline in federal funding given to local health department operations—it dropped from $15 million (19 percent of the total spent by local health departments) in 1947 to $9 million (5 percent of the total) in 1956, so that the brunt of expenditures fell increasingly on states and, especially, localities. This decline in federal contribution came in spite of increased local outlays, from $54 million to $127 million, and increased state contributions, from $10 million to $40 million, during the same period. The relative decline in federal money, therefore, was even greater than the absolute reduction (12).

Public Policy Implications

The federal government's criticism of the adaptive abilities of local public health departments was reflected in its mechanisms for giving grants to local governments. This issue is discussed in greater detail later, but it is appropriate to mention it here. The federal grants-in-aid to states that had been used since 1936 largely to help local health departments develop their traditional functions—the so-called formula grants for general health purposes—declined, while the categorical formula and the project grants increased (13). The last two, especially the project grants, were aimed at promoting carefully focused demonstration projects to encourage innovative approaches to expanding public health functions in directions desired by the federal government. Many articles and speeches by public health figures and federal analysts, and the changing positions being taken in the policy statements of the APHA, showed that changing social conditions were placing demands on local health departments in large metropolitan areas that were perceived in Washington as not being met. These demands centered on medical care for the poor, enforcement of local environmental health conditions in the ghettos (particularly housing conditions), and regional environmental control, demanded primarily by sections of the middle classes. None of these demands was met to any great degree, despite the infusion of federal and state funds, policy statements by public health organizations, and the writings of professional public

health administrators, academics, journalists, and a wide assortment of general pundits. Why were adequately substantial changes in scope of function not being made?

Solving these rapidly growing problems involved tackling adversaries for which the local health department was no match politically. Eliminating the unhealthy conditions of ghetto life meant fighting slum landlords, urban redevelopers, and urban political machines to obtain adequate and meaningful inspection and enforce compliance, and to alter the balance of power controlling local planning and development agencies. This meant taking on the entire problem of the deterioration of the inner city. Providing adequate medical care for the poor in the cities involved tackling the entire system of medical care distribution, including the traditional treatment of the public medical care sector as a residual, second-class track. The fundamental problems of the health delivery system and the inner cities could not be solved by local public health departments, although vigorously and skillfully led ones could do more than others. The problem of environmental decay that was troubling the middle class was not amenable to local solution. The large corporations and their polluting activities, as well as the attendant problems of automobile transportation and housing sprawl, could scarcely be tackled by the states, let alone the local government. Thus, despite suggestions for policy changes appearing in APHA resolutions and goading by speeches and writings of commentators— and that of officers of the federal government and grant mechanism manipulation—the local health department as an institution, departed little from its well-beaten path.

Also, the problem of medical care for low-income groups was shifting to a national focus, and the battle to preserve the environment was shifting to the state and federal arenas. Local health departments continued to perform the six basic functions and reacted to developments in medical care needs and environmental control in a variety of ways, depending on local conditions. In some areas, they became the local agents of new federal programs for operating neighborhood and migrant health centers and became actively involved in fostering federally and state-financed systems of medical care for low-income people. In most areas, they did not.

State Public Health Agencies: 1946–1965—Trends in Organization and Functions

The previously discussed Mountin study of 1946 (9), analyzing the effects of 10 years of Social Security Act compliance on the expansion of local health department activity, also addressed these effects on state health department activities. Mountin found that expenditures of the 48 states for health departments increased from $12.9 million in 1930 to $18.7 million in 1940 to $37.0 million in 1946. The breakdown of these expenditures by category showed that "such activities as communicable disease control (including tuberculosis and venereal disease control), sanitation, laboratory services, and maternal and child hygiene—which accounted for a majority of State expenditures in 1930—still received more than half of the funds available in 1946." (9) At the same time, "the growth of newer programs is illustrated by such figures as these for dental hygiene: 37,000 in 1930, 227,000 in 1941, and 708,000 in 1946.

These data represented real services and were not all due to price increases, as is shown by the corresponding increase in full-time personnel from 4672 in 1930 to 10,128 in 1940 to 12,414 in 1946. An additional indication given by Mountin that the expansion in the years 1935–1946 was real, and not merely a reflection of general price increases, is the number of activities reported as "identified projects" by state health departments. Although this sort of measure taken alone does not necessarily imply an increase in total service volume, it was used by Mountin as an indicator of expanding scope function. Of the 46 states reporting, 39 listed communicable disease control projects for 1935, 43 in 1940, and 45 in 1946. The number of states reporting tuberculosis control programs rose from

19 in 1935 to 32 in 1940 and 45 in 1946: Virtually all of the traditional public health functions showed similar increases in the number of states involved in them. Mental hygiene and cancer control, however, were listed by only seven and 27 states, respectively, in 1946. (It should be noted, however, that at the time of Mountin's report, the states were heavily involved in psychiatric care, maintaining large censuses in state mental hospitals. But these functions were generally lodged in state hospital departments or special departments of mental hospitals. The organizational separation of what is today called *mental health* from *public health* is still true.)

Planning, chronic disease work, and other more modern functions did not appear as identified projects at all. If they were in effect in any state, they were subsumed in the statistics under the catchall category "other central services." Thus the increased scope of function was not mainly in the areas new to public health but represented expansion into standard areas by departments that had not engaged in them before.

A noteworthy exception was the striking increase in the number of states operating industrial hygiene programs. In 1935 this activity was listed as an identified project by only four states, compared with 26 states listing it in 1940 and 38 in 1946. The two states that did not respond to the question regarding identified projects did, in fact, have industrial hygiene units in both 1940 and 1946. In addition, New York and Massachusetts provided industrial hygiene units through their departments of labor. Thus by 1946, 42 states had such units covering 96 percent of the country's labor force. The services most commonly supplied by such units were "general surveys or inspections of plants for occupational health hazards with recommendations for improvement" (8). As early as 1946, state health departments had begun to inspect for occupational health hazards; this was one of the relatively few new areas they had entered. (It was not until 1970 that the federal government established the Occupational Safety and Health Administration.)

By 1946, then, the post-Social Security Act state health department was well established in most states. It may be characterized as a supervising, coordinating, equalizing, and mediating agency, whereas the local health department was the principal agency carrying the responsibility for the day-to-day operations of public health programs. There were exceptions. In some states the state health department conducted all the local public health work functions, with no local government health departments involved (These cases are discussed later.) Generally, however, the state agency provided a complete set of personal public health services directly only when local organization was lacking or inadequate, and then only as an interim measure pending local organization. More often, it provided only selected special services, if any. Many of the types of public health services provided by local health departments were among those also assigned most frequently by state law to the state health department, again with the difference that the state health department's actual functions have been mostly supervisory rather than involved with direct delivery of services. Examples of such functional areas are sanitation and maternal and child health. In addition, because of the breadth of the state's police powers, many state health departments engaged in health-related functions that were never or rarely practiced by local public health departments, such as licensing and accreditation of health professionals and health facilities, setting standards for automobile safety devices, and supervising the quality of public medical payment programs such as Medicaid.

A 1961 study by Shubick and Wright (14) summarized in Hanlon (15) listed the principal activities of state health agencies in terms of how many of the 50 states were actually practicing them. Table 4-1 lists a few of the most frequently encountered activities and the number of states in which they were carried on. It should be noted that these activities are, for the most part, either the traditional programs or the programs that were categorically funded by the federal government. On the other hand, newer programs such as "program planning,

development, and evaluation" appeared as activities in only seven state health departments, "radiologic health" in 11, and "heart disease control" in 25. Other programs that were frequently encountered, such as "professional registration and licensure," appearing in only three states, represent the type of program generally administered by a special licensing body of the state, organizationally independent of its health department.

The state health functions considered appropriate for state health departments were outlined in a policy statement of governing council of the APHA adopted at its 96th annual meeting on November 13, 1968 (16). These may be summarized as 1) health surveillance, planning, and program development; 2) promotion of local health coverage; 3) setting and enforcement of standards; 4) and providing health services. (The complexity of the monitoring and supervision that results from local programs operating with both state and federal support and supervision is treated in greater detail in a later discussion of the federal role.) The quality of local public health work throughout a particular state has been strongly influenced by the quality of the state health department leadership, as constrained by its budget, and the responsibilities assigned to it by the state government. This is particularly true outside the big cities and highly urbanized counties. In urban areas, the local health department has often depended less on the state health department, has had more direct ties with Washington, and indeed has often been lax in reporting to the state health agency.

A study of the composition of state boards of health by Gossert and Miller (17), completed in 1972, revealed that the standards set by Lemuel Shattuck in 1850 or by the updating policy statements of the APHA were far from being met. Alaska and Rhode Island had no statutory boards. In Illinois and Delaware, there was statutory provision, but no board was currently appointed in Illinois and the Delaware board consisted solely of two state officials. In 16 states, the health function was combined with at least one other agency, and four states had a conglomerate human resources agency.

TABLE 4-1. Sixteen Most Frequently Conducted Activities of State Health Departments, 1961

Rank	Activity	Number of States
1	Environmental health	50
2	Health education	50
3	Maternal and child health	50
4	Nursing	50
5	Vital statistics	49
6	Laboratories	47
7	Dental health	46
8	Communicable diseases	45
9	Engineering	43
10	Tuberculosis control	43
11	Hospital survey, planning, and construction licensure	42
12	Local health services	42
13	Industrial health	36
14	Personnel	34
15	Cancer control	31
16	Chronic disease control	30

SOURCE: Shubick, H. J., & Wright, E. O. (1961). *Composite study of fifty health department organizational charts representing forty-nine states and the District of Columbia.* Unpublished report cited in reference 22 (p. 224).

Of the 46 states with functioning boards, 32 of these boards include as one third of their memberships medical doctors. In 12 doctors constituted a majority of the board. In two states, Alabama and South Carolina, the state medical society was the board of health. Shattuck had warned in 1850 against domination of the board of health by any one profession. In 1972 only 12.5 percent of the 433 seats in 46 states were occupied by individuals identified as consumers. Appointments to the board were almost always made by governors, with some form of legislative approval being required in half the states. The trend was toward merging state health departments with other departments. In 1969, eight states had done this; in 1972 16 had.

The previously described trends in changing attitudes regarding the functions of local health departments also occurred at the state level. Over time, there had been a shift away from a conception of function restricted to a few communitywide preventive measures toward one of responsibility for making the total system of health care available to all citizens of the state. However, a comparison of the 1968 APHA statement of policy with the actual activities of state health departments in later years reveals that the traditional functions continued to be paramount—with the newer ones of community coordination for total health care, particularly medical care—becoming less evident.

A More Recent Picture: The ASTHO Data

Since 1970, annual statistics on the operation of state health departments have been assembled via questionnaire under the auspices of the Association of State and Territorial Health Officers (AS-THO). The organizational entity established by AS-THO to carry out this task in 1970 was called the National Public Health Program Reporting System (NPHPRS). In 1981, its successor, the nonprofit ASTHO Foundation was established to monitor developments in public health and facilitate the exchange of information. Its ASTHO Reporting System (ASTHO/RS) continued collection and publication of public health data that the NPHPRS had been assembling and in November of 1985, the name of the ASTHO Foundation was changed to the Public Health Foundation.

Because promotion of local public health department activities is such an important part of the state health agency's functions, these data also include much information about the local health departments (or LHDs, as they are referred to in these reports). Fiscal 1974 was the first year of publication of these data and with the publication of the report for fiscal year 1988 fifteen consecutive years of comprehensive data became available. Most of the following remarks about the 1988 status of these departments, state health agencies (SHAs), as they are called in these reports, are based on the June 1990 reports (18).

In fiscal year 1988, there were 55 SHAs in 50

states and five territories. Only the Northern Mariana Islands and the Trust Territory had no SHAs, although they had in prior years. The state health agencies of one state (Montana) and three territories (American Samoa, Puerto Rico, and the Virgin Islands) did not submit data for fiscal year 1988. The Public Health Foundation estimated data for these four jurisdictions.

In 1988 the 55 reporting SHAs spent a total of $8.3 billion for public health, of which $6.0 billion, or 75 percent, was allocated to personal health services and the remainder to other categories such as environmental health, health resources, laboratory, and general administration. The data indicate a substantial transfer of funding source from state and local to federal. In 1974, 25.5 percent of the funding of SHA expenditures was of federal origin. By 1978 this proportion had risen to 34.8 percent and in 1988, it was 36.3 percent. It is worth noting that in 1988, total public health expenditures by state and local public health agencies in the 55 reporting states was $11.0 billion, indicating that the SHAs spent 75 percent of this amount. In 1978, by contrast, this ratio was only 65 percent. Despite the widespread discussion of the need to pay greater attention to public health, only 2.8 percent of the total $388 billion spent for health services in calendar year 1988 was spent for public health (19), and only a bit more than 1.5 percent of this total was spent by SHAs.

The principal functions being performed by SHAs generally continue to emphasize those areas that Mountin found predominant in 1946, in terms of both the relative distribution of the dollar and the number of SHAs involved. Comparison of the state health department functions cited by Mountin for 1930, 1940, and 1946—on the one hand, with the number of states presently reporting SHA programs, and with the 1961 tabulations shown in table 4-1, on the other hand—indicates that the scope of activities has not been significantly enlarged. In 1988 nearly all SHAs were concerned with maternal and child health, communicable disease control, chronic disease, dental health, public health nursing (including home visits), nutrition,

consumer protection, sanitation, water quality, health statistics, and diagnostic laboratory tests. However, the amounts spent for these functions varied widely, with maternal and child health comprising 35 percent, chronic disease 3.0 percent, and dental health 0.7 percent.

Local consumer protection and sanitation are still the leading environmental functions and maternal and child health continues to represent the mainstay noninstitutional activities of most state health departments in the area of personal services. After maternal and child services (excluding institutional operations), the order of SHAs expenditures for personal health is as follows: communicable disease control, handicapped children's services, alcohol and drug abuse, supporting personal health services (e.g., health education, home health care, public health nursing), chronic disease, mental health and dental health. The "newer" function of chronic disease that Mountin stressed is now shown as a function of 46 of the 51 reporting SHAs, but only 2 percent of the total personal health expenditures (3.3 percent of the noninstitutional expenditures) went for this function.

The dominance of a single functional area, maternal and child health, is striking. Expenditures for these programs comprise one-third of the total expenses and 47 percent of personal health expenditures (59 percent of noninstitutional personal health program expenditures.) The percentages are even higher if one includes handicapped children programs. The dominant position of maternal and child health program expenditures is, in turn, also largely due to a single item, Women and Infant Care (WIC) nutrition, a diet supplement program supported by the U.S. Department of Agriculture. In 1988 $1,729 million of the $2,945 million in maternal and child health (MCH) expenditures, or 59 percent, came from the Department of Agriculture, presumably for this single program.

The predominance of the MCH and handicapped children's programs, even without the WIC component, raises provocative questions about the future. If a national medical care program, with universal eligibility and comprehensive benefits, were ever implemented, it presumably would include prenatal care, mother and infant care, and care of handicapped. It would, parenthetically, also include much of the care now provided under categorical programs for venereal disease, dental health, chronic disease, and other personal health programs. The personal health care functions of the SHAs might then be reduced, in which event the environmental, planning, and monitoring functions would be likely candidates to become the most important functions. It is interesting, therefore, to look at the status of these program categories in SHAs in 1988.

The organization of the environmental protection function within state government exemplifies an important trend in recent years—the widespread use of agencies other than SHAs for health protection functions. In the District of Columbia all environmental services are provided by agencies other than the SHA. In 45 reporting SHAs, these services were provided in varying degrees, with at least 26 percent of the $381 million in expenditures going for consumer protection and sanitation programs. At least another 23 percent was spent on water quality programs. However, most of the environmental activities were of the standard type.

The 1978 ASTHO report stated:

All of the SHAs reporting environmental health programs provided *consumer protection and sanitation* [emphasis in original] services, including food, or milk control, substance control and product safety, sanitation of health care facilities and other institutions, housing and recreational sanitation, or vector and zoonotic disease control. *Water quality* services, provided by 51 SHAs, were usually related to public drinking water, individual water supply, and individual sewage disposal. Public water pollution control services were more often provided by an agency other than the SHA. *Radiation control* services were offered by 45 SHAs. Fewer SHAs provided other environmental health services: *occupational health and safety and related services* (38 SHAs), *waste management* (34 SHAs), and *air quality* [emphasis added].

These sorts of questions were not discussed in later reports. Environmental health expenditures of state health agencies were funded predominantly (61 percent) by the state, almost 25 percent came

from federal sources, and the rest originated from local government and other sources. However, the Environmental Protection Act of 1970 called for the governor and/or the legislature of each state to designate a "lead environmental agency" with overall responsibility for environmental activities. There are three generally recognized models for such agency selection: an SHA, a specialized state environmental protection agency, and a state natural resources agency (20). In only 10 of the 55 states and territories were SHAs designated as lead environmental agencies.

Turning to the role of SHAs in statewide health planning, the picture has been similar to, but not quite the same as, that in environmental health. In many states, other agencies are mainly responsible for health planning, but more SHAs have been given this function than in environmental health. Under the Health Planning and Resource Development Act of 1974 (PL 93-641), each state was to appoint a single agency as the State Health Planning and Development Agency (SHPDA). Of the 55 states and territories, 32 designated their SHAs as the SHPDA in 1984 (similar to the number that did so under the Comprehensive Health Planning Act of 1966). The data for 1988 were not given.

One of the most important activities of state health departments is the development of local public health departments and the supervision and monitoring of their work. The ASTHO definition of a local public health department (and therefore, the definition of the presence or absence of public health coverage for a particular locality) has been somewhat relaxed as compared to previous definitions in that it no longer requires medical leadership. The 1988 ASTHO definition asserts a local health department to be:

An official governmental public health agency which is, in whole or in part, responsible to a substate governmental entity or entities. An entity may be a city, county, city-county, federation of counties, borough, township, or any other substate governmental entity. A local health department must: have a staff of one or more full-time professional public health employees (e.g., public health nurse, sanitarian); deliver public health services; serve a definable geographic area and have identifiable expenditures and/or budget in the political subdivisions which it serves [18].

ASTHO is now defining local health departments even more liberally than the full-time public health department was defined in the older literature of Ferrell, Mountin, and Emerson. Relaxation of the previous requirement for a medically trained health officer to head the agency is not merely a compromise with reality. Some of the literature in the intervening period (21,22) has reported the belief—and often strong advocacy—that it is not merely expedient but desirable, to discontinue this requirement. The health officer position has been seen by some as largely involving administration and policy analysis and requiring a grasp of overall public health knowledge and principles of administration, rather than one of medicine. And in the last decade the concept of community leadership skills in developing more effective public health action programs has been accorded increasing importance.

In the fiscal 1975 report, three types of local public health departments (LHD) were identified: an LHD operated by the SHA as part of a centrally directed state system of local public health agencies; a largely autonomous LHD receiving some technical assistance and consultation from the SHA; and a partly autonomous LHD that shares control with the SHA, which has direct operating authority in some areas. In 1988 there were 2,884 LHDs meeting the definition of the Public Health Foundation. Forty of the 55 states (the Public Health Foundation uses the word "states" to mean "states, territories, and the District of Columbia" unless the context indicates otherwise) had LHDs. Arkansas, Delaware, the District of Columbia, Rhode Island, Vermont, American Samoa, and the Virgin Islands had none. Twelve "states" reported that only portions of their population were served by their SHAs. (This includes three states with greater than 95 percent coverage.) These ranged from New Mexico with 1 percent through Illinois with 94 percent. Twelve states reported portions of their populations

receiving direct services from SHAs rather than from LHDs. Principal among these were New Mexico (where 99 percent of the population was served by local units of the state health agency), Maine with 89 percent, Louisiana with 87 percent, New Hampshire with 82 percent, Pennsylvania with 63 percent, and Alaska with 55 percent. Only three states reported any part of their population having no local public health services, either SHA or LHD (6 percent in Illinois and North Dakota and 1 percent in Kansas).

About 21 percent of SHA money ($1.7 billion) spent on public health went to LHDs in the 49 states reporting for 1988. Most of this money was allocated for personal health programs (such as public health nursing, health education, maternal and child health, chronic disease, etc.). A little more than half of the money (55 percent) originated within the state itself, and 31 percent ($529 million) was federal money which was transmitted to the local government via the SHA.

Although 55 percent of the funding of the LHDs originated from the SHAs, some of this SHA money granted to the LHDs came, in turn, from the federal government. In terms of the *ultimate* source of LHD expenditures, 28 percent came from state money, 7 percent from federal, 35 percent from local funds, and the rest from fees collected and other sources. The percentage coming from local sources varied greatly from state to state, as it always has. In California, Kansas, Pennsylvania, and 18 other states, none of the LHD expenditures originated from local sources. In Texas, 63 percent was estimated to have originated locally. In other states, the percentage varied within the 0 to 63 percent range. Tables 4-2 and 4-3 summarize the patterns of LHD sources of funds, and tables 4-4 and 4-5 show the pattern of the combined SHA and LHD expenditures by source of funds.

Some Public Policy Implications of Recent Trends

At the beginning of this section, it was noted that the state's responsibilities for health protection are much broader than those of the local government.

TABLE 4-2. Expenditures of Local Health Departments by Program Area, Fiscal Year 1988 (amounts in millions of dollars)

Program Area	Total LHD Expenditures		SHA Intergovernmental Grants to LHDs		Additional LHD Expenditures	
	Amount	Percentage of Total	Amount	Percentage of Total	Amount	Percentage of Total
Personal health	$2,291.0	57.6	$1,244.9	72.2	$1,046.3	46.4
Environmental health	$ 352.6	8.9	$ 99.2	5.8	$ 253.4	11.2
Health resources	$ 294.4	7.4	$ 204.1	11.8	$ 90.2	4.0
Laboratory	$ 32.8	0.8	$ 8.4	0.5	$ 24.3	1.1
General administration	$ 168.5	4.2	$ 47.1	2.7	$ 121.4	5.4
Unallocated to program areas	$ 839.4	21.1	$ 120.3	7.0	$ 719.1	31.9
Total	$3,978.7	100.0	$1,724	100.0	$2,254.7	100.0

SOURCE: Public Health Foundation. (1990). *Public health agencies 1990: An inventory of programs and block grant expenditures.* Washington, DC: Public Health Foundation.

TABLE 4-3. Expenditures of Local Health Departments by Ultimate Source of Funds, Fiscal Year 1988 (amounts in millions of dollars)

Source of Funds	Total LHD Expenditures		SHA Intergovernmental Grants to LHDs		Additional LHD Expenditures	
	Amount	Percentage of Total	Amount	Percentage of Total	Amount	Percentage of Total
State funds	$1,113.8	27.8	$ 950.0	54.5	$ 163.8	7.2
Federal grant and contract funds	$ 665.4	16.7	$ 529.1	30.6	$ 136.3	6.0
Local funds	$1,395.5	35.4	$ 126.4	7.3	$1,268.1	56.2
Fees and reimbursements	$ 558.2	14.0	$ 91.1	5.2	$ 467.1	20.6
Other sources	$ 71.9	1.8	$ 27.4	2.4	$ 44.5	2.3
Sources unknown	$ 174.2	4.3	—		$ 174.2	7.7
Total	$3,979.0	100.0	$1,724.0	100.0	$2,254.0	100.0

SOURCE: Public Health Foundation. (1990). *Public health agencies 1990: An inventory of programs and block grant expenditures.* Washington, DC: Public Health Foundation.

Consequently, there is a wider range of possible functions that could appear in the list of programs engaged in by any particular state health department. Despite this greater breadth of choice, the number of functions carried on by different state governments and the ones assigned to the health agency vary markedly from state to state. Responsibility and control are shared with other agencies. The reasons for the wide variation among the states in the number and types of health functions assigned to their SHAs are complex. They reflect a growing tendency since 1960 to assign health problems to agencies other than health departments.

Although much rhetoric ascribes the "need" to choose another agency to the alleged fact that the SHAs is technically inadequate or managerially inefficient or both, there is reason to believe that various special interest groups seek such a choice because they believe it to be advantageous to

TABLE 4-4. Combined Expenditures of the Nation's State Public Health Agencies and Local Health Departments, by Program Area, Fiscal Year 1988 (amounts in millions of dollars)

Program Area	Total SHA and LHD Expenditures	Direct SHA Expenditures	SHA Inter-Governmental Grants to LHDs	Additional Expenditures of LHDs
Personal health	$ 7,305	$5,013	$1,245	$1,046
Environmental health	$ 717	$ 365	99	$ 253
Health resources	$ 811	$ 516	$ 204	$ 90
Laboratory	$ 303	$ 270	$ 8	$ 24
General administration	$ 593	$ 424	$ 47	$ 121
Not allocated to program areas	$ 839		$ 120	$ 719
Total public health	$10,568	$6,588	$1,723	$2,253

SOURCE: Public Health Foundation. (1988). *Public health agencies 1988.* Washington, DC: Public Health Foundation.

TABLE 4-5. Expenditures of the Nation's State Public Health Agencies and Local Health Departments, by Source of Funds, Fiscal Year 1988 (amounts in millions of dollars)

Source of Funds	Total SHA and LHD Expenditures	Direct SHA Expenditures	SHA Inter-Governmental Grants to LHDs	Additional Expenditures of LHDs
State funds	$ 4,764	$3,650	$ 950	$ 164
Federal grant and contract funds	$ 3,152	$2,487	$ 529	$ 136
Local funds	$ 1,410	$ 14	$ 126	$1,269
Fees, reimbursements and other sources	$ 1,068	$ 438	$ 119	$ 512
Source unknown	$ 174	—	—	174
Total	$10,568	$6,589	$1,724	$2,255

SOURCE: Public Health Foundation. (1988). *Public health agencies 1988.* Washington, DC: Public Health Foundation.

them. Whatever factors are actually most influential, the trend away from assigning major health-related programs to SHAs is unmistakable. This issue will be further addressed in the discussion of the federal role, but it is so important in terms of the future development of SHAs that it is worth pausing to review the evidence corroborating this trend as fact.

One of the principal functions of the SHA, especially after the passage of the Social Security Act, has been that of liaison and administrative agent for the distribution and supervision of federal grants among local health agencies within the state. Use of the SHA health agency was generally explicitly mandated by the early post-1935 legislation. Later, beginning in the 1950s, the SHA began to be bypassed with increasing frequency as the state agency chosen to distribute federal monies to localities for health activities and to supervise their implementation. Project grants for local services given directly by the federal agency to the local grantee became increasingly prevalent. For example, the Comprehensive Health Planning Act of 1966 specified only that *a* single state agency in each state was to administer federal grants to that state under this act; 23 states placed this function in agencies other than their SHAs. Under the provision of the 1975 Planning Act, in 1978 36 states designated the SHA as their state health planning and development agencies (SHPDAs); the remaining 21 naming other agencies.

Under the Medicaid Act, only eight SHAs are the designated state agency for administering Medicaid, despite the fact that nearly all SHAs have their own general ambulatory care programs, and in 1988, 16 SHAs spent a total of $1.2 billion for SHA-operated institutions, including general, mental, and chronic disease hospitals; institutions for the mentally retarded; and skilled nursing facilities. Other examples could be cited, but these will suffice to support the assertion that SHAs have often been bypassed since 1950 as chief administrators of new statewide health programs. This tendency has been widespread, even in the area of health planning, despite the fact that public health professionals and others have long advocated that areawide and state health planning should be *the* basic function of state and local health departments. In 1984, only 32 of the 55 "states" designated their SHAs as their official planning agency, and in its tabulation of 1988 statistics (18), the Public Health Foundation does not give this type of information at all. (Only the amounts spent for "general health resources," a conglomerate category including "emergency medical services, planning, development, regulation, and other" are shown.)

Federal Role in State and Local Public Health Services After 1935: 1936–1945

It was previously noted that passage of the Social Security Act of 1935 heralded the beginning of a major program of federal grants-in-aid to the states for health purposes, and that the portions of the act that affected public health departments were Title V (Section I) and Title VI. Administration of these two titles comprised the major public health activities of the federal government in the 1930s.

Selected details of the original provisions of these titles, especially Title VI, are presented here to illustrate some of the characteristics of revenue-sharing grants discussed earlier.

Under Title V, federal grants could be given to the states for "promoting the health of mothers and children" (7). The funds were distributed by the Children's Bureau to the SHAs to be used for supporting these services in state and local health agencies (These programs were subsequently expanded. Amendments passed in 1965 as part of the Medicare Act later provided for project grants to state and local health agencies for comprehensive maternity care to high-risk mothers and for the development of high-quality, comprehensive health services to children and youths of school or preschool age. The operating agency could be a public or appropriate nonprofit private agency. Amounts were subsequently also appropriated for research projects "relating to maternal and child health and crippled children's services." Expanded federal support of maternal and child health activities by state and local health departments continued until 1981, when these grants were consolidated with six other programs into a Maternal and Child Health Services Block Grant. This action was part of the reduction in social programs during the Reagan administration embodied in the Omnibus Budget Reconciliation Act of 1981, which is discussed in further detail later.) Title VI of the act directly addressed the buildup of state and local health departments, and the monies appropriated under it have been administered by the PHS. In the original act, federal funds were appropriated annually, under a block grant formula, for the years 1936–1940. "For the purpose of assisting states, counties, health districts and other political subdivisions of the states in establishing and maintaining adequate public health services" (7).

In 1944 Title VI, with some changes, was transferred from the Social Security Act to Section 314 of the newly constituted Public Health Service Act. The original act required that funds be allocated among the states on the basis of a formula to be promulgated by the U.S. Surgeon General, taking into account three factors: 1) the state's population size, 2) the state's relative economic status, and 3) the prevalence of special health problems in the state. Each state health department was required to file an acceptable plan with the U.S. Surgeon General indicating how the grant was to be used, and a report at the end of the year detailing how it had actually been used.

Several aspects of the allocation and administrative provisions of Title VI set important precedents for future federal government policy: 1) all funds were to be administered nationally by a general health agency; 2) the system of tax sharing was partially a per capita redistribution of federal tax revenues and partly an attempt to equalize relative local and state tax burdens among the states; 3) the filing of state plans and the requirement of annual reports was a modest attempt to achieve quality control and encourage statewide planning; and 4) the funds went directly to a single state agency, which was mandated to be the state health department, to be redistributed within the state.

Public Health in the Period 1946–1968

The previous discussion of local public health departments noted that public health professionals, some members of Congress, and the Democratic presidents came to believe that the state and local health departments were being inordinately slow to enter the newer fields of public health work. These concerns, dealing principally with primary care in medically underserved areas, chronic disease abatement, and control of the more recent environmental threats, were being defined by students of personal health care organization and environmental control as a major concern of the local health department. It was also mentioned that attempts by the federal government to nudge local health departments toward these special programs led to increased use of categorical grants, as opposed to general-purpose formula grants (13). The categorical grants were still formula grants and required matching—usually on a one-to-one basis—but, as opposed to block formula grants, they

were intended to stimulate spending for specific activities that the federal government deemed desirable nationally rather than to support the general budget of the health department.

From 1950 on, the federal grant structure was increasingly framed to encourage state and local public health agencies to move more aggressively into areas defined by the federal government as national health priorities. The number of categorical formula grants increased over the years, as did the proportion of dollars of formula grants that was so earmarked. By 1965, out of about $50 million in formula grants, only $10 million, or about 20 percent, was allocated for general health: the rest was designated for specific categories (23). Some states and localities found the earmarking to be inappropriate for the types of programs needed in their areas.

After 15 years of continued unsuccessful efforts to promote greater activity in chronic disease control, pollution abatement, medical care services, and similar programs through the use of earmarked (categorical) formula grants, the federal government attempted in 1966 to discontinue the use of earmarked grants funneled through state governments for accomplishing these goals. The Comprehensive Health Planning and Public Health Service Amendments of 1966 (PL89-749) abolished all categorical earmarking of formula grants (24). These amendments are discussed in further detail in the next section.

Growth of Project Grants

One of the factors inhibiting the development of programs being promoted by the federal government via categorical formula grants was the conflict between large metropolitan centers and their state governments (25). Many state legislatures were so structured that the influence of rural sections was out of proportion to the size of their populations. These states had been slow to assign comprehensive health care and wide ecological control responsibilities to their state health departments. The populations and organizations in the large municipal centers and their suburbs, on the other hand, had increasingly attempted to expand such activities. Unable to prevail in the state capital, these states turned to Washington for direct aid. These factors, among others, led to the emergence of project grants as an increasingly important segment of federal grants in the 1960s.

Project grants were not a new phenomenon. Such grants for rural sanitation projects had been made as far back as before 1935, but in very modest amounts. After 1935, the first project grant to be administered by the Public Health Service was made in 1946 for venereal disease control (9), and between 1947 and 1959, the project grant program for this purpose remained unique. But "The first half of the 1960s was marked by a flood of new project grant programs" (22). Formula grants (including both block and categorical grants) were 77 percent of the $76 million total in health grants in 1963; they only accounted for 48 percent of the $105 million distributed in 1965. In the latter years, the proportion of total grants-in-aid for project grants exceeded that for formula grants for the first time.

The overall emphasis of the 1966–1967 amendments to Section 314 of the Public Health Service Act was not only on removing the categorical earmarking from formula grants but also on establishing the project grant as a permanent form of aid, and at the same time meeting the various objections to the disintegrative effects of project grants on planning. All formula grants were now block grants with no categorical formula grants included in the 1966 act. (The formula public health grants that were continued as block grants in subsequent years came to be known as "314d" monies, after the section of the Public Health Act that provided for them.) The federal government's attempts to encourage local public health departments and other agencies to act on its high-priority targets were to be continued and intensified, but this was done only by the use of project grants, which were by their very nature well suited to promoting categorical programs.

Despite the 1966 legislation, which intended that formula grants to public health departments be of the block type, Congress was apparently unable to resist the pleas of various advocates of specific programs. Categorical programs continued to proliferate in effect (via the use of numerous project grants), while the block 314d money continued to dwindle.

The continued inability of the federal government structure to bring state and local public health departments more into line with federal priorities led to a number of subsequent reorganizations that weakened the Office of the Surgeon General, the head of the U.S. Public Health Service. The status of that office and the role of the PHS remained in a state of flux for a number of years, with the position of the U.S. Surgeon General actually being abolished for a time during the reorganization of the PHS during the Nixon administration in 1973. The position was later reinstated under the Carter administration and its incumbent attempted to strengthen the role and prestige of the PHS with an emphasis on prevention.

Public Health in the Period 1969–1980

Following the inauguration of Richard Nixon as president in 1969, the executive branch began to reverse certain aspects of the relationship that had been developing, mainly since the passage of the Social Security Act in 1935, among the federal, state, and local governments. This tripartite arrangement has often been called federalism, the federal partnership, or the federal system. In this formulation the term "federal" refers to the system of intergovernmental relationships among the national [i.e., federal], state, and local levels of government in the United States. The clarity of the expression "federal system" has been compromised by the growing tendency to write "federal" with a lower-case "f" even when the meaning intended is the "Federal" or national government. Because I am constrained to adopt the newer usage of the spelling of "federal", I shall refer to the federal government as the "national" government whenever the meaning is otherwise ambiguous.) This attempted change was directly pertinent to public health policy because of the federal grant system for supporting public health programs. The main goal of this policy, dubbed the "New Federalism" by his administration, was summarized by President Nixon early in 1969: "After over a century and a half of power flowing from the people and the local communities and from the states to Washington, D.C., let's get it back to the people and to the cities and to the states where it belongs" (26). Of the three principal legislative and organizational changes that the administration expected to use to translate the goals of the New Federalism into action (27), the main one was to place greater reliance on state and local governments in the operation and administration of federal grant programs. Categorical grants were to be eliminated as far as possible in favor of global block grants (revenue sharing). It should be noted that the term "block" here meant a lump sum granted to a state or a local government for all purposes, health included. The amount of the grant to be used for health and how it would be used would be decided solely by the state or local government.

On October 20, 1972, general revenue sharing was enacted into law (PL 92-512) as the State and Local Fiscal Assistance Act of 1972. A total of $30.2 billion was appropriated to the states and localities to be distributed over a five-year period beginning January 1, 1972. About one third of the money went to the states and two-thirds to local governments. (The program was extended in 1977 for five years, through 1981. The budget program proposed by President Ronald Reagan for 1983 envisaged a continuation of the revenue-sharing program, at least through 1986, at slightly increased levels over those of 1981 and 1982 (28). It was discontinued in 1987.)

The revenue-sharing programs were of great potential importance for state and local public health programs. Block grants provided to states and localities subsequently increased state and local decision-making power—a power that could be used to reduce or augment public health programs in relation to other spending areas. Nationally, this potential was only modestly realized, but in such areas as Oakland, California, it was an important source of funding for local community centers.

While agreeing to the president's revenue-sharing proposals, Congress opposed the elimination of appropriations for many ongoing categorical programs that had been funded in the past. President Nixon's 1974 budget had called for discontinuing many of these programs and cutting others substantially (29). It also proposed cancellations totaling about $550 million, appropriated in 1973, which the administration had not spent (recissions). An apparent truce in the administration/ Congress battle over the federally funded programs was declared when the president, in June 1973, signed a law extending expiring health programs for one year.

Further contest between President Nixon and the Democratic Congress was ended with Mr. Nixon's resignation on August 9, 1974 and the succession of Gerald R. Ford to the presidency. President Ford generally continued Nixon's health policies. The principal emphasis included overall reduction of health budgets and consolidation of existing categorical programs into block formula grants. In his last State of the Union Address, President Ford called for budgetary consolidation of 16 health programs, including such programs as formula grants (314d), immunization, rat control, lead paint poisoning prevention, maternal and child health, state health grants, and family planning. Because the states were not required to match the federal funds under this budget proposal, they could have offset reductions in federal funds by reducing their own expenditures and curtailing programs. The proposal seemed clearly tied to a reduction of health services, and was opposed by Congress. In January 1977, President Jimmy Carter was inaugurated, and certain health policies began to change.

The Carter administration discontinued Ford's attempts to consolidate most public health categorical grants into a single block grant. However, the total sum allotted for health programs in the Carter budget for 1977–1978 was only slightly higher than it had been in the Ford budget (29). Throughout the Carter administration, three major goals were emphasized in public health: expansion of preventive and some treatment services for poor children; health promotion and prevention for the entire population; and mental health services, especially in the community.

The measures suggested to expand services for children were embodied in a proposal called Comprehensive Health Assessment and Treatment for Poor Children (CHAP). It was to have reached 1.8 million children in addition to the 12 million who were already eligible for such services through Medicaid. During 1977, CHAP bills were introduced in both the Senate and the House of Representatives and throughout President Carter's term of office, this proposal was pushed in Congress but failed to pass. A leading factor in its defeat was an antiabortion amendment that was attached by legislators opposed to abortion, a tactic that split congressional support.

The health promotion and disease prevention program consisted of stepped-up national campaigns to inform people about the importance of health matters such as smoking, proper diet, and exercise. The program was the centerpiece of the agenda of Dr. Julius Richmond, the surgeon general of the PHS. Appointed in July 1977, he set out to revitalize the PHS largely by assertively promoting the idea of prevention and health maintenance. In documents issued in 1979 and 1980, which may reasonably be construed as PHS "position papers," the importance of disease prevention and health promotion was carefully delineated and national achievable goals for 1990 established. The publications called for allocating a greater proportion of the health dollar to prevention. The 1980 report set targets for the following priority areas: high blood pressure control, family planning, pregnancy, infant health, immunization, sexually transmitted diseases, toxic agent control, occupational safety and health, accident prevention and injury control, fluoridation and dental health, surveillance and control of infectious diseases, smoking and health, misuse of alcohol and drugs, physical fitness and exercise, and control of stress and violent behavior (30).

Using extant research writings, the reports concluded that of deaths due to the 10 leading causes of mortality in 1976, 50 percent were due to unhealthy behavior or life-style, 20 percent to environmental factors, 20 percent to human biologic factors, and 10 percent to inadequacies in the existing health care system (31,32). The so-called position papers argued that the facts clearly indicated that changing unhealthy behavior was the most important way of preventing or controlling the diseases that were the leading causes of death.

In October 1980, a reorganization changed the Communicable Disease Center to the Centers for Disease Control. The new organization had six bureaus: the Center for Preventive Services, the Center for Environmental Health, the National Institute for Occupational Safety and Health, the Center for Health Promotion and Education, the Center for Professional Development and Training, and the Center for Disease Investigation and Diagnosis.

Thus was the campaign to establish disease prevention, with chronic disease as a major component—as a priority of the federal health agency—organized along lines analogous to those of previous campaigns to prevent communicable disease. Included were the identification of health threats, determination of probable causes and methods for combating them, and an organizational structure with which to help lead the campaign. The early public health measures of sanitation and quarantine had often been successful even though they were based on as yet imperfectly understood causes of acute disease and the method of their transmission. Indeed, referring to these early efforts, one historian of public health wrote, "The program of the sanitary reformers was based to a large extent on a structure of erroneous theories, and while they hit upon the right solution, it was mostly for the wrong reasons" (5). It seemed reasonable to hope that a public health campaign to curb the ravages of chronic and degenerative disease might also result in partial, but significant, successes. Even though the precise mechanisms of the chronic disease processes were still only imperfectly understood, the association of their incidence with certain risk factors was applied as a guide to proper preventive measures. (With the appearance of the HIV/AIDS epidemic, it has become abundantly clear that the days of having to fight highly infectious fatal disease armed only with risk factor scientific knowledge, and relying on changing health behavior to control, are far from over.)

Not all public health writers fully agreed with Dr. Richmond. There were those who, while agreeing with the importance of making greater efforts to change human health behavior in the overall effort to improve the public's health, cautioned that too one-sided an effort in that direction was unwise and was not as unequivocally indicated by research results as was being claimed. They argued that ascribing the causes of death and disease more heavily to personal health behavior than was warranted contributed a form of victim blaming (33) that detracted from proper attention to the need to control the rapid growth of environmental health hazards. Furthermore, at present, and for a long time to come, people will continue to get sick and when they do, they need medical care. Poor people get sick more often and more seriously than do nonpoor (34), and the only reason they often do not receive appropriate treatment is that they are socially and economically disadvantaged. Single-minded emphasis placed on the behavioral causes of illness without offering care to those who succumb can reinforce a public apathy, or even antipathy, to ensuring medical care for the poor who become ill. Therefore, the medical care problems must be solved, they argued, before real political support could be mustered behind prevention.

People facing imminent financial ruin because of impending medical bills could not be expected to concentrate on preventing illness in the future. The various ramifications of this rift, especially its political repercussions in Congress and within the Democratic Party leadership, inhibited unified support for President Carter's health proposals in Congress. It may fairly be said that *financial* support for public health did not advance substantially under Carter, despite his avowed commitment to improving public health. In fact, considering inflation, it retrogressed. Carter's own budgets for fiscal years 1980 and 1981 mandated cuts in public health funds. The principal positive contribution was the substantial *theoretical leadership* provided by the U.S. Surgeon General in beginning to define more completely what a modern program of disease prevention might look like.

The Reagan administration took office in January 1981 determined to slash all government social programs, cutting appropriations for others, and turning as many as possible back to the states. President Reagan hoped to eventually consolidate all remaining federal money for public health given to the states into one block grant.

The first major legislative result of the new administration was the Omnibus Budget Reconciliation Act (PL 97-35), passed on August 13, 1981, specifying the appropriations for the fiscal year ending in 1982. The Reagan administration did not obtain its full request that 26 public health programs be combined into two block grants for public health, but it did succeed in getting 20 programs combined into four block grants. Six programs remained categorical. The block grants were set up as a new section of the Public Health Service Act, Title XIX. The folding in of the program into block grants consisted of the following:

1. Preventive Health and Health Services (PHS) Block Grant. The programs folded in were (a) rodent control, (b) fluoridation, (c) hypertension control, (d) health services and centers (rape crisis centers), (e) old 314d money, (f) home health services, and (g) emergency services. The grants were to be distributed among the states according to a formula based on population and other factors deemed appropriate by the secretary of Health and Human Services (HHS). Each state had to apply for these grants.
2. Alcohol Abuse, Drug Abuse, and Mental Health Block Grant. The programs folded in were (a) Community Mental Health Centers Act; (b) Mental Health Systems

Act; (c) Comprehensive Alcohol Abuse and Alcoholism Prevention, Treatment, and Rehabilitation Act of 1970; and (d) Drug Abuse Prevention, Treatment, and Rehabilitation Act.

3. Primary Care Block Grant. This section consisted of the Community Health Centers. States could begin to take them over beginning in fiscal year 1983.

4. Maternal and Child Health (MCH) Block Grant (amends Title V of the Social Security Act). The programs folded in were (a) maternal and child health and crippled children's services of Title V of the Social Security Act, (b) supplementary security income to provide rehabilitation services for blind and disabled children, (c) lead-based paint poisoning prevention, (d) genetic disease service, (e) sudden infant death syndrome (SIDS), (f) hemophilia treatment, and (g) adolescent pregnancy under the Health Services and Centers Amendment of 1978. The SHA was designated the administering agency, and the formula for fiscal years 1982 and 1983 was based on the number of low-income children. Alternative bases for the formula in the future were to be submitted to Congress by the secretary of HHS by June 1982. The states had to contribute three dollars for every four dollars of federal funds received.

The six programs left as categorical grants were 1) childhood immunization, 2) tuberculosis control, 3) family planning, 4) migrant health centers, 5) venereal disease control, and 6) an amount equal to 15 percent of the total Maternal and Child Health Services Grant that was to be set aside for use by HHS to fund projects of "regional or national significance" in training and research, genetic disease testing, and information development and comprehensive hemophilia diagnostic and treatment centers. In addition, the Women, Infants, and Children (WIC) nutrition program funded by the Agriculture Department was also left categorical. As has been noted, this food supplement program is important LHD activity. Thus six programs were left categorical and the remaining 20 were folded into four block grants, instead of all being folded into two block grants, because of vigorous lobbying in Congress by advocates of the varying programs.

The block grants were not simply being turned over to the states to administer; total funding for the programs in each block grant was reduced by 21 percent. After accounting for inflation, the actual reduction in resources was expected to be even higher, perhaps 30 percent. Taking into account the simultaneous reduction in state and local tax revenues because of the recession of the early 1980s and the tax revolt of the late 1970s and early 1980s, it is clear that local and state public health services faced a severe financial shortfall. For 1983, President Reagan's budget proposals had requested further reductions in federal grants for public health, to be accomplished by further folding remaining categorical grants into blocks and reducing the total. In his State of the Union Address, he had called for turning over 43 federal programs to the states by 1984 and giving them the choice of continuing them or not. By then, however, the congressional consensus that had so quickly passed the Omnibus Budget Reconciliation Act had weakened considerably, and the request for further cuts was met with substantial opposition in Congress.

After the reduction for fiscal year 1982 contained in the Omnibus Budget Act, most of the federal money for state and local public health department work was not further substantially eroded, and in some cases, was later raised to fiscal year 1982 or earlier levels. For example, the MCH block grant federal obligations for fiscal year 1982 were $374 million and for 1985, $478 million (34). Adjusting for inflation would bring the new amounts into approximate equality in terms of resources they would command. Similar remarks apply to other Block Grants.

The appropriations for fiscal years 1986 and 1987 each provided $478 million for the Maternal and Child Health Block Grant and $89.5 million for the Preventive Health and Health Services Block Grant. From 1982 to 1990, inflation-adjusted appropriations for the Prevention Block Grant decreased from approximately $79 million to $64 million [35].) The Alcohol, Drug Abuse, and Mental Health block grant for 1987 received $720 million, an increase of $225 million over 1986, reflecting the prevailing emphasis on drug abuse control in Congress and the Reagan administration in 1986.

Appropriations for disease prevention were also increased over prior years, providing $75 million for childhood immunization grants, $7 million for tuberculosis protection, and $50 million for control of sexually transmitted diseases. In addition to the last item, $400 million was appropriated for 1987 to finance the fight against AIDS, an increase from $234 million appropriated for 1986 (36).

Public Policy Implications

The Reagan program stood for a reversal in U.S. federal policy in health, but it is important to recognize that the essentials of Reagan administration policies, insofar as they deal with public health services, were largely continuations of policies first formulated by presidents Nixon and Ford. What, then, were the essential features of these policies, insofar as they have important implications for public health in the United States?

First, they called for an end to federal grants to the states and localities for public health services. During a transition period money was to be given to the states for public health and ambulatory care services on a block grant basis, with little or no categorical restrictions on how it was to be spent by programs. Federal government regulation of operations would be minimal.

Second, direct federal health activities would be limited to a few programs that are clearly national in scope, such as research. Environmental protection activities would be sharply reduced.

Third, federal income taxes would be substantially reduced so that individuals would have more disposable income. Thus citizens could vote for more state or local taxes if they wanted particular public health programs.

Finally, federal grants would go to the states and direct federal-local government contact would be avoided wherever feasible. The SHA would be the administering agency for Maternal and Child Health Services Block Grants.

Persons favoring this program argued that the federal government had become too large and its influence too pervasive in state and local activities (and other activities, as well). Local requirements and needs were not well determined in distant Washington, D.C., and should be decided locally. The massive amount of federal regulation had made most programs inefficient; they were top-heavy with administrative personnel and procedures, and stifled innovative initiatives for effective operation. Many of the environmental and workplace protections have been extreme and have hurt the growth of the economy, which is basic to national welfare. Furthermore, many programs did not achieve their purpose. The mechanisms of the marketplace, if unfettered by aggressive regulation, will see to it that industry's operations in a competitive world serve the American people in the best manner. In particular the Reagan program would revitalize industry and result in an increased tax base for states and localities. They would then be able to decide for themselves what programs they want and be able to raise the taxes to pay for them.

Those opposing the Reagan program pointed to the American economy's shift from a local to a regional and national one. These developments led to a centralization of tax revenue in the federal government, while the responsibility for public health services remained with the states and localities. This divergence led to ever-growing disparities between needs and available tax bases in states and among localities within states. Everyone, especially children and youth, should have equal—or as nearly equal opportunity as possible—to develop their potential (37), regardless of the state or locality in which they were born or reared. This belief requires either that programs be run entirely out of Washington or that federal tax money be redistributed among states and localities according to measures of need. These advocates also point to the fact that the American economic system is increasingly consolidating and centralizing its control. The organization needed to protect the public interest, they would argue, also needs to be increasingly centralized to correspond to this changing system. In the public health field, the emergence of chronic and degenerative diseases as the leading health threats points to nationwide causation and the need for nationwide preventive measures. Local agencies cannot act to control activities of national and international combines. Returning environmental control to the states, for example, could result in competition among the states to offer the fewest environmental controls possible in an effort to attract national industry.

This is not to say that maximum control and administration from Washington is desirable. There should be as much local administration as possible, but with goals and aims coordinated on a national basis. That was the central idea for the federal partnership system, as differentiated from presidents Nixon's and Reagan's New Federalism.

Finally, the federal partnership system grew in a typically American way: it developed as a series of responses to specific problems. The Reagan program, its opponents argue, is based on abstract ideology and consists merely of a set of assertions stemming from theoretical assumptions about the functioning of the market. The reply of Reagan policy supporters is that the federal partnership really became a federal dictatorship and that its programs have not worked. Something else must be tried.

Where Do We Stand?

What does the future hold for public health? After almost 50 years of proceeding in one direction, a reversal of cooperative federalism was attempted by the Nixon and Ford administrations and was pushed further by the Reagan administration. The question is whether this "counterrevolution" is an aberration or a harbinger. The long-term answer is unlikely to be decided by either ideology or empirical developments alone. If history is any guide, the American pattern will be to adopt solutions based on dominant ideological beliefs strongly modified by programmatic responses perceived to be required by circumstances.

With respect to the organization and content of public health services, an overriding fact is the changed nature of the major threats to health—

the chronic degenerative diseases as well as the appearance of AIDS. It may be that public health now stands with respect to those diseases where it stood with respect to acute infectious diseases in the mid–1850s. We are beginning to know something about the determinants or risk factors of these diseases, and, therefore, certain preventive measures can reasonably be advocated. For these measures to be as effective as public health measures became against acute infectious diseases after 1915, considerable more epidemiologic and biological research is needed. As the results of this research continue to be revealed, and as the smoke settles from the political battles being waged over the future structure of our federal system, decisions will have to be made about the structure of our public health system.

The structure and roles of local, state, and federal public health agencies and that of other agencies performing health-related work will need to be determined. Again, if history is any guide, these relationships and functions will be worked out in a combination of theoretical formulation, pragmatic experiments in administrative accommodation, and political battles. After a period of change and turmoil, an attempt will be made to codify the existing arrangements into a comprehensive federal law. If this process of realignment is to be as painless as possible, the nation will need public health leaders who keep up with the findings and have the political and administrative ability to incorporate the pioneering ones into public health practice, not only as experiments in individual places but also as national and state policy. The foremost leaders will need to have a good grasp of health problems and what is known about solving them—both preventive and curative. They will need to understand the political, social, and historical background of health services and society as a whole. They will also need to understand what kind of community leadership skills local public health administrators need to organize the community to battle against existing health threats as well as how such leaders can be trained.

A number of developments in the federal role in

public health have not been addressed here. These include the Food and Drug Administration (FDA), the Occupational Safety and Health Act (OSHA), the federal Community Mental Health Act, the Alcohol and Drug Abuse Act, and the Environmental Protection Act of 1970. These are extremely important to the total understanding of government's public health roles, but aside from the community mental health legislation, they deal with direct national regulation by the federal government, whereas this chapter has addressed public health activities of the federal government only from the viewpoint of the federal system of public health agencies— the PHS, SHAs, and local health departments.

References

1. Last, J. A. (Ed.). (1980). *Maxcy-Rosenau public health and preventive medicine* (11th ed.). New York: Appleton-Century-Crofts.

2. Dubos, R. (1959). *The mirage of health.* Garden City, NY: Doubleday.

3. Dubos, R. (1965). *Man adapting.* New Haven, CT: Yale University Press.

4. Shyrock, R. (1979). *The development of modern medicine.* Madison, WI: University of Wisconsin Press.

5. Rosen, G. (1958). *A history of public health.* New York: MD Publications.

6. Grad, F. P. (1970). *Public health law manual: A handbook on the legal aspects of public health administration and enforcement.* Washington, DC: American Public Health Association.

7. Mustard, H. S. (1945). *Government in public health.* New York: Commonwealth Fund.

8. Ferrell, J. A., Wilson, G. S., Covington, P. W., et al. (1929, April 1). *Health departments of states and provinces of the United States and Canada* (Public Health Bulletin No. 184). Washington, DC: U.S. Public Health Service, U.S. Department of the Treasury.

9. Mountin, J. W., Hankela, E. K., & Druzin, G. B. (1947). *Ten years of federal grants-in-aid for public health, 1936–1946* (Public Health Bulletin No. 300). Washington, DC: U.S. Public Health Service.

10. Emerson, H. (1945). *Local health units for the nation.* New York: Commonwealth Fund.

11. Greve, C. H., & Campbell, J. R. (1961 revision). *Organization and staffing for local health services* (U.S. Public Health Service Publication No. 682). Washington, DC: U.S. Government Printing Office.

12. Sanders, B. S. (1957). Local health departments: Growth or illusion? *Public Health Reports. 74.* 13–20.

13. Kenadjian, B. (1966). Appropriate types of federal grants for state and community health services. *Public Health Reports. 81.* 9.

14. Shubick, H. J., & Wright, E. O. (1961). *Compositive study of fifty health departments' organizational charts representing forty-nine states and the District of Columbia.* Unpublished report. (Cited in reference 22, p. 22.)

15. Hanlon, J. J. (1969). *Principles of public health administration.* St. Louis, MO: Mosby. (See also the ninth edition for additional information.)

16. American Public Health Association. (1968, November 13). *The state health department policy statement of the governing council of the Association.* Unpublished statement. (A condensed version of the statement appeared in *American Journal of Public Health.* [1969]. *59.* 158–159.)

17. Gossert, D. J., & Miller, C. A. (1973). State boards of health, their numbers and commitments. *American Journal of Public Health. 63.* 486–493.

18. Public Health Foundation. (1990, June). *Public health agencies, 1990.* Washington, DC: Author.

19. Levit, K. R., et al. (1985). National health expenditures, 1984. *Health Care Financing Review. 7.* 1–35.

20. *Book of states, 1976–1977.* (1977). Washington, DC: Council of State Governments.

21. Shonick, W. (1980). Mergers of public health departments with public hospitals in urban areas: Findings of 12 field studies. *Medical Care. 18 (suppl.).* 1–50.

22. Cameron, C. M., & Kobylarz, A. (1980). Nonphysician directors of local public health departments: Results of a national survey. *Public Health Reporter. 95.* 386–397.

23. Zwick, D. (1977). Project grants for health services. *Public Health Reporter. 82.* 131–138.

24. Cavanaugh, J. H. (1967). Comprehensive Health Planning and Public Health Service Act of 1966 (PL 89-749). *Health Education and Welfare Indicators.* 9–18.

25. Ingraham, H. S. (1965). Federal grants manage-

ment: A state health officer's view. *Public Health Reporter. 80.* 670–676.

26. Executive Office of the President. (1971, June). *Restoring the balance of federalism.* Washington, DC: Office of Management and Budget.

27. Office of the Secretary, U.S. Department of Health, Education and Welfare. (1972, June). *Federal assistance review: A special report from the Department of Health, Education and Welfare* (DHEW Publication No. [OS] 72-38). Washington, DC: U.S. Government Printing Office.

28. Palmer, J. L., & Sawhill, I. W. (Eds.). (1982). *The Reagan experiment: An examination of economic and social policies under the Reagan administration.* Washington, DC: Urban Institute Press.

29. *Washington Report on Medicine and Health.* Washington, DC: McGraw-Hill. February 1973, February 1977, February 1982.

30. *Promoting health/preventing disease.* (1980, Fall). Washington, DC: U.S. Department of Health and Human Services.

31. Office of the Assistant Secretary for Health and Surgeon General, U.S. Public Health Service. (1979). *Healthy people, the U.S. Surgeon General's report on health promotion and disease prevention* (DHEW Publication No. [PHS] 79-05571A). Washington, DC: U.S. Government Printing Office.

32. Office of the Assistant Secretary for Health and Surgeon General, U.S. Public Health Service. (1979). *Healthy people, the U.S. Surgeon General's report on health promotion and disease prevention* (DHEW Publication No. [PHS] 79-05517A). Washington, D.C.: U.S. Government Printing Office.

33. Crawford, R. (1977). You are dangerous to your health: The idealogy and politics of victim blaming. *International Journal of Health Services. 7*(4). 663–680.

34. Hurley, R. (1971). The health crisis of the poor. In H. P. Dreitzel (Ed.). *The social organization of health* (pp. 83–122). New York: Macmillan.

35. Public Health Foundation. (1990, July). *1990 prevention block grant chart book.* Washington, DC: Author. Figure 1.

36. U.S. Office of Management and Budget. (1987). *Budget of the United States, 1987.* Washington, DC: U.S. Government Printing Office. Appendix, Section I–K.

37. Tobin, J. (1981, December 3). Reaganomics and economics. *The New York Review of Books.* Pp. 11–14.

Chapter 5

Ambulatory Health Care Services

Stephen J. Williams

This chapter presents a brief overview of the scope and history of ambulatory care services. Office-based practice is discussed, including both solo and group practice. Institutional providers of ambulatory care services are also presented, as are noninstitutional and government-sponsored providers. Most important, the role of ambulatory care services in structuring the health care system is discussed in considerable detail.

Traditionally ambulatory care services have been viewed as the primary source of contact that most people have with the health care system. Although there are few concise definitions of ambulatory care, these services can be defined as care provided to noninstitutionalized patients. Sometimes ambulatory care is termed for the "walking patient." Ambulatory care includes a wide range of services, from simple routine treatment to surprisingly complex tests and therapies.

The role of ambulatory care services in organizing and rationalizing the health care system has been greatly enhanced by the rapid growth of managed care, by the changing nature and role of hospitals and hospital systems, and by enhancement of the gatekeeper and coordinating function of front line providers of care. The increasing shift of many services that had been traditionally performed on an inpatient basis, such as many surgical services, patient maintenance care that is now provided in the home rather than the hospital, and other practical and technological changes, has also heightened interest in ambulatory care. Finally, the increasing consolidation and vertical integration of the health care system is greatly increasing the linkages between ambulatory care and other services. Many of these changes and trends are discussed in other chapters of this book; their relevance to ambulatory care and ambulatory care's enhanced role in the system are discussed in this chapter. Ambulatory care has long had a central role in health care, a role that is now increasing in scope and importance, and a long and interesting history characterizes the evolution of these services.

Historical Perspective and Types of Care

Ambulatory care originated with the healing arts themselves. In primitive societies and for many years thereafter, until the advent of institutional care, all care was provided on what might be referred to as an *ambulatory care basis*. Of course, the types of care given then have little resemblance to today's health care, but the history of civilization demonstrates a consistent commitment to caring for the sick, using whatever knowledge has been available at the time. Remarkable forms of medical practice occurred in Greece, Rome, and other relatively sophisticated societies. In fact, many primitive societies had, and most, if not all, countries still have, their own indigenous practitioners such as religious healers and medicine men.

In more recent times, ambulatory care was provided in many new settings by a variety of more advanced practitioners. In Europe, and later in the United States, many of these services were given to wealthy patients in their homes, and poor people were cared for in dispensaries and public clinics. With the improvements in hospital care more patients of all social classes received both inpatient and outpatient care in hospital settings. In the United States the poor have always been more likely than wealthier people to obtain care from the hospital versus a private physician.

In the United States, ambulatory care services were traditionally provided by individual medical practitioners working in their offices and in patients' homes and by public clinics operating primarily for poor and indigent patients. The limited technological armament that physicians required allowed them to travel easily, carrying with them their principal equipment and supplies. Thus home care was common, especially among wealthier patients. Physicians' offices were frequently located in their homes or in other small buildings, as opposed to today's medical office buildings or large medical centers (1). The general practitioner who made house calls, provided guidance, and offered available treatments was typical of the primary care provided before World War II.

Since World War II, however, an explosion of medical knowledge has led to increasing specialization, more complex technology, and rapid changes in the setting and nature of services. Fewer physicians are able or willing to travel to the patient's home, and many can no longer carry with them either the equipment and supplies or the specialized personnel available in an office. The growth of technical specialization in particular, has led to the rapid expansion of new settings for providing care, such as group practices and hospital clinics, both of which are discussed further below. Increased knowledge has led to the partial phasing out of the "traditional" general practitioner.

For the poor, in both Europe and the United States, care, when available, was often limited to public or philanthropic clinics or dispensaries. Private practitioners may have given their time to serve the poor, but their devotion to the patient was probably limited, as was the availability of care and the facilities in which services were provided.

Early efforts to link ambulatory care services and integrate them formally with inpatient care were promoted in this country and in Europe, in part, through the concept of regionalization. In Great Britain, the concept was presented in the Dawson Report (2), which eventually led to the National Health Service. In the United States, however, centralization of authority under government of the health care system has not been accepted as a politically viable alternative.

The increasing sophistication of insurance mechanisms and the use of ambulatory care services as a control mechanism on the use of all services has led to an increase in the degree of structure of the health care system over the past few years. This increasing structure has primarily been in the private, nongovernmental sector. The concept of social and economic regulation of the system through governmental intervention, carried to a high level of sophistication in the Dawson Report, has largely been abandoned, at least for the foreseeable future. Integration of services will largely focus on multiple independently organized systems of care that are competitive with one another, especially as discussed in Chapter 13 in the section on managed care.

Table 5-1 demonstrates some of the diversity of services, providers, and facilities involved in ambulatory care today. Many of these services and organizations are discussed in this chapter. Particular attention is directed toward rapidly expanding and innovative settings, such as group practice, and integration of settings and services through organized systems of care. The role of ambulatory care is further discussed in other chapters of this book, especially those dealing with insurance and organizational arrangements.

Levels of Ambulatory Care Services

Ambulatory care services can be differentiated into a number of distinct levels or types of care. Primary prevention seeks to reduce the risks of illness or morbidity by removing disease-causing agents from our society. These activities include efforts to eliminate environmental pollutants that are suspected to cause diseases such as cancer. Other examples of primary prevention include encouraging people to use automobile seat belts, treatment of water and sewage, and sanitation inspections in restaurants. Preventive health services are more direct interventions to detect and prevent disease. Examples of these services include hypertension, diabetes, and cancer screening clinics and immunization programs. The combination of primary prevention and preventive services is our first line of defense against disease.

Medical care that is oriented toward the daily, routine needs of patients, such as initial diagnosis and continuing treatment of common illness, is termed *primary care* (3). This care is not highly complex and generally does not require sophisticated technology and personnel. The vision of the general practitioner of bygone days, traveling from house to house and ministering to the sick, represents the traditional role of primary care which is replaced in today's society by considerably better skilled practitioners in relatively complex facilities.

In addition to providing services directly, the primary care professional should serve the role of patient advisor, advocate, and system "gatekeeper." In this coordinating role, the provider refers patients to sources of specialized care, gives advice regarding various diagnoses and therapies, and provides continuing care for chronic conditions. In many organized systems of care, such as managed care programs, this role is very important in controlling costs, utilization, and the rational allocation of resources.

The evolution of technology and medicine's increasing ability to intervene in illness have led to greater specialization of health care services. These more specialized services, termed *secondary* and *tertiary care,* are provided in both ambulatory and inpatient settings. The content of secondary and tertiary care practices is usually more narrowly defined than that of the primary care provider. Subspecialists, who provide the bulk of secondary and tertiary care, also often require more complex equipment and more highly trained support personnel than do primary care providers.

In recent years the evolution of health care services has led to greatly expanded provision of secondary care on an outpatient, or ambulatory care, basis. Numerous surgical services of increasing complexity have been shifted to the ambulatory arena; recent advances in the use of laparoscopic and other technologies suggest that this trend will continue. Diagnostic and therapeutic procedures that used to require hospitalization are also increasing by being performed in ambulatory settings.

There are no clear dividing lines for primary versus secondary and secondary versus tertiary care. Secondary services include routine hospitalization and specialized outpatient care. These services are more complex than those of primary care and include many diagnostic procedures as well as more complex therapies. Tertiary care includes the most complex services, such as open heart surgery, burn treatment, and transplantation, and is provided in inpatient hospital facilities. Most of the care discussed in this chapter involves primary care and those secondary services that can be provided in such settings as office-based practice,

TABLE 5-1. Typical Ambulatory Care Services

Settings	Principal Practitioners	Level or Type of Service
Private office-based solo and group practice	Physicians, dentists, nurses, MEDEX, therapists	Primary and secondary care
Hospital clinics	Physicians, dentists, nurses, MEDEX, therapists	Primary and secondary care
Hospital emergency rooms	Physicians, nurses	All types
Ambulatory surgery centers (hospital-based and freestanding)	Surgeons, nurses, anesthesiologists	Surgical secondary care
Communitywide emergency medical systems	Technicians, nurses, drivers	Emergency transportation, communications, and immediate care
Poison control centers, community hotlines	Physicians, technicians, nurses	Emergency advice
Neighborhood health centers, migrant health centers	Physicians, dentists, nurses	Primary care
Community mental health centers	Psychologists, social workers	Primary health services
Federal systems—Veterans Administration, Indian Health Service, Public Health Service, military	All types	All types
Home health services	Nurses	Primary care
School health services	Nurses	Primary and preventive care
Prison health services	All types	Primary care
Public health services and clinics	Physicians, nurses	Targeted programs (e.g., family planning, immunization, inspections, screening programs, health education); primary care
Family planning and other specialized clinics (nongovernmental)	Physicians, nurses, aides	Specialized services; primary care
Industrial clinics	Physicians, nurses, environmental health specialists	Preventive, primary, and emergency care
Pharmacies	Pharmacists	Drugs and health education
Vision care	Opticians Optometrists Ophthalmologists	Examinations, screening, prescriptions filled
Medical laboratories	Technicians	Specialized laboratory services
Indigenous	Chiropractors, medicine men, naturopaths	Primary and supportive care

hospital outpatient departments, or community clinics.

The differences between the types of services provided within the ambulatory care sector are an important concern throughout this book since one objective of improving or rationalizing the health services system is to match the capabilities of providers or levels of care, with the needs of consumers. As different settings for providing ambulatory care are presented, one must consider the advantages and disadvantages of each to patient care needs and the optimal relationships that should be developed between the different levels of care. Similarly, one needs to regard the importance of these considerations as they relate to the managers of organized health care systems.

Settings for the Provision of Ambulatory Care

Office-Based Practice

Historically, and at the present time, most ambulatory care services are provided in solo and group practice, office-based settings. Institutional settings for care, primarily the hospital, although an important component of the health care system, remain less prominent. However, overlap between office-based practice and institutional settings is increasingly common as the dividing lines between various components of the health care system continue to blur (4). Managed care programs especially tend to integrate these services.

An indication of the distribution of ambulatory care visits by type of setting is contained in table 5-2 which presents survey results on utilization patterns, based on national data, representative of the entire U.S. population. The data in this table are taken from the National Health Interview Survey, a national survey of Americans' use of health care services, and complement the utilization data presented in Chapter 3.

Relatively little quantitative data is available on the utilization of ambulatory care services. Most utilization data is available from survey research

results. However, in an attempt to obtain more detailed information on health care use in physician office settings, the federal government has conducted an ongoing survey of private, office-based physicians—the National Ambulatory Medical Care Survey (NAMCS) (5). This survey involves a random sample of the nation's office-based, nonfederal physicians. Physicians are asked to complete a data collection form for each patient treated during a two-week interval.

Tables 5-3 and 5-4 list the most common reasons and the principal diagnoses for all office visits, respectively. The relative prominence of routine care, of follow-up or ongoing care, and of relatively simple primary care is rather striking and reflects the predominance of "routine" day-to-day needs of patients seeking ambulatory care services.

Further understanding of the nature of the visits is available from additional data regarding the services provided to patients and the interactions shared between patients and physicians. Table 5-5 represents the diagnostic services provided to patients, excluding the prescription of drugs. Most visits entail relatively limited examination and some degree of testing. Table 5-6 presents certain therapeutic services, much of which is focused on counseling. This further reinforces the widely recognized importance of the primary care role of patient advising. The drugs prescribed during these visits are listed in table 5-7. The majority of drugs prescribed comprise anti-infection agents, cardiovascular drugs, and central nervous system (CNS) agents.

Finally, Table 5-8 suggests that the majority of office-based care requires relatively short periods of contact between patients and physicians; nearly three-fourths of all visits required 15 minutes or less. A high percentage of visits concluded with the recommendation that the patient return at a specified time interval for a follow-up visit.

The National Ambulatory Medical Care Survey thus provides some insight into the nature of office-based ambulatory care. Much more extensive documentation of the survey and results for various types of services, providers, and patient character-

TABLE 5-2. Physician Contacts, According to Place of Contact and Selected Patient Characteristics: United States, 1989

Characteristic	Physician Contacts *Number per Person*	Place of Contact				
		Doctor's Office	Hospital Outpatient Department[1]	Telephone	Home	Other[2]
		Percent Distribution				
Total[3,4]	5.3	59.6	13.2	12.3	1.4	13.4
Age						
Under 5 years	6.7	61.4	9.8	15.5	0.5	12.8
5–14 years	3.5	63.0	13.8	13.4	0.4	9.4
15–44 years	4.6	58.1	13.5	11.4	0.6	16.3
45–64 years	6.1	59.0	14.4	12.5	1.6	12.5
65–74 years	8.2	58.4	15.5	10.0	4.0	12.1
75 years +	9.9	61.1	10.4	8.7	12.0	7.9
Sex[3]						
Male	4.8	58.1	15.0	11.2	1.2	14.5
Female	5.9	60.5	12.1	12.9	1.6	12.9
Race[2]						
White	5.5	60.9	12.2	12.9	1.4	12.7
Black	4.9	50.6	20.4	9.3	2.0	17.6
Family income[3,5]						
Under $14,000	6.3	48.5	18.0	10.8	2.4	20.3
$14–$24,999	5.2	58.9	14.3	12.9	1.4	12.5
$25–$34,999	5.5	61.0	12.1	12.4	0.8	13.7
$35–$49,999	5.2	63.1	12.1	12.9	0.6	11.4
$50,000+	6.0	64.4	10.7	13.6	1.7	10.7
Geographic region[3]						
Northeast	5.3	59.8	16.0	12.8	1.4	10.0
Midwest	5.4	57.6	13.3	12.9	1.7	14.5
South	5.3	62.5	11.1	12.3	1.6	12.5
West	5.5	57.4	13.8	11.3	0.9	16.5

[1] Includes hospital outpatient clinic, emergency room, and other hospital contacts.
[2] Includes clinics or other places outside a hospital.
[3] Age adjusted.
[4] Includes all other races not shown separately and unknown family income.
[5] Family income categories for 1989. Income categories for 1984 are: less than $10,000; $10–$18,999; $19–$29,999; $30–$39,999; and $40,000 or more.

SOURCE: Division of Health Interview Statistics, National Center for Health Statistics: Data from the National Health Survey.

TABLE 5-3. NAMCS, Most Common Reasons for Office Visits, 1990

Rank	Most Common Principal Reason for Visits	Number of Visits in Thousands	Percent Distribution
	All visits	704,604	100.0
1	General medical examination	30,341	4.3
2	Cough	25,740	3.7
3	Routine prenatal examination	25,296	3.6
4	Symptoms referable to the throat	18,866	2.7
5	Postoperative visit	17,523	2.5
6	Earache, or ear infection	14,633	2.1
7	Well baby examination	14,534	2.1
8	Back symptoms	12,497	1.8
9	Stomach pain, cramps, and spasms	12,054	1.7
10	Skin rash	11,562	1.6
11	Fever	11,500	1.6
12	Vision dysfunctions	11,397	1.6
13	Hypertension	10,391	1.5
14	Headache, pain in head	10,203	1.4
15	Knee symptoms	9,755	1.4
16	Chest pain and related symptoms (not referable to body system)	9,684	1.4
17	Head cold, upper respiratory infection (coryza)	8,557	1.2
18	Nasal congestion	8,546	1.2
19	Blood pressure test	7,922	1.1
20	Neck symptoms	7,006	1.0
	All other reasons	426,597	60.5

SOURCE: Schappert SM. National Ambulatory Medical Care Survey: 1990 Summary. Advance data from vital and health statistics; no 213. Hyattsville, Maryland: National Center for Health Statistics. 1992.

istics are available from the federal government. The survey data are an aid to planning health services in the ambulatory care setting and provide perspectives on national patterns of utilization. The applicability of the data to setting standards of performance in prepaid settings or under contracted agreements for service, however, is limited because of the many variables that could not be adequately measured.

The National Ambulatory Medical Care Survey aggregates physicians in private practice regardless of the specific setting in which they function. In reality, significant differences exist among phy-

sician practice settings and these are discussed in the following sections of this chapter. The two primary noninstitutional settings for the provision of ambulatory care are solo and group practice. Each of these settings may be components of larger systems of care through such integrating mechanisms as referral arrangements, insurance contracts, and direct ownership of practices. An organized system of care can, in turn, be comprised of various settings or types of ambulatory care providers.

Although the solo practice of medicine has traditionally attracted the greatest number of practi-

TABLE 5-4. NAMCS, Most Common Principal Diagnoses for Office Visits, 1990

Rank	Most Common Principal Diagnosis	Number of Visits in Thousands	Percent Distribution
	All visits	704,604	100.0
1	Essential hypertension	27,310	3.9
2	Normal pregnancy	23,561	3.3
3	Suppurative and unspecified otitis media	21,043	3.0
4	General medical examination	20,555	2.9
5	Acute upper respiratory infections of multiple or unspecified sites	18,676	2.7
6	Health supervision of infant or child	15,676	2.2
7	Diabetes mellitus	15,303	2.2
8	Allergic rhinitis	12,123	1.7
9	Bronchitis, not specified as acute or chronic	12,098	1.7
10	Acute pharyngitis	11,536	1.6
11	Chronic sinusitis	11,141	1.6
12	Neurotic disorders	9,531	1.4
13	Diseases of sebaceous glands	8,346	1.2
14	Disorders of refraction and accommodation	7,288	1.0
15	Cataract	7,282	1.0
16	Glaucoma	7,234	1.0
17	Asthma	7,137	1.0
18	Sprains and strains of other and unspecified parts of back	6,951	1.0
19	Other forms of chronic ischemic heart disease	6,429	0.9
20	Osteoarthrosis and allied disorders	6,358	0.9

SOURCE: Schappert SM. National Ambulatory Medical Care Survey: 1990 Summary. Advance data from vital and health statistics; no 213. Hyattsville, Maryland: National Center for Health Statistics. 1992.

tioners, group practice and institutionally based services are now expanding dramatically, continuing a trend that has been building over the past 30 years. Changing life-styles, the cost of establishing a practice, personal financial pressures on practitioners, contracting and affiliation opportunities, and the burdens of government regulations have enhanced the attractiveness of group practice for many physicians. With sharp increases in the number of physicians beginning practice, the growths of alternative settings, and especially of group practice, has been dramatic. Although solo practice remains an important avenue for providing ambulatory care services, these other settings have rapidly assumed a more prominent and visi-

ble role in the health care system, particularly as they provide a further mechanism for the integration, management, and control of health care services.

Solo Practice

Solo practitioners are difficult to characterize for a number of reasons. First, there are little data available on their practice patterns and activities. Some of the early studies focused on specific questions, such as referral patterns or quality of care, and do not provide a comprehensive picture of what the solo practitioner does (6). The studies that do

TABLE 5-5. NAMCS, Diagnostic Services Provided, 1990

Diagnostic and Screening Services[1]	Number of Visits in Thousands	Percent		
		Both Sexes	Female	Male
All visits	704,604	100.0	100.0	100.0
None	254,305	36.1	32.5	41.6
Pap test	33,898	4.8	7.9	0.0
Pelvic exam	51,422	7.3	12.0	—
Breast palpation	39,509	5.6	9.2	0.0
Mammogram	11,773	1.7	2.8	—
Visual acuity	45,291	6.4	6.2	6.8
Blood pressure	271,390	38.5	42.9	31.8
Urinalysis	89,904	12.8	15.2	9.0
Chest x-ray	20,293	2.9	2.7	3.2
Digital rectal examination	25,823	3.7	3.9	3.4
Proctoscopy or sigmoidoscopy	3,057	0.4	0.4	0.5
Stool blood examination	17,480	2.5	2.6	2.3
Oral glucose tolerance	3,421	0.5	0.6	0.3
Cholesterol measure	26,155	3.7	3.8	3.5
HIV serology	1,280	0.2	0.2	0.2
Other blood test	94,009	13.3	13.7	12.9
Other	176,390	25.0	24.6	25.6

[1] Total may exceed total number of visits because more than one service may be reported per visit.

SOURCE: Schappert SM. National Ambulatory Medical Care Survey: 1990 Summary. Advance data from vital and health statistics; no 213. Hyattsville, Maryland: National Center for Health Statistics. 1992.

contribute to a more complete understanding of the activities of solo practitioners are based on physicians in one geographic area or a particular specialty, and the results of these studies, although interesting and useful, may not be applicable to other practices or areas. The second problem in attempting to characterize solo practitioners is their heterogeneity; they include many types of health care professionals and provide an immense array of services.

The available evidence indicates that physicians in private solo practice generally work hard, although they often earn less, on average, than their counterparts in group practice. Many solo practitioners are subspecialists who provide secondary care primarily on referral from primary care practitioners. These practitioners include allergists, dermatologists, and surgeons. Some subspecialists provide both primary and secondary care since they have insufficient work in their own specialty to achieve desired income levels.

Many solo practitioners, including those trained in general and family practice, internal medicine, pediatrics, and obstetrics and gynecology, provide primary care services. There is some controversy and competition among practitioners concerning which specialists should be providing primary care. The specialty of family practice, in particular, represents a challenge to internal medicine in providing adult primary care and to pediatrics in child care, although the role of family practice is now firmly established, especially in health maintenance organizations (HMOs) (7).

Little detailed information exists on how the individual practitioner's time during the workday is allocated among various activities. Most solo prac-

TABLE 5-6. NAMCS, Therapeutic Services Provided, 1990

Therapeutic Service[1]	Number of Visits in Thousands	Percent Distribution
All visits	704,604	100.0
Medication therapy[2]		
Drug visits[3]	424,587	60.3
Number of medications ordered or provided by the physician		
None	280,017	39.7
1	230,716	32.7
2	110,865	15.7
3–5	83,007	11.8
Counseling and advice[1]		
None	442,833	62.8
Weight reduction	44,378	6.3
Cholesterol reduction	22,566	3.2
Breast self-exam	16,174	2.3
Smoking cessation	14,937	2.1
HIV transmission	1,740	0.2
Other	198,607	28.2
Other nonmedication therapy[1]		
None	566,077	80.3
Psychotherapy	26,922	3.8
Physiotherapy	16,572	2.4
Ambulatory surgery	14,203	2.0
Corrective lenses	9,580	1.4
Other	75,338	10.7

[1] Total may exceed total number of visits because more than one category may be reported per visit.
[2] Medications include prescription drugs, over-the counter preparations, immunizing agents, desensitizing agents, etc.
[3] Drug visits are visits at which one or more medication is ordered or supplied by the physician.

SOURCE: Schappert SM. National Ambulatory Medical Care Survey: 1990 Summary. Advance data from vital and health statistics; no 213. Hyattsville, Maryland: National Center for Health Statistics. 1992.

titioners perform a number of functions in the office, including patient care, consultations, and administration and supervision of office staff. Exactly how much time each of these activities requires is difficult to assess, but the requirements for administration and for supervision of personnel have been increasing in recent years.

Solo practice is often associated with an increased feeling that the provider cares about the welfare of the patient, possibly resulting in a stronger patient-provider relationship than occurs in other settings. There is some evidence that this situation, where it occurs, is a result of the lower level of bureaucracy or organizational complexity in solo

practice (8). Since there is also some evidence that the relationship between patient and physician is related to patient compliance with medical regimens, patients who perceive that they are receiving more personalized care may respond to the care process more positively (9). Solo practitioners are also not as restricted in referrals to specialists as are providers in some other settings, such as group practice, where organizational loyalties intervene. Finally, the solo practitioner may feel a greater identification with the community served since there is a more direct relationship between patient and provider. Organizational forms, especially managed care, that incorporate solo practitioners into

TABLE 5-7. Number and Percent Distribution of Drug Mentions by Therapeutic Categories: United States, 1990

Therapeutic Class [1]	Number of Mentions in Thousands	Percent Distribution
All drug mentions	759,406	100.0
Antimicrobial	125,275	16.5
Cardiovascular-renal	109,171	14.4
Respiratory tract	86,562	11.4
Pain relief	77,355	10.2
Hormones and related agents	67,544	8.9
Dermatologic	43,558	5.7
Psychopharmacologic	46,188	6.1
Metabolic and nutrient	29,238	3.9
Gastrointestinal	31,139	4.1
Ophthalmic	30,375	4.0
Immunologic	19,337	2.5
Neurologic	14,111	1.9
Hemotologic	9,914	1.3
Other and unclassified	69,639	9.2

[1] Therapeutic class based on the standard drug classification used in the *National Drug Code Directory, 1982 Edition.*

SOURCE: Schappert SM. National Ambulatory Medical Care Survey: 1990 Summary. Advance data from vital and health statistics; no 213. Hyattsville, Maryland: National Center for Health Statistics. 1992.

larger systems of care may be decreasing some of this physician-patient bond, especially as providers are forced to discount fees, increase productivity, and focus on the cost-effectiveness of their practice.

From the provider's perspective, solo practice offers an opportunity to avoid organizational dependence and to be self-employed; there is also no need to share resources or income with other providers. Philosophically, solo practice is most closely aligned with the traditional economic and political orientations that have characterized medicine; younger physicians faced with discounting, contracting, and networks for care may no longer identify with the more traditional perspectives, however.

All of the increasingly complex problems of administering a practice must be dealt with in solo practice unless a professional manager is hired. Furthermore, competitive pressures in the health care industry are leading many practitioners to question the feasibility and desirability of going it alone. Thus solo practice offers distinct opportunities and has philosophical and emotional appeal but is far from devoid of problems and constraints, especially in light of the realities of medical practice today.

Group Practice

Office-based practice includes, in addition to solo practice, group practice. This form of practice has been growing in popularity in recent years, especially as the increasing pressures of practice have led many providers to seek alternative settings in which to work.

Group practice is an affiliation of three or more providers, usually physicians, who share income, expenses, facilities, equipment, medical records, and support personnel in the provision of services through a formal, legally constituted organization (11). The formal definition of group practice, developed by the American Medical Association and the Medical Group Management Association, is three or more physicians formally organized to provide medical care, consultation, diagnosis, and/or treatment through the joint use of equipment and personnel, and with income from medical practice distributed in accordance with methods previously determined by members of the group. Although definitions of a group practice vary somewhat, the essential elements are formal sharing of resources and distribution of income.

Traditionally, group practice has meant participation and ownership by physicians. Increasingly, however, as new and more diversified models for the provision of services are developed, other practitioners will participate in group practices. In some communities, for example, group practices of nurse practitioners may be the only sources of health services. Dentists, optometrists, podiatrists, and other

TABLE 5-8. NAMCS, Characteristics of Office Visits, 1990

Disposition [1]	Number of Visits in Thousands	Percent Distribution
All visits	704,604	100.0
No followup planned	68,310	9.7
Return at specified time	437,530	62.1
Return if needed	159,101	22.6
Telephone followup planned	27,207	3.9
Referred to other physician	22,939	3.3
Returned to referring physician	7,210	1.0
Admit to hospital	6,802	1.0
Other	11,513	1.6

Duration	Number of Visits in Thousands	Percent Distribution
All visits	704,604	100.0
0 minutes [1]	8,262	1.2
1–5 minutes	63,383	9.0
6–10 minutes	199,086	28.3
11–15 minutes	217,608	30.9
16–30 minutes	167,690	23.8
31 minutes and over	48,575	6.9
Mean duration: 15.9 minutes		

[1] Represents office visits in which there was no face-to-face contact between the patient and the physician.

SOURCE: Schappert SM. National Ambulatory Medical Care Survey: 1990 Summary. Advance data from vital and health statistics; no 213. Hyattsville, Maryland: National Center for Health Statistics. 1992.

specialized personnel are also increasingly developing group practices.

History of Group Practice

Some of the earliest group practices in the United States were started by companies that needed to provide care to employees in rural sites where medical care was unobtainable. For example, the Northern Pacific Railroad organized a practice in 1883 to provide care to employees building the transcontinental railroad. This industrial clinic was one of a number of such clinics founded in the 19th century. Even more significant, however, was the establishment of the Mayo Clinic in Rochester, Minnesota—the first successful nonindustrial group practice. The Mayo Clinic, originally organized as a single-specialty group practice in 1887 and later broadened into a multispecialty group, demonstrated that group practice was feasible in the private sector. The Mayo Clinic also represented a reputable model for group practice in a national atmosphere of fierce independence where group practice was viewed with skepticism and distrust. By the early 1930s there were about 150 medical groups throughout the country, many of which were located in the Midwest. Most included or were started by someone who had practiced or trained at the Mayo Clinic.

In 1932 a national committee—the Committee on the Costs of Medical Care—was established to assess health care needs for the nation. It issued a report that suggested a major role for group practice in the provision of medical care. The committee recommended that these groups be associated with hospitals to provide comprehensive care and that there be prepayment for all services (11). The report strongly supported the concept of regionalization that eventually gained wide recognition in the establishment of the British National Health Service, our own military health care systems, and other national models of organized health service systems.

Other constituencies, including some unions, also developed group practices. After World War II, a number of pioneeering groups were established. In New York City, the Health Insurance Plan of New York was organized to provide prepaid medical care to the employees of the city—an idea promoted by Mayor Fiorello LaGuardia. On the West Coast, the Kaiser Foundation Health Plan was established to provide health care to employees of

Kaiser Industries; Kaiser is an affiliation of plans and providers that is now serving millions of Americans across the nation. In Seattle, a revolutionary development included the establishment of Group Health Cooperative of Puget Sound, a consumer-owned cooperative prepaid group practice, which now provides comprehensive care to more than 200,000 people. It was founded by progressive individuals who were dissatisfied with the private medical care available to them in the late 1940s.

Developments in medical practice also spurred the group practice movement. Perhaps most notable was the increasing specialization of medicine and the rapid expansion of technology. This increasing sophistication meant that no individual practitioner could provide all the expertise that patients would require. It also meant that more complex and expensive facilities, equipment, and personnel were needed to care for patients. Group practice provided a formal structure for sharing these costs among providers. Many people believed that resources would be used more efficiently in groups. In addition, multispeciality groups, encompassing more than on specialty, could provide patients with more of their health care under one roof and, hence, reduce problems of physical access to care and coordination of services.

Group practice was also thought to promote higher-quality care since most of the different specialists that a person required would be practicing together and would thus have the opportunity to discuss patient problems among themselves, share a common medical record, and be more able to ensure the quality and continuity of care. Therefore, group practice was viewed by many as being advantageous for the physician—offering opportunities such as easily developed referral arrangements, sharing of after-hours coverage, greater flexibility in working hours, and less financial risk—while also benefiting the patient.

Opposition to group practice has occurred mostly for political and philosophical reasons. The American Medical Association and local medical societies have, at times, opposed group practice. Many early group practices had difficulties when physicians were denied admitting privileges in local hospitals. Community-based specialists sometimes refused to treat patients referred by group practice physicians. In more recent years, however, opposition to group practice has lessened dramatically and restrictive laws have been challenged. The need to form affiliations for contracting under reimbursement programs and for achieving efficiencies in organizing health services more generally has resulted in little remaining formal opposition to group practice.

Survey of Group Practice

The American Medical Association has conducted surveys of physician-oriented medical group practices in the United States on a periodic basis since 1965. These surveys represent the most comprehensive data available concerning the growth and characteristics of group practice in this country. Group practices that qualified within the American Medical Association's definition were identified from a variety of data sources and were then surveyed through a mail data collection instrument. Numerous items of information were collected regarding the nature of the practice and its facilities and relationships to other entities (12).

The dramatic increase in popularity of practices is reflected in table 5-9. The number of group practices nearly doubled during the period from 1975 to 1988. There are now over 16,000 group practices in the United States, two-thirds of which are single-speciality groups.

Even more dramatic is the growth in the number of physicians practicing in a group-practice setting. Over 155,000 physicians in the United States are now working in group practices, which represents a marked increase from 67,000 in 1975 and 88,000 in 1980. A higher percentage of all physicians in group practice work in multispecialty-oriented groups as compared to the percentage of total groups that are multispecialty, largely because the average multispecialty group is substantially larger than the average single-specialty group. The average size of all group practices in the United

TABLE 5-9. Number of Medical Groups and Number of Physicians in Group Practice by Specialty Orientation of Group, United States, Selected Years

Year	Single Specialty	Multispecialty	Family or General Practice	Total
		Number of Groups		
1969	3,169	2,418	784	6,371
1975	4,601	2,976	906	8,488
1980	6,156	3,552	1,054	10,762
1984	10,635	2,781	1,770	15,186
1988	11,709	3,168	1,618	16,495
		Number of Physician Positions in Group Practice		
1969	13,053	24,349	2,691	40,093
1975	23,572	39,311	3,959	66,842
1980	29,456	4,122	4,712	88,290
1984	59,917	69,371	9,839	139,127
1988	71,861	75,760	8,007	155,628

SOURCE: Havlicek, P. L. (1990). *Medical groups in the U.S., 1990 edition. A survey of practice characteristics.* Chicago: American Medical Association.

States in 1988 was about nine physicians, an increase from 1980. These data reflect only physician "positions" and exclude other medically related professionals such as nurse practitioners.

Most group practices are professional corporations. The dramatic shift toward professional corporations since 1969 is primarily a result of changes in federal and state laws pertaining to taxation, the increasing size and complexity of the practices themselves, and interrelationships among physicians participating. Changes in federal tax law may result in further shifts in patterns of legal organizational forms.

Specialty distribution of physicians in group practice has not changed dramatically over the past 10 years. The specialties that account for the largest percentage of physicians participating in group practice include family and general practice, internal medicine, anesthesiology, obstetrics and gynecology, pediatrics, and radiology, many groups are now involved in managed care contracting.

Relatively few groups account for a significant percentage of all physicians in group practice as presented in table 5-10. There are relatively few

groups that employ more than 15 physicians. As would be expected, most of the larger groups are multispecialty, while the predominance of the smaller groups are single specialty.

The geographic distribution of group practice in the United States is dominated by seven states, which account for 40 percent of all groups. These states are California, Pennsylvania, New York, Texas, Illinois, Florida, and Ohio. The origin, growth, and current distribution of group practice and group practice physicians are not homogeneous throughout the various regions, which reflects a greater acceptance of group practice in some regions as well as a varied distribution of larger urban population centers in the country. As might be expected, physician groups and group-practice physicians are substantially more prominent in metropolitan areas than in nonmetropolitan areas of the country. The development of prepaid group practice also varies by region.

Interestingly, most group practices employed a business manager or administrator, although far fewer had an identifiable medical director. Multispecialty groups were more likely to employ a

TABLE 5-10. Total Groups and Group Physician Positions by Size of Group, 1988

Size of Group	Groups		Group Physician Positions	
	Percent	Number	Percent	Number
3	28.0	4,547	8.8	13,641
4	22.3	3,618		14,472
5–6	22.0	3,569	12.3	19,166
7–9	11.4	1,850	9.2	14,385
10–15	7.8	1,266	9.7	15,098
16–25	4.1	672	8.4	13,109
26–49	2.5	403	8.9	13,872
50–75	0.9	147	5.7	8,915
76–99	0.3	51	2.8	4,367
100 or more	0.7	118	24.8	38,603
Total	100.0	16,241[a]	99.9[b]	155,628

SOURCE: Havlicek, P. L. (1990). *Medical groups in the U.S., 1990 edition. A survey of practice characteristics.* Chicago: American Medical Association.

[a]Includes 107 groups with fewer than three physicians who qualified, per the AMA definition of group, in other important respects.
[b]Includes 185 physician positions in groups with fewer than three physicians.
[c]Excludes 784 groups whose size was unknown.

group administrator, and, as might be expected, larger groups were much more likely to employ administrators and have medical directors than were smaller groups. Nearly all the larger groups did employ an administrator. The market for trained group-practice administrators has grown substantially over the past few years, and its growth is likely to continue as the number of group practices increases.

An Assessment of Group Practice

A critical assessment of group practice yields distinct advantages and disadvantages for both patients and providers as compared to other modalities for providing ambulatory services. Some of these are summarized in table 5-11. Specific advantages and disadvantages vary from group to group, and table 5-11 also lists major considerations generally associated with group practice. Some of the topics listed under patient or provider perspectives could readily pertain to both.

The advantages of group practice from the perspective of the provider include shared operation of the practice, joint ownership of facilities and equipment; centralized administrative functions; and, in larger groups, a professional manager. The professional manager can provide expertise in areas often lacking among the providers such as billing; personnel management; patient scheduling; ordering of supplies; and, recently, of particular importance, negotiating, contracting, and related matters.

Financially, the group relieves the provider of the heavy initial investment often required to establish a practice. In most groups, however, co-ownership requires that new members buy into the group through purchase of a share of the group's capital over a period of time.

The burden of operating costs is also lessened

TABLE 5-11. Some Advantages and Disadvantages of Group Practice[a]

Advantages	Disadvantages
From Perspective of Health Services Provider	
Availability of professional manager	Less individual freedom
Organizational responsibility for patient	May lead to excess use of specialists
Less physician administrative time	Fewer outside consultants
Shared capital expense	Possible reduced identity with patient and community
Shared financial risk	
Improved contracting and negotiating ability	Group rather than individual decision making
Better coverage and shared on-call shifts	Share all problems
More flexible working hours	Must work with others
More peer interaction	Less individual incentive and more security-oriented
Increased access to specialists	
Broader array of ancillary services	Income limitations
Stable income for providers	Income distribution arguments
No direct financial concerns with patient	
Lower initial investment	
More time for continuing education	
More flexible vacation time	
Generally excellent benefits	
Possible efficiencies of scale	
Use of nonphysician practitioners	
From Perspective of Group Practice Patient	
Care under one roof	Possible lessening of provider–patient relationship
Availability of specialists, laboratories, etc.	
Improved coverage and emergency care	Possible overuse of ancillary services
Medical and administrative records centrally located	Possible high provider turnover
	Heavy patient loads and waiting times may be increased
Referrals simplified	
Peer interaction among providers	Less provider incentive for care
Better administration of group	More bureaucracy
Efficiency may be promoted in patient care	

[a]Some advantages and disadvantages could be included under both provider and patient categories.

for any individual member of a group. Rather than having to independently absorb the ups and downs of a practice, as do sole practitioners, those involved in a group practice share the income and expenses within the group, allowing for moderation of those fluctuations experienced in individual practices. For example, a solo practitioners who becomes ill may have no practice income aside from disability insurance, whereas a group member's income may continue during a short period of illness since other providers are simultaneously generating revenue. However, the provisions of income distribution plans vary substantially among groups.

The participation of physicians in group practice also has a significant advantage in facilitating the development of definitive arrangements for contracting and negotiating. The group can support increased levels of participation, has a knowledge group practice administrator to manage the contracts, and can respond to the market with a wider range of services. Even single-specialty groups, with shared on-call services and subspecialization of group members, will be able to offer more to the market on a contractual basis than the individual practitioner. Having a professional manager to negotiate on behalf of the group further enhances the relative attractiveness of group practice, particularly for physicians who lack experience in interpreting and negotiating contracts.

Patient care responsibilities are also shared in group practice. This sharing results in greater flexibility of working hours for the provider, as well as more time for vacation and continuing education, without sacrificing the quality of care for the patient. For example, providers cover for each other during vacations and after normal working hours. Although most practitioners in solo practice arrange for patient care coverage, the continuity of care and the extent of coverage are probably greater in group practice since the patients' medical records and the full resources of the group are always available, even if specific providers are not working.

Sharing of patient care may have some other potential benefits. These include more peer interaction as a result of informal discussions and referral of patients among providers. The inclusion of more providers also results in the availability, by necessity, of a wider range of specialists and ancillary services, which represents a convenience for both providers and patients as well as a source of added revenue for the group.

Does the sharing of administrative and patient care activities within group practice produce better care at lower cost? Although many people believe that effective group management uses resources more efficiently than solo practice, the evidence is mixed. Some evidence tends to refute these beliefs, but more analytical research indicates some economies of scale, or efficiencies, attributable to the grouping of resources for smaller groups but possibly less so for larger and more bureaucratic groups (13). The use of personnel may be more advantageous in group than solo practice. Receptionists, medical records specialists, laboratory and radiology technicians, nurses, and other types of personnel may be used more efficiently and in the specialized areas of their training in many medium- and larger-sized groups. In addition, there is some question as to whether any savings that are achieved will be returned to consumers or simply represent higher income for providers. Further, the increasing supply of physicians may reduce the desirability of employing mid-level practitioners, except in certain prepaid settings.

The effect of groups on patient care, especially on the quality of care, has been investigated more extensively in the prepaid, as opposed to fee-for-service, setting. In prepaid group practices the incentives are substantially different since providers are paid a salary and consumers pay "in advance" for all care. Sharing of medical records, peer interaction, easy referrals and consultations with specialists, more sophisticated and accessible ancillary services, and more skilled and diversified support personnel are all arguments suggested in support of higher-quality care in group practice.

Group practice also offers advantages to patients and their communities. For the patient, the group offers a wide range of services under one roof so that travel between providers is reduced and access increased. A unified medical record can contribute to continuity of care and less duplication in diagnosis and treatment. Some groups also own or operate hospitals and thus further extend the integration and scope of the services that they provide, an especially important consideration in negotiating with employers and insurers.

Group practices usually offer more accessible care after normal working hours. Some groups also offer emergency services through their own emergency rooms or clinics. Groups with a broader community perspective may even be involved in programs such as school health services and community immunization efforts.

The use of a professional manager should benefit the patient through more efficient scheduling and patient flow and improved overall management of the practice. Billing is simplified since all care received can be included on one statement.

On a communitywide basis, group practice may offer a means of attracting providers to areas with inadequate numbers of medical care personnel. By offering peer interaction, support services, and other advantages, groups may increase the appeal of practicing in rural or inadequately served urban centers.

There are also distinct disadvantages to group practice for providers, patients, and communities. From the perspective of the provider, practicing in a group implies less individual freedom, with a variety of restrictions imposed through the sharing of a practice. Ideologically, the limitations of a group in this regard may be difficult for some people to accept since medicine has traditionally been an individualistic enterprise. In addition to reduced freedom, group practice entails sharing responsibilities and problems with others. The interpersonal requirements for working out these responsibilities may not appeal to all practitioners. Older individuals who have been working in solo practice may be especially unlikely to adapt readily to group practice.

The financial advantages for group practice are a trade-off against some restrictions on income generation and the necessity of complying with the group's income distribution and practice pattern requirements. Thus there often is more security and less risk but also less incentive and reward for individual initiative and production.

The shift of some patient care responsibilities from the individual practitioner to the group also may adversely affect the patient-provider relationship by introducing a degree of impersonalization. If a group has high physician turnover, which is rare, the patient may have to change providers frequently. Groups that have too few providers for the number of patients they serve, a common occurrence when excess capacity is being avoided, will also have waiting times for appointments in the office that the patient may believe to be excessive. The group may impose greater restrictions on referral practices, consequently limiting the practitioner's willingness to use the expertise of other specialists in the community.

From a community perspective, groups may reduce the geographic dispersion of providers and thus increase difficulties of physical access to care. In addition, groups may reduce competition in the health care marketplace by consolidating what would otherwise be competing providers. Consolidation may eventually reduce the ability of insurers, employers, and other plan sponsors to negotiate favorable terms for contracted care.

The changing organizational structure of the health care system is also changing some aspects of the role of ambulatory care services from the perspectives of providers, consumers, and the community. Ambulatory care is assuming a much greater role in the rationing of care, especially for primary care, and in the control of referrals and use of specialty, laboratory, and other services. These changes are especially notable in managed care and for hospital-sponsored systems of care as discussed elsewhere in this book. Ambulatory care is substantially affecting other provider organizations, especially the hospital, as more and more care is provided on an ambulatory basis. There are important fiscal, organizational, and utilization implications for all components of the system as a result of these changes.

The implications of these structural changes in the provision of health care are profound. Consumers are affected in terms of where and how they receive services. Providers are affected by changes in their affiliations, referral patterns, incentives, and practice characteristics. And, finally, the community is obviously affected by the changing organization of services, by the formation of alliances, and by shifts in the economic and political clout of various providers.

Institutionally Based Ambulatory Services

In addition to solo and group practice in the traditional private sector, many institutions have expanded their involvement in ambulatory care. These institutionally based settings, especially those associated with hospitals, are discussed next.

The hospital has evolved from an institution for poor people who could not be cared for at home to a provider of a full range of health services from primary to tertiary care. As technological advances have brought more services into the hospital and expanded the scope of care provided, the hospital has assumed an especially important role in the provision of highly complex health services. At the same time, an increasing number of people have sought primary care from hospitals, sometimes as a result of lack of access to other sources of care.

Outpatient and Ambulatory Care Clinics

The increased demands placed on hospitals for care taxed the ability of many facilities to respond with appropriate and adequate resources. The result was overcrowded facilities: the wrong mix of services, equipment, and personnel to respond to patient needs; and extremely dissatisfied consumers and providers. Most hospitals have now successfully responded to these demands by expanding outpatient services and hiring full-time providers to staff redesigned hospital ambulatory facilities.

Traditional hospital outpatient services have been provided in clinics and emergency rooms. In many hospitals, clinics have had second-class status as compared to complex and expensive inpatient services. However, as hospitals are increasingly recognizing the important role of primary care, especially in contracting, and are seeking to expand the base of patients who are potential users of inpatient and ancillary services, more attention is being directed toward improving clinic operations and services.

Hospital clinics include both primary care and specialty clinics. Many hospitals differentiate between clinics for walk-in patients without appointments and those for scheduled visits. Specialty clinics are usually organized by department and provide services such as ophthalmology, neurol-

ogy, and allergy care. In teaching hospitals, clinics serve as important settings in which house staff members provide ongoing care to patients and follow up after hospitalization. Increasingly, clinics also provide an opportunity to expose medical students and house staff to ambulatory care services in order to complement the traditionally more extensive experience with inpatient care. In teaching hospitals, there may be more than 100 different clinics reflecting the diversity of subspecialties. In nonteaching hospitals, there are fewer specialty clinics, and there may be more emphasis on primary care.

Many hospital primary-care clinics evolved from an orientation of service to the poor and were staffed by physicians who served without reimbursement in exchange for staff privileges. The level of commitment to the patient under such circumstances was, not surprisingly, less than desirable. Many hospitals now employ physicians and other practitioners as full-time clinic staff. Some hospitals have established primary-care group practices to complement other outpatient services and to assume the burden of providing primary care to patients who seek most of their care from the hospital.

The development of a group practice has advantages for both consumers and the hospital by providing comprehensive and accessible care and by removing primary-care patients from facilities that are not designed to serve their needs, such as emergency rooms. Development of these group practices also has the potential of increasing use of the hospital's inpatient and ancillary services, an advantage if occupancy is low (14). Hospitals with ambulatory care resources can negotiate contracts for providing a wide range of both inpatient and outpatient services. They are subsequently also able to more effectively control the use of services and thus costs. However, questions have been raised concerning the ability of hospitals to compete effectively in an arena in which they have not been overly successful in the past (15). But the increasingly competitive nature of the hospital and the health care marketplace is forcing many hospitals to enter this area of practice even if they are uncertain about doing so.

Ambulatory Surgery Centers

A further innovation in hospital-based care has been the development of ambulatory surgery centers. Originated in hospitals in Washington, D.C., Los Angeles, and elsewhere, these organized hospital units provide one-day surgical care. Patients are usually screened for acceptability by their personal surgeon and then report at an assigned date and time for surgery. The surgeon is supported by the unit's facilities, equipment, and personnel, and the patient is discharged one to three hours after surgery when recovery from anesthesia is sufficiently complete.

In the early 1970s, freestanding ambulatory surgery centers were opened; one of the first was in Phoenix, Arizona. These facilities are independent of hospitals and usually provide a full range of services for the types of surgery that can be performed on an outpatient basis. Community surgeons are granted operating privileges and can perform surgery in these facilities when the patient agrees and when there are no medical contraindications.

Other facilities are also used for ambulatory or outpatient surgery. Many physicians traditionally performed surgery in their offices, although this practice has declined in some specialities as a result of malpractice concerns and the increasing availability of better-equipped and -staffed alternative facilities. Other specialities, such as oral surgery, plastic surgery, and ophthalmology extensively use office-based facilities.

Freestanding emergency centers have also opened in many cities, paralleling the success of ambulatory surgery centers. These emergency centers sometimes provide a wide range of primary care in addition to responding to urgent problems. The future of specialized ambulatory centers, in both hospitals and as freestanding facilities, will probably include further expansion into other areas of health care, ranging from sports medicine to women's health care.

Even greater innovation has occurred in recent years. Freestanding postsurgical recovery centers for short nonhospital stays of one to three nights are under development to provide a less intensive recovery setting for less complex surgical cases. Mobile diagnostic facilities with sophisticated imaging equipment have been operational for a number of years. Even mobile physician vans are now in use to return the house call to more frequent clinical use by transporting the physician along with his or her office to the patient's home without sacrificing technological capabilities. The challenge for the future remains to identify economically feasible and innovative approaches to providing patient care that expedite the care process and are accepted by consumer, providers, and payors (16).

Emergency Medical Services

The emergency room, like other hospital departments, has undergone transformation in recent years. The emergency room has expanded in the range of services offered and in complexity. An especially important long-term trend has been the increasing use of the emergency room for primary care. Since the emergency room requires sophisticated facilities and highly trained personnel and must be accessible 24 hours a day, costs are high and services are not designed for nonurgent care. To reduce the burden on the emergency room and to meet patient need more effectively, many hospitals treat patients on a triage basis. In this process, often performed by a nurse, the patient's health care needs are determined and the patient is referred to a more appropriate source of care within the hospital. Misuse of the emergency room has received considerable attention over the past 20 years.

Emergency medical services have also been increasingly integrated with other community resources. Included are drug and alcohol treatment programs, mental health centers, and voluntary agencies. Most major urban centers have developed formal emergency medical systems that incorporate all hospital emergency rooms as well as transportation and communication systems. In these communities, people needing emergency care either transport themselves or call an emergency number (such as 911). An ambulance is dispatched by a central communications center that also identifies and alerts the most appropriately equipped and located hospital. In many communities, regional hospital-based trauma centers have been built with extremely sophisticated capabilities. Specialized ambulance services, including mobile coronary care units and shock-trauma vans, are also increasingly prevalent.

The Red Cross and other voluntary agencies have administered programs for many years to train people to respond to accidents, drownings, and other emergencies. In Seattle, a program was initiated—now expanding to other cities—to augment emergency capabilities by teaching as many people as possible to respond to heart attacks by administering cardiopulmonary resuscitation (CPR). Because accidents and heart attacks are major sources of mortality, these programs have the potential of contributing to reductions in deaths.

Government Programs

In addition to private sector and institutionally initiated efforts, government programs have been designed to increase the availability of health care resources in many communities. These programs have adapted some of the concepts of private institutional settings, especially those of group practice.

Neighborhood health centers were funded starting in 1965. Originally intended to serve approximately 25 million people, this federal program never reached its initial objectives. The program was designed to provide primary medical care with a family orientation. It was targeted for population groups in need of services, as reflected by such indicators as disease prevalence and income level. At the same time, the centers were intended to employ people from the communities they serve in positions that would offer opportunities for training and advancement. Responsiveness to community needs was to be ensured by a community board or advisory panel. The centers were to recognize that the broad attributes of a community, such as housing and employment, contributed to health and illness.

Most of the neighborhood health centers are freestanding group practices, although some are affiliated with other institutions such as hospitals, medical schools, or community associations. The majority of centers are located in urban areas. There is considerable diversity in the types of service provided by the centers, but all give primary care and most offer pharmacy, laboratory, radiology, and, to a lesser extent, dental services. Some centers also provide transportation for patients and social services to address broader health needs.

Although these health centers were originally intended to serve the poor, changes in federal policy that encouraged them to collect fees from patients and from third-party insurers have broadened the socioeconomic mixture of patients obtaining care. However, the centers still predominantly serve the medically indigent. Sources of funding have been broadened to include local government as well. Pressures for achieving self-sufficiency have been very powerful in recent years.

A related category of provider, the "free clinic," evolved from a strong social commitment but has had to face similar financial realities. The combination of "former" free clinics, neighborhood health centers, public agency clinics, and some hospital clinics and groups now form an informal "safety net" of providers for individuals who lack private insurance or access to other sources of care, or simply need care from an available, sympathetic provider. Many of these providers now contract on their own or in coalitions with other providers to provide care to various individuals under government entitlement programs as well.

Neighborhood health centers were subjected to

considerable criticism, especially from traditional medicine. These centers were often noted as having low productivity and substandard care as compared to the private sector, unwarranted federal intervention in the provision of health services, and high administrative costs. Although it is not possible to generalize across all the centers, some probably had high costs and low productivity. This circumstance was, at least, partially attributable to several factors, including their goals of employing and training local residents, occasionally inexperienced management, constraints imposed by the federal government, and local politics. Neighborhood health centers also had difficulty finding adequate facilities, had problems in physician recruitment, and experienced high staff turnover. There have been practical problems in designing family-oriented comprehensive care for clients used to receiving few services and only episodic care. Studies designed to measure the quality of care provided in these centers have generally concluded that the centers met acceptable standards and, in some instances, provided a higher quality of care than did local practitioners on average; succeeded in increasing access to care under difficult circumstances; and served as an interesting experimental model for the provision of ambulatory care (17).

Other community health centers that have been funded by the federal government included migrant health centers serving transient farm workers in agricultural areas and rural health centers. The National Health Service Corps supported practitioners who were placed in urban and rural areas with shortages of medical resources. Other innovations, such as mobile health vans in rural areas, have also been used to expand the scope of services. The Community Mental Health Center program was established to provide ambulatory mental health services in underserved areas. Community mental health centers were intended to provide outpatient services and emergency care and to work with other community agencies to foster action and concern for mental health.

In recent years community health centers have generally evolved into larger practices with multiple sources of support, including increasing reliance on patient fees and private donations. Many of these centers have become more businesslike in their operations. Yet most still face serious problems in attracting adequate financing, in attracting and retaining physicians, and in diversifying their patient mix, especially with regard to patients with insurance or the ability to pay for services on their own. Conflicts exist in some centers over the historical mission of serving the medically indigent versus the need for enhanced fiscal diversity and adopting a more business-oriented approach to operations.

Other Federal Government Programs

The federal government, in addition to supporting a variety of community-based health services organizations, directly operates many health facilities. The Veterans Administration includes the largest health services system under a unified management structure in the United States with more than 170 hospitals and clinics. This system provides needed care to millions of veterans throughout the nation. The military services also provide health care to millions of individuals in the armed forces and have developed extensive regionalized facilities throughout the world.

The government has a special responsibility for providing health care to a number of groups within the country. The Indian Health Service is charged with ensuring access to medical care on Indian reservations and in certain other locations. Although the difficulties of operating a largely rural system are immense, the Indian Health Service has succeeded in bringing modern medicine to many people.

Noninstitutional and Public Health Services

As noted in the introduction to this chapter, there are many ways in which ambulatory and community health services are provided. Although only the most prevalent types of provider and service are discussed here, each helps to meet the many health care needs of a community. The list is nearly endless, and a number of services warrant further discussion.

Home health services, discussed in more detail in Chapter 7, are provided by visiting nurse associations, proprietary companies, some hospitals, public health departments, and other agencies. These services allow people to remain in their homes and yet receive essential health services, thereby reducing costs and increasing the quality of life for many.

Rural health care has required unique and innovative solutions in many communities especially in the absence of adequate supplies of physicians and facilities. In rural Alaska, many towns are served by physicians and other professionals who regularly fly in to treat patients. Satellites are used to facilitate communications with specialists in urban medical centers since even ordinary communications in remote areas may be difficult. Rural health care in many areas remains a challenging test of the ingenuity and resourcefulness of the health services system and community residents.

Other community health services not discussed in detail here include—but are not limited to—school health services; prison health services; vision care; dental care provided by solo, group, and institutionally based practitioners; foot care from podiatrists; and drug dispensing from pharmacists, who often also extensively advise and educate consumers. Voluntary agencies also provide health care services such as cancer screening clinics and health education. Finally, many indigenous health practitioners offer their services in this country and abroad. These practitioners include chiropractors, "medicine men," naturopaths, and others. The supportive and sometimes curative role of these individuals is often underestimated.

Among the most important contributions to reductions in mortality and morbidity in the twentieth century have been such public health measures as the improvement of sanitation, ensurance of potable water supplies, and upgraded housing. In recent years there has also been an increased awareness of the need to control air and water pollution, to reduce exposure to carcinogens, and to improve and ensure the quality of the environment. The contribution of these efforts to health far exceeds, dollar for dollar, efforts to treat illness once it occurs (18). Their importance to ambulatory care is mentioned here, however, because public health agencies have responsibility for a remarkable range of relevant services.

And in this context it is important to emphasize that health care and ambulatory care services must also successfully interact with other aspects of our society. These other areas include social and welfare services, accident prevention in industry and in transportation, protection of the environment, improvement of food and water supplies, and even the general economic well-being of society since health is directly correlated to employment and income security.

Organization of Ambulatory Care Systems

The changing structure of the health services system has had tremendous implications for ambulatory care services. The increased movement toward integrated systems of care, such as managed care, has led ambulatory care services to assume a central role in the design and operation of many insurance and delivery programs. In addition, those paying for health services, including employers and insurers, have increasingly focused attention on the role that ambulatory care services can provide in improving the coordination and control of care as well as in reducing costs through the reduction of duplication and shifting of services to lower-cost settings.

Finally, those organizations constructing large-scale, integrated systems of care are continuing to seek existing ambulatory care structures, or are building new ones, as a means to complete their systems. In particular, insurers, hospitals, and other organizational entities are developing or purchasing ambulatory care resources such as medical practices, clinics, and other existing networks. Gov-

TABLE 5-12. Design Criteria for Ambulatory Care Systems

Criteria Topics	Criteria Requirements
Community criteria	
Availability and distribution of resources	Adequate number of facilities and practitioners
	Geographic dispersion
	Adequate transportation
Use of resources	Integration of community resources
	Effective referral network
	Appropriate mix of services
	Constrained excess capacity (few underused services)
Consumer criteria	
Convenience and satisfaction	Physical access assured
	Availability (hours of operation, after-hours coverage) ensured
	Efficient scheduling (appointments, follow ups, waiting times)
	Financial access (insurance coverage, reasonable prices)
	Caring providers
Quality services	Continuity and coordination of care (medical records, follow ups, etc.)
	Comprehensive services
	Technical quality of care ensured
	Multilingual staff and other special needs ensured
	Health education and instruction provided
Provider criteria	
Work environment	Pleasant and humane
	Appropriate roles for all providers
	Adequate income
	Productivity encouraged
	Personnel duties match skills and training
Patient care services	Efficient use of resources (personnel, capital, and technology)
	Use of most appropriate personnel
	Adequate support services available
System concerns	Technological progress readily adopted
	Development of owned or contractual systems of care
	Competitive delivery of services

ernment units, such as the military, have long recognized the key attributes of ambulatory care in coordinating and controlling the overall utilization of services and, then, the cost and quality of care. These trends are likely to continue.

There are many key design attributes of ambulatory care that are essential for both the effective operation of ambulatory services and for the full integration of these services into larger systems of care. Table 5-12 lists many of these criteria.

Ambulatory care is important in providing access to care, particularly within larger integrated systems. Access considerations include scope of services provided and hours of operation as well as distribution of resources throughout a geographic region populated by the target group of consumers. Physical access to facilities must also be assured, including such considerations as parking, access to public transportation where appropriate, and access to physical facilities for the handicapped.

The scope of services provided must respond to population needs. These needs differ depending on whether the population is prepaid or fee-for-service. How the population is served differs substantially in each situation. For both situations, however, decisions must be made concerning the type of care to be provided on an ambulatory versus an inpatient basis.

Marketing advantages can be achieved in the ambulatory care setting by recognizing the special needs of consumers, such as having multilingual staff available where appropriate. The friendliness of the staff and the attractiveness of the physical facilities can have dramatic effects on patient attitudes and satisfaction, with not only the ambulatory care provider but the larger system of care as well. Thus ambulatory care provides an influential marketing function in any system of care. Ambulatory care services generally also provide an opportunity for educating the consumer in terms of both health behaviors and "appropriate" use of the system. This educational role can contribute to cost containment by having patients help in "managing" their use.

Ambulatory care can provide a key role in the overall provision of coordinated and continuous care. By accepting the gatekeeper role of the primary-care physician, using medical records and other administrative tracking of patients, and avoiding duplication of services and unnecessary care, the ambulatory care setting can contribute handsomely to the overall effectiveness of all care provided to the patient. Physician payment incentives can facilitate an enhanced coordinating role for ambulatory care (19). Centralization of responsibility for patient care thus must be clearly assigned. Mechanisms for monitoring patient and provider behavior to ensure compliance with health system

operating guidelines are essential. There is also evidence that more effective continuity of care is associated with higher levels of patient compliance regarding medical regimens, which, in turn, may lead to better health outcomes and eventually lower subsequent utilization rates. Patient satisfaction is generally greater when continuity and coordination of care are achieved—both effective marketing and cost containment tools.

The quality of care should reflect not only adequate medical skills but also a caring attitude on the part of the provider (20). Consumers in ambulatory care are capable of detecting some aspects of the technical quality of care, but they are even more aware of provider and system attitudes and behavior. Responding to the consumer is increasingly important in the competitive environment (21,22).

The challenge in ambulatory care is to effectively shift from a traditionally reactive set of providers, attitudes, and operational approaches, to the proactive leadership role needed in today's competitive environment. Ambulatory care once meant a largely unaffiliated and unstructured set of small providers responding as business walked in the door. Now ambulatory care is a key vital element in the structuring of large-scale systems. These systems require financial and contractual arrangements with providers, and these ties are critical to all parties concerned.

The system's structure itself vitally affects the role of ambulatory care services; ambulatory care can, in turn, be vital to the success of the system. Whether services are organized on a fee-for-service, prepaid, or combined fee-for-service—prepaid basis, success in the provision of services mandates building the delivery of care around ambulatory care providers. In increasingly competitive markets, this is especially important (23). In managed care systems such as HMOs, fee-for-service systems, and particularly in aggressively contracted and discounted arrangements such as preferred provider organizations (PPOs), the ability to control providers and consumers—and hence costs—depends on structuring the system based on the controlling role of ambulatory care and performing needed services through ambulatory delivery vehicles where feasible, while also maintaining quality (24). Ideally, quality, access, and health status will attain acceptable minimum levels under any delivery system, and controls will be built in to monitor both (25,26).

From a health care delivery perspective, as opposed to the financial focus of other chapters, the demands on ambulatory care to provide a marketing, integrating, controlling, and organizing function are great. At the same time, services must retain the attributes of high quality, meeting specific patient needs, and offering a stimulating and rewarding environment for the providers as well. This is no small challenge.

References

1. Roemer, M. (1981). *Ambulatory health services in America.* Rockville, MD: Aspen Systems Corporation.
2. United Kingdom Ministry of Health. (1920). *Dawson report, interim report on the future provision of medical and allied services.* London, UK: His Majesty's Stationery Office.
3. Noble, J. (Ed.). (1976). *Primary care and the practice of medicine.* Boston: Little, Brown.
4. Roemer, M. (1975). From poor beginnings, the growth of primary care. *Hospitals. 49*(5). 38–43.
5. DeLozier, J. E., & Gagnon, R. O. (1991). *1989 summary: National Ambulatory Medical Survey. Advance data from vital and health statistics,* No. 203. Hyattsville, MD: National Center for Health Statistics.
6. Peterson, O. L., Andrews, L. P., Spain, R. S., et al. (1956). An analytical study of North Carolina general practice 1953–1954. *Journal of Medical Education. 31(Part2).* 1–165.
7. Petersdorf, R. (1975). Internal medicine and family practice, controversies, conflict and compromise. *New England Journal of Medicine. 293.* 326–332.
8. Mechanic, D. (1976). *The growth of bureaucratic medicine.* New York: Wiley.
9. Becker, M. & Maiman, L. (1975). Sociobehavioral determinants of compliance with health and medical recommendations. *Medical Care. 13.* 10–24.
10. Ross, A., Williams, S. J., & Schafer, E. L. (1991). *Ambulatory care management* (2nd ed.). Albany, NY: Delmar Publishers, Inc.
11. Rorem, R. (1931). *Private group clinics.* Chicago: University of Chicago Press.
12. Havlicek, P. L. (1990). *Medical groups in the U.S. 1990 edition. A survey of practice characteristics.* Chicago: American Medical Association.
13. Kimball, L. & Lorant, J. (1977). Physician productivity and returns to scale. *Health Services Research. 12.* 367–379.
14. Williams, S., Shortell, S. Dowling, W., et al. (1978). Hospital sponsored primary care group practice: A developing modality of care. *Health and Medical Care Services Review. 1.* 1–130.
15. Williams, S. J. (1983). Ambulatory care: Can hospitals compete? *Hospital and Health Services Administration. 28.* 22–34.
16. Burns, L. A. (1984). *Ambulatory surgery: Developing and managing successful programs.* Rockville, MD: Aspen Systems.
17. Morehead, M., Donaldson, R., & Seravalli, M. (1971). Comparison between OEO neighborhood health centers and other health care providers of ratings of quality of health care. *American Journal of Public Health. 61.* 1294–1306.
18. McKinlay, J., and McKinlay, S. (1977). The questionable contribution of medical measures to the decline of mortality in the United States in the twentieth century. *Milbank Memorial Fund Quarterly. 55.* 450–528.
19. Hsiao, W. C., Braun, P., Kelly, N. L., & Becker, E. R. (1988). Results, potential effects and implementation issues of the resource-based relative value scale. *Journal of the American Medical Association. 260*(28). 2429–2438.
20. Benson, D. S., Townes, M. D., & Townes, P. G., Jr. (1990). *A practical guide to developing effective quality assurance programs.* San Francisco: Jossey-Bass.
21. Cunningham, L. (1991). *The quality connection in health care: Integrating patient satisfaction and risk management.* San Francisco: Jossey-Bass.
22. Albrecht, K. G., & Bradford, L. J. (1990). *The service advantage: How to identify and fulfill customer needs.* Homewood, IL: Dow Jones-Irwin.

23. Iglehart, J. K. (1984). The twin cities' medical marketplace. *New England Journal of Medicine. 311.* 1505–1510.

24. Manning, W. G.; Leibowitz, A., Goldberg, G., et al. (1984). A controlled trial of the effect of a prepaid group practice on use of services. *New England Journal of Medicine. 310.* 1505–1510.

25. Ware, J. E., Jr., Brook, R. H., Rogers, W. H., Keeler, E. B., et al. (1986, May 3). Comparison of health outcomes at a health maintenance organization with those of fee-for-service care. *Lancet. 1*(8488). 1017–1022.

26. Cunningham, F. C., & Williamson, J. W. (1980). How does the quality of health care in HMOs compare to that in other settings? An analytic literature review: 1958 10 1979. *Group Health Journal. 1.* 4–25.

Chapter 6

The Hospital

Claudia L. Haglund
William L. Dowling

The modern hospital is the key resource and organizational hub of the American health care system, central to the delivery of patient care, the training of health personnel, and the conduct and dissemination of health-related research. The hospital represents the community's collective investment in health care resources, presumably available for the benefit of all, and it is often the first place people think of when they need medical care. Since the turn of the century, hospitals, the indispensable workshop of the physician, have become even more the economic and professional heart of medical practice as the accelerating pace of advances in medical knowledge and technology continues. In recent years, hospitals have expanded beyond their inpatient role in an effort to become comprehensive, vertically integrated community health systems. As highly advanced, scientific institutions, hospitals manifest the complexity and detached efficiency of a clinical laboratory. As human service organizations, they are charged with the emotions of life and death of triumphs and tragedies. Hospitals are frequently the caregivers of last resort for many of the nation's poor who have nowhere else to turn for health care.

Hospitals are also big business. Collectively, they are among the largest industries in the United States in terms of the number of people they employ. By far the largest part of the health care system, hospitals employ about three-fourths of all health care personnel and consume 38 percent of the nation's health expenditures. About 53 percent of all federal health expenditures and about 40 percent of all state and local government health expenditures are for hospital care (1).

It is ironic that the magnitude of the hospital sector and the central role hospitals play in the delivery of health services now place hospitals at the root of many of the health care system's most pressing problems—cost increases, duplication of services, bed surpluses, overemphasis on specialized services versus primary care, depersonalization of care, and so forth. Furthermore, as community or quasi-public institutions heavily dependent on public dollars, hospitals are open systems, subject to influence from outside forces and, therefore, susceptible to the efforts of community groups, external agencies, business coalitions, and insurance carriers to use them as instruments of social change and health system reform (2).

The hospital system is a mix of public and private for-profit and not-for-profit institutions. Hospitals range from small institutions in less-populated communities and isolated rural areas providing basic medical care to large regional referral centers providing a comprehensive range of sophisticated, highly specialized services. Many hospitals have expanded their roles to include an array of outpatient services, including primary-care clinics, home care, health promotion, and long-term care services. Other hospitals have reorganized to develop for-profit enterprises or to sponsor managed-care systems.

The purpose of this chapter is to characterize the hospital system in the United States, emphasizing major issues and trends. Because the character of the modern hospital reflects its past, this chapter begins with a discussion of the historical development of hospitals. The second section describes the hospital system as it exists today. The third section describes the internal organization of hospitals. The final section discusses a number of major issues now confronting hospitals. It should be noted that while the discussion of hospitals in this chapter focuses primarily on their inpatient role, hospitals now play an increasingly important role in the provision of outpatient care and are evolving toward a new role as providers of a comprehensive and integrated continuum of health services (3). To illustrate, outpatient services, virtually nonexistent until the 1960s, today claim about 22 percent of total hospital revenue, and if the present trend continues, will exceed inpatient revenue by the year 2003 (4). Today, fully 85 percent of the nation's community hospitals have organized outpatient departments, 94 percent have emergency departments, 95 percent have ambulatory surgery units, 77 percent have health promotion programs, and 36 percent offer home health services (5).

Historical Development of Hospitals

The history of hospitals in this country (figure 6-1) can be traced back to the almshouses and pesthouses that existed in some form in almost all cities of moderate size by the mid–1700s (6,7). Almshouses, also called *poorhouses* or *workhouses*, were established by city governments to provide food and shelter for the homeless poor, including many aged, chronically ill, disabled, mentally ill, and orphaned people. Medical care was a secondary function of the poorhouse; however, in some facilities, those who became ill were isolated in infirmaries where care, such as it was before the advent of modern medicine, was provided, typically by other residents. Not until the late 1800s did the infirmaries or hospital departments of city poorhouses break away to become medical care institutions on their own—the first public hospitals.

Pesthouses were operated by local governments as isolation or quarantine stations in seaports where it was necessary to isolate people who contracted contagious diseases aboard ship. During epidemics, these institutions were used to isolate victims of cholera, smallpox, typhus, and yellow fever. Their primary purpose was to control the spread of infectious diseases by removing infected individuals from the community. As in almshouses, medical care was a secondary function—in this case, secondary to protecting the community from outbreaks of contagious disease. Pesthouses were often established during epidemics and discontinued or closed down when the threat of disease subsided. These institutions were the predecessors of the contagious disease and tuberculosis hospitals that later emerged.

Almshouses and pesthouses were maintained for the poor and the homeless and were avoided by everyone else. These institutions were dismal places: crowded, unsanitary, and poorly heated and ventilated. Nutrition was often inadequate, nursing care incompetent, and separation of different types of patients minimal. The contagious, the disabled, the dying, and the mentally ill were often crowded

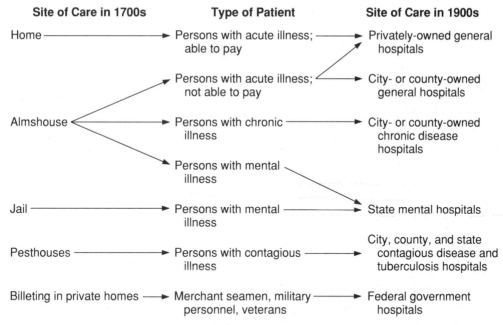

Figure 6-1. Evolution of institutional care sites.

together. Cross-infection was rampant and mortality high. All those who could be were cared for at home or in the homes of neighbors.

The first community-owned or voluntary hospitals in this country were established in the late 1700s and early 1800s, often at the urging of influential physicians trained in Europe who needed facilities to practice obstetrics and surgery in the manner in which they had been taught, and also to provide preceptor-type instruction for medical students. These early hospitals depended on philanthropy, and contributions were solicited from both private citizens and the local government. Voluntary hospitals generally preceded both religious and public hospitals in the United States, representing a departure from patterns in England and Europe. Voluntary hospitals admitted both indigent and paying patients. For example, in its first year of operation (1751), the Pennsylvania Hospital admitted 24 paying patients and 40 poor patients. These hospitals were supported by community contributions and philanthropy, rather than by a church or the state. Except in the largest cities, where the concentration of poor was too great, the early voluntary hospitals cared on a charitable basis for people in their communities who were unable to pay, drawing on philanthropy and donations of time by members of the medical staff (6,8).

The first hospitals of this type were the Pennsylvania Hospital, Philadelphia, 1751; New York Hospital, New York City, 1773; Massachusetts General Hospital, Boston, 1816; and New Haven Hospital, New Haven, Connecticut, 1826. Additional voluntary hospitals were established in Savannah, Georgia, in 1830; Lowell, Massachusetts, in 1836; and Raleigh, North Carolina, in 1839. Voluntary hospitals cared for patients with acute illnesses and injuries but did not admit persons with contagious diseases or mental illness. Isolation of these unfortunates from the rest of the community was seen as a government responsibility. Therefore, during the same period, a number of city, county, and state mental hospitals were established. These included hospitals in Williamsburg, Virginia, 1773; Lexington, Kentucky, 1817; Columbia, South Carolina, 1829; Worcester, Massachusetts, 1832; Augusta, Maine, 1834; Brooklyn, New York, 1838; and Boston, Massachusetts, 1839.

Although voluntary hospitals provided better accommodations and care for the sick than had the poorhouses that preceded them, the efficacy of care improved little, and it was not until the late 1800s that hospitals became accepted by persons of all economic strata as the best setting for the care of serious illness and injury. In 1873, there were only 178 hospitals with 35,604 beds in the United States. By 1909, the number of hospitals had increased to 4,359, with 421,065 beds, and by 1929, to 6,665 hospitals with 907,133 beds. This rapid growth was brought about by advances in medical science that rapidly transformed the hospital's role from a custodial institution in which to isolate and shelter the poor to a curative institution in which communities concentrated their health care resources in support of the practicing physician for the benefit of all (8,9). Starr (10) has characterized this redefinition of the hospital as a transformation from a social welfare facility to an institution of medical science, from a charitable organization to a business, and from an orientation toward patrons and the poor to a focus on professionals and patients.

Forces Affecting the Development of Hospitals

Six major developments in health care were particularly significant in transforming hospitals into the institutions of today: advances in medical science increased the efficacy and safety of hospitals; the development of technological sophistication and specialization necessitated the institutionalization of medical care; the development of professional nursing brought about more humane treatment of patients; advances in medical education added teaching and research to the hospital's role; the

health insurance industry grew; and the role of government increased (6,8,10,11,12).

Advances in Medical Science

Most notable in terms of their impact on hospitals were the discovery of anesthesia and the rapid advances in surgery that followed, and the development of the germ theory of disease and the subsequent discovery of antiseptic and sterilization techniques. By the early 1800s, enough was known about anatomy and physiology that surgeons were able to perform a variety of fairly complex surgical procedures; however, the inability to deaden pain meant that surgery had to be carried out with extreme speed. In addition, infection from surgery was common. Ether was first used as an anesthetic in surgery by Long in 1842 and then by Morton in 1846, and its use then spread rapidly. Great advances in the efficacy of surgery followed.

Before the formulation of the germ theory of disease, a few scientists, most notably Holmes in the United States and Semmelweis in Vienna, had observed and reported that fever, infection, and mortality could be reduced through cleanliness. Both concluded that childbed fever, which was the cause of high maternal mortality, was an infection transmitted by physicians, midwives, and medical students to women in labor. In 1861, Pasteur proved that bacteria were living, reproducing microorganisms that could be carried by air or on clothing and hands. It became clear that germs were the cause rather than the result of infection and could be destroyed by chemicals and heat. Lister built on Pasteur's work and, in 1867, introduced carbolic acid spray in operating rooms as an antiseptic to keep air and incisions clean. In 1886, steam sterilization was introduced, providing a means of freeing medical equipment from microorganisms. Surgical infection rates fell. Advances in surgery led to the need for skilled preoperative and postoperative care and operating room facilities, which could be provided only in hospitals. By 1900, 40 percent of all hospitalizations were for surgery.

Development of Specialized Technology

By the late 1800s, medical technology began to proliferate. The first hospital laboratory opened in 1889, and X-ray films were first used for diagnosis in 1896. These developments greatly increased the diagnostic effectiveness of hospitals. The discovery of blood types in 1901 made blood transfusions safe; the electrocardiogram (EKG) was first used in 1903 and the electroencephalogram (EEG) in 1929. In addition to increasing the efficiency of medical care, these advances in technology affected the site and the organization of care. Since the tools of the new technology could no longer be carried around in the physician's black bag, hospitals became the central resource where the equipment, facilities, and personnel required by modern medicine were housed. In addition, since one person could no longer be competent in all areas of medical practice, specialization began to occur within medicine, and new professional and technical occupations began to emerge. Again, the hospital became the place where physicians and support personnel came together to provide patient care.

Development of Professional Nursing

Humane treatment of patients awaited the development of professional nursing. Before the late 1800s, humane nursing care was provided primarily by Catholic sisters and Protestant deaconesses, who were dedicated to caring for patients. Some religious orders established their own hospitals, and occasionally they were called on by city officials to provide nursing services in public institutions. Almshouses used untrained female residents to provide nursing care, and hospitals relied on poorly paid, unskilled labor.

The transformation of nursing into a profession is credited to Florence Nightingale, who completed four months of nurses' training in a deaconess school in Germany. In 1854, Nightingale and 38 nurses were sent by the British government to the Crimea to take charge of nursing care for wounded soldiers. The nurses found conditions deplorable and instituted cleanliness and sanitation, dietary reforms, simple but humane care, discipline, and organization. As a result, mortality dropped dramatically. On her return to England, Nightingale wrote of her experiences in the Crimea and on the contributions of sanitation to the recovery of wounded and ill patients. In 1860, she founded the Nightingale School for Nursing in England.

In the United States, President Abraham Lincoln called on Catholic religious communities to provide nursing care for the wounded during the Civil War, but more nurses were needed. Dorothea Dix was appointed Superintendent of Nursing for the Union Army. She began a recruitment program and encouraged a one-month hospital training program for new nurses. By the end of the war, there were 2,000 lay nurses in the United States. The first permanent schools of nursing were established at Bellevue Hospital, New Haven Hospital, and Massachusetts General Hospital in 1873. Although there was some initial reluctance on the part of hospital administrators and trustees to establish nursing schools, the benefits of good nursing soon became apparent. In addition, student nurses provided better care and were less expensive than the untrained women previously employed to do this work. By 1883, there were 22 nursing schools and 600 graduates; by 1898, these totals had grown to 400 schools with 10,000 graduates.

Advances in nursing contributed to the growth of hospitals in two ways: 1) increased efficacy of treatment, cleanliness, nutritious diets, and formal treatment routines all contributed to patient recovery; and 2) considerate, skilled patient care made hospitals acceptable to all people, not just the poor. The public's fear of hospitals began to give way to an attitude of confidence and respect.

Advances in Medical Education

Changes in medical education brought about by the Flexner report (13) in 1910 had a major impact on the development of hospitals. Before 1900, there was a great variation in the nature and quality of medical education. There were no standards of academic training for physicians. Most medical schools were proprietary and were not connected with universities. They were dominated by influential practitioners, and most instruction was through didactic (often unscientific) lectures. Apprenticeship practices varied greatly. There was little clinical or laboratory instruction and little research.

The Flexner report led to changes in the content and methods of instruction to emphasize the scientific basis of medicine. The standards of education established by the Flexner report led to changes in the content and methods of instruction to emphasize the scientific basis of medicine. The standards of education established by the Flexner report were widely accepted by both the profession and the public; as a result, schools that did not meet the standards were forced to close. State laws were established requiring graduation from a medical school accredited by the American Medical Association as the basis for a license to practice medicine. A four-year course of study at a medical school based in a university became standard, as did clinical training in the wards of a hospital.

These changes expanded the role of the hospital to include education and research as well as patient care. The hospital's role in education became even more prominent as specialization in medicine led to a proliferation of internships and residencies in the 1920s and 1930s. The requirements of medical education necessitated the expansion of hospital facilities and services and the addition of equipment and personnel. Hospitals were called on to assume a greater responsibility for coordinating and organizing these resources. Quality of care improved through advances in medical education, especially for patients with complex and serious illnesses. On the other hand, specialization led to a fragmentation of care among different physician specialists and ancillary personnel and a lack of interest in chronic, routine, and other "uninteresting" medical conditions.

Thus the growth of hospitals in the United States

was a direct result of advances in medical science that made hospitals effective and safe. These advances, particularly the discovery of sulfa drugs in the mid–1930s and antibiotics in the mid–1940s, changed the prevalent causes of death from acute, infectious diseases to the diseases of old age, particularly heart disease, cancer, and stroke. Hospitals have not been quick to respond to the chronic health care problems of an aging population. There resources continue to be concentrated on curable, short-term illnesses that respond quickly to medical treatment, rather than on chronic, long-term illnesses that must be managed over long periods of time. Hospitals are just now beginning to expand their role to include extended or skilled nursing care units, inpatient or outpatient rehabilitation programs, day care, home care, and other nontraditional services (14).

Growth of Health Insurance

Another factor that has significantly affected the development of hospitals is the growth of the health insurance industry. Private insurance for hospital care grew rapidly, especially between 1940 and 1960, increasing both the proportion of the population with insurance and the adequacy and scope of coverage. Today, the out-of-pocket cost of hospital care at the time of use is relatively modest for most people, because most of the bill is covered by some third-party purchaser—either government or private health insurance.

A variety of factors led to the growth of hospital insurance. From the consumer's perspective, of course, a hospital stay is sufficiently expensive to warrant the purchase of insurance protection. The hospital industry's interest in insurance began with the Great Depression of the 1930s, when the number of patients who could not pay their bill increased markedly and hospital use declined. The financial solvency of many hospitals was threatened, and the number of hospitals dropped from 6,852 in 1928 to 6,189 in 1937. Furthermore, a study of nonprofit hospitals in 1935 revealed that total income was 3 percent less than total expenses. As a result, acting through the American Hospital Association, hospitals took the initiative in actively encouraging the development of hospital insurance plans, primarily Blue Cross (11, 15).

The growth of health insurance has had a substantial impact on hospitals. First, ensuring the financial stability of hospitals, insurance subsequently provided the flow of funds that made possible the great expansion of facilities and services and the prompt implementation of new medical technology that have characterized the hospital industry since the end of World War II. Insurance also contributed to the increased demand for health services. Historically, hospital services have been better covered by insurance than services provided outside the hospital, so patients have been reluctant to substitute less expensive out-of-hospital services. This attitude resulted in a bias toward hospital use versus the use of ambulatory care services, home care programs, or nursing care facilities as sources of care and a general overuse of expensive hospital services (16). In recent years, however, concern over the rising costs of hospital care and inappropriate hospital admissions has reversed this trend. Insurance carriers are now actively promoting nonhospital alternatives for medical care and stringent control over inpatient admissions. The belief that hospital admissions are unwarranted in many instances was underscored in a Rand Corporation study based on a sample of hospital records from 1974 to 1982. The study concluded that 23 percent of the admissions studied were inappropriate and another 17 percent could have been avoided through the use of ambulatory surgery (17).

Another problem in the hospital industry can be traced at least partially to cost-based reimbursement, the method of payment used until recently, by Medicare, Medicaid, and most Blue Cross plans. Cost reimbursement does not provide hospitals with an incentive to contain costs. The result has been inefficiency, duplication of services, and overbuilding. To stem rising hospital costs, public and private payors have experimented in recent years with a number of regulatory and competitive approaches to cost containment (18). Regulatory approaches to cost containment—most notably certificate-of-need (CON) review for new hospital equipment, services, and beds—and hospital rate regulation, were initiated in the 1970s. As hospital costs continued to rise, however, economists, business coalitions, and policy makers began suggesting that true market competition would provide greater incentives for controlling health care spending (19). As a result, the 1980s witnessed a weakening of regulatory approaches to hospital cost containment and a growing emphasis on competition. One hallmark of the competitive model is the centrality of the buying power of major purchasers of hospital care such as Blue Cross, Medicare, and Medicaid. These purchasers have taken swift action to replace payment systems based on retrospective costs with one based on competitive prices and prospective rates.

A major step toward the introduction of market power occurred when the Tax Equity and Fiscal Responsibility Act of 1982 (PL 97-248) converted Medicare reimbursement to a prospective per case system based on diagnosis-related groups (DRGs). In turn, several states revised their Medicaid programs and now pay hospitals on a prospective basis. In addition, managed care programs, included health maintenance organizations (HMOs) and preferred provider organizations (PPOs), which emphasize strict utilization controls over hospital admissions, began to proliferate in the private health insurance sector. Hospitals now find themselves competing on the basis of price and discount for patients covered by health insurance plans. While cost reimbursement is widely blamed as the root cause of runaway hospital costs, it nevertheless has allowed hospitals to keep up to date with advances in medical technology and demands from their communities and physicians for access to a broad range of services. A key public policy issue yet unresolved is how to guarantee the poor and disadvantaged a decent standard of care in a system driven by competitive forces.

Role of Government

Government's role in the hospital industry has changed substantially in both form and level. During colonial times, government involvement was mainly at the local level through ownership of almshouses and pesthouses and grants to help construct and support voluntary hospitals. State government limited its role to running hospitals for merchant seamen, military personnel, and veterans. Gradually, the forms of involvement have multiplied and the balance has shifted to the federal level.

The initial thrust of federal involvement began in 1935, with federal categorical grants-in-aid to state and local governments to assist in the establishment of traditional public health programs: public health departments; communicable disease programs; maternal and child health programs; and public assistance for specific groups such as crippled children, the aged, the blind, the disabled, and poor families with dependent children. These programs were part of the general social reform movement that developed during the Depression with the recognition that state and local government and voluntary efforts were not sufficient to meet social needs.

Direct federal involvement in the hospital industry began in 1946 with the Hill-Burton (Hospital Survey and Construction) Act. Few hospitals had been constructed during the Depression and World War II, and by the end of the war, a severe shortage of hospitals existed. The Hill-Burton program was enacted to help states and communities plan for and construct hospitals and other health facilities by providing federal grants on a matching basis to supplement funds raised at the community level. Although the initial emphasis of the program was to provide funds for the construction of new hospitals, priorities changed over time from construction to modernization and from inpatient to outpatient facilities. Funds were available through the program for the construction of nursing homes as well.

The Hill-Burton program assisted in the construction of nearly 40 percent of the beds in the nation's short-term general hospitals and was the greatest single factor in the increase in the nation's bed supply during the 1950s and 1960s. Another positive impact of the program is that hospital facilities are more evenly distributed across rural and urban areas and high- and low-income states than they would have been without the program. However, the program also contributed to the overbuilding of hospitals and to the preponderance of small rural hospitals existing today.

From assisting with the financing of hospital construction, the federal government's involvement in the hospital industry has expanded to financing the provision of care and regulating the construction, operation, and use of hospitals. Fifty-three percent of hospital expenditures are now made by government programs, primarily Medicare and Medicaid, which puts the federal government in a position to exercise a great amount of control over the operations of hospitals.

Characteristics of the Hospital System

The hospital industry is complex and diverse and, therefore, difficult to describe simply. Hospitals can be classified generally in one of three ways: according to length of stay, predominant type of service provided, and ownership. In terms of length of stay, the most common type of hospital is the short-stay or short-term hospital, in which most patients suffer from acute conditions requiring hospital stays of less than 30 days. The average length of stay in short-term hospitals is about seven days and has declined significantly over the last 10 years. In long-term hospitals, most of which are chronic disease, psychiatric, or tuberculosis hospitals, the average length of stay ranges from three to six months (5).

The second method of classification is by type of service. Predominant is the general hospital, offering a wide range of medical, surgical, obstetric, and pediatric services. Specialty hospitals, on the other hand, provide care for a specific disease or population group. Examples of specialty hospitals are children's hospitals, maternity hospitals, chronic disease hospitals, psychiatric hospitals, and tuberculosis hospitals. During the first part of the 20th century, a number of specialty hospitals were established as a result of philanthropists responding to the initiative of prestigious physician specialists who wanted to develop their own hospitals. Because of financial difficulties and advances in medical science that make general hospitals more appropriate and efficient, specialty hospitals are less common today. Most have either closed down or converted to general hospitals.

The third method of classifying hospitals is according to form of ownership: government or public ownership, private for-profit (proprietary) ownership, and private nonprofit (religious or voluntary) ownership.

Public Hospitals

Public hospitals are owned by agencies of federal, state, or local government. Federally owned hospitals are maintained primarily for special groups of federal beneficiaries: Native Americans, merchant seamen, military personnel, and veterans. State governments have generally limited themselves to the operation of mental and tuberculosis hospitals, reflecting government's early role of protecting the healthy by isolating the mentally ill and persons with contagious diseases from the rest of society. Most local government hospitals are short-term general hospitals. These institutions constitute 27 percent of the nation's short-term hospitals and accommodate 17 percent of all admissions and 20 percent of all outpatient visits to short-term hospitals (table 6-1). Local government hospitals can be divided into two types. The first is city, county, or hospital district institutions, mostly small or moderate in bed size, with medical staffs consisting of private physicians and serving both indigent and paying patients. These hospitals tend to be located in small cities and towns. Their costs are met primarily through third-party reimbursement, and they receive little tax support. For all practical purposes, they function the same as com-

munity-owned hospitals. The second type is large city or county hospitals in major urban areas. These hospitals serve mostly the poor, near poor, and minorities. They are generally staffed by salaried physicians, mostly residents. Most are affiliated with medical schools. Their costs usually exceed their patient revenues, and so their deficits must be made up through tax subsidies.

Large urban public hospitals play an important role in the health care system. They are the place of last resort for the poor, both because they care for all patients regardless of ability to pay and because they provide services that private hospitals cannot finance or do not wish to offer: burn and trauma care, alcohol and drug abuse treatment, psychiatric services, care for persons with chronic and communicable diseases, treatment of persons with AIDS, abortion and family planning services, and so forth. They are located in areas where health resources, especially private physicians, are in short supply, and their outpatient departments are often the only accessible source of ambulatory care, for many inner-city residents. Large urban public hospitals average about 13 outpatient visits per inpatient admission, compared to nine outpatient visits per admission in privately owned hospitals with more than 500 beds (5). In addition, these large public hospitals play a major role in medical education; most are affiliated with a medical school and offer residency training programs. More than half of all practicing physicians receive at least some of their training in public hospitals.

It was thought that enactment of Medicare and Medicaid would greatly reduce the demand on public hospitals by giving the aged and the poor the means to purchase care from other sources. The expected exodus did not occur, however, probably because the gatekeepers of the community hospitals, private practitioners, are in short supply in inner-city areas. In addition, some of those who are located close enough to be accessible limited the number of welfare patients they would accept. Cultural and social barriers also discouraged the poor from approaching community hospitals. As a result, inpatient and outpatient

TABLE 6-1. Hospitals, Beds, Admissions, and Outpatient Visits by Ownership and Type of Service, 1990

	Hospitals		Beds		Admissions		Outpatient Visits	
	Number	Percent	Number	Percent	Number	Percent	Number	Percent
Total—all hospitals	6,595	100	1,200,056	100	33,750,172	100	365,803,133	100
Federal	337	5	98,255	8	1,759,058	5	58,527,091	16
Nonfederal								
Psychiatric	739	11	148,980	12	719,875	2	5,379,365	1
Tuberculosis	4	<1	470	<1	1,849	<1	16,863	<1
Long-term	131	2	24,991	3	88,344	<1	1,551,052	<1
Short-term	5,384	81	927,360	76	31,181,046	92	301,328,762	82
Short-term hospitals								
Nongovernmental								
Not-for-profit	3,191	59	656,755	71	22,878,443	73	221,073,380	73
Investor-owned, for-profit	749	14	101,377	11	3,066,198	10	20,109,508	7
State and local governmental	1,444	27	169,228	18	5,236,405	17	60,145,874	20

SOURCE: *Hospital statistics*. (1991). Chicago: American Hospital Association.

use of public hospitals dipped only slightly in 1967, the first full year of operation of both Medicare and Medicaid, and then continued a steady upward climb. A disproportionate share of charity care, nearly 90 percent, is provided by public hospitals (20).

Given the increasing demand that large urban public hospitals are called on to satisfy, their problems are great. Characteristically, these hospitals are old and outmoded. They tend to be underequipped, underfinanced, and understaffed. They have difficulty attracting physicians and rely heavily on interns, residents, and foreign-trained physicians. Their administration is constrained by the bureaucratic red tape and rigidity of city or county government. Public hospitals have responded to these difficulties in a variety of ways. Most are affiliated with medical schools to attract faculty as supervisory physicians and to facilitate the recruitment of residents. In some areas, a special agency or commission has been created to run the public hospital in order to buffer it from government bureaucracy. In some cases, the agency is com-

pletely separate from city or county government but is empowered by enabling legislation to borrow, issue bonds, and tax, much like a school district. In other instances, public hospitals have entered into contract management agreements with private organizations, most notably investor-owned hospital systems. A number of public hospitals are attempting to improve their position by becoming the source of highly specialized tertiary services such as regional trauma services, burn care, neonatal intensive care, or kidney dialysis. Other aspects of this strategy include opening the medical staff to private physicians, adding amenities, and improving facilities to encourage physicians to bring their private patients to the public hospital, at least for more specialized services.

For-Profit Hospitals

For-profit, investor-owned, or proprietary hospitals are operated for the financial benefit of the individual, partnership, or corporation that owns the institution. Around the turn of the century, more than

TABLE 6-2. Characteristics of Proprietary Short-Term Hospitals in the United States, Selected Years

Year	Number of Hospitals	Number of Beds	Admissions
1950	1218	42,000	1,661,000
1960	856	37,000	1,550,000
1970	769	53,000	2,031,000
1975	775	73,000	2,646,000
1980	730	87,000	3,165,000
1985	805	104,000	3,242,000
1990	749	101,377	3,066,198

SOURCE: *Hospital statistics.* (1991). Chicago: American Hospital Association.

one-half of the nation's hospitals were proprietary. Most of these hospitals had been established by one or a small group of physicians who wanted a place to hospitalize their own patients, and most were quite small (21). Gradually, these institutions were closed or sold to community organizations. The number of proprietary hospitals declined steadily through 1972, although the number of beds in proprietary hospitals began to increase around 1960 as the better-situated proprietary hospitals expanded to accommodate population increases and as new proprietary hospitals, typically larger than those that were closing, were built (table 6-2). As of 1985, proprietary hospitals comprised 14 percent of the nation's short-term hospitals, with 10 percent of the beds and 6 percent of the outpatient visits (table 6-1) (5).

The most significant trend over the past few years is not the number of proprietary hospitals per se but the building or acquisition of a substantial number of hospitals by large, investor-owned corporations to form multiunit, for-profit hospital systems. In 1990 investor-owned corporations owned or leased about 824 hospitals totaling 107,958 beds. These corporations manage another 311 hospitals, totaling 30,000 beds (22). After several years of spectacular increases, the rate of growth for investor-owned hospital chains has slowed. Hospitals owned, leased, or managed by for-profit firms increased by 72 percent between 1980 and 1985, but fell by 6 percent between 1985 and 1990.

Investor-owned hospital corporations claim that they are able to earn a profit by operating their hospitals more efficiently than nonprofit hospitals. They point to the availability of management specialists, the application of modern management techniques, cost savings in construction and maintenance, economies of scale, and group purchasing as the key factors enabling them to control costs sufficiently to make a profit and pay taxes without compromising quality. Investor-owned hospital systems have also been able to respond promptly to population shifts because of their ability to raise capital quickly. Critics of for-profit hospitals claim that they undermine traditional medical values and that their profits are attributable to the practice of "cream skimming"—admitting only patients with less serious medical conditions and patients who are able to pay the full costs of their hospitalization (23,24). By not admitting unsured patients, for-profit hospitals can avoid bad debts, which may run as high as 10 percent of total patient charges in nonprofit and public hospitals in certain locations. By not admitting seriously ill patients, for-profit hospitals can avoid providing expensive or unprofitable services. The quality of care in for-profit hospitals has also been criticized. The lower employee:bed ratio in these hospitals, for example, is pointed to as an indicator of lower quality and less sophisticated services rather than more efficient management. Another criticism is that even if for-profit hospitals are more efficient, their costs savings are not passed on to patients.

There is a growing body of research that focuses on the comparative analysis of for-profit and nonprofit hospitals. One study (25) that compared economic performance between 80 matched pairs of nonprofit and investor-owned chain hospitals concluded that total charges adjusted for case mix and net revenues per case were significantly higher in investor-owned chain hospitals, primarily as a result of higher charges for ancillary services. Investor-owned hospitals were found to be more profitable but incurred higher administrative costs; they also had fewer employees per occupied bed but paid higher salaries. The authors concluded that investor-owned chain hospitals realized greater profits primarily through more aggressive pricing and not through greater efficiencies. These results concur with the findings of earlier studies (26,27), but by no means reflect universal opinions within the health care industry. By contrast, another report (28) asserts that for-profit hospitals provide greater worth to society because they require virtually no social investment to keep them afloat, are more efficient, reinvest earnings in newer plants and equipment, and offer an equally broad range of services to patients, including the medically indigent.

Furthermore, it has been noted that the behavior of many nonprofit hospitals barely can be distinguished from that of their investor-owned competitors. As a result, the tax-exempt status of nonprofit hospitals may be challenged in the future (29). It is true that many nonprofit hospitals have adopted new legal structures that allow them to operate for-profit subsidiary corporations. Nonprofit hospitals are also evaluating and implementing numerous management techniques from the private sector.

In all fairness, the cream skimming that does occur in for-profit hospitals is likely to be attributed more to the location of the for-profit hospitals (e.g., in rapidly growing suburban areas) than to the actual turning away of patients who cannot pay. The refusal to admit patients with complex conditions requiring sophisticated services and the lack of high-cost, low-use specialized technology are cited by for-profit hospitals as examples of the methods they use to avoid duplication by referring outpatients requiring costly services—a longtime goal of those who would reform the health care system. It seems appropriate to conclude that the implications of the recent growth of investor-owned hospitals are still unclear. The current debate about for-profit health care is fueled as much by values as by evidence. Perhaps the greatest challenge is to determine how for-profit and nonprofit hospitals can effectively and successfully coexist in a future that holds challenges for both of them. It is likely, however, that the increasingly competitive health care environment will make the relationship between the two quite strained.

Nonprofit Hospitals

Fifty-nine percent of the nation's short-term hospitals are nonprofit or voluntary institutions owned and operated by community associations or religious organizations. These hospitals accommodate more than two-thirds of all short-term hospital admissions and outpatient visits (table 6-1).

Community Hospitals

Taken together, nonfederal short-term hospitals, whether for-profit, nonprofit, or public, are commonly referred to as "community hospitals" because they are typically available to the entire community and meet most of the public's needs for hospital services. Community hospitals represent more than 80 percent of the nation's hospitals. They provide care for more than 90 percent of all patients admitted to hospitals each year and accommodate over 80 percent of all outpatient visits. In 1990 there were 5,384 short-term community hospitals with 927,360 beds (table 6-1). The average length of stay in these hospitals is 7.1 days, down from 8.4 days in 1967, shortly after Medicare and Medicaid went into effect. The steady decline in length of stay since then is due to changing styles of medical practice, the emphasis placed on utilization review in hospitals, and the shift to prospective per case reimbursement by Medicare and other payors.

The major role of community hospitals is to provide short-term inpatient care for patients with acute illnesses and injuries. However, their outpatient role has been growing in importance and accounted for over 20 percent of gross hospital revenues in 1990. In that year there were 86,692,505 emergency room visits and 214,636,259 outpatient department visits and ancillary service visits by patients referred to departments such as laboratory, X-ray, or physical therapy for diagnostic or therapeutic procedures. Taken together, these types of outpatient visit totaled 301,328,762 or 9.7 outpatient visits for every inpatient admission and represented a 38 percent increase over 1985 (5).

Community hospitals are experiencing pressures to expand their roles even more to become true community health systems (30). The fundamental rationale is that these hospitals represent their community's collective investment in health resources, assembled in one place and financially supported by all. Hence, access to these resources should not be limited to patients who happen to need inpatient hospitalization. More recently, diversification has also been undertaken for competitive and economic reasons.

Community hospitals are seeking to play a more central and substantial role in planning and coordinating the entire range of community health services. For a variety of reasons in the past, including a lack of physician interest, health insurance coverage biases, poor reimbursement for out-of-hospital services, the small size of the average community hospital, and resistance by nursing homes and other community health agencies to hospital encroachment, hospitals were slow to expand their roles. Now, however, the traditional role of the hospital as provider of inpatient care is changing rapidly. Many hospitals, especially the larger institutions, have added services in areas such as ambulatory care, which indicate a movement in the direction of a broadening role (table 6-3). It appears that the persistent rise in the pub-

lic's use of community hospitals has finally peaked, motivating many hospitals to search for new diversified services they might offer. Perhaps this development, more than the underlying rationale, will finally give impetus to the several-decades-old concept of the hospital as a community health center.

Forty-five percent of all community hospitals have fewer than 100 beds; in 1990 the average size was 172 beds (5). Small hospitals tend to care for less seriously ill patients than do larger hospitals. Their average length of stay is shorter and their care less intensive and less specialized. Small hospitals cannot support as broad a range of services as can larger hospitals and find it difficult to keep abreast with developments in medical technology. They also cannot support the range of management specialists found in larger hospitals. Several hundred smaller hospitals have closed since the early 1970s. During the ten-year period between 1980 and 1990, a total of 446 community hospitals with 61,000 beds closed in the United States. (5). Of these, 415 were rural hospitals. An even greater number of small community hospitals have become part of multiunit hospital systems. In fact, the rapid growth of multihospital systems, both for-profit and nonprofit, is one of the most significant trends in the hospital field today.

Multihospital Systems

A total of 306 nonfederal multihospital systems, defined as corporations that own, lease, or manage two or more acute care hospitals, accounted for 2,571, or 48 percent, of the nation's community hospitals in 1990 (22). These system hospitals contain 460,622, or 50 percent, of the nation's community hospital beds. Of the 306 multihospital systems, 72, or 24 percent, are Catholic; 25, or 5 percent, have other religious affiliations; 765, or 54 percent, are secular nonprofit; and 54, or 18 percent, are investor owned (table 6-4). Although they represent only 18 percent of the nation's multihospital systems, the investor-owned systems tend to be large, averaging 21 hospitals and 2,543 beds

TABLE 6-3. Trends in Selected Hospital Facilities and Services (Community Hospitals), United States, 1960, 1990

Facility or Service	Percent of Hospitals with Facility or Providing Service		
	1960	1990	1990
		All hospitals	300–400-bed hospitals
Ambulatory care:			
Emergency service	91	94	98
Outpatient department	54	85	92
Outpatient hemodialysis	NA[a]	27	66
Outpatient psychiatry	NA	20	43
Outpatient rehabilitation	NA	52	76
Outpatient surgery	NA	95	99
Inpatient care:			
Intensive care unit (all)	10	NA	NA
Neonatal care unit	NA	14	36
Pediatric care unit	NA	6	16
Cardiac care unit	NA	22	60
Mixed/other	NA	79	98
Trauma center	NA	13	24
Home care program	3	36	48
Long-term care and rehabilitation			
Physical therapy	41	85	97
Occupational therapy	9	40	70
Skilled nursing care unit	NA	21	22
Inpatient rehabilitation unit	7 (1962)	13	34
Geriatric care unit	NA	10	20
Mental Health care:			
Inpatient unit	11	28	62
Outpatient unit	NA	20	43
Partial hospitalization program	NA	13	28
Emergency psychiatric services	NA	34	64
Education	NA	22	48
Other:			
Hospice	NA	16	28
Magnetic resonance imaging	NA	18	40
Social work	15	78	98
Women's health center	NA	21	43
Reproductive health	NA	42	55
Alcohol/drug dependency	NA	21	37
Speech therapy	NA	46	76
Health promotion	NA	77	92
CT scanners	NA	70	97
Open heart surgery	NA	17	51

SOURCE: *Hospital statistics.* (1990). Chicago: American Hospital Association.

[a] NA—not available, not applicable, or none.

TABLE 6-4. Hospitals and Beds in Nonfederal Multihospital Systems by Type of Ownership and Control, 1980 and 1990 (as a percentage of all systems in parentheses)

Ownership Control	Number of Systems			Hospitals and Beds in Systems[a]						
	1980	1990	Percent Change 1980–1990	1980		1990		Percent Change 1980–1990		
				H	B	H	B	H	B	
Catholic Church-related	124 (46.4)	72 (24.0)	−41.9	533 (29.7)	139,767 (40.9)	531 (20.6)	123,959 (26.9)	−0.4	−11.3	
Other church-related	20 (7.5)	15 (4.9)	−25.0	137 (7.6)	20,590 (6.1)	99 (3.8)	19,248 (4.2)	−27.7	−6.5	
Other not-for-profit	88 (33.0)	165 (53.9)	+87.5	426 (23.7)	91,356 (26.7)	806 (31.3)	180,097 (39.1)	+89.2	+97.1	
Investor-owned	35 (13.1)	54 (17.6)	+54.3	701 (39.0)	89,635 (26.3)	1,135 (44.2)	137,318 (29.8)	+61.9	+53.2	
All systems	267 (100)	306 (100)	+14.6	1,797 (100)	341,348 (100)	2,571 (100)	460,622 (100)	+43.1	+34.9	

SOURCES: Adapted from *Data book on multihospital systems* 1980–1981. (1981). Chicago: American Hospital Association; and *AHA guide*. (1991).

[a]Includes hospitals (H) and beds (B) owned, leased, sponsored, or managed by multihospital systems.

per system, compared to only six hospitals and 1283 beds per nonprofit system. As a result, investor-owned systems contain 44 percent of all system hospitals, representing 30 percent of all system beds.

Two fundamental motives seem to underlie the multihospital system movement that is so dramatically changing the character of the hospital sector—organizational survival and organizational growth. Survival applies to the freestanding, single-ownership institution and explains why such a hospital decides to relinquish its autonomy and become part of a system. Organizational growth, on the other hand, applies to the system itself and explains why it seeks to build, buy, lease, or manage additional hospitals. For the single institution, today's increasingly complex, fast-changing, demanding, and even hostile health care environment has made survival of the fittest a stark reality. Competition, financial pressures, regulation, and other external forces so weaken or threaten many solo institutions that they turn to systems for the strength to survive, albeit under different ownership. For the established systems, acquisition of additional hospitals is a means to grow—to add new services, enter new markets, establish new referral patterns, or build more financial and political power.

Another associated trend is the recent proliferation of hospital alliances, which are defined as formally organized groups of hospitals or hospital systems that have come together for specific purposes, have specific membership criteria, and are controlled by independent and autonomous member institutions. In 1991 there were 18 major hospital alliances ranging in size from 8- to 1,155-member institutions. Hospital alliances differ from multihospital systems in that they are generally voluntary affiliations of hospitals that have joined together to reap the benefits of joint activities such as group purchasing and shared product development, without relinquishing their independent identity and autonomy. Alliances lack the corporate control found in multihospital systems.

Patterns of Financing and Ownership

Patterns of hospital financing and ownership differ from country to country. Most countries recognize health care as an essential service in which government should have a major role. In Great Britain and many other industrialized nations, government owns and operates most of the hospitals and employs the physicians who work in them. In other countries, the government limits its role to financing care provided by private hospitals and private practitioners, but in countries such as Canada, where comprehensive national health insurance is in effect, hospitals operate primarily on public funds and hence are essentially controlled by the government even though many are not government-owned. In the United States, by contrast, government's role has been generally limited to financing care for needy groups such as the aged, the poor, and the disabled. This role has grown, however, to the point where hospitals now receive 55 percent of their income from government sources (primarily Medicare and Medicaid). The rest comes from private health insurance (35 percent), direct payments by patients (5 percent), and other private sources (5 percent) (1). In short, the United States has a pluralistic public–private financing system with largely privately owned hospitals. However, as the portion of hospital income financed by government has increased (from about 25 percent in 1960 to 55 percent today), so has the amount of regulation.

The limited role of government in the ownership of hospitals in the United States has been shaped by four major forces. First, the government was still relatively weak in the 1800s, when the short-term hospital as it exists today was evolving as a result of advances in medical science. Innovations and progress generally came from the private sector. At that time, poverty was not so severe (or was not perceived as so severe) that the needy could not be cared for through charity and philanthropy in private hospitals. It was generally believed that the private sector could provide care for the poor as well as those who could pay. The exception was in major cities with large concentrations of the poor. There, public hospitals were established to care for the needy.

Second, government responsibility for the public's health was viewed narrowly before the Depression of the 1930s and was limited mainly to public safety (i.e., protecting healthy citizens from persons with communicable diseases and mental illnesses); to providing care for special groups such as merchant seamen, military personnel, and veterans; and to assisting the needy. State government operated hospitals for its beneficiary groups, and city and county governments in large urban areas operated hospitals for the poor.

Third, our strong tradition of reliance on the private sector means that government becomes involved only when the private sector clearly fails to provide a critical service. For example, chronic disease, mental, and tuburculosis hospital care would have been difficult to finance privately. The long stays that previously prevailed would have been expensive and not readily insurable. Hospitalization generally meant loss of one's job and income, especially since the incidence of hospitalization for these conditions was greatest among the poor. As a result, these areas of care have traditionally fallen to the public sector. The private sector proved better able to finance short-term hospital care through direct payments and private health insurance, and so the government's role has been supplementary. For example, the government helped to finance the construction of hospitals through the Hill-Burton program beginning in 1946 and finance care for the groups that could not afford to pay, primarily the aged and the poor.

Fourth, government involvement has been resisted by the medical profession. Physicians represent a particularly powerful group in the United States and have long been concerned that government involvement in the health care system would compromise their economic and professional interests (31).

Internal Organization of Community Hospitals

From the outside, a community hospital appears as one organization with a clear goal of providing high-quality patient care to which the efforts of the professional and technical groups working there are devoted. From the inside, it is apparent that there are at least two different organizations with two distinct set of goals: the administrative organization, which is responsible for the efficient management and operation of the institution as a whole; and the medical staff organization, which is responsible for the patient care provided by individual physicians.

Furthermore, there are three loci of authority within a hospital—the governing board, the medical staff, and the administration—and much balancing goes on among them (32). Each authority group has a distinct responsibility. The board is ultimately responsible for everything that goes on in the hospital, both administratively and professionally. It oversees the operation of the hospital and carries out its responsibility by: 1) adopting policies and plans to guide the hospital's operation; 2) selecting and delegating responsibility for the day-to-day management of the hospital administrator and supervising that person's performance; and 3) appointing physicians to the medical staff, approving the medical staff's organization for governing itself and for supervising the professional activities of its members, and delegating responsibility to the medical staff for the provision of high-quality patient care.

In practice, the three areas of authority are not this clear or distinct. For example, it might seem that there is a clear distinction between governance and the medical staff's responsibility for patient care. Court decisions have made it clear, however, that the hospital as an institution has a corporate responsibility or legal liability for ensuring that patients receive high-quality patient care. Therefore, the governing board must make sure that only qualified physicians practice in the hospital and that quality review mechanisms are established and working (33). However, only the medical staff has the expertise to assess the qualifications and care provided by physicians. Although the medical staff is clearly subordinate to the governing board in terms of authority for the affairs of the institution, physicians are independent of strict control by the board because the board does not share their expert knowledge and special skill.

Employees of the hospital working in clinical areas often find themselves in the middle when physicians' actions conflict with hospital policy. Legally, they should follow hospital policy; however, professionally they are expected to follow the physicians' orders regarding patient care, and their day-to-day working relationships are with the medical staff. A substantial degree of physician independence from the hospital exists because most are in private practice and not employed by the institution. On the other hand, physicians must have access to a hospital to practice modern medicine, and only the governing board has the power to grant them the privilege of practicing there. This unique relationship between physicians and hospitals is not without stresses and strains, and it makes the governance and management of hospitals a challenging responsibility (34).

The distinction between adopting policies to guide hospital operations and managing operations on a day-to-day basis is not always clear, either. Problems arise when the governing board becomes involved in administrative matters, such as acting directly on employee grievances that come to their attention rather than referring them to the administrator. On the other hand, the administrator may make decisions that go beyond board policies. Thus the community hospital is not a united front, but rather an organization with at least two separate lines of authority—administrative and medical—and with some ambiguity between what is governance and what is management. Power at the top is shared, both because the board depends on the expertise of the medical staff and because of the independent contractor status of physicians. Administrators have also become very influential be-

cause of their expertise in dealing with the increasingly complex operational and regulatory issues confronting hospitals (35). Since the internal powers do not always agree among themselves on priorities and programs, hospitals often experience internal tensions and find it difficult to respond in a systematic way to environmental conditions and changing community needs.

The Governing Board

The governing board of the community hospital has evolved in function and structure as the hospital itself has developed new roles. During the late 1800s and early 1900s, when advances in medical science were transforming hospitals from custodial institutions for the sick poor to sources of effective and safe care for the entire community, board members were mostly wealthy benefactors who made substantial donations to establish and equip the hospital and meet its deficits. The primary function of the board at that time was trusteeship, that is, preserving the assets that they and others like them donated. The trustees' job was seen as providing the facilities and equipment the medical staff needed to care for their patients. There was little trustee involvement in medical matters. The administrator was essentially a clerk, and administrative duties were divided among the board members.

After World War I, the complexity and size of hospitals grew to the point where board members could no longer administer and financially support the hospital. Business managers were hired to handle administrative and financial matters; the business manager, along with the superintendent of nurses, reported to the board, and the board coordinated work between the two. As the complexity of the hospital and the competence of managers increased, the business manager gradually assumed responsibility for overseeing nursing and all other departments as well, so that only one person reported directly to the board. The manager's title became "superintendent." The board of trustees moved into an oversight role, relinquishing day-to-day management matters to the superintendent (36).

The governing board's role changed further as hospitals continued to grow, as management decisions took on greater complexity and significance, and as philanthropy yielded to patient revenue as the primary source of financial support. The board's role became one of overall policy making and planning, and board membership was used to augment and supplement the skills of the administrative staff. Boards began to be composed of fewer philanthropists and more individuals with specific management skills, such as business executives, attorneys, bankers, architects, and contractors (36). Even so, community hospital boards remained relatively closed to external scrutiny, with their membership consisting essentially of self-perpetuating groups of community influentials (37,38). Board decisions were mostly in the areas of finance, personnel, and physical plant and their areas of expertise, and boards typically deferred to the medical staff on medical and patient care matters, delegating fully the responsibility for the qualifications and quality of care provided by the medical staff.

During the 1960s four major factors caused further changes in the governing board's role: 1) continuing advances in medical science, the proliferation of medical technology, and the rapid growth in the size and sophistication of hospitals gave rise to public concern about the cost of hospital care, while making the hospital even more central in the delivery of health care and valuable to the public; 2) public expectations regarding the hospital's responsibility to the community changed, so that hospitals began to be viewed as community resources with a definite obligation to respond to community needs; 3) regulation of hospital construction, costs, quality, and use, as well as labor relations, became more and more stringent, particularly following the establishment of Medicare and Medicaid; and 4) court decisions established the concept of corporate or institutional responsibility for ensuring the quality of patient care (34, 39).

As a result of these forces, the governing board's role broadened and became even more demanding. Boards grew active in environmental surveillance, becoming knowledgeable about community concerns and external trends and interpreting their significance for the hospital (40). External pressures forced hospitals to reexamine their priorities and programs, and boards found it necessary to provide clearer direction and stronger leadership in long-range planning. Boards have also assumed an active role in seeing that community concerns and interests are brought into hospital decision making, and many have expanded community representation within their membership. The board has found itself in the role of balancing and mediating between the demands and pressures on the hospital from the community and external agencies, on one hand, and from the medical staff, employees, and other internal groups, on the other hand. Finally, boards have been forced to take a more active role in quality control, rather than abdicating this responsibility to the medical staff. Although the function of quality monitoring is still delegated to the medical staff, the board is now being held accountable for how well this function is carried out. The board is responsible for ensuring that the mechanisms for evaluating the credentials of physicians and monitoring the care they provide are established and working. Courts have held the board and the hospital responsible in malpractice cases in which reasonable precautions were not taken to ensure 1) careful selection of the medical staff; 2) establishment of high standards of care; 3) monitoring and supervision of care; and 4) enforcement of policies, rules, and regulations. In practice, board control over medical staff performance remains limited and depends more on the commitment of the medical staff, the character of hospital–medical staff relations, and moral sanctions than on formal sanctions such as suspending or terminating a physician's privileges, an action that is very rare.

As governing boards became more actively involved in medical and patient care matters, in both determining the hospital's role and relationships with other institutions and overseeing quality assurance mechanisms, physicians began to seek more involvement in hospital planning and policy making. At the same time, boards felt a greater need for more direct physician participation in their deliberations to address issues related to quality, medical staff privileges, and changing medical technology and practice patterns (41). As a result, an increasing number of boards have added physicians to their membership. More than half of all community hospital boards now include physicians. Less frequent but emerging is the tendency of the administrator to serve on the board, generally with a change in title to "president" or "executive vice president," in a corporate type of structure.

A new issue for the hospital field concerns the structure and functions of governance within multiple hospital systems. Three models for structuring governance in multiple hospital systems have been described (42, 43). In the parent holding company model, governing bodies exist at both the system and institutional levels. Some systems have adopted a variation of the parent holding company model in which there is a system-level governing board, but boards at the institutional level serve in only an advisory capacity. The responsibilities of the advisory boards are generally limited to community relations and monitoring quality of care (44). The third or corporate model occurs when only a system-level governing board exists to carry out all the governance activities of a multihospital system. A recent study of 159 multihospital systems revealed that 41 percent used the parent holding company model, 22 percent the modified parent holding company model, and 23 percent the corporate model (43). This study also revealed that regardless of the governance model, corporate-level boards are likely to retain responsibility for decisions regarding the transfer or sale of assets, the formation of new companies, purchase of assets greater than $100,000, changes in hos-

pital by-laws, and appointment of local board members. For other activities, the governance model affects the locus of decision-making authority. In general, the more decentralized the governance model, the more likely it is that activities such as service development, strategic planning, capital and operating budget approval, medical staff privileges, and appointment and evaluation of the hospital chief executive officer will be under the authority of the local board. A major agenda item for future research on governance of multihospital systems pertains to the relationship between governance structure and operational efficiency and effectiveness. The corporate model has the advantage of structural simplicity and clear lines of authority while holding company models provide for greater input and involvement at the community level. Further examination of the advantages and disadvantages of these approaches to system-level governance will become more important as hospitals grow both horizontally and vertically in the future.

Today, governing boards are being challenged and scrutinized as never before. They are being called on to demonstrate their effectiveness in ensuring that the hospitals they govern meet community needs and provide high-quality care while at the same time functioning efficiently within a complex structure of guidelines and regulations, all in an environment of constant change. Not all boards are capable of performing this task. Boards have been criticized as too inward-looking, passive, uninformed, reluctant to become involved in medical matters, and unwilling to change the status quo. Recent legal decisions have found hospital board members personally liable for making hasty, ill-informed decisions (45). It appears, however, that the pressures discussed above are causing boards to take active steps to broaden and strengthen their membership, educate themselves more fully, and streamline their structure so that they will be better equipped to provide the strong leadership that will be required in the future (46, 47).

Hospital Administration

Hospital administration has grown in importance and status as hospitals have grown in size and sophistication. The job of implementing board policy and responsibility for the day-to-day management and supervision of the hospital is delegated by the board to the hospital administrator. The administrator has responsibility for managing the hospital's finances, acquiring and maintaining equipment and facilities, hiring and supervising hospital personnel, and coordinating hospital activities. The breadth of the administrator's responsibility is illustrated by a typical community hospital organization chart (Figure 6-2). A key aspect of the administrator's job is to coordinate and serve as the channel of communication among the governing board, medical staff, and hospital departments. Another is strategic planning for the future development of the hospital's services. Large hospitals have several assistant administrators who are responsible for nursing, professional services, support services, and hospital finance.

In addition to financial, personnel, and physical plant matters, administration plays an important role in patient care. For example, administration is responsible for coordinating the patient care departments with each other and with the support

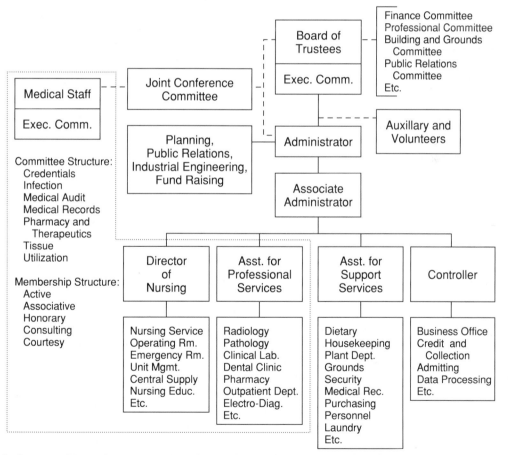

Figure 6-2. Prototypical hospital organization chart. (SOURCE: Reprinted with permission from Chamber of Commerce of the United States. [1974]. *A primer for hospital trustees.* Washington, DC: Author.)

departments, ensuring that they are adequately equipped and staffed and technically up to date, and ensuring that they function smoothly. Administration must make sure that physician orders for the treatment of patients are carried out correctly and promptly by hospital personnel and also that orders do not conflict with governing board policies or hospital rules. The administrator is also actively involved in planning for new patient care services and in ensuring that the hospital meets accreditation, licensure, and other standards. Because the medical staff is not employed by the hospital, the administrator must establish a cooperative working relationship with the members in order to effectively handle the many tasks that involve both administration and medical questions. Finally, the administration acts as the liaison with the community and with external agencies, both bringing information from these sources into hospital decision making and planning and representing the hospital to these outside parties. Because of the increasing impact of external and regulatory pressures on hospitals, this boundary-spanning role has become one of the most important aspects of the administrator's job.

Hospital administration has advanced rapidly as a profession. Schulz and Johnson (48) describe the transition as moving from business manager (1920s–1940s), to coordinator (1950s–1960s), and now to corporate chief (with full authority for directing all aspects of the hospital's operation) and management team leader (promoting participative decision making by board, medical staff, nursing staff, and administrative representatives). Administrators are now full participants in the development of policies and plans, as well as in their implementation and in the external and internal affairs of the hospital. It has been suggested that in order to survive the challenges encountered by hospitals in the current competitive environment, the successful administrator must develop new skills and priorities, including the ability to innovate, value-based management, concern for patient satisfaction, and a willingness to accept entrepreneurial risk (49, 50).

Hospital Medical Staff

The governing board delegates responsibility for the provision of high-quality patient care to the medical staff, which is formally organized to carry out this responsibility and is accountable for it to the board (40). Unlike in many advanced countries, where hospital medical staffs are composed of salaried physicians, the medical staffs of community hospitals in the United States are composed mostly of private practitioners who are not employees of the hospital. The relationship between the hospital and its medical staff is a mutually dependent and sometimes stressful one. The hospital is dependent on the medical staff to admit and care for patients and monitor the quality of patient care. In a sense, the clients of the hospital are the physicians, since it is they who admit patients, decide how long the patients will stay, and order hospital services. On the other hand, physicians are dependent on hospitals because, in order to practice modern medicine, they must have access to the diagnostic and therapeutic services of the hospital. This is particularly true of specialties such as obstetrics and surgery. Thus a quid pro quo relationship exists; physicians agree to abide by hospital policies and medical staff rules and to devote time to the medical staff's quality monitoring activities (in the past, they also contributed time to care for patients who could not pay), in return for the privilege of using the community's hospital to care for their private patients.

Different categories of appointment for the medical staff carry different privileges and responsibilities (51):

Active medical staff have full hospital privileges and provide most of the medical care in the hospital. They are responsible for the administrative activities of the organized medical staff. They can vote, hold office, and serve on committees.

Associated medical staff may consist of physicians and dentists who are being considered for advancement to the active medical staff. The period to be served in the associate medical staff status is defined in the medical staff by-laws. At the end of this period, frequently one to two years, the associate member is considered for advancement through the mechanism established in the by-laws.

Courtesy medical staff is composed of physicians who are eligible for active membership on the staff but who admit patients to the hospital only occasionally (usually because they are on the active staff of another hospital). They are not involved in any administrative functions.

Consulting medical staff includes physicians and dentists who are recognized for their professional expertise and who are willing to act as consultants to the hospital's medical staff, although they practice primarily in other hospitals.

Honorary staff consists of physicians or dentists who are recognized for their noteworthy contributions and/or outstanding service to the hospital. Honorary status is often attained at a certain age as defined in the medical staff by-laws.

Provisional status are initial appointments to the medical staff, except honorary and consulting, that are provisioned for a period of time designated in the medical staff by-laws. If at the end of the provisional period an individual has not satisfied the requirements for staff eligibility, provisional status automatically terminates.

House staff are interns and residents who form the house staff of a hospital. They function under the supervision of attending physicians but are employees of the hospital.

In carrying out its delegated responsibility for ensuring the quality of care, the medical staff governs itself, establishes qualifications for appointment to the staff and for clinical privileges, establishes standards of care and rules and regulations to guide the provision of care, and supervises the professional performance of its members. These duties are accomplished within the medical staff by-laws, which set forth the form, functions, and responsibilities of the medical staff. The by-laws must be approved by both the medical staff and the governing board (51).

The administrative head of the medical staff organization is the president or chief of staff. The chief of staff is responsible for 1) acting as a liaison among the governing board, the administrator, and the medical staff; 2) chairing the executive committee of the medical staff and serving as an ex-officio member of all committees and usually of the governing board; 3) establishing medical staff committees and appointing their members; 4) enforcing government board policies; 5) enforcing medical staff by-laws, rules, and regulations; 6) maintaining standards of medical care in the hospital; and 7) providing for continuing education for the medical staff.

Although the chief of staff is usually elected by the medical staff for a one- or two-year term, this position is also in a sense part of the hospital's administrative structure, directly accountable to the hospital's governing board. As such, the chief of staff is consulted by the board for advice on medical matters, as well as for assurance that the medical staff's responsibilities are being carried out. Administration of medical staff affairs can be a time-consuming job, but in most community hospitals the chief of staff fills this role in addition to pursuing a busy private medical practice. Larger hospitals often hire a full-time salaried medical director to carry out many of the administrative duties of the chief of staff; this trend is spreading although not without controversy (52).

Most of the organizational responsibilities of the medical staff are carried out by committees (51, 53). The "executive committee" is the key administrative and policy-making body of the medical staff. It governs the activities of the medical staff, and all other committees are advisory to it. It is composed of the chief of staff, the chiefs of the clinical departments, and members at large elected by the active medical staff. The "joint conference committee" is the formal liaison between the governing board and medical staff and includes members from both groups plus the administrator. This committee is a forum for discussing medical administrative matters of mutual concern. The "credentials committee" reviews the qualifications of applicants to the medical staff and makes recommendations regarding appointments, annual reappointments, and clinical privileges. Recommenda-tions are transmitted through the executive committee of the hospital's governing board, which has final decision-making authority regarding medical staff membership and privileges.

A second type of medical staff committee ad-vises or oversees specific functional areas or de-partments; examples include emergency room, nursing, pharmacy, special care, and disaster com-mittees. A third type of committee is the evaluative or quality assurance committee responsible for monitoring the patient care provided by individual physicians. These include medical audit, utilization review, and tissue committees. Finally, a continu-ing education committee plans education pro-grams for the medical staff. In larger hospitals, most of these committee functions are duplicated in each clinical department.

There is a small but growing body of empirical evidence in support of the presumption that the structure of the medical staff affects quality and other aspects of hospital performance (54, 55, 56, 57). Roemer and Friedman (53) studied the extent to which the degree of structure of the medical staff influences the costliness, quality, and scope of hospital services and found that a relationship does exist. They concluded that a fairly highly structured medical staff organization functions bet-ter than does one with a low or moderate structure. They found that effectiveness is enhanced by a core of full-time salaried physicians within the medical staff; a comprehensive department and committee structure; clearly specified policies, rules, and regulations; and thorough documentation of medical staff activities. This type of organization pattern offers the private physicians who use the hospital the benefits of full-time, hospital-based physicians who provide administrative support and supervision and take the leadership in developing standards of care and educational programs. An interesting finding is that a core of full-time salaried physicians tends to stimulate the other physicians to take their quality monitoring responsibilities more seriously. The mix of both salaried and private practice physicians tends to provide an environ-ment conducive for change and improvement. An-other study (57) concluded that physician partici-pation in hospital decision making was the single most important variable associated with lower pa-tient mortality for acute myocardial infarction and that active physician participation in hospitalwide decision-making bodies is strongly associated with overall quality of care.

It is apparent that hospitals are moving slowly, but surely, and not without conflict, toward more highly structured forms of medical staff organiza-tion that can be held more directly accountable for quality. At the same time, medical staff officers are being asked to participate more actively in govern-ing board and management decision making. Re-cent shifts in reimbursement toward prospective payment methodologies have significantly changed the financial incentives for hospitals. To a greater extent than ever before, hospitals now must assure that hospital admissions are justifiable, that length of stay does not exceed accepted norms, and that treatment regimens are medically appropriate. The reality is, however, that much of the care provided to patients in hospitals is under the control of physicians. As a result, hospitals are faced with the formidable task of attempting to change physician practice patterns. Possible methods of changing physician behavior include education, peer review and feedback, administrative changes, participa-tion in hospital activities, and penalties and rewards (58). It is clear that the need for hospitals to exer-cise greater control or influence over physician behavior represents a significant threat to physi-cians' traditional autonomy and may result in in-creased tension and conflict between hospital ad-ministration and medical staffs. Methods used by hospitals to influence physician behavior to achieve greater cost containment include direct appeals for assistance, joint ventures, limits on physician priv-ileges, and employment of physicians (59). While direct appeals are the least threatening to physician autonomy and employment is the most threaten-ing of all these approaches are likely to be adopted by some hospitals in the future. There has been particular interest most recently in joint venture arrangements in which hospitals share the risks and benefits of new activities such as technology acquisition or clinic development with members of their medical staffs. Joint ventures also provide a means of fostering hospital–physician bonding in an era of stress and competition. Clearly, the hospital–physician relationship of the future will be different from what it was in the past.

Trends and Issues in the Hospital Industry

The high and persistently climbing cost of hospital care, combined with increasing disenchantment with regulatory efforts to reduce health costs, has led to a new emphasis on marketplace competition for hospitals. Although the overall annual rate of inflation for hospitals has declined from a high point of nearly 15 percent in 1982, health care costs in general and hospital costs in particular, continue to increase at a rate far in excess of the consumer price index (CPI). The obvious conclusion is that while inflationary pressures have been controlled for the general economy, hospitals have not been as successful in containing their costs. There are several reasons for this, including prior commitments to expensive building and construction projects by many hospitals, the growing role of sophisticated technology and computers in hospital care, the power of unions, and the hospital's limited ability to control the practice patterns of physicians. As a result of their continuing high costs, hospitals tend to be the prime target of the cost-containment efforts of both public and private payors.

The mid-1980s witnessed dramatic changes in hospital utilization patterns—changes strongly influenced by the introduction of prospective payment methodologies by Medicare and tremendous growth in managed health care plans such as HMOs and PPOs. Average hospital occupancy rates declined by nearly 11 percent between 1980 and 1990 (5). Lower occupancy has led to a widespread perception that hospitals are a mature, if not declining, industry. Declining occupancy com-

bined with pressure to contain costs has resulted in a new competitive mind-set for hospitals that are actively pursuing diversification strategies, product-line management, marketing, and advertising. The long-term effects of this competitive approach to health care delivery continue to be debated with many deeply concerned about the impact it may have on hospitals' public service commitment to the poor.

These trends present special problems for small and rural hospitals whose difficulties in attracting resources, keeping up to date with advances in medical technology, and maintaining financial viability raise questions about their future survival and how they should relate to larger institutions offering the specialized services that they are not able to provide. Another challenge for hospitals concerns ethical issues, including those related to termination of life-support services, nutrition and hydration for terminally ill patients, care for unsponsored patients, and allocation of resources to expensive and contested medical procedures such as artificial heart transplantation. These trends, their impact on hospitals, and the issues they raise are discussed in this section.

Hospital Cost Containment

The nation's health expenditures have been increasing dramatically, with hospital spending leading the way. On a per capita basis, hospital expenditures increased from $50 per person in 1960 to $975 per person in 1990 (1). This $975 was double the per capita spending for physicians' services, five times what was spent for nursing home care, and more than six times what was spent for drugs or dental services. Because the cost of hospital care has been increasing so much faster than other elements of health care, hospitals are consuming a larger and larger share of the nation's health expenditures. About 38 percent of our health expenditures now go for hospital care, compared to about 33 percent in 1960 (1).

In 1980, $102 billion was spent for care in community hospitals. By 1990, this figure had *why few no restric. on quantity?*

reached $256 billion, a 150 percent increase in 10 years. This increase occurred even though overall utilization of inpatient hospital services in 1980 (33,774 million admissions) was lower than in 1980, (38,892 million admissions) (5). This leveling off of hospital admissions was a direct result of efforts to shift more care from an inpatient to an outpatient setting. Hospital admissions reached their lowest point in 10 years in 1989, although the overall population of the United States increased by 25 million from 1980 to 1990. Thus it is clear that the continuing high rate of inflation in hospital costs cannot be explained by increases in utilization. Instead, hospital cost increases are more likely attributable to changes in the nature of hospital output (i.e., in the intensity, scope, sophistication, and quality of hospital care)—which, in turn, cause hospitals to employ more and better labor inputs (accounting for 54 percent of all community hospital expenditures in 1990) and more and better nonlabor inputs.

Hospital services are continuously increasing in intensity, scope, and sophistication as a result of advances in medical science and community and physician demands for the widest possible range of the most up-to-date services. The average hospital stay now costs about $5,000 (5).

Regarding intensity, patients today receive more laboratory, X-ray, and other diagnostic and therapeutic services than did patients treated for the same conditions a few years ago. Several factors have contributed to the increased intensity. Advances in medical science have made more diagnostic and therapeutic procedures available, and both patients and physicians want to take advantage of all that modern medicine has to offer. The nature of physician training in sophisticated hospitals may lead them to order more procedures. Another factor is the fear of malpractice suits, which leads to defensive medical practice. Physicians are inclined to order the extra laboratory tests or X-ray procedure "just to make sure." The shortening length of stay has resulted in patients receiving more services each day than if the same services were spread over a longer period of time.

Many experts believe that a major factor is that physicians are not directly affected financially by the costs of the services they order on behalf of their patients. A most important factor again is hospital insurance, which has led patients to want the best of care regardless of cost. Only recently have insurance companies begun to implement tough utilization review protocols for hospital admissions and ancillary service use.

Regarding the broadening scope of services offered by community hospitals, advances in medical science have created new diagnostic and treatment technology not dreamed of a few years ago. Fetal monitoring, diagnostic radioisotope procedures, computed tomography, magnetic resonance imaging, lithotripsy, open heart surgery, organ transplants, laser and microscope surgery, radiation therapy, renal dialysis, and other complicated procedures require expensive equipment, expensive facilities, and skilled personnel. Communities and physicians alike have come to expect a wide range of services to be available in their local hospitals. As a result, there has been an increase in the scope and sophistication of services being offered by even relatively small community hospitals serving limited populations.

The increased investment by hospitals in equipment and facilities is reflected by a substantial increase in assets per bed. In 1960, the capital investment per bed in community hospitals was about $17,000. This figure is now well over $100,000. Expenditures for equipment, facilities, and supplies have been increasing faster than expenditures for personnel. As a result, nonpayroll expenses as a portion of total expenses increased from 38 percent in 1960 to 46 percent in 1990. However, the use of personnel has increased, as well. It is interesting to note that hospital full-time-equivalent personnel (FTEs) have not declined as rapidly as patient admissions. In addition, the skill levels of hospital personnel have increased, and more hospitals are employing physicians. The average hospital salary increased by 721 percent between 1960 and 1985, from $3,239 to $26,590 (5).

Another cost-increasing factor is debt financing of capital projects. In the past, hospital construction projects were financed mostly by community fund-raising drives, philanthropy, and government programs such as Hill-Burton. As these sources of capital declined in importance, hospitals have been forced to borrow a larger proportion of the funds needed for capital projects, adding interest expense to the cost of these projects (60).

A final and increasingly significant factor is the administrative cost of complying with regulations. Programs now exist to regulate hospital construction, rates, reimbursement, quality, use, plant safety, and labor relations, to name only a few. The array of complex and often conflicting requirements hospitals must comply with contributes substantially to increased costs. The current situation is approaching the point where the solution is becoming part of the problem: hospitals must spend money to comply with regulations, which adds to the costs that regulations are designed to control. As a result, there has been a marked shift away from regulatory controls over health care providers in favor of a competitive marketplace approach to cost containment. In 1986 the federal government terminated funding for the nation's health systems agencies (HSAs), the major source of regulatory review for hospital construction, services, and equipment, and it is expected that many states will follow the lead of California in all but abandoning certificate-of-need (CON) requirements for hospital services.

The prices hospitals charge private-pay patients have increased even faster than total costs because of the difference between what hospitals charge to meet their full financial needs and what Medicare and Medicaid actually pay. These allowances, or discounts, along with the charity care and bad debts that hospitals incur but Medicare and Medicaid do not reimburse, are passed on to private-pay patients and their insurance carriers in the form of higher prices. This "cost shifting" explains why hospital charges or prices have been increasing at a considerably faster rate than hospital costs. Private insurance carriers in recent years, however, have taken steps to limit the amount of cost shifting they have traditionally absorbed. Seizing the initiative inherent in PPOs, carriers have begun to initiate selective contracts with hospitals that grant them discounts or preferred rates. Individuals insured under such plans are given financial incentives for using the "preferred" hospitals. The hospitals are caught in a "catch-22" position, either they offer carriers discounted rates or face lower patient volume. Since hospital admissions have been declining, most hospitals are willing to compete for patients through competitive bidding on selective contracts. This is a dangerous scenario for many hospitals that could produce financial crisis in the future.

Clearly, the problem of hospital cost inflation is complex, and complex problems call for multifaceted solutions. It would seem that any solution must first encourage prudent hospital use consistent with good medical practice. There is empirical evidence that perhaps as many as one-fourth of all patient days provided by hospitals between 1974 and 1982 were not medically necessary (17). The public's use of hospitals may be constrained by building higher copayment and deductible provisions into health insurance policies and limiting benefits, although the arguments against shifting more of the economic burden to the consumer are many. Other strategies include 1) attempting to counterbalance the physicians' inclination to use the hospital by changing their financial incentives and developing more managed care plans such as HMOs and PPOs; 2) attempting to strengthen external review of the appropriateness of hospital use through public and private utilization review organizations; 3) encouraging the development of more ambulatory care, day care, home care, skilled and intermediate nursing care, and other out-of-hospital care programs and improving insurance coverage for them; and 4) interjecting greater marketplace competition into purchase of hospital services.

The question of how to deal with the increasing complexity and intensity of hospital care is equally difficult. It is physicians, not hospitals, who decide what diagnostic and therapeutic services to order for patients. Hence, changes in physician incentives and training must be part of the solution. Again, HMOs would seem to provide an appropriate set of incentives in this regard. Another approach would be to control malpractice insurance premiums and pressures that apparently cause physicians to practice defensive medicine. Finally, the financial incentives inherent in hospital reimbursement can be modified, as in the case with prospective payment, so as to discourage overuse of services.

Both public and private purchasers of health care services have recognized that prospective payment schemes as opposed to cost-based reimbursement introduce powerful incentives for health care providers to contain costs. The single most significant change in health care financing in the United States occurred when the Tax Equity and Fiscal Responsibility Act of 1982 (PL 97-248) established Medicare per case payment rates for hospitals based on 468 diagnosis-related groups (DRGs). Under this payment system hospitals are reimbursed a flat fee for the entire episode of hospitalization of a patient in a given DRG, regardless of the actual costs incurred in the care of that patient. DRG rates have moved from a blend of hospital-specific costs and national averages toward a national average over several years. If a hospital treats a patient for less than the DRG payment rate, it may retain the difference. If a patient requires more resources than allotted by the DRG, the hospital must absorb the loss. Adaptation to this new payment system has important implications for hospital organization and management including greater emphasis on efficient staffing, greater attention to discharge planning, and movement toward vertical integration (61).

Hospital Responses to Competition and Prospective Payment

Hospitals are actively adapting to the new competitive environment. Prospective payment and price competition create a strong incentive for hospitals to achieve efficient staffing levels since labor represents approximately 54 percent of the average hospital's costs. Hospitals are looking at ways to utilize nurses more efficiently (62), considering substitution of licensed practical nurses for registered nurses or aides for practical nurses in some cases, or moving to an all R.N. staff in other instances. Hospitals are also attempting to increase productivity standards for hospital employees and investigating opportunities to cross-train employees to fill multiple positions. Unfortunately, this emphasis on cost containment and productivity is likely to create new conflicts between hospital administration and unions that are attempting to upgrade the professional status and salaries of their members.

Hospitals are investigating other methods of increasing their profitability, including product- or service-line management. The practice of analyzing hospital programs and services as strategic business units (SBUs) in order to identify and enhance profitable services and turn around or eliminate unprofitable services is being advocated by many as a more businesslike approach to hospital management (63). The concern is that some hospitals may discontinue unprofitable services that are needed by the community. Many argue that defining health care as a commodity and rationing it based on ability to pay is unacceptable if our society holds that health care is a basic right (64). Still, a positive aspect of product-line management is the development and organization of services to meet the special needs of certain segments of the population. Examples include women's health centers and sports medicine clinics. It can be argued that competition is forcing hospitals to be much more sensitive to the needs and desires of people for convenient, specially tailored services.

Under the Medicare per case prospective payment system there is also a strong incentive for hospitals to discharge patients as soon as medically warranted; therefore, Medicare prospective payment has done a great deal to foster the effectiveness of discharge planning. The role of the discharge planner is critical in ensuring that patients receive proper care after leaving the hospital. For elderly patients in particular, rapid rehospitalization may result unless proper discharge instructions and support services are received (65). In many instances the elderly patient cannot be discharged from the hospital until placement in a nursing home is secured or arrangements are made for home care. The necessity of ensuring that patients receive proper postdischarge treatment has heightened the interest of many hospitals in operating their own skilled nursing units and home care programs. One major concern of the Medicare program and its professional review organizations (PROs) is that hospitals may be discharging patients too soon in some instances. Hospitals are under great pressure to deliver exactly the right amount of care to Medicare patients since too much care may result in reimbursement denials and too little care can result in penalty assessments or lawsuits. As a result, hospitals are placing more emphasis on complete documentation of patient treatment records.

Vertical Integration

The increasingly stringent economic environment has also spurred the interest of hospitals in vertical integration. Vertical integration represents a response by hospitals to capture and control more of the factors that lead to inpatient hospitalization. The ultimate goals of vertical integration include 1) increasing a hospital's market and financial position; 2) enhancing the hospital's overall cost effectiveness; 3) improving continuity of care; and 4) responding to changing consumer preferences. Vertical integration in a health enterprise involves linking together different levels of care and assembling the human resources needed to render that care. Vertical integration may be distinguished from diversification efforts in that vertical integration involves the development of new nonhospital services to support and enhance the hospital base while diversification involves the development of distinct new business lines that are independent from the hospital and have profit as their primary

objective (66). Vertical integration has historically proceeded in two directions. As industrial firms integrated forward (toward the ultimate consumer of the firm's product), they either bought out the distributors of their goods or created their own distribution systems to bring their products to market. As they integrated backward (toward the supply of raw materials), they purchased either raw materials or the primary producers of the goods needed to manufacture their products (30).

Backward integration involves all of the activities in which a firm engages to secure an adequate supply of the raw materials needed to produce its particular product. In the health care setting, the product is a human service, patient care; therefore, backward integration involves the equipment, supplies, and human resources required to care for patients. The most critically scarce resources of a hospital are its professionals: physicians, nurses, technicians, and other health personnel. Efforts to secure adequate supplies of these individuals are essential to a health care provider's ability to function. Many hospitals have developed linkages with educational institutions, providing a source of new recruits by serving as training sites. Some hospitals have considered integrating backward into medical supplies and other goods needed to operate; however, these organizations may be entering very competitive markets dominated by large firms.

Since the hospital is the most highly organized form of production of health services, efforts by the hospital to provide those forms of care rendered to the patient prior to hospitalization can be considered forward integration—reaching out toward the patient. A major form of forward integration for a hospital involves development of ambulatory care systems. In health care a distribution or "feeder" system is that set of pathways which result in bringing the patient to the hospital. The feeder system of a hospital includes all of those settings in which the potential patient receives ambulatory services, or diagnosis, as well as the transportation systems and physician referral relationships that ultimately lead to hospitalization (30). The principal feeder system for most hospitals is a network of private physician offices and group practices. One way hospitals have moved to integrate physician practices is by providing office space on the hospital campus, assisting new physicians in starting practices, and helping to market physician services. Physician practice support services, such as office training, management, billing, and referral services, are also activities that build a feeder system and further develop forward integration.

Many hospitals have recognized the importance of a feeder system in building the name recognition of the facility and promoting patient accessibility. As a result, hospitals are engaging in more marketing and advertising activities that increase the visibility of their institutions including direct-mail advertising, use of billboards, and broadcasting on radio and television. There are three channels through which advertising may assist hospitals in increasing their market share: 1) hospitals may influence the choice of patients who are admitted through emergency departments of outpatient clinics; 2) patients may influence the choice of physicians with admitting privileges at multiple institutions; and 3) patients may actually choose a physician affiliated with a particular hospital, especially if they use a hospital referral service (67).

Vertical integration has particular significance for hospitals because it gives them the potential to package a broad range of health care services at a competitive price. There are distinct advantages to such integration if economies of scale result, and the hospital is able to control a broad range of referral services. Vertical integration focuses on hospitals being in the business of health rather than being oriented almost exclusively toward acute care services.

Vertical integration strategies for hospitals experiencing declines in census include several options (68). First, underused acute inpatient facilities can be converted to long-term care, substance abuse, mental health, or other services. Second, hospitals can focus on developing a coordinated and integrated delivery system whereby local residents can obtain most health care services through the programs, services, and facilities managed by one hospital. Third, many institutions have developed physicians' office buildings and ambulatory surgery, diagnostic, and primary care centers through joint ventures with their medical staff in order to improve their market penetration. Fourth, hospitals that are able to contract directly with HMOs, PPOs, third-party payors, and major corporate interests to provide a full range of preacute, acute, and postacute care services at a highly competitive price will place themselves in an excellent market position.

To date, there is relatively little empirical research that assesses the impact of vertical integration on hospital performance. There is one recent study that suggests hospital development of primary care group practice has a positive effect on hospital use and market share (69). During a four-year period (1976–1982), hospitals that sponsored such group practices experienced a 9.0 percent increase in patient days, an 8.2 percent increase in admissions, and an average increase in market share for patient days and admissions of 4.9 percent and 3.6 percent, respectively.

Despite these advantages, the movement toward vertical integration by hospitals may be slowed in the future because of difficulties such as a loss of institutional identity and autonomy, fear of domination by the larger players in the integrated system, uncertainty of roles within an umbrella corporation, and possible imbalances in political power at the governing board, medical staff, or management level (68). Furthermore, vertical integration presents additional problems for hospitals related to controlling the flow of patients among components of a coordinated system, acquiring the requisite expertise to manage new ventures, and maintaining traditional values and character. In order to remain viable and successful, individual institutions must examine the concept of vertical integration further and attempt to apply the knowledge attained in the business world to the health care industry.

Patient Satisfaction

As a result of growing competition, the satisfaction of hospital patients has become more salient to hospital administration in recent years. In the past, hospitals concentrated on satisfying members of their medical staffs in order to increase their market share, but now more attention is being given to the patient and patient preferences for care. Many suggest that hospitals should adopt a continuous quality improvement approach to providing services that actively considers the opinions and preferences of patients (70, 71). In response, many hospitals have begun to routinely administer patient satisfaction surveys while others have initiated programs based on techniques used in hotels and other consumer-oriented service organizations. In many respects it is rather surprising that hospitals have paid so little attention to patient satisfaction in the past. It has been noted that the hospital environment can be very unpleasant and that patients are often fraught with apprehension and anxiety (72, 73). Furthermore, negative aspects of hospital care have been linked with poor compliance with medical treatment protocols and even delayed physical recovery (74). Thus it is desirable to identify, and within reasonable limits, alter those factors that contribute to negative experiences within the hospital. Evaluation of patient satisfaction provides important information on the patients' perception of the quality of medical care and allows the patient as a consumer to have a greater voice in the design and delivery of health services.

Small and Rural Hospitals

In part because Hill-Burton priorities in the early years channeled funds to thinly populated rural areas, the United States is a nation of many small hospitals: about 45 percent of all community hospitals have fewer than 100 beds. These hospitals face a number of problems that threaten their future viability. First, they are losing patients. Admissions to community hospitals with fewer than 100 beds have declined, as has their average daily census (table 6-5). Between 1989 and 1990, the number of community hospitals with fewer than 100 beds fell from 2,750 to 2,424 or almost 12 percent (5). Labor requirements are high in small

TABLE 6-5. Change in Average Daily Census by Hospital Size, United States, 1980–1990

Bed Size	Average Daily Census		Percent Change
	1980	1990	
6–24	2,308	1,431	−38
25–49	19,806	14,645	−26
50–99	67,630	48,617	−28
100–199	137,774	112,987	−18
200–299	133,391	120,469	−10
300–399	111,144	97,212	−13
400–499	95,559	72,642	−24
≥500	179,254	151,272	−19

SOURCE: *Hospital statistics.* (1991). Chicago: American Hospital Association.

TABLE 6-6. Selected Indicators by Hospital Size, United States, 1990

Hospital Bed Size	Full-Time-Equivalent Personnel per 100 Adjusted Census	Percent Occupancy
6–24	437	32.3
25–49	398	41.3
50–99	350	53.8
100–199	373	61.5
200–299	404	67.1
300–399	441	70.0
400–499	446	73.5
≥500	478	77.3

SOURCE: *Hospital statistics.* (1990). Chicago: American Hospital Association.

hospitals for the services offered, and small hospitals tend to operate at less efficient levels of occupancy than larger hospitals (table 6-6). These efficiency limitations, coupled with the limited financial means of some rural populations, have caused many small hospitals to incur substantial operating losses. Small hospitals offer a more limited range of services than larger institutions, because they have neither the patient volume nor the physicians or specialized personnel to support much beyond the basic essential services. Small hospitals are often located in areas where they have a difficult time attracting qualified personnel. Furthermore, the federal government's initial decision to adopt separate wage scales for urban and rural institutions under the Medicare prospective pricing system (PPS) resulted in rural hospitals receiving about 20 percent less reimbursement than their urban counterparts (75). In 1989, Congress directed the U.S. Department of Health and Human Services to eliminate the urban–rural payment differential by 1995. Together, these problems may lead to difficulty in achieving accreditation, and in meeting hospital certification and licensure standards, or may even threaten survival.

Small hospitals also find it especially difficult to keep up with and respond to the increasingly complex and demanding regulatory environment without the range of management specialists common to larger institutions, and as a result, many are contracting with hospital systems or larger hospitals to take over their management. It would appear that the future viability of small hospitals will depend on adapting their mission and the services they offer to fit available resources, establishing relationships with other institutions, and seeking additional resources to support new programs to broaden their role in health care delivery in the communities they serve (76–78).

Because it is especially difficult for smaller hospitals to assemble the array of equipment and personnel or attain the patient volume needed to support a broad range of services, it is critical to consolidate around the small hospital to the greatest extent possible whatever health resources do exist in the community. Ideally, the hospital building or campus might include physicians' offices, facilities for public health nurses and health-related community organizations, a nursing home, and so forth. Consolidation would enable limited health resources to be stretched further and provide opportunities for jointly supporting personnel such as a home care nurse, laboratory technician, or physician assistant. The hospital need not own all of these facilities; merely grouping the community's health-related activities together would be an important step.

The key to the future of smaller rural hospitals still seems to lie in the concept of regionalization or networking, the much discussed but little implemented idea of formally relating small hospitals with larger urban hospitals (79, 80). Regionalization begins with the concept that each level of hospital—small basic service hospitals, moderate-size community hospitals, and large regional referral centers—should provide only those services that they can offer efficiently and at a high level of quality. Communities would be ensured access to a full range of services, not by each hospital attempting to provide every service, but rather by the development of closer relationships among networks of hospitals and their medical staffs to encourage the referral of patients to the institutional setting most appropriate to their needs. Such relationships could range from informal agreements to formal affiliations, jointly provided programs, or mergers of institutions into multihospital systems.

The specific objectives of regionalization include: 1) a two-way flow of patients, with patients referred to larger hospitals for specialized services and returned to smaller hospitals for convalescent, long-term, follow-up, and home care; 2) continuing education for physicians, nurses, and other personnel from the small hospitals through participation in the educational programs of the larger hospital; 3) assistance from administrative, nursing, and professional department heads and specialists from the larger hospital representing skills not available in the small hospitals; 4) consolidation (in the larger hospital) and sharing of services the small hospitals cannot provide as efficiently or at the same level of quality as larger hospitals; 5) regularly scheduled visits by physician specialists from the larger hospitals to conduct clinics and serve as consultants in the small hospitals; 6) sharing of personnel; and 7) joint purchasing (81).

The success of regionalization depends on the support of the community, the governing board, and the medical staffs of both the small and larger hospitals. There are few examples of effective regional relationships. In part, this situation reflects community and professional pride and a desire for independence. It also partially reflects the difficulty of working out the essential elements of regionalization: 1) the movement of referrals in both directions so that the small hospitals do not lose patients but maintain their census by providing basic, convalescent, and follow-up care; 2) reforming reimbursement to recognize a different distribution of patients among large and small hospitals; 3) granting physicians from the small hospitals privileges in the larger hospital and making them feel welcome to admit and treat their patients there when they need the specialized services of the larger hospital; and 4) broadening the role of the small hospital to include convalescent and follow-up, long-term, and home care, and so forth. In the long run, regionalization may preserve rather than threaten the independence and viability of smaller hospitals.

Unionization of Hospital Personnel

The number of health care unions has increased steadily in recent years, rising by 6 percent between 1980 and 1985 and bringing union representation to about 20 percent of all workers in health care institutions (82). This has occurred even though union representation in all industries dropped from 23 percent to 18 percent during the same period. These trends reflect both aggressive pursuit of white-collar service industries by labor unions and current upheavals in the health care field because of cost containment pressures (83). Prospective payment, downsizing, and mergers have created new tensions for health care workers; as a result, their values are shifting such that they regard unions more favorably than in the past. Major issues for nurses and other hospital employees include job security, quality standards, and staffing levels as well as wages. Perhaps the most revealing change in the attitudes of health professionals toward unionization is the growing movement to establish collective bargaining capability for the house staff physicians in hospitals. California and the industrialized eastern states have the greatest number of unionized hospitals, and unionization is most common in metropolitan areas. In addition, there tend to be more unionized hospitals in states that had labor laws before 1974.

When Congress began to consider bringing hos-

pitals under Taft-Hartley, hospitals pressed for special protection against strikes, priority for National Labor Relations Board action on disputes, and mandatory mediation requirements. Hospitals also wanted to limit the number of bargaining units, with one each for professional, technical, clinical, and maintenance and service workers (84). In 1974 hospitals became subject to Taft-Hartley, but with special provisions. A hospital or union must give 90 days' notice to the other party of a desire to change an existing contract. The Federal Mediation and Conciliation Service (FMCS) must be given 60 days' notice, and 30 days' notice if an impasse occurs in bargaining for an initial contract after the union is first recognized. A cooling-off period of at least 10 days is required before a strike can occur to enable the hospital to plan for the care of patients. The FMCS may appoint a board of inquiry to mediate among the parties if it determines that a strike would impair delivery of health care to the community. Neither the hospital nor the union are required to accept the board's recommendation, although they must provide information and witnesses called for by the board (85).

With the exemption from Taft-Hartley removed, several factors have rendered the hospital industry more vulnerable to unionization. First, many hospitals lag behind industry in personnel practices. A substantial number have no professional personnel director, and policies for resolving grievances, discipline, promotion, seniority, overtime, and night-shift work are often poorly spelled out. Wages and fringe benefits in hospitals also appear to have lagged behind those of other industries.

Second, supervisory training is often insufficient. Department heads and supervisors are commonly promoted because of their professional or technical skills rather than their managerial or supervisory capabilities. In addition, supervisors and professional department heads may have divided loyalties between being part of hospital management, on one hand, and members of professional associations that act as unions on the other hand.

Third, the reluctance of professional workers to unionize has diminished. The change in attitude is attributable, in part, to the fact that their professional associations act as their unions. Professional associations are more acceptable than national trade unions. In addition, the professional associations point to collective bargaining not only as a means of improving wages but also as a way to negotiate over staffing standards and work prerogatives that could affect the quality of patient care. The underlying issue of the balance between administrative and professional control regarding work and the work setting is especially important in institutions such as hospitals and adds a unique dimension to unionization in this industry. Also unique is the fear that a strike could harm patients (86, 87).

Regulation of Hospitals

In spite of the recent promotion of marketplace competition for health care providers, hospitals remain a highly regulated industry. External regulation of hospitals has grown rapidly since the mid–1960s. There are external controls over: 1) institutional quality standards (licensure, certification, accreditation); 2) construction and expansion of facilities and services (Section 1122 of the 1972 Social Security Amendments, state certificate of need;) 3) costs or rates (Blue Cross, Medicare, state rate regulation); and 4) use (Blue Cross, Medicare, Medicaid, PROs). Hospital regulations derive from both public agencies and private organizations. Many federal controls are tied to Medicare and Medicaid as conditions for participation or payment: certification, utilization review, and capital expenditure review, to name a few. The major private sector organizations that exert control over hospitals include Blue Cross plans and the Joint Commission on Accreditation of Hospitals (JCAHO) (88). Regulations that most directly affect hospitals are discussed below.

Controls on Quality

The regulatory structure for controlling quality includes state licensure, federal certification, and voluntary accreditation. Licensure is a state function, generally carried out by the department of health,

whereby minimum standards are established and enforced regarding the equipment, personnel, plant, and safety features an institution must have to operate. Licensing agencies are empowered to set standards, conduct inspections, issue licenses, close down facilities that cannot comply with the agency's standards, and provide consultation services. In many states, however, these agencies are underfinanced and understaffed; therefore, standards are not enforced stringently. In addition, there is a tendency to focus on fire, safety, and physical plant standards rather than standards for medical services.

Hospitals must be certified by the designated state agency in order to participate in Medicare and Medicaid. The purpose of certification is to ensure that care for beneficiaries of these programs is purchased only from institutions that can meet acceptable minimum quality requirements. In most states, the U.S. Department of Health and Human Services (DHHS) contracts with the health department to carry out the actual inspection process. Virtually all community hospitals are certified, so it can only be concluded that the administration of this program is not very stringent.

Accreditation is a professionally sponsored, voluntary process carried out by the JCAHO, a private organization formed in 1951 as a joint effort of the American College of Physicians, the American College of Surgeons, the American Hospital Association, and the American Medical Association. The JCAHO establishes quality standards and surveys hospitals that choose to seek accreditation voluntarily. Standards relate to the structure and process aspects of quality, as well as outcome measures, and considerable emphasis is given to the organization of the medial staff. About three-fourths of the nation's community hospitals, and more than 95 percent of those with more than 200 beds, are accredited. Accreditation is designed to encourage institutions to maintain the highest possible levels of performance rather than just minimum standards. Accredited hospitals are deemed to meet DHHS's certification requirement. Although the relevance and rigor of the JCAHO's standards and survey procedures are not above challenge, there is little question that from a historical perspective the JCAHO has been a major force in elevating institutional standards.

Controls on Facilities and Services

Areawide hospital planning began with Hill-Burton in 1946 (89). States were required to define hospital service areas and inventory existing facilities, and identify the areas of greatest need as determined by bed:population ratios. Voluntary areawide planning was promoted by the American Hospital Association and the U.S. Public Health Service (PHS) beginning in 1959. In 1965, the Regional Medical Program was established to encourage regional planning in treatment of heart disease, cancer, and stroke. Federally sponsored health planning began in earnest in 1966 with the Comprehensive Health Planning Act. State planning agencies (A agencies) and areawide, private, nonprofit planning agencies (B agencies) were set up with federal aid to coordinate the development of health facilities and services and to discourage overbuilding and duplication. These agencies had little economic or political power, however, and no legal means of stopping capital projects, and it is generally agreed that few were effective (90).

The 1972 Social Security Amendments (Section 1122) added clout to facility and services regulation by authorizing denial of Medicare and Medicaid reimbursement for building and depreciation expenses for capital projects over $150,000 not approved by the designated state agency. Proposed projects were reviewed by area comprehensive health planning (CHP) agencies, but approval powers remained with the state. There is some evidence that Section 1122 and state CON programs have contained the growth in beds but not in equipment and other capital investments (91). The National Health Planning and Resources Development Act of 1974 established a network of state and area planning agencies. This program linked federal funding more closely with state regulation and required states to establish certificate of need programs that require prior approval by state agencies of plans to build or modernize facilities or add new services (92). Findings of a study of certificate of need experience with computed tomographic scanners suggest that these programs have not been successful in either controlling the introduction of new technology or ensuring equitable distribution of equipment among hospitals (93). Evidence that CON review is costly, time-consuming, and only marginally effective in restraining hospital investments in new technologies and services led Congress to terminate funding for health planning beginning in 1986. Federal withdrawal from the health planning arena means that the fate of health planning agencies will not be a state issue. It is expected that many states will abandon CON review and rate regulation in favor of more competitive approaches to cost containment.

Cost Controls

Programs to control hospital costs or regulate hospital rates were introduced by federal and state agencies and by private third-party purchasers as a result of their concern over the rapid rise in their expenditures for hospital care. Public involvement in cost controls and rate regulation began in earnest after the rapid post-Medicare inflation in hospital costs in the late 1960s. Medicare had adopted cost-based reimbursement and, like Blue Cross, was directly affected by cost increases. Section 223 of the 1972 Social Security Amendments authorized Medicare to set upper limits on routine inpatient service costs for reimbursement purposes, and Section 1122 limited Medicare reimbursement for capital expenditures made without approval of the designated state planning agency.

The Economic Stabilization Program (ESP), which President Nixon imposed in 1971 to deal with economywide inflation, limited the amount by which hospitals could raise their rates from year to year. Hospitals were subject to ESP until 1974. It appears that this stringent program did slow rate increases and, to a lesser degree, cost increases during the

1971–1974 period, although costs soared dramatically as soon as the controls were removed. In the late 1970s, the Carter administration pushed without success for the reestablishment of federal cost and revue controls for the hospital industry (94).

In addition to federal efforts, about a dozen states concerned with controlling their Medicaid expenditures have empowered state agencies or special public utility-type commissions to regulate hospital rates. In general, these agencies approve prospectively the rates hospitals may charge for their services based on budget review or formula methods for projecting hospital costs or financial needs for the coming year. Hospitals are then reimbursed at these rates rather than on the basis of the costs they actually incur. Thus hospitals are at risk to keep their costs below the prospectively set rates. Evidence regarding the effectiveness of state prospective rate-setting programs in containing costs is sparse but suggests that this strategy may have some potential. The critical question may well be whether this cost containment potential can be exploited with enough care and sensitivity so that the quality and financial viability of the hospital system are protected (95, 96).

Recent federal cost containment efforts have been directed toward the Medicare program. Annual expenditures for Medicare increased from $4.9 billion in 1967 to $108.9 billion in 1990. The Tax Equity and Fiscal Responsibility Act of 1982 established Medicare inpatient cost per case reimbursement limits based on DRGs. Within the hospital industry there is substantial controversy concerning the ability of DRGs to reflect true hospital costs since they do not adequately measure severity of illness or compensate for regional differences in costs or practice patterns (97). Since enactment of the Medicare prospective payment legislation, average length-of-stay and admission rates for Medicare patients have declined significantly. Hospitals have also acted to reduce staffing levels and overall expenses (98). Because prospective payment gives hospitals an incentive to provide less care, some have expressed concern regarding its

possible effects on quality. From the hospital perspective there is also great concern regarding the inequities of a national payment rate and failure of DRG price increases to parallel increases in the cost of hospital operations. At this time Congress has not yet adopted a mechanism for incorporating capital costs into DRG payment rates, although a graduated system for including capital payments in prospective payment rates is anticipated in the near future. In spite of hospital complaints about the DRG system, a study of Medicare cost reports for 892 hospitals in nine states (Alaska, California, Connecticut, Florida, Illinois, Minnesota, Oregon, Texas, and Washington), found an average profit margin for Medicare services of 14.1 percent in 1984, although there is great controversy over the way Medicare-related costs were measured in this study (98). While hospital profits appear to be declining in subsequent years of the DRG program, it is clear that there will probably be extensive revisions and fine tuning of Medicare's prospective payment system in the years ahead to maximize its cost savings potential for the federal government.

Control of Utilization

The most recent form of regulation in the hospital industry is the attempt to control utilization. Medicare first required that hospitals and extended-care facilities establish utilization review programs as a condition for participation. Physician committees were to review the medical records of discharged Medicare patients to determine the necessity of the hospital care provided. This requirement was seen as a way to discourage inappropriate admissions and unnecessarily long lengths of stays and, hence, as a means of keeping Medicare and Medicaid expenditures down. However, utilization review raises a number of sensitive issues, because establishing standards and monitoring physician practices with regard to hospitals may be seen as infringing on professional judgment regarding patient care.

Building on the utilization review requirements, the 1972 Social Security Amendments established professional standards review organizations (PSROs) to strengthen the appropriate monitoring process (99). PSROs were established as non profit organizations to review the quality and appropriateness of the care provided Medicare and Medicaid patients in all institutions under contract with DHHS. PSROs established standards of treatment against which utilization could be judged. Although the Reagan administration had originally targeted PSROs for extinction, the program was resurrected through the Tax Equity and Fiscal Responsibility Act of 1982, which requires implementation of utilization and quality control peer review organizations (PROs). PROs, which began operation in October 1983, are closely modeled after the original PSROs in terms of staffing and operational authority. One significant difference, however, is that the new PROs are private organizations and are capable of making utilization review contracts with the business community as well as Medicare and Medicaid.

Despite the widespread advocacy for greater competition in the hospital industry, a complex regulatory environment already exists. That environment is fragmented because a great number of individual regulatory programs have evolved as specific responses to specific problems. Attempts to coordinate and rationalize the multiplicity of regulatory programs to impact on the entire delivery system in a positive manner are relatively recent. Regulation has become expensive for hospitals as well, calling for more careful cost-benefit analysis of regulatory requirements. On the other hand, some argue that the forces currently giving rise to a much more competitive health care environment will make extensive regulation unnecessary.

Ethical Issues for Hospitals

Increasingly, hospital decision making is affected by ethical issues. Within the hospital setting these ethical concerns touch on a variety of administrative and patient care duties, including respect for patient privacy and confidentiality, informed consent, continuation of life support services to ter-

minally ill patients, resource allocation decisions, and care for the poor (100). Many hospitals have constituted institutional ethics committees to provide ethical guidance on both clinical decision making and administrative problems. Because they are the focal point of the most complex applications of modern medicine, hospitals are naturally at the center of many of the most difficult and painful bioethical decisions of our generation. One of the most critical decisions relates to patient competency and the right to refuse treatment. While the right of competent patients to refuse medical care is well established, the desires of incompetent or comatose patients present a great ethical dilemma. Treatment decisions for terminally ill patients who are not able to express their own wishes are often shared among family members, legal guardians, and/or health care providers.

Understandably, health care providers are often reluctant to discontinue medical intervention because it violates their ethical commitment to sustain life, and also because they fear legal repercussions. No less challenging is the ethical issue surrounding the definition of extraordinary or artificial medical intervention for the purpose of sustaining life. For example, medical and legal experts differ on the controversial issue of withdrawing nutrition and hydration supplied through artificial means to a dying patient (101). No less difficult are treatment decisions for severely handicapped newborns as illustrated by the federal government's "Baby Doe regulations," which attempted to establish procedures and guidelines for the care of such infants and to assure that they receive equal protection under the law (102). The challenge for hospitals is to ensure that such decisions are made in a responsible manner, that family and physician viewpoints are exchanged, and that legal guidelines are understood and upheld. Frequently, it is the role of the hospital to serve as facilitator in the ethical decision-making process—a role that requires extreme sensitivity to the interests of all parties.

On December 31, 1991, the Patient Self-Determination Act of 1990 (PSDA) went into effect. The law applies to all health care facilities receiving Medicare or Medicaid funds, including hospitals, and requires them to provide all patients on admission with written information that describes the patient's rights to make decisions regarding medical care, to refuse treatment, and to formulate advance directives. Advance directives refer to the patient's wishes regarding continuation of treatment directives, such as living wills stating treatment preferences and durable power of attorney appointments indicating proxy decision makers.

The intent of the statute is to establish a procedure that ensures increased clarity about the patient's wishes, while creating an environment that makes it more likely that health care professionals will honor the patient's directives. Concerns about the law on the part of health care providers include: 1) possible insensitivity in the process of requiring patients to indicate advance directives, thereby unnecessarily inducing patient anxiety; 2) patients may lack sufficient information about treatment options; 3) the statute requires special training for health care workers; 4) advance directives may overrule other actions in the patient's best interest; and 5) the patient may change his or her mind at a later point in the care process (103). In spite of these concerns, the PSDA represents an important step in integrating patients into medical decisions with significant ethical overtones.

Summary

This chapter has reviewed the historical development and contemporary challenges faced by America's hospitals. Our hospitals are part of a dynamic and changing health care system. They face significant challenges in their dual or competing roles as charitable institutions to serve the poor and businesses functioning within a difficult financial environment (104). They also play important roles in community and professional education. At present, hospitals face new challenges as they expand beyond their traditional boundaries as providers of short-term, acute care to assume growing responsibilities for the delivery of a wide range of health services that correspond to community needs.

Current trends in health care, including the need to provide humane and respectful treatment for acquired immune deficiency syndrome (AIDS) patients, care for the growing elderly population, the health needs of unsponsored patients, and the application of new technological breakthroughs, particularly in the area of genetic engineering, will act to increase the hospital's central role in ethical decision making for health care in the years ahead. This challenge to provide compassionate, quality care that respects the privacy and dignity of all patients will be a critical focus for hospitals and their trustees.

References

1. Levit, K. R., Lazenby, H. C., Cowan, C. A., & Letsch, S. W. (1991). National health expenditures, 1990. *Health Care Financing Review. 13.* 29–54.
2. Shortell, S. M. (1977). Organization of hospital resources. In *Hospitals in the 1980s*. Chicago: American Hospital Association.
3. Williams, S., Shortell, S., Dowling, W., et al. (1978). Hospital sponsored primary care group practice: A developing modality of care. *Health and Medical Care Services Review. 1.* 1–13.
4. Philip, J. (1990, Fourth Quarter). Standard indicators of hospital activity have failed to keep pace with changes of hospitals and in the practice of medicine. *HMO.* 14–17.
5. *Hospital statistics.* (1991). Chicago: American Hospital Association.
6. MacEachern, M. T. (1957). *Hospital organization and management* (3rd ed.). Chicago: Physicians Record Company.
7. Rosenberg, S. (1971). The hospital in America: A century's perspective. In *Medicine and society* (publication 4). Philadelphia: American Philosophical Society Library.
8. Rosen, G. (1963). The hospital—historical sociology of a community institution. In E. Freidson (Ed.). *The hospital in modern society* (pp. 1–36). New York: The Free Press.
9. Corwin, E. H. (1946). *The American hospital* (pp. 193–213). New York: Commonwealth Fund.

10. Starr, P. (1982). *The social transformation of American medicine* (pp. 145–179). New York: Basic Books.

11. Commission of Hospital Care. (1947). Expansion of hospitals, 1840–1900. In *Hospital care in the United States* (pp. 454–526). Cambridge, MA: Harvard University Press.

12. Davis, K. (1962). The hospital's position in American society. In J. Owen (Ed.). *Modern concepts in hospital administration* (pp. 6–16). Philadelphia: Saunders.

13. Flexner, A. (1910). *Medical education in the United States and Canada* (Bulletin No. 4). New York: Carnegie Foundation for the Advancement of Teaching.

14. Coile, R. C., Jr. (1986). *The new hospital: Future strategies for a changing industry*. Rockville, MD: Aspen Publishers.

15. Starr, P. (1982). *The social transformation of American medicine* (p. 290–334). New York: Basic Books.

16. Feldstein, M. (1971). *The rising cost of hospital care*. Washington, DC: Information Resource Press.

17. Siu, A. L., Sonnenberg, F. A., Manning, W. G., et al. (1986). Inappropriate use of hospitals in a randomized trial of health insurance plans. *New England Journal of Medicine. 315*. 1259–1266.

18. Luft, H. S. (1985). Competition and regulation. *Medical Care. 23*. 383–400.

19. Havighurst, C. C. (1986). Changing the locus of decision making in the health care sector. *Journal of Health Politics, Policy and Law. 11*. 697–735.

20. Ohsfeldt, R. L. (1985). Uncompensated medical services provided by physicians and hospitals. *Medical Care. 23*. 1338–1344.

21. Stewart, D. A. (1973). The history and status of proprietary hospitals. *Blue Cross Reports* (Research Series 9). Chicago: Blue Cross Association.

22. Statistics for multihospital health care systems. (1991). *AHA guide*. Chicago: American Hospital Association.

23. Relman, A. S. (1980). The new medical–industrial complex. *New England Journal of Medicine. 303*. 963–970.

24. Relman, A. S. (1985). Selling to the for-profits: Undermining the mission. *Health Progress. 66*. 81–85.

25. Watt, A. J., Derzon, R. A., Renn, S. C., et al. (1968). The comparative economic performance of investor-owned chain and not-for-profit hospitals. *New England Journal of Medicine. 314*. 89–96.

26. Lewin, L. S., Derzon, R. A., & Margulies. (1981). Investor-owned and non-profits differ in economic performance. *Hospital. 55*. 52–58.

27. Pattison, R. V., & Katz, H. M. (1983). Investor-owned and not-for-profit hospitals: Comparison based on California data. *New England Journal of Medicine. 309*. 347–353.

28. Herzlinger, R. E., & Krasker, W. S. (1987). Who profits from nonprofits? *Harvard Business Review. 65*. 93–105.

29. Gray, B. H., & McNerney, W. J. (1986). For-profit enterprise in health care: The Institute of Medicine study. *New England Journal of Medicine. 314*. 1523–1528.

30. Goldsmith, J. C. (1981). *Can hospitals survive?* Homewood, IL: Dow Jones-Irwin.

31. Starr, P. (1982). *The social transformation of American medicine* (pp. 79–144). New York: Basic Books.

32. Georgopoulos, B. A. (Ed.). (1973). *Organizational research in hospitals*. Ann Arbor, MI: University of Michigan Press.

33. Southwick, A. (1973). The hospital as an institution—expanding responsibilities change its relationship with the staff physician. *California Western Law Review. 9*. 429–467.

34. Perkins, R. (1975). The physician's view of the hospital: A love-hate relationship. Parts 1 and 2. *Hospital Medical Staff. 4*. 1–7, 10–14.

35. Perrow, C. (1963). Goals and power structure: A historical care study. In E. Freidson (Ed.). *The hospital in modern society*. New York: The Free Press.

36. Johnson, E. L. (1970). Changing role of the hospital's chief executive officer. *Hosp. Admin. 15*. 21–34.

37. Blankenship, L. V., & Elling, R. H. (1962). Organizational support and community power structure: The hospital. *Journal of Health and Human Behavior. 3*. 257–369.

38. Burling, T., Lentz, E. M., & Wilson, R. N. (1956). The board of trustees. In *The give and take in hospitals* (pp. 39–50). New York: G. P. Putnam's Sons.

39. *Darling v. Charleston Community Memorial Hospital*. (1965). 33 Illinois, 2d. 236 211 ME 2d. 253.

40. Totten, M. K., Orlikoff, J. E., & Ewell, C. M. (1990. *The guide to governance for hospital trustees.*

Chicago: The Hospital Research and Education Trust, American Hospital Association.

41. Guest, R. (1972). The role of a doctor in institutional management. In B. Georgopoulos (Ed.). *Organizational research in health institutions.* Ann Arbor, MI: University of Michigan Press.

42. Reynolds, J., & Stunden, A. E. (1978). The organization of not-for-profit hospital systems. *Health Care Management Review. 3.* 23–36.

43. Morlock, L. L., & Alexander, J. A. (1986). Models of governance in multihospital systems: Implications for hospital and system-level decision-making. *Medical Care. 24.* 1118–1135.

44. Johnson, R. L. (1980). Boards are remodeled and hospitals merge. *Hospitals. 54.* 101–105.

45. Blues, S. M. (1987). New legal standards for trustee performance. *Health Progress. 68.* 60–63, 95.

46. Umbdenstock, R. J. (1987). Refinement of boards' role required. *Health Progress. 68.* 44–49.

47. Bader, B. S. (1986). *Three waves of change: Hospital board responsibilities in the new health care environment.* Rockville, MD: Bader & Associates, Inc.

48. Schulz, R., & Johnson, A. C. (1976). *Management of hospitals* (pp. 147–164). New York: McGraw-Hill.

49. Brozovich, J. P., & Shortell, S. M. (1984). How to create more humane and productive health care environments. *Health Care Management Review, 9.* 43–53.

50. Coile, R. C., Jr., & Pointer, D. D., (1985, May–June). The new age CEO. *Hospital Forum. 28.* 390–41.

51. Accreditation manual for hospitals (pp. 89–104). (1983). Chicago Joint Commission on Accreditation of Hospitals.

52. Harvey, J. D. (1978). The hospital medical director: An administrator's view. In J. S. Rakish and K. Darr (Ed.). *Hospital organization and management* (pp. 132–136). New York: Spectrum Publications.

53. Roemer, M., & Friedman, E. (1971). *Doctors in hospitals.* Baltimore: Johns Hopkins University Press.

54. Shortell, S. M. (1974). Hospital medical staff organization: Structure, process and outcome. *Hospital Administration. 19.* 96–107.

55. Scott, W. R., Flood, A. B., & Ewy, W. (1979). Organizational determinants of services, quality, and cost of care in hospitals. *Milbank Memorial Fund Trustee Quarterly. 57.* 234–264.

56. Shortell, S. M., Becker, S. W., & Neuhauser, D. (1976). The effects of management practices on hospital efficiency and quality of care. In S. M. Shortell & M. Brown (Eds.). *Organizational research in hospitals.* Chicago: Blue Cross Association.

57. Shortell, S. M., & LoGerfo, J. P. (1981). Hospital medical staff organization and quality of care. Results for myocardinal infarction and appendectomy. *Medical Care. 14.* 1041–1056.

58. Eisenberg, J., & Williams, S. (1981). Cost containment and changing physicians' practice behavior. *Journal of the American Medical Association. 246.* 2195–2201.

59. Glandon, G. L., & Morrisey, M. A. (1986). Redefining the hospital-physician relationship under prospective payment. *Inquiry. 23.* 166–175.

60. Grimmelman, F. J. (1981). Are not-for-profit hospitals experiencing a revolution in capital resources? *Topics in Health Care Financing. 7.* 45–55.

61. Newscomer, R., Wood, J., & Sankar, A. (1985). Medicare prospective payment: Anticipated effect on hospitals, other community agencies and families. *Journal of Health Politics, Policy and Law. 10.* 275–282.

62. Kovener, R. J., & Palmer, M. (1983). Implementing the Medicare prospective pricing system. *Health Care Financial Management. 13.* 74–78.

63. Ruffner, J. K. (1986). Product line management: How six healthcare institutions make it work. *Healthcare Forum. 29.* 11–14.

64. Nutter, D. (1984). Access to care and the evolution of corporate, for-profit medicine. *New England Journal of Medicine. 311.* 919.

65. Robinson, B. C., & Barbaccia, J. C. (1982). Acute hospital discharge of older patients and extended control. *Home Health Care Services Quarterly. 3.* 29–57.

66. Placella, L. E. (1986). Choosing a growth strategy. Diversification versus vertical integration. *Trustee. 39.* 26–28.

67. Folland, S. T. (1985). The effects of health care advertising. *Journal of Health, Politics, Policy and Law. 10.* 329–345.

68. Weil, T. P. (1984). Vertical integration: The wave of the future? *Health Care Strategic Management. 4–* 11.

69. Wheeler, J. R. C., Wickizer, T. M., & Shortell, S. M. (1986). Hospital-physician vertical integration. *Hospital and Health Services Administration. 31.* 67–80.

70. Lathrop, J. P. (1991, July/August). The patient-focused hospital. *Healthcare Forum Journal*. 17–20.

71. Casalou, R. F. (1991). Total quality management in health care. *Hospital & Health Administration*. 36. 134–146.

72. Taylor, S. (1975). Hospital patient behavior: Reactance, helplessness or control? *Journal of Social Issues*. 35. 156–184.

73. Ben-Sira, Z. (1983). The structure of a hospital's image. *Medical Care*. 21. 943–954.

74. Wartman, S. A., Morlock, L. L., Malitz, F. E., et al. (1983). Patient understanding and satisfaction and predictors of compliance. *Medical Care*. 21. 886–891.

75. *Washington Report on Medicine and Health*. Washington, DC: McGraw-Hill, February 2, 1987, Vol. 41: p. 2.

76. *Delivery of health care in rural America* (pp. 38–61). (1977). Chicago: American Hospital Association.

77. Health care in rural America: The Crisis unfolds. (1988, May). *National Rural Health Association Report*.

78. Murrin, K. L. (1982). Laying the groundwork: Issues facing rural primary care. In G. H. Bisbee, Jr. (Ed.). *Management of rural primary care concepts and cases* (pp. 1–27). Chicago: The Hospital Research and Education Trust.

79. Rannels, H. W., Ross, D. E., & Waxman, C. R. (1975). The community hospital and regional health care responsibilities—how to do it! *Medical Care*. 13. 885–896.

80. Grim, S. A. (1986). Win/win: Urban and rural hospitals network for survival. *Hospital and Health Services Administration*. 31. 34–36.

81. McNerney, W. J., & Riedel, D. *Regionalization and rural health care* (Research Series No. 2). Ann Arbor, MI: University of Michigan Press.

82. McCormick, B. (1986). Union activity on the rise, new AHA report states. *Hospitals*. 60. 73.

83. Schanie, C. F. (1984). Unionization and hospitals: Causes, effects, and preventive strategies. *Hospital and Health Services Administration*. 29. 68–78.

84. *Taft-Hartley amendments: Implications for the health care field, Report of a symposium*. (1976). Chicago: American Hospital Association.

85. Pointer, D., & Metzger, N. (1975). *The National Labor Relations Act: A guidebook for health care facility administrators* (pp. 41–60). New York: Spectrum Publications.

86. Kilgor, J. G. (1984). Union organizing activity in the hospital industry. *Hospital and Health Services Administration*. 29. 79–90.

87. Wilmor, I. G. (1976). Management's viewpoint. In *Taft-Hartley Amendments: Implications for the health care field* (pp. 78–94). Chicago: American Medical Association.

88. Somers, A. R. (1969). *Hospital regulation: The dilemma of public policy*. Princeton, NJ: Princeton University, Industrial Relations Section.

89. Somers, A. R. (1971). *Health care in transition: Directions for the future* (pp. 132–161). Chicago: The Hospital Research and Education Trust.

90. Bureau of Health Planning and Resource Development, Health Planning Information Service. (1976). *Trends affecting the U.S. health care system* (DHEW Publication No. [HRA] 76-14503). Washington, DC: U.S. Government Printing Office.

91. Salkever, D. S., & Bice, T. W. (1978). Certificate-of-need legislation and hospital costs. In M. Zubkoff, E. Raskin, & R. S. Hanft (Eds.). *Hospital cost containment: Selected notes for future policy* (pp. 429–460). New York: Milbank Memorial Fund.

92. U.S. Congress Public Law 97-35. The Omnibus Budget Reconciliation Act of 1981. Washington, DC: U.S. Government Printing Office.

93. Pardini, A. P., Cohodes, D. R., & Cohen, A. B. (1980). *Certificate of need and high capital cost technology: The case of computerized axial tomographic scanners* (report to the Bureau of Health Planning, HRA DHHS, HRA Contract No. 231-77-1004). Cambridge, MA: Urban Systems Research and Engineering.

94. Dunn, W., & Lefkowitz, B. (1979). The hospital cost containment act of 1977: An analysis of the administration's proposal. In M. Zubkoff, E. Raskin, & R. S. Hanft (Eds.). *Hospital cost containment: Selected notes for future policy* (pp. 166-214). New York: Milbank Memorial Fund.

95. Dowling, W. L. (1976). Prospective rate-setting—concept and practice. *Topics in Health Care Financing*. 2. 1–37.

96. Sloan, F. (1983). Rate regulation for hospital cost control. Evidence from the last decade. *Milbank Memorial Fund Trustee Quarterly*. 61. 195–217.

97. Horn, S. D., Horn, R. A., Sharkey, M. S. (1986).

Severity of illness within DRGs: Homogeneity study. *Medical Care. 24.* 225–235.

98. Iglehart, J. K. (1986). Early experiences with prospective payment of hospitals. *New England Journal of Medicine. 314.* 1460–1464.

99. Goran, M. J., Roberts, J. S., Kellogg, M., et al. (1975). The PSRO hospital review system. *Medical Care. 13 (Suppl.).* 1–33.

100. Darr, K., Longest, B. B., Jr., & Rakish, J. S. (1986). The ethical imperative in health services governance and management. *Hospital and Health Services Administration. 31.* 53–66.

101. Bresnohan, J. F., & Drane, J. F. (1986). A challenge to examine the meaning of living and dying. *Health Progress. 67.* 32–37, 98.

102. Reiser, S. J. (1986). Survival at what cost? Origins and effects of the modern controversy on treating severely handicapped newborns. *Journal of Health Politics, Policy and Law. 11.* 199–214.

103. Wolf, S. M., et al. (1991). Sources of concern about the Patient Self-Determination Act. *New England Journal of Medicine. 325*(23). 1666–1671.

104. Stevens, R. (1989). *In sickness and in wealth: American hospitals in the twentieth century.* New York: Basic Books.

Chapter 7

The Continuum of Long-Term Care

Connie J. Evashwick

Long-term care is one of the greatest challenges facing the health care delivery system. In terms of population need, consumer demand, resource consumption, financing, and system organization, long-term care will be a dominant issue during the coming decades. The components of long-term care each have grown during the past decade. Integration is beginning to occur. In order for the limited available resources to meet increasing demand, the system that currently exists—an under-financed disarray of fragmented services—must evolve into a well-organized, efficient, client-oriented continuum of care.

A case study illustrates the current issues and problems of long-term care.

Mr. Jackson is a 66-year-old successful businessman who lives alone in a third-story suburban apartment. He is generally healthy, but has mild hypertension and is diabetic. One night during the winter he slips on the ice while carrying groceries up the front steps of his building and breaks his hip. A neighbor calls the 911 emergency number and eventually an ambulance arrives. The ambulance takes Mr. Jackson to the emergency room of the nearest hospital. Mr. Jackson cannot be admitted because he does not have proof of insurance, his Medicare care, credit cards, or even his checkbook on hand, and his condition is determined not to be life-threatening. He is thus transferred to another hospital. Mr. Jackson's only physician is an internist who cannot handle a fracture, so Mr. Jackson is operated on by the surgeon on call.

After the surgery, Mr. Jackson spends two weeks in the hospital, one on the surgical floor and one on a step-down unit. His physician stops by to visit, but his care is the responsibility of the surgical residents who change on an undetermined schedule. His employer has recently reduced the health benefits that his group policy covers. His insurance covers only the first 30 days of hospital care, and Medicare picks up some of the uncovered expenses. Nonetheless, he has a daily copay, so he is anxious to be discharged as quickly as possible. The physician recommends that Mr. Jackson go to a rehabilitation hospital. However, the nearest one is in the next town. Instead, Mr. Jackson agrees to spend a week or two at a nursing home until he is able to move about more easily. Mr. Jackson knows that he will be responsible for all payments, since he has no insurance for nursing home care, and Medicare will not cover his convalescence in the nursing home because he does not meet the rather stringent criteria of requiring

177

24-hour nursing care. Despite the cost, he does not feel strong enough to go home alone.

Mr. Jackson hates the nursing home because the staff are always irritable and hurried, and the pleasant ones seem to resign the day after he gets to know them. Most of the patients are quite elderly—i.e., in their late 80s—and little is done to encourage them to become more independent in hopes of going home.

At home, Mr. Jackson must recuperate before he is able to get around easily. He is unable to go down the stairs, let alone to the grocery store, post office, or pharmacy. A neighbor who is a nurse arranges for a homemaker from a local agency to come in three days a week for two hours each day to help him. He is not quite ill enough to qualify for home health care as defined by the regulations of his health insurance or Medicare, i.e., "homebound," thus he pays the home-maker directly. A colleague from work offers to stop by the pharmacy and pick up a prescription for him. As a bachelor, he was accustomed to eating meals out, and never cooked much for himself. A friend arranges for Meals on Wheels to deliver a hot meal at lunch and a cold snack for dinner. However, no food comes on the weekends. Meanwhile, bills begin to flood in from the emergency room, the hospital, the nursing home, several different physicians, and the home health agency. He is not sure what his private insurance will pay, what Medicare will pay, and what he must pay himself.

Mr. Jackson returns to the hospital outpatient department for rehabilitation therapy, but he must depend on one of his neighbors being home to help him get up and down the stairs. He cannot drive, so he calls a cab, which does not always come to the suburbs on time and is expensive. The therapists at the outpatient department are different from those in the hospital or at the nursing home, and Mr. Jackson feels as though no one quite knows what has clinically happened to him. His insurance does not cover outpatient rehabilitation, but the office clerks tell him that Medicare Part B may cover the services.

Mr. Jackson struggles along for several weeks and eventually is able to return to work. He believes that the medical care and therapy he received have been of good quality. However, he also comes out of the experience with huge bills and negative feelings about the imper-sonality of the health care system, the high costs and low insurance coverage for long-term care, the frag-mentation of services and payment, and the frustrating helplessness—even on the part of professionals—in mo-bilizing resources to facilitate the simple functions of daily living. He realizes that if he were 20 years older, were no longer covered by his employer's insurance, had spent much of his savings, and lived in an isolated two-story house rather than in an apartment complex filled with friends and neighbors, his experience would have been far worse.

The implications? The existing formal system of providing care to persons with long-term, complex problems is both complicated and inadequate. With some notable exceptions, the LTC system func-tions due to individual and informal relationships. On a broad scale, it is disorganized, underfunded, highly regulated, too costly, and most of all, it does not consistently meet the needs of consumers or providers. The demand for long-term care, as de-scribed below, will grow exponentially during the coming years. The Baby Boom generation will swell the population of older adults early in the next decade and consumer interest in arranging services will likely soar. This growth, in turn, will exacerbate the forces that are already prompting change in the organization and financing of the health care delivery system.

This chapter describes the various facets of long-term care as they exist in the 1990s. It also presents a conceptual framework for understanding how the ragged pieces can be molded into a rational system for the future.

What Is Long-Term Care?

Long-term care refers to health, mental health, social, and residential services provided to tem-porarily or chronically disabled persons over an extended period of time with a goal of enabling them to function as independently as possible. There is no single regulatory or academic defini-tion of long-term care. The several definitions be-low collectively convey the concept. Long-term care has been defined as:

The array of medical, social, and support services for individuals in nursing homes or in the community, who, for an extended period of time, are dependent on others for physical assistance (1).

A wide range of services that address the social, custo-dial, and medical needs of individuals who lack some capacity for self-care and whose continuing incapacity will necessitate the provision of care for a relatively long, indefinite period of time (2).

Those services designed to provide diagnostic, preventive, therapeutic, rehabilitative, supportive, and maintenance services for individuals of all age groups who have chronic physical and/or mental impairments, in a variety of institutional and noninstitutional settings, including the home, with the goal of promoting optimum levels of physical, social, and psychological functioning (3).

One or more services provided on a sustained basis to enable individuals whose functional capacities are chronically impaired to be maintained at their maximum level of health and well-being (4).

A range of services that address the health, personal care, and social needs of individuals who lack some capacity for self-care. Services may be continuous or intermittent but are delivered for a sustained period to individuals who have a demonstrated need, usually measured by some index of functional dependence (5).

Health and social services provided within or outside institutions over extended periods to chronically ill, functionally impaired persons, most of whom are elderly (6).

- long-term care is targeted at those with *functional disabilities.* The basis for these disabilities may be physical or mental, temporary or permanent;
- the goal is to promote or maintain health and *independence in functional abilities* and quality of life. For the terminally ill, the goal is to enable them to die peacefully and with dignity;
- the multiple services required, the professions involved, and the settings of care span *a broad spectrum;* and
- care is orchestrated around the unique needs of the individual and family.

Who Needs Long-Term Care?

The primary consumers of long-term care are persons who have chronic or long-term, complex health problems and functional disabilities. Clients can thus be divided into two types: those requiring shorter term care and those requiring longer term or permanent long-term care (7).

The first group includes those who have relatively short-term problems but ones that require orchestration of a complex set of services. This group includes those with acute injury or illness who ultimately will achieve complete recovery or independence but who require an extended period of convalescence or treatment. People with specific diseases, not necessarily characterized initially by functional disability, may also require complex, comprehensive care for a prolonged period of time. For example, those suffering from cancer, cataracts, hip fractures, or accident trauma may use, for a shorter period of time, some of the same long-term care services as those with permanent functional disabilities.

The second group is the traditional long-term care population: those who have ongoing *(chronic)* and multiple health, mental health, and/or social problems and who are unable to care for themselves *(functionally disabled)* and thus require nursing or supportive health care for a longer period of time.

Chronic usually connotes permanent, or at least indefinite. For technical data collection purposes, chronic is defined by the National Health Interview Survey as any condition that lasts three months (or 90 days) or more. Chronic conditions may be as life-threatening as coronary artery disease or as harmless as mild arthritis.

Functional ability has been described as a person's ability to perform the basic activities of daily living. Initially defined by Katz and colleagues, commonly accepted measures and scales of functioning are the product of years of research. These are referred to as activities of daily living (ADL) (8) and instrumental activities of daily living (IADL) (9). Activities of daily living include the ability to eat, dress, perform personal care and grooming, transfer from bed to chair, bathe, walk, and maintain bowel and bladder continence. The instrumental activities of daily living include handling monetary affairs, telephoning, grocery shopping, housekeeping, doing chores, and arranging for transportation. Functional disability increases with age. Of those age 65–74, less than one in six, or 14 percent, is disabled, while nearly three out of five, or 58 percent, of those age 85 and older are disabled (10).

Chronic illness and functional disabilities are interrelated and both increase with age. The majority of chronic problems are permanent, and thus the prevalence of chronic conditions increases with age. Of persons age 65 and older, 80 percent have at least one chronic health problem, and the majority have multiple problems. Table 7-1 shows the prevalence of the top 10 chronic conditions among older adults. Chronic diseases are accompanied by functional disabilities. The older one gets, the greater the likelihood of functional disabilities. Table 7-2 shows the prevalence of functional disabilities by age. Disabilities may be due to physical or mental problems. Estimates are that 25 percent of those age 85 and older have Alzheimer's or a related dementia (12). The number of persons with Alzheimer's disease and other dementias will also increase as the population ages, to as many as 6 million by 2040 (12).

The changing demographic composition of the United States will make long-term care an increasingly significant aspect of the health care system. The number of people over the age of 65 will increase from 32 million in 1990 to 65 million in 2030 (figure 7-1) (11). The very old—those over age 85—will increase the most rapidly in terms of numbers and percentage. As stated above, the very old are the most disabled and those who most need long-term care. As the number of old and very old people increases, the need for long-term care will rise (table 7-3).

Because women outnumber men among the very old, long-term care is often associated with women. However, men, too, need long-term care. The Veterans Administration (VA) is facing the challenge of caring for aged veterans, the vast majority of whom are men (13,14,15). In 1988, of the 27.3 million total veterans, 5.7 million, or 24 percent, were age 65 or older. By the year 2000, 8.9 million, or 37 percent of veterans, will be seniors, and by 2020, 7.7 million, or 45 percent of living veterans, will be age 65 or above (assuming there are no new major wars) (16). The VA, which has its own health care services, faces the same challenge as the public and private sectors in trying to construct an efficient, integrated system to care for those with multifaceted, chronic illnesses and functional dependencies.

The total demand for long-term care will include

TABLE 7-1. Top Ten Chronic Conditions Among Older Adults Prevalence per 1000 People

	Adults Age 65+	Adults Age 45–64
Arthritis	480	285
Hypertension	394	251
Hearing impairment	296	136
Heart conditions	277	123
Orthopedic impairment	173	162
Sinusitis	169	187
Cataracts	141	21
Diabetes	98	64
Visual impairment	95	46
Tinnitus	85	49

SOURCE: National Center for Health Statistics. (1987, October). Current estimates from the National Health Interview Survey, United States, 1986. *Vital and Health Statistics.* Series 10. *164.*

TABLE 7-2. Functional Disability Among Older Adults

Age	Needs Help with One or More Activities of Daily Living* (Percent)	Needs Help with One or More Instrumental Activities of Daily Living** (Percent)
65–69	14.7	19.9
70–74	21.1	24.7
75–79	24.1	29.2
80–85	34.4	40.0
85+	49.8	55.2

*Activities of daily living include bathing, dressing, eating, getting in and out of bed and chairs, walking, going outside, and toileting.
**Instrumental activities of daily living include preparing meals, shopping for personal items, managing money, using the telephone, doing heavy housework, and doing light housework.
SOURCE: Adapted from Dawson, D., Hendershot, G., & Fulton, J. (1987, June 10). Aging in the eighties: Functional limitations of individuals 65 and over. *Advance Data. 133.* (National Center for Health Statistics.)

younger people who are disabled. Additional population groups requiring long-term care include those with mental conditions, neurological diseases or degenerative neurological conditions, ac-

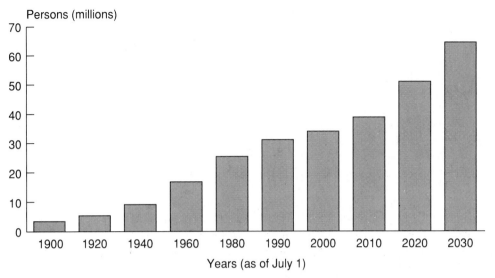

Figure 7-1. Number of persons 65+: 1900 to 2030 (in millions) (NOTE: Increments in years on horizontal scale are uneven.) (SOURCE: U.S. Bureau of the Census, Current Population Reports, Direct Communication.)

TABLE 7-3. Three Projections of the Disabled Elderly or Elderly Using Long-Term Care Services

	Total Using Care	Setting	
		Home	Institution
Brookings Institution Projections of Elderly Using Long-Term Care Services, 2018			
Baseline	10.38	6.36	4.02
Low Disability	8.91	5.88	3.03
High Disability	12.90	7.88	5.02
Urban Institute Projections of the Disabled Elderly, 2030			
Baseline	23.49	19.17	4.32
Low Mortality	27.39	22.09	5.29
Low Mortality/Disability	25.15	20.90	4.26
Duke University Projections of Disabled Elderly, 2020			
Baseline	12.68	10.13	2.55
Low Mortality	13.70	10.93	2.77
Low Disability	10.10	8.10	2.36

SOURCES: General Accounting Office. (1991). *Long-term care: Projected needs of the aging baby boom generation* (Appendix II and III) (GAO Publication No. [HRD] 91-86). Washington, DC: U.S. Government Printing Office. For a complete explanation and details, see original references: Rivlin, A., et al. (1988). *Caring for the disabled elderly: Who will pay?* Washington, DC: The Brookings Institution; Zedlewski, S., et al. (1990). *The needs of the elderly in the 21st century.* Washington, DC: The Urban Institute; Manton, K. (1989). Epidemiological, demographic and social correlates of disability among the elderly. *The Milbank Memorial Fund Quarterly. 67.* Suppl 2, Pt 1, pp. 13–58.

cidents resulting in paralysis, children with chronic congenital abnormalities, paralyzing strokes, end-stage cancer, blindness, early Alzheimer's disease, and acquired immunodeficiency syndrome/AIDS-related complex (AIDS/ARC). For example, nearly a half-million people are blind (17). An additional 11.5 million are visually impaired. One and a half million people have serious vision handicaps, such as being unable to read, that they may not be able to do the instrumental activities of daily living. Nearly 50,000 people lose their sight each year; half of these are seniors. However, one in 20 children also has a serious vision problem. The blind require assistance with the functions of daily living and, when ill, require all the more help.

The number of people who are HIV-positive, and thus likely to become AIDS/ARC victims, had grown to almost 200,000 in 1991 (18). Unless a cure or vaccine is found, these numbers will continue to grow during the decade of the 1990s. The majority of HIV-positive people will need long-term care at some stage of their illness.

People with functional disabilities need help to perform the ADLs and the IADLs; the majority of this care is provided by family and friends on an informal basis. Determining the population requiring formal care mandates an understanding of the terms and subsets of the population and the expected growth of each, tempered by projections of advances in biomedical technology, changes in the work force, and other demographic and clinical factors.

Several groups have attempted to estimate the number of people who will require long-term care in the future. Projections vary based on the definition of "disabled," population projections, and expectations about whether changes in biomedical technology will increase life while decreasing disability or increase life and thereby increase disability. Of the populations requiring long-term care listed above, two-thirds are elderly (19). Projections of the number of disabled elderly range from as low as 8.9 million in 2018 to as high as 27 million in 2030. Table 7-3 compares three disability pro-

jections from three sources, breaking down the total number of disabled elderly into the location of residence where they will receive care. An additional 50 percent can be added to the projections to take into account the younger population that will also require care.

The consumer demand for long-term care must include caregivers and employers, as well as the disabled themselves. Caregiving, which has always existed, became recognized as a health care issue during the 1980s. For the first time in history, the average American family had more parents than children (20). In the late 1980s, it was estimated that women spend an average of 17 years of their lives caring for their children and 18 years caring for their parents (20). Trends toward increasing number of women working and smaller families mean that in the future, the United States will face a significant decline in available family caregivers at the same time that the population in need of help increases dramatically.

The average caregiver for older adults is a married woman in her late 40s or 50s (20,21). Twenty-five to 35 percent of caregivers for the elderly are over age 65 themselves, and 10 percent are over age 75 (20).

Caregivers are susceptible to health problems. The physical and emotional demands of caregiving can be extensive. When caregivers can no longer meet the needs of the functionally disabled person, they often turn to a nursing home. The health care system has begun to accommodate this situation by organizing services for caregivers, such as respite, educational programs, counseling, and support groups.

Employers have recognized that caregiving adds to their costs both in the health consequences for caregivers and the days of work lost due to caregiving responsibilities. The Travelers Company was one of the first businesses to study the prevalence of caregiving. In a 1985 survey, the company found that 28 percent of its employees age 30 or older cared for an aged parent an average of 10 hours a week (22). The productive time lost by employees in caring for elderly relatives is estimated to cost American businesses $10–15 billion each year (23).

As a result, employers have set up programs to facilitate caregiving, thereby reducing stress and time lost while enabling employees to fulfill their responsibilities to their family members. A well-organized system of long-term care is sought not only by those suffering from complex chronic illnesses but by family, friends, employers, providers, and payors.

How Is Long-Term Care Organized?

Eighty to 90 percent of long-term care is provided by friends and family (24). The formal system of providing long-term care has no single structure or financing. Rather, each community has its own combination of available resources, funding sources, and organization. A distinct arrangement is made for each individual and is usually more informal than formal. A major dilemma in long-term care is the incongruence between ideal long-term care services and how they actually are.

As described above, long-term care is designed for people who require multiple and ongoing health, mental health, and social support services over an extended period of time and whose needs are likely to change. The ideal system is thus one that provides comprehensive, integrated care on an ongoing basis and offers various levels of intensity that change as a client's needs change. The goal is to provide the medical and related support services that enable a person to maximize his or her functional independence. This contrasts with the goal of acute care, which is to "cure" the patient of an illness. Many clients may use only select components of the system and may remain involved with the organized system of care for a relatively short period of time; others may use only a limited and stable set of services over a prolonged period of time.

This ideal system of long-term care is referred to throughout the remainder of this chapter as the *continuum of care*. A continuum of care is defined as:

a client-oriented system composed of both services and integrating mechanisms that guides and tracks patients over time through a comprehensive array of health, mental health and social services spanning all levels of intensity of care (25).

The continuum of care concept extends beyond traditional definitions of long-term care. A continuum of care is a comprehensive, coordinated *system of care* designed to meet the needs of patients with complex and/or ongoing problems efficiently and effectively. A continuum is more than a collection of fragmented services. It includes mechanisms for organizing those services and operating them as an integrated system.

The goal is to facilitate the client's access to the appropriate services at the appropriate time quickly and efficiently. Ideally, a continuum of care:

- Matches resources to the patient's condition
- Monitors the client's condition and changes services as the needs change
- Coordinates the care of many professionals and disciplines
- Integrates care provided in a range of settings
- Streamlines patient flow
- Maintains a comprehensive record incorporating clinical, financial, and utilization data

By doing the above, a true continuum of care should: 1) achieve cost-effectiveness by maximizing the use of resources; and 2) enhance quality through appropriateness and continuity of care.

Services in the Continuum

More than 80 distinct services could be identified in the complete continuum of care. For simplicity, the services are grouped into seven categories: extended care, acute inpatient care, ambulatory care, home care, outreach, wellness, and housing. Table 7-4 lists the major services within these categories. This chapter approaches the contin-

TABLE 7-4. Services of the Continuum of Care

EXTENDED
__Skilled nursing facilities
__Step-down units
__Swing beds
__Nursing home follow up

ACUTE
__Med/sur inpatient unit
__Psychiatric inpatient unit
__Rehabilitation inpatient unit
__Interdisciplinary assessment team
__Consultation service

AMBULATORY
__Physicians' offices
__Outpatient clinics
__Interdisciplinary assessment clinics
__Day hospital
__Adult day care
__Mental health clinic
__Satellite clinics
__Psychosocial counseling
__Alcohol and substance abuse

HOME CARE
__Home health—Medicare
__Home health—private
__Hospice
__High technology
__Durable medical equipment
__Home visitors
__Home-delivered meals
__Homemaker and personal care

OUTREACH & LINKAGE
__Screening
__Information and referral
__Telephone contact
__Emergency response system
__Transportation
__Senior membership program

WELLNESS & HEALTH PROMOTION
__Educational programs
__Exercise programs
__Recreational and social groups
__Senior volunteers
__Congregate meals
__Support groups

HOUSING
__Continuing care retirement communities
__Independent senior housing
__Congregate care facilities
__Adult family homes
__Assisted living

Reprinted with permission from: Evashwick, C. (1987). Definition of the continuum of care. In C. Evashwick & L. Weiss (Eds.). *Managing the continuum of care*. Rockville, MD: Aspen Publishers, Inc., p. 28.

uum of care from the perspective of health care. In theory and practice, the continuum concept also applies to the social service and mental health spheres. Thus, additional services could be included, such as legal counseling, retirement planning, and guardianship.

In brief, the seven categories represent the basic types of health care assistance that a person would need over time, through periods of both wellness and illness.

Extended inpatient care is for people who are so sick or functionally disabled that they require ongoing nursing and support services provided in a formal health care institution, but who are not so acutely ill that they require the technological and professional intensity of a hospital. The majority of extended-care facilities are referred to as nursing homes, although this is a broad term that includes many levels and types of programs.

Acute inpatient care is hospital care for those

who have a major and acute health care problem. For the majority of people, a typical hospital stay of five to eight days is the intensive aspect of a longer spell of illness, preceded by diagnostic testing and succeeded by follow-up care.

Ambulatory care services are provided in a formal health care facility, whether a physician's office or the outpatient clinic of a hospital, and provide a wide spectrum of preventive, maintenance, diagnostic, and recuperative services for people who manifest a variety of conditions, from those who are entirely healthy and simply want an annual checkup to those with major health problems who are recuperating from hospitalization.

Home care represents a variety of nursing, therapy, and support services provided to people who are homebound and have some degree of illness but who are able to satisfy their needs by bringing services into the home setting. Home health programs range from formal organizations providing skilled nursing care to relatively informal networks that arrange housekeeping for friends.

Outreach programs make health and social services readily available in the community rather than within the formidable walls of a large institution. Health fairs in shopping centers, senior membership programs, and emergency response systems are all forms of outreach. They are targeted at the healthy or mildly ill to keep them connected with the health care system.

Wellness programs are provided for those who are basically healthy and want to stay that way by actively engaging in health promotion. Wellness programs include health education classes, exercise programs, and health screenings.

Housing for frail populations increasingly includes access to health and support services and, conversely, recognizes that the home setting affects health. Housing incorporating health care ranges from independent apartments affiliated with a health care system that sends a nurse to do weekly blood-pressure checks, to assisted living with nursing and social services provided around the clock on site.

The order of the categories and the services comprising them can vary. The categories can be appropriately reordered on the basis of the dimension being considered: duration of stay, intensity of care, stage of illness, disciplines of professionals, type of facility, and availability of informal support. Within each category are health, mental health, and social services, potentially provided by professional clinicians, provider organizations, families, and/or patients themselves. A more accurate diagram would be a multidimensional matrix showing the interrelationship of all of these factors in caring for a single individual and family. Such a matrix would be dynamic, not static, for the relationships would be different for each individual client and would change over time as the client's needs changed.

Within the categories, as well as between them, the services of the continuum are distinct. Each has different regulatory, financing, target population, staffing, and physical requirements. Each has its own admission policies, patient treatment protocols, and billing system. Each organization has its own referral and discharge networks. A primary reason for ongoing services into a continuum is to achieve integration; yet the differences among services make unified planning and operations quite difficult. One challenge faced by administrators in the initial creation of a continuum of care is that each service must be dealt with separately and brought into a cohesive whole.

The continuum of care is so extensive that it is unlikely that any single organization can offer a complete continuum for all of its clients. The goal of the provider should be to facilitate *access* for clients to the services they need. In brief, an organization need not have all services under its direct ownership or control. Rather, it may have a variety of formal and informal relationships with other providers in the community.

The trend in the 1980s was for organizations to broaden the scope of the services provided and lay the groundwork for the continuum of care to be created during the 1990s. Some organizations bought others, some started new entities, some simply added new staff and new divisions. The incentives were several and continue as present trends:

- Tight funding in all sectors of health care prompted organizations to diversify, thereby adding new streams of revenue. Conversely, those organizations too small or too financially troubled to make it on their own often joined larger organizations that offered complementary rather than duplicative services.
- Hospitals, the dominant provider organizations, reacted to the prospective payment system imposed in the early 1980s by adding less acute services to their sphere of control as a way to maximize payment (or minimize loss) from Medicare.
- Those organizations attuned to the changes in consumer demand realized that patients and families want comprehensive care rather than fragmentation and will choose providers accordingly.
- Employers have become more directly involved in health care and have sought both comprehensive and cost-effective care for their employees, often negotiating directly with providers rather than through third-party insurers.
- Managed care emerged as a strong, if not dominant, payor for the future. Asking providers to share in the risk is becoming common. Providers have realized that the more services they can offer and control, the more they can profit.
- As the population ages, all industry sectors have begun to realize the demands of older adults and to restructure their services and products to appeal to older consumers. Hence, retirement communities, insurance companies, health care providers, as well as commercial companies and other service providers, are seeking to meet expectations of older consumers and their families. Health care organizations are beginning to acknowledge that older adults are a large segment, if not the majority, of their clients, and they no longer accept the high costs and fragmentation of the past.

In brief, the 1980s and early 1990s saw the expansion of long-term care services and the recognition that fragmented services do not meet the need of those with multifaceted, chronic conditions. This groundwork of service availability, collaboration, and consumer responsiveness is a prerequisite for a continuum of care.

Integrating Mechanisms for the Continuum

By definition, a continuum of care is more than a fragmented collection of services. It is an integrated system of care. To gain the system benefits of efficiencies of operation, smooth patient flow, and quality of service, integrating mechanisms are essential. Four integrating management systems are essential: interentity structure, care coordination, information systems and financing.

Interentity structure means that management arrangements and operating policies are in place to enable services to coordinate care, facilitate smooth patient flow, and maximize use of professional staff and other resources. Examples include product line management organization, joint planning committees, transfer arrangements, and negotiated budgeting.

Care coordination refers to the coordination of the clinical components of care, usually by a combination of a dedicated person and established processes that facilitate communication among professionals of various disciplines at multiple sites.

Integrated information systems refer to one patient record that combines financial, clinical, and utilization information to be used by multiple providers and payors across multiple sites.

Integrated financing removes barriers to continuity and appropriateness of care by having adequate financing for long-term care as well as acute care, preferably paid by a capitated system.

Figure 7-2 presents a schematic diagram of the services and integrating mechanisms of the continuum. The following sections describe in detail select services and the four basic integrating mechanisms.

Hospitals and Long-Term Care

The common vision of the acute hospital is one of complicated machines, bustling staff, and patients arriving and then departing quickly, cured of their ailments. In reality, the hospital plays a significant role in providing the continuum of long-term care.

Of the 6,649 hospitals in the United States in 1990, 508, or nearly 8 percent, were long-term (26). By definition, these hospitals care for patients who have an average length of stay longer than 25 days. The characteristics are shown in table 7-5.

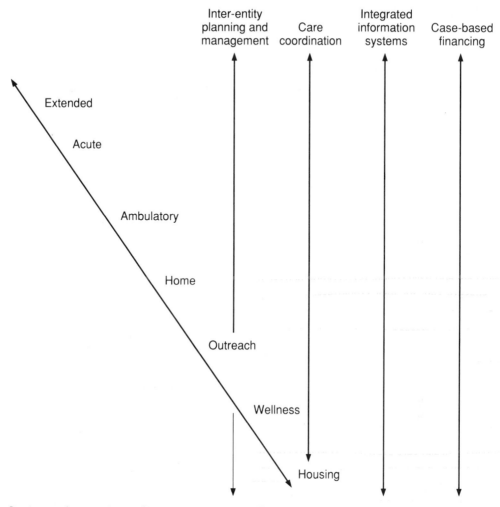

Figure 7-2. Continuum of care services and integrating mechanisms. The seven categories and sixty-plus services of the continuum of care can be ordered on several dimensions; the order thus can vary. The integrating mechanisms are management systems that encompass and coordinate services of all categories. (Reprinted with permission from: Evashwick, C. (1987). Definition of the continuum of care. In C. Evashwick & L. Weiss. *Managing the continuum of care*. Rockville, MD: Aspen Publishers, p. 25.)

A high proportion of long-stay hospitals are psychiatric and are integral parts of the continuum of care for the mentally ill. Long-term hospitals represent 13.6 percent of the annual admissions to hospitals. On any given day, 17.6 percent, or nearly one in five, of the people in a hospital are in a long-term hospital. Thus the importance of long-term hospitals as providers of care cannot be ignored.

In addition to long-term hospitals, community hospitals provide many of the services of the continuum of care. Nationwide surveys conducted in 1981 (27) and 1985 (28) to ascertain the activities of hospitals in long-term care and geriatrics demonstrated that hospitals provide a wide array of programs and services that reach patients and families before and after a stay in the inpatient unit. Hospital activities for the older and long-term care populations received considerable attention during the decade of the 1980s (29,30,31) and are likely

TABLE 7-5. Long-Term Hospitals in the United States, 1990

	Hospitals	Beds	Admissions	Occu.	Avg. Daily Census
All U.S.	6,649	1,213,000	33,774,000	69.5	844,000
Short-term	6,141	1,047,851	33,301,614	76.0	702,156
Long-term	508	165,476	471,960	85.6	141,568
General	31	11,599	80,225	78.4	9,093
Psychiatric	382	131,356	3,428,578	86.1	113,103
TB	3	355	638	65.4	232
All other	125	22,166	72,519	86.3	19,140

SOURCE: Adapted from *AHA hospital statistics, 1991–2 edition* (table 1, 2A, 2B). (1991). Chicago: American Hospital Association.

TABLE 7-6. Long-Term Care Services Offered by Hospitals, 1990

	Number (N = 6,105)	Percent (100.00)
Adult day care	427	7.0
AIDS/ARC unit	146	2.4
Alcohol/drug abuse outpatient services	1,508	24.7
Alzheimer's diagnostic assessment services	570	9.3
Arthritis treatment center	418	6.8
Cardiac rehabilitation program	2,148	35.2
Chronic obstructive pulmonary disease services	3,647	58.7
Comprehensive geriatric assessment	1,202	19.7
Emergency response systems	1,853	30.4
Geriatric care unit	666	10.9
Geriatric clinics	461	7.6
Geriatric psychiatry	1,652	27.1
Respite care	1,005	16.5
Senior membership programs	1,159	19.0
Home health services	1,921	31.5
Hospice	868	14.2
Outpatient rehabilitation	2,924	47.9

SOURCE: Adapted from *AHA hospital statistics, 1991–92 edition* (table 12A). (1991). Chicago: American Hospital Association.

to continue during the 1990s (32,33). Table 7-6 shows some of the geriatric and chronic care services offered by hospitals at the beginning of the decade.

Many hospitals also own, contract with, or operate freestanding nursing homes and hospital-based step-down units. These enable the hospital to continue to care for patients who are not yet ready to be discharged into the community but whose needs can be met in an institutional setting less intense than that of the acute hospital. In 1990, 1,321 hospitals, or nearly one of every five short-term, nonfederal hospitals, had a hospital-based skilled nursing unit (34).

Rehabilitation is yet another long-term service offered by hospitals. Patients who are discharged quickly from a short-term inpatient stay often continue to receive therapy for months. They may transfer to a rehabilitation hospital or unit for intense therapy; be transferred to skilled nursing to regain their strength, then transferred to a rehabilitation unit; or sent home and return as an outpatient to the hospital or a freestanding outpatient rehabilitation center. In 1990, the United States had 128 rehabilitation hospitals and an additional 781 rehabilitation units in other general and special hospitals, with a total of 28,940 beds (35).

Federal hospitals, short-stay as well as long-stay, include Veterans Administration (VA) facilities. The VA operates its own continuum of care for veterans, which is "the largest coordinated system of health and long-term care services in the world" (36). VA complexes often include short-stay hospitals, long-stay hospitals or units within the acute hospital, geriatric evaluation units (GEUs), skilled nursing facilities or units, adult day care, hospice, home health, residential care homes, and respite (37). The VA has also been in the forefront of developing geriatric research, education, and clinical centers (GRECCs). Since 1975, the VA has established 15 GRECCS, which are based in VA hospitals throughout the nation. Previously, the largest proportion of the VA budget was for hospital care. As noted earlier, by 2020, 45 percent of veterans will be age 65 or older. Thus, in the future, the most rapidly increasing portion of the VA health care budget will be for long-term care (38).

The rationale for hospitals to be involved in long-term care is clear. Nationally, 34 percent of hospital discharges and 46 percent of hospital inpatient days are for persons age 65 and older (39). One in four older adults is admitted to the hospital each year, and, of those admitted, more than 50 percent are readmitted at least once. As noted above, the health problems of seniors are characterized as chronic and multifaceted. For hospitals to provide high-quality care to seniors, they must address the needs of these patients beyond the few days spent in the hospital. As the older population grows in number and proportion, hospitals will be faced with an increasing demand for comprehensive, coordinated, continuing care by senior consumers and their families.

The trend toward outpatient care also contributes to the hospital's role in providing long-term care. Futurists project that by the year 2000 more than half of a hospital's income will derive from outpatient services (40). The more that can be done on an outpatient basis, the more patients who are admitted are those with multiple and/or long-term conditions who need multifaceted, continuing care.

A third trend prompting hospitals' involvement in the continuum of care is financial. As comprehensive, capitated, and managed care payment systems grow, the acute hospital finds it financially advantageous, and essential from a marketing standpoint, to provide a spectrum of services. To ensure viable financial performance, the hospital must manage access to services beyond those of acute inpatient care. Diversification of owning and operating multiple levels of service may also contribute to the hospital's revenues.

Today's hospital cannot realistically expect to remain in business by providing only short-term, curative care. The 1980s saw the beginning of hospital diversification into a wide array of services, including long-term care. The 1990s has seen the refinement of hospitals developing comprehensive continuums of care that combine not only services but integrating mechanisms as well (41). Hospitals with vision will concentrate on refinement and expansion of the integrating mechanisms during the 90s to give their patients access to care over time.

Nursing Homes

Nursing home is a broad term than encompasses a wide spectrum of facilities ranging from three-bed privately-owned adult residential care homes to 20-bed units of acute community hospitals to 1,200-bed government-operated institutions. *Convalescent home, retirement center, long-term care facility care center,* and other similar terms have no specific meaning. Nursing homes may be freestanding, units of hospitals, or integral parts of a

TABLE 7-7. Characteristics of Nursing Homes, 1973–74 and 1985

	1973–74	1985
Number of homes	15,700	19,100
Beds	1,177,300	1,624,200
Full-time-equivalent employees	485,400	793,600
FTE/s per 100 beds	41.2	48.9
Current residents	1,075,800	1,491,400
Annual discharges	1,077,500	1,223,500
Annual admissions	1,110,800	1,299,200
Occupancy	86.5	91.6

SOURCE: Strahan, G. (1987, March 27). Nursing home characteristics, preliminary data from the 1985 National Nursing Home Survey. *Advance data from vital and health statistics* (DHHS Publication No. [PHS] 87-1250). Hyattsville, MD: Public Health Service, National Center for Health Statistics.

campus of care retirement centers. Many facilities have a combination of skilled nursing care and personal-care beds. The common feature is that a person who is not able to remain at home alone due to physical health problems, mental health problems, or functional disabilities resides at the facility. They are thus called "residents" rather than "patients." Residents may stay for a few days or an indefinite period of time.

Each state licenses long-term care facilities, and each has its own licensing requirements, reimbursement policies, governing regulations, classification systems, and terminology. As part of the regulatory process, each state establishes its own definitions of nursing homes and related long-term care institutions.

For data collection purposes, the National Center for Health Statistics defined nursing homes in 1985 as "facilities with three beds or more with nursing or personal care available to the residents." The most recent NCHS survey was done in 1985 (42). This survey reported 19,100 nursing homes with 1,624,200 beds. Table 7-7 gives key characteristics. The data do not include some step-down units of hospitals, intermediate care facilities for the mentally retarded, or supportive-living residences licensed by some states.

The findings of the 1985 study describe the nursing home component of the continuum of care (43). Three-fourths of nursing homes are proprietary; 20 percent are nonprofit; and the remaining 5 percent are owned and operated by federal, state, or local governments. Two-fifths of nursing homes belong to a chain; about half are independent. Nursing homes tend to be small: one-third have fewer than 50 beds; one-third have 50–99 beds; only 6 percent have 200 beds or more. Homes that are part of a chain have a larger average number of beds. Table 7-8 shows select characteristics of nursing homes.

As is evident from table 7-7, the nursing home field has grown during the past two decades. From the 1973–74 survey to the 1985 survey, the number of nursing homes increased by 22 percent and the number of beds increased 38 percent. The number of residents increased, as did the average occupancy. The demand for nursing home care is expected to increase further in the future as the population ages.

Nursing homes may be certified by Medicare (federal) and Medicaid (state) to accept patients whose care is paid for by the respective program (table 7-8). To be certified by Medicare, a nursing home must qualify under Medicare's regulations for a "skilled nursing facility" (SNF). The former certification categories for Medicaid of "skilled nursing facility (SNF)" and "intermediate care facility (ICF)" have been combined. Medicaid now recognizes one category of "nursing facilities." In 1985, three-fourths of all nursing homes were certified for Medicare or Medicaid. The remaining 25 percent were smaller in bed size and represented only 11 percent of total nursing home beds. In addition, most step-down units of acute-care hospitals are certified for participation in Medicare.

Nursing homes operate on a very tight margin; high occupancy is critical. Compared to hospitals, which had an average occupancy in 1990 of less than 63 percent, the vast majority of nursing homes must stay at higher than 90 percent occupancy to maintain financial viability.

In 1990, the average cost of nursing home care

TABLE 7-8. Characteristics of Nursing Homes, 1985

| | Nursing Homes | | Nursing Home Beds | | Beds Per Home |
	Number	Percent	Number	Percent	
Total Number of Homes	19,100	100	1,624,200	100	85.0
Ownership					
Proprietary	14,300	74.9	1,121,500	69.0	78.4
Voluntary nonprofit	3,800	19.9	370,700	22.8	97.6
Government	1,000	5.2	131,900	8.1	131.9
Certification					
Certified	14,400	75.4	1,441,300	88.7	100.1
Not Certified	4,700	24.6	182,900	11.3	38.9
Bed Size					
Less than 50 beds	6,300	33.0	151,100	9.3	23.9
50–99 beds	6,200	32.5	444,300	27.4	71.7
100–199 beds	5,400	28.3	702,100	43.2	130.0
200 beds or more	1,200	6.3	326,700	20.1	272.3
Census Region					
Northeast	4,400	23.0	371,100	22.8	84.3
North Central	5,600	29.3	531,700	32.7	94.9
South	6,100	31.9	488,300	30.1	80.0
West	3,000	15.7	233.100	14.4	77.7
Affiliation					
Chain	7,900	41.4	800,000	49.3	101.3
Independent	10,000	52.4	680,700	41.9	68.1
Government	1,100	5.8	131,900	8.1	119.9
Unknown	100	.5	11,600	0.7	116.0

SOURCE: Strahan, G. (1987, March 27). Nursing home characteristics, preliminary data from the 1985 National Nursing Home Survey. *Advance data from vital and health statistics* (table 2). (DHHS Publication No. [PHS] 87-1250. Hyattsville, MD: Public Health Service.

ranged from $2,000 to $4,000 per month, depending upon the state and type of facility. Payment for nursing home care (44) is made primarily by Medicaid (45 percent) and private individuals and families (48 percent). Medicare pays only about 2 percent of the annual costs of nursing home care. Veterans Administration, private insurance, and other payors account for the remainder. The heavy dependence on state Medicaid payments poses a financial challenge for nursing homes. In some states, expenditures for the nursing home component of Medicaid is the largest, single expense in the budget. As states look for ways to control their budgets, funding for nursing home care is heavily scrutinized. States have used certif-

icate of need (CON) authorities to limit the number of nursing home beds allowed in the state, thereby limiting state spending.

Payment methods for nursing homes vary by state. A variety of payment systems have been tried. Most states now have some form of prospective payment and a cap on per diem rates. Efforts to implement case-mix payment systems are underway at both state and federal levels.

Nursing homes are highly regulated. Concern about quality is juxtaposed with the limited budgets of state Medicaid agencies and private families. The 1987 Nursing Home Reform Act, incorporated into the Omnibus Budget Reconciliation Act of 1987 (OBRA 87), made significant changes in how

WI moratorium

TABLE 7-9. Nursing Home and Personal Care Home Residents Age 65 and Older, by Age, Sex, and Race, 1985

	Residents	Residents/ 1,000 U.S. Population
All Ages	1,318,400	46.2
65–74 year	212,100	12.5
75–84 years	509,000	57.7
85 years and older	597,300	220.3
Males	334,500	29.0
65–74 year	80,600	10.8
75–84 years	141,300	43.0
85 years and older	112,600	145.7
Females	983,900	57.9
65–74 year	131,500	13.8
75–84 years	367,700	66.4
85 years and older	484,700	250.1
White	1,227,400	47.7
Black, Other	91,000	35.0

SOURCE: National Center for Health Statistics. (1991). *Health, United States, 1990* (table 80). Hyattsville, MD: Public Health Service.

nursing homes operate and how they are evaluated (45). The survey process was changed from one that focused on physical and task criteria to one that focuses on the caring process, resident feelings, and patient care outcomes.

The majority of employees of nursing homes are unskilled or low-skilled: nurses aides and housekeeping, maintenance, and food service workers. Even in skilled nursing facilities that meet Medicare requirements, a registered nurse must be on duty only eight hours per day. On evening and night shifts, the highest professional staff may be a licensed vocational nurse. Other health care professionals who work with nursing homes include physicians; pharmacists; nutritionists; occupational, physical, speech, and respiratory therapists; and medical social workers. Except in very large homes, these professionals will work at the home on a part-time basis and are likely to associate by contract rather than as paid employees.

Table 7-9 characterizes nursing home residents

at the time of the most recent national survey. Nursing homes serve the very old, frail elderly. In 1985, 88 percent of the 1.4 million nursing home residents were age 65 and older; 40 percent were age 85 and over. The median age was 81. Three out of four residents were women, and nine out of ten were white.

The lifetime chance of ever being in a nursing home is nearly one in two: 49 percent probability for women and 47 percent probability for men. However, the likelihood increases with age. Of people age 65–74, only one in 10 is in a nursing home. Of those age 85 and above, 20 percent reside in a nursing home (46). Contrary to popular belief, most people do not spend many years in a nursing home (47). Nearly one-third of those admitted to a nursing home are discharged within 90 days; an additional 20 percent are discharged within one year. Nineteen percent of women and 12 percent of men stay in a nursing home more than five years.

The primary diagnoses of nursing home residents are circulatory system disorders (33 percent), mental disorders (22.2 percent), and diseases of the nervous system (11 percent) (48). Nearly half of nursing home residents (47 percent) have two or three major diagnoses, and two out of five (40 percent) have three or more diagnoses.

Functional dependence is high among nursing home residents. Many have suffered debilitating strokes and have not fully recovered mentally or physically. As many as one-third to two-fifths of nursing home residents has some type of mental disorder (49), most often organic brain syndrome or senile dementia. As the population ages, the number of people with Alzheimer's disease will increase, and many of these people ultimately go into a nursing home. Table 7-10 delineates the dependency status of nursing home residents and also shows how the level of dependency has increased over time.

The reasons people are admitted to nursing homes tend to be functional dependency rather than diagnosis. Research has shown that for every person in a nursing home, two equally ill people live at home, cared for by family and friends. Admission to a home usually occurs because friends and family can no longer provide the level of support required. Night wandering and incontinence are two problems that frequently stress a family beyond its caregiving capacity and result in the frail person being admitted to a nursing home. People who are single and do not have strong social support systems are also more likely to be in a nursing home.

Use of nursing homes will continue to grow in the future. As indicated in table 7-3, as the population grows older, there simply will be more people with the characteristics of those who enter nursing homes. The rate of nursing home use may decline as more community-based options become available. However, the increase in numbers is likely to outweigh any decrease in the use rate. National expenditures for nursing home care are expected to climb from $53 billion in 1989 to $86 billion in 1995 to $131 billion in 2000 (50,51).

Home Health

Home health care is one of the oldest components of the continuum of care. A number of home health agencies across the nation have celebrated their centennial. Today, home health care is one of the most exciting and rapidly growing areas of health care.

Expansion of this field began in the early 1980s and is expected to continue during the 1990s. It reflects the convergence of five major factors:

- desire by both consumers and payors to minimize health care costs by substituting less intense alternatives to institutional care,
- financial pressures of hospitals to diversify and to control patient flow under capitated and prospective payment systems,
- an increase in demand due to the growing number of older people,
- preference of patients and families for care in their own home, and
- advances in technology that enable therapies, which formerly would have been provided only in hospitals or doctors' offices by health care professionals, to be

TABLE 7-10. Dependency Status of Nursing Home Residents

	1977	1985
Type of Dependency: Requires Assistance with:		
Bathing	86.3	88.7
Dressing	69.4	75.4
Using bathroom	52.6	60.9
Mobility or transferring	66.1	70.7
Difficulty with bowel/bladder control	45.3	51.9
Eating	32.6	39.3
Number of Dependencies		
None	9.6	8.2
One	12.4	9.3
Two	12.9	10.4
Three	10.7	9.2
Four	13.5	14.3
Five	17.6	19.5
Six	23.3	29.1
Average	3.5	3.9

SOURCE: Hing, E. (1989, October). Nursing home utilization by current residents; United States, 1985. (table F). *Vital Health Statistics. 13* (102).

provided safely and effectively in the home by home-care professionals or patients and family members.

Home care consists of several types of services: skilled nursing care and therapies, homemaker/home health aide care, high technology home therapy, and durable medical equipment (DME) suppliers. The services may all be provided by one agency, or an agency may specialize in only one aspect of home care. However, high-technology home therapy and DME companies are likely to be distinct organizations and are discussed separately.

Skilled Home Health and Homemaker Services

Skilled home health services include:

- nursing care, provided by a registered nurse or licensed vocational nurse, ranging from patient education and basic nursing procedures to highly complex care;

• physical, occupational, and speech therapy;
• respiratory therapy;
• medical social service; and
• nutrition counseling.

Often, several services are provided to a single patient by a multidisciplinary team. However, each provider may visit the patient at a different time. Patients are those who are recovering from an acute episode of illness, require rehabilitation, suffer from chronic illnesses that need ongoing monitoring or intense attention, are undergoing special short-term therapies, or are in the last stages of life. All patients are homebound, i.e., unable to leave their homes safely to get the care they need.

Homemaker/home health aide care includes:

• personal care,
• bathing and grooming,
• meal preparation,
• shopping,
• transportation,
• select household chores, and
• other tasks that do not require trained health care professionals.

Patients are often those who are functionally impaired on a short-term or permanent basis and require assistance with the activities of daily living.

The agencies providing home health and homemaker care take an array of organizational forms. The Health Care Financing Administration has developed a classification system that involves ownership, control, and tax status. The categories are (52):

Hospital-based—operated as an integral part of a hospital, such as a department.

Visiting nurse associations—voluntary, nonprofit organizations governed by a community-based board of directors and usually financed by tax-deductible contributions as well as by earnings. (The term earlier had a more specific meaning and referred to home care agencies that were named Visiting Nurse Associations and shared a common history.)

Government agencies—sponsored by a state, county, city, or other unit of local government, such as public health department, having a major responsibility for prevention of disease and for community health education. These are sometimes referred to as "public" or "official" agencies.

Proprietary agencies—for-profit. These range from single agencies owned by individuals to large nationwide chains.

Private nonprofit—privately developed, governed, and owned nonprofit agency.

Home health agencies are licensed in most states, and a few states require a certificate of need. The Joint Commission for the Accreditation of Healthcare Organizations and the Community Health Accreditation Program of the National League For Nursing accredit home health agencies; and the National Homecaring Council accredits homecare aide organizations.

Medicare-Certified Home Health Agencies

Home health agencies that meet stringent federal standards can be certified by Medicare to care for clients enrolled in Medicare Part A or Part B. The agency is shaped by federal requirements and serves almost exclusively patients whose payors are Medicare, Medicaid, workers' compensation, or private insurance. Medicare limits participation to home care agencies that are primarily engaged in providing skilled nursing services and other therapeutic services. Homemaker/home health aide organizations are not certifiable.

The number of Medicare-certified home health agencies doubled during the mid-1980s, from 2,858 in 1980 (53) to 5,831 in 1991 (52). The field changed from primarily Visiting Nurses Associations and government agencies to hospital-based and private for-profit or nonprofit agencies. Table 7-11 shows this transition from 1967, when Medicare first certified home health agencies, to 1991. Although a home health agency may be part of a larger health care organization, it is typically structured as a distinct department or organization in order to maximize the financial benefits under Medicare. Home health agency productivity and size are measured by number of visits.

To be eligible for home health coverage by

TABLE 7-11. Number of Medicare-Certified Home Health Care Agencies by Auspice, 1967, 1987 & 1991

Auspice	1967		1987		1991	
	No.	*Percent*	*No.*	*Percent*	*No.*	*Percent*
VNA	642	36.7	551	9.5	525	9.0
Government	939	53.6	1,073	18.5	932	16.0
Proprietary	0	0	1,846	31.9	2,016	34.6
Nonprofit	0	0	766	13.2	683	11.7
Hospital	133	7.6	1,439	24.9	1,558	26.7
Other	39	2.2	110	1.9	117	2.0
Total:	1,753	100.0	5,785	100.0	5,831	100.0

SOURCE: *Basic statistics about home care—1991.* (1991). Washington, DC: National Association for Home Care.

Medicare, a client must be homebound; be capable of improvement; and require short-term, intermittent nursing care, physical therapy, or speech therapy. The patient must show the ability to improve. Home health agencies may also provide occupational therapy, medical social work, and home health aide services. Medicare will pay for these, but only if the client first meets the preceding criteria and receives one or more of the primary services. All services must be prescribed by a physician. The duration of services is limited. In 1990, those served received an average of 40 visits per person.

Like the number of agencies, the number of individuals who receive home health care from Medicare-certified agencies has increased. The number of Medicare enrollees served suggests the magnitude of growth. In 1987, approximately 1.5 million Medicare recipients received home health care. A 1985 projection estimated that 2.1 million people would receive formal home health care by the year 2000 (54). However, by 1990 1.67 million Medicare patients had been served (54). As shown in table 7-3, by 2018, the number of people receiving home care including Medicare beneficiaries could grow to as many as 6 to 8 million. Due to the changes in technology and an increase in use of home care for younger persons, the use of home care will no doubt exceed the population-based projections.

The majority of clients served by Medicare-certified agencies are age 65 and older. For many agencies, seniors are 80 percent or more of their patients. The single largest group are patients being discharged from hospitals who required short-term follow-up to complete their recovery. Hospitals are the predominant referral source. Of the 33 million individuals enrolled in Medicare in 1990, the 1.67 million receiving home care represent about 7 percent of the total (54). In contrast, about 20 percent of Medicare enrollees age 65 or older are hospitalized each year.

Despite the growth of home health care, total funds spent on it are relatively small. In 1990, Medicare spent $4.3 billion on home care of its total $105 billion budget, or about 3 percent (54). Medicaid spent an additional $2.6 billion, or 4.7 percent of its total $55 billion budget (54). The Brookings Institution projects that home care spending just for those age 65 and older may reach $22 billion by 2020 (55).

The average charge for a visit from a Medicare-certified agency was $70 in 1991 (52). The charge varies according to the type of professional service rendered and the geographic area. For patients covered by Medicare, Medicaid, local government programs, private insurance, or other third parties, the agency bills insurance directly on behalf of the patient. Since the great majority of business is with Medicare, a growing number of agencies are electronically linked with their Medicare intermediary and submit claims at the end of each day.

Medicare currently pays on a cost-reimbursement basis, thereby limiting the amount of profit an agency can make. There is thus no strong financial incentive to establish services (such as homemaker care) or clients beyond those of Medicare and other government programs. The Health Care Financing Administration is exploring a prospective payment system based on severity of illness. A change in Medicare's payment system may occur in the mid–1990s.

Private Home Health Agencies

Private home health agencies serve primarily private-pay and contract patients. These agencies are not certified for payment by Medicare, and concomitantly, are not bound by Medicare regulations. Although they must be licensed as health care providers in some states, in many other states, these agencies operate with only a business license. Noncertified agencies emerged during the 1970s and grew during the 1980s to fill the demand for home care by patients who do not qualify for Medicare or Medicaid.

The agencies offer the same professional services provided by Medicare-certified agencies, plus numerous others. Services include skilled nursing, physical therapy, occupational therapy, speech therapy, medical social work, home health aides, homemakers, high-technology home infusion therapy, ventilator care, high-risk pregnancy monitoring, and neonatal care, among others. In contrast to Medicare-certified agencies, which Medicare authorizes to provide only intermittent and skilled visits, noncertified agencies provide 24-hour care, daily care, and specialty services. Private agencies also offer homemaker/home health aide care such as personal grooming, bathing and shaving, housekeeping, transportation, shopping, meal preparation, and home repair.

Private home health agencies are staffed differently from Medicare-certified agencies. Private agencies tend to draw from a large pool of home health aides and homemakers. Staff often work on an on-call basis and may work for several agencies. Professional staff are also likely to work on an as-needed basis rather than as full-time employees. The challenge for many private home care providers is to keep a minimum number of staff on full-time payroll and a large enough cadre of staff available on-call to meet demand. The loose association with staff makes quality control particularly important.

Clients of these agencies comprise a broader group than those served by Medicare-certified agencies. While the latter receive the majority of their referrals directly from hospitals of patients who are being discharged, private home care agencies engage in active marketing to secure clients of many types. Clients range from young accident victims who require 24-hour nursing care, to workers' compensation clients who need rehabilitation before returning to work, to seniors living alone who have no severe health problems but do have functional disabilities. Depending on the payment source, private home care does not necessarily require a physician's prescription; thus, clients come from many sources. Social service agencies, Medicare-certified home health agencies, relatives, friends, and the yellow pages all serve as referrals to private home care. Some private agencies pursue contracts with various government agencies to be the preferred provider for particular types of patients.

Because private home care agencies are not reimbursed or certified by any federal agencies, no single source maintains comprehensive national statistics. The National Association for Home Care identified at least 5,500 private home care agencies in 1991 (52). This suggests that the total number of private agencies equals the number of Medicare-certified ones. The great majority of private home health agencies are proprietary; the few operated by churches or social service agencies are non-profit. Several large nationwide chains characterize the private home care field, in contrast to Medicare-

TABLE 7-12. Cost per Month of Hospital Care Compared to Home Care, Selected Conditions

Condition	Cost of Hospital Care	Cost of Home Care	Dollar Savings
Infant born w/breathing & feeding problems	$60,970	$20,209	$40,761
Neurological disorder w/respiratory problems	17,783	196*	17,587
Ventilator-dependent patient care	22,569	1,766	20,803
Nutrition infusions	23,670	9,000	14,670
Antibiotic infusions	7,290	2,070	5,220
Patient requiring respiratory support	24,715	9,267	15,448
Quadriplegic patient w/spinal cord injury	23,862	13,931	9,931
Cerebral palsy patient	8,425	4,867**	3,558

*After initial cost of equipment.
**In extended-care unit of hospital.

SOURCE: National Association for Home Care. (1991). *Basic statistics about home care—1991*. Washington, DC: National Association for Home Care.

certified agencies, which are typically independent of each other and more likely to be affiliated with a hospital or local multihealth care system.

Private home care agencies charge by the hour, rather than by the visit. Often a minimum number of hours is required. Charges tend to be less than Medicare-certified agencies, even for the same service, because private agencies are not required to have comparable staffing, which adds to overhead. The trade-off is that some professional services, such as medical social services, may not be available from a private agency, and quality control may not receive the same attention as that enforced by government regulation unless the agency chooses optional accreditation.

Private home care agencies have many private pay patients. Other payors include private insurance and government contracts. Worker's compensation, Title XX of the Social Security Act, the Older Americans Act, state and local mental health department funds, child welfare department programs, and local block grants may contract with a home care agency to care for clients who are eligible for the particular program. Such contract-

ing is often done with the nonprofit private home care agencies.

Through the 1980s, private and Medicare-certified agencies tended to be separate and, hence, to compete with each other for some types of cases. The current trend is for companies to offer both services. Even if housed in the same office, the two programs must operate as separate businesses because of Medicare regulations.

High-Technology Home Therapy

High-technology home therapy appeared in the early 1980s. Cost-containment initiatives squeezing hospitals, and advances in drug and equipment technology, made it possible to deliver services in the home that had formerly been available only to patients in hospitals. A major advantage of providing high-technology therapy in the home is that it is much less expensive than providing the same care in a hospital or nursing home (56,57). Cost comparisons are shown in table 7-12. The expansion of ambulatory care, especially ambulatory surgery, during the late 1980s further abetted the trend to move services out of the hospital and into home settings.

High technology services now provided in the home include:

- intravenous antibiotics,
- oncology therapy,
- pain management,
- parenteral and enteral nutrition,
- ventilator care,
- high-risk pregnancy, and
- infant monitoring.

High-technology home therapy typically involves pharmaceuticals and equipment that are expensive, require special staff expertise to use and monitor, and are available only from select sources. The total volume of patients requiring high-technology care is small, and the protocols can vary on an individual basis much more than for basic home care.

High-technology home therapy is provided by many Medicare-certified and private home health agencies. In addition, some agencies specialize only in providing high-technology home care. The cost for each patient can be quite high, and reimbursement is often unconventional. For example, Medicare will pay for the equipment for enteral nutrition, but not for the nutrients or drugs. Companies with the requisite expertise have found that they can thrive just by specializing in this one component of home care (57). Experts project expansive growth in the high-technology arena in the future (57,58).

Durable Medical Equipment

Durable medical equipment (DME), ranging from walkers to electric beds, is frequently provided in conjunction with home health care (59). The home health agency often assumes responsibility for arranging for equipment. The agency may have a formal or informal affiliation with a local durable medical equipment company to provide the needed equipment. If the equipment is to be paid for by Medicare, it must be prescribed by the patient's physician.

During the 1980s, the durable medical equipment business was a fast-growing area of home health care less regulated and more lucrative than other areas of health care delivery. Joint ventures were initiated, multihealth care systems were acquired or started, and DME businesses and home health conglomerates were tried, bringing all aspects of home health care together into one parent company. In the mid– and late 1980s, Medicare tightened its regulatory and payment policies, and the DME field has since stabilized. In the 1990s, DME remains an essential, distinct component of home health care.

Precise data on durable medical equipment companies are not maintained by any single national source. The number of medical equipment dealers is estimated at between 6,000 and 7,000 (55). The vast majority are for-profit agencies. In 1991, approximately $4 billion was spent on durable medical equipment (55). Of this, Medicare paid for about half.

While expecting growth in numbers of clients, the home care field is beginning to reach maturity. The number of agencies has leveled off, federal regulations are fairly clear and fairly stringent, management systems have become standardized, and the distinct split between Medicare-certified and uncertified agencies is blurring. Medicare is examining a prospective payment system for home care, but implementation is not likely until the mid–1990s. With a stable organizational structure and predictable payments, home care advances in the near future are likely to be in new technologies and new types of clients.

Hospice

Hospice is the concept of providing care for the terminally ill. It began as a formal program in Great Britain and spread to the United States during the 1970s. The philosophy of hospice is that terminally ill individuals should be allowed to maintain life during their final days in as natural and comfortable a setting as possible. Every attempt is made to enable the person to remain at home; other

TABLE 7-13. Hospice Program Characteristics

*Organizational Auspice of Hospice
Programs in the United States, 1990*

Independent	40 percent
Hospital-based	30 percent
Home-health agency	24 percent
Nursing home and other	6 percent

Growth in Hospice, 1986–1990

	1986	1990
Number of hospices	1,500	1,800
Number of Medicare-certified hospices	275	1,200
Number of patients	100,000	200,000

SOURCE: National Hospice Organization.

services are brought in as needed. All aspects of hospice emphasize quality, rather than length, of life.

Elements common to all hospices include (60,61):

- Service availability, including medical and nursing care, to home care patients and institutional inpatients on a 24-hour-per-day, seven-day-per-week, on-call basis
- A full complement of skilled and homemaker home care service
- Inpatient care as needed
- Respite care for the family provided in the home, hospital, or nursing home
- Control of physical symptoms, including use of palliative drugs
- Psychological, social, and spiritual counseling for patient and family
- Physician direction of services
- Central administration and coordination of services; collaboration among provider organizations (home health agencies, hospitals, nursing homes)
- Multidisciplinary team of care providers
- Use of volunteers as an integral part of the health care team
- Treatment of the patient and family together as a unit
- Bereavement follow-up for family and friends.

Hospice is an approach to care and as such can be offered through a variety of organizational settings. As shown in table 7-13, hospice programs vary in their organizational auspices. In 1990, the United States had about 1,800 formal hospices.

This was a 20 percent increase over 1986, indicating that the hospice movement is still growing. Both Medicare and the Joint Commission for the Accreditation of Healthcare Organizations accredit hospices. In 1990, about 1,200 hospices were accredited. Table 7-13 also shows the growth of hospices over time.

To participate in a hospice program, a person must generally have a diagnosis of terminal illness fatal within 90 to 180 days. The patient and the family must be willing to acknowledge the imminence of death and desire palliative care. The majority of hospice patients are victims of cancer. Some hospice programs require the clients to have a caregiver; others care for patients who live alone and have no designated caregiver. The number of people cared for annually by hospices was estimated in 1990 to be 200,000.

The concept of hospice and its implementation received considerable national attention during the late 1970s and 1980s. Federally funded demonstration projects tested the impact of hospice on patient and family quality of life and on cost-effective use of resources. Ultimately, service criteria and payment authorization by Medicare were included in the Tax Equity and Fiscal Responsibility Act of 1982 and were extended in 1986. Payment benefits were revised in 1991. By the 1990s, hospice has become a common and accepted component of the continuum of care.

Under Medicare Hospital Insurance (Part A), defined hospice benefits are covered when provided by a Medicare-certified agency. Blue Cross, Blue Shield, and many private insurance companies recognize and pay for hospice care. Hospice services not organized as a special program may nonetheless be paid for as separate home health, hospital, or nursing home care.

Adult Day Care

Adult day care is a daytime program of nursing care, rehabilitation therapies, supervision, and socialization that enables frail, often elderly, people to remain in the community. By attending adult day care, people who are functionally disabled and/or moderately ill and are not in need of 24-hour nursing care can remain in their homes at night with their families and friends while receiving the care they need during the day. The goal is to foster the best possible health and maximum independence in functioning for each client as well as the optimum combination of caregiving and respite for each family. For many, if a supportive home environment and adult day care are not available, the only alternative is to enter a nursing home.

Adult day care proliferated during the 1980s. Before 1975, fewer than 100 centers were identified (62). The number had grown to 1,200 in 1985 (62). By 1989, in excess of 2,100 adult day-care centers existed, providing care to nearly 42,000 people each week day (63). Two out of every five adult day-care centers opened between 1985 and 1989. By the 1990s, although adult day care was not universally available, it could be found in all states and in most cities. Adult day care has become an accepted and integral component of the continuum of care, and more development is being encouraged during the 1990s (64).

No comprehensive reporting mechanism captures adult day-care programs for the entire United States. The National Institute on Adult Daycare (NIAD) of the National Council on Aging (NCOA) periodically surveys adult day-care programs in conjunction with the Health Care Financing Administration. Nationwide surveys were conducted in 1980 (65), 1985 (62), and 1989 (63). The data in this discussion come from the 1989 survey.

The services adult day-care programs provide include nursing, activities of daily living assistance, personal care, meals, recreation, nutrition counseling, social services, physical therapy, occupational therapy, medical assessment and treatment, family counseling, and transportation. Forty percent of adult day-care centers provide all of the above services; the remainder provide select services. Some adult day-care centers focus on a particular target population and tailor their services accordingly. Most adult day-care programs operate Monday through Friday, from 8 a.m. to 4 p.m.

Adult day-care centers may be freestanding or sponsored by and housed in a parent organization. Of the centers existing in 1989, 20 percent were affiliated with a nursing home, 15 percent with a multipurpose senior center, and 10 percent with a hospital. Other sponsors include community social services agencies, government agencies, and church groups. Only 11 percent were for-profit entities. Nearly three-fourths (72 percent) were nonprofit; one in five (17 percent) was run by city or county government.

The costs of adult day care range from $21–$40 per day, depending on the range of services offered. Client fees average $20 per day for private-pay patients and $34 per day for public programs, such as Medicaid. Many centers use a sliding fee scale to accommodate family incomes. Average costs are $34–$38. Most adult day-care centers cannot cover their costs, and more than half (52 percent) operate at a loss. Adult day-care centers depend heavily on philanthropy, volunteers, and in-kind contributions. The rationale for their existence is clearly to meet a service need, not to generate excessive revenues.

Despite the fact that most of the clients are over age 65, Medicare does not pay for adult day care. The largest single payer is Medicaid. Fees paid directly by clients and families are the second largest source. Most adult day-care centers patch together funds from several sources, including Title III of the Older Americans Act, Title XX Social Service Block grants, state and local mental health and development disability programs, United Way, private foundation grants, and fund-raising activities.

Reflecting the growth and evolution of adult day-care centers, many states now license them. Each state sets its own licensing requirements and definitions. Adult day-care centers may also be certified by a given payor to offer services to authorized clients. California, for example, recognizes three types of adult day-care programs. Two-fifths of such adult centers are certified by two or more public agencies; one-fifth are not certified by any public payors.

Average attendance at an adult day-care center is 37 people per day, with 50 the maximum capacity for most centers. Those attending are primarily the frail elderly. The average age of participants is 76 years. Two-thirds of all participants are women; two-thirds of participants live with a spouse, adult children, other family, or friends; and one-fourth live alone. Two-fifths of the participants qualify for Medicaid.

Those who attend adult day-care centers are typically in fragile mental or physical condition. About half suffer from cognitive impairment; an additional one-third have Alzheimer's disease or related disorders. Nearly 60 percent require assistance in two or more activities of daily living. One-fourth rely on a cane or walker; many are wheelchair-bound. The majority of participants come for an indefinite period of time; however, some come during the recuperative period of an acute episode of illness until they have regained independence in physical or mental functioning.

About 12 percent of adult day-care centers are certified to care for those who suffer from mental retardation or have developmental disabilities. These centers tend to have younger clients and offer a different spectrum of services.

Functional and personal client characteristics suggest that adult day-care centers do indeed offer an alternative to nursing home care for people who would be unable to function alone but who are able to live with family or friends, provided that respite and daily supervision are available.

Integrating Mechanisms

For a continuum of care to function as a system of care rather than as a fragmented collection of services, integrating mechanisms are essential. As described above, these include an internal organization that coordinates the operations of various services; a management information system that integrates clinical, utilization, and financial data and follows clients across settings; a case management/care coordination program that works with clients to arrange services; and a financing mechanism that enables pooling of funds across services.

These integrating mechanisms are in various stages of development; few comprehensive systems that include all of these components exist. However, proposals in the early 1990s for national health care reform recognize the need for integrating mechanisms to achieve the financial and patient care benefits of a well-organized system of care (66,67).

Interentity Structure

Interentity planning and administration must be structured both within an organization and across organizations. Patient services are not likely to be coordinated unless the units that are providing the services are coordinated administratively, particularly when budgeting and financial issues arise (68).

Practicing in a continuum of care creates changes in traditional roles. New roles and responsibilities develop in relation to patients and families, providers and payors, and other professionals (69). The human component is an essential dimension of the continuum of care for the patient and practitioner; thus, staff interactions and attitudes must be managed, as well as financial and structural issues.

Administrative structures are necessary to 1) ensure channels of communication and cooperation; 2) establish clear lines of authority, accountability, and responsibility for patient care services; 3) negotiate budgets and financial trade-offs; and 4) present a cohesive, consistent message in interactions with external agencies and the community. Administrative mechanisms within an organization include:

- committees that cut across service areas;
- a multilevel structure and designated senior administrator responsible for decisions that affect several different departments or units;
- an integrated budget that recognizes the contribution of each unit to the performance of the whole, including losses in one unit that produce larger gains in another unit;

- interdisciplinary team conferences for clinicians;
- clinical liaisons assigned to service programs that have frequent patient referrals;
- multidepartment planning teams;
- multidisciplinary and multidepartmental task forces focusing on specific short-term issues; and
- product line management organization.

Between and among agencies, agreements regarding affiliation and patient transfer may be put in place. Managed-care organizations that already have preferred provider networks offer an organizational base from which to add long-term care providers.

The organizational issues inherent in operating an efficient continuum of care are only beginning to be articulated (70) and implemented (71). Organizations that exemplify continuum structure in the early 1990s are ones that have evolved over time with gradual modifications. Only as the other integrating mechanisms have evolved to the stage of being practical realities have organizations realized that they must implement administrative structures in order to maximize the benefits of comprehensiveness, continuity, and integration.

Integrated Information Systems

Integrated information systems are necessary for efficient management of the continuum. Many health and social service organizations still maintain separate clinical, financial, and utilization data systems. Many, particularly social service agencies and small health care companies, are not computerized. Nursing homes have only recently been forced to computerize patient records due to reporting requirements specified in OBRA (Omnibus Budget Reconciliation Act) of 1987. Very few health care organizations maintain data on patients as they move from one service to another, such as from acute hospital care to home care. Yet, financing of health care and social services is increasingly dependent on prepaid and/or capitated systems encompassing a comprehensive service package. In order to implement quality assurance and utiliza-

tion review programs, assess efficiency of operations, and track and aggregate patient experiences, comprehensive and integrated data systems and accompanying management reporting systems are imperative.

The ideal information system for a continuum of care was conceived in the mid-1980s (72). However, the computer technology to make such a system feasible and affordable depended on the development of new computer chips with expanded capacity and networking technology, both of which occurred during the latter part of the 1980s. In the 1990s, the individual services of the continuum are upgrading their information systems to combine clinical, financial, and utilization data. Local area networks (LANs) are being tried, particularly in linking physicians with hospitals. Senior membership programs are realizing the need to track the array of health and social support services used by seniors with complex, changing, chronic illnesses. Information systems that combine the financial, clinical, or utilization aspects of a patient's care across settings are being considered. Payors and utilization review companies are enhancing their data bases and tracking programs to evaluate the cost of caring for a patient through an episode of illness. Once these information systems are in place, they can be combined to the degree required for the ideal continuum.

Care Coordination

Care coordination is also referred to as service coordination, case management, and occasionally, by other terms. The purpose of care coordination is to work directly with clients and families over time to assist them in arranging and managing the complex set of resources that the client requires to maintain health and independent functioning. Care coordination seeks to achieve the maximum cost-effective use of scarce resources by helping clients get the health, social, and support services most appropriate for their needs at a given time. It guides the client and family through the maze of services, matches service need with funding authorization, and coordinates with clinicians and provider organizations.

Applebaum and Austin distinguish long-term care coordination from the short-term service arrangement provided by many health care professionals. The key features of long-term care coordination are intensity, breadth of services encompassed, and duration (73).

Care coordination began through public programs, often with social workers in the public welfare department, caseworkers in mental health, or nurses in public health departments. For years, care coordination struggled for identity. The most frequent locus in the private sector was in social service agencies. During the late 1970s and continuing through the mid–1980s, demonstration projects examined the benefits and costs of care coordination and tried to classify models. The findings on cost savings were mixed.

In the latter part of the 1980s, care coordination began to be recognized as necessary to streamline care and negotiate the maze of long-term care services. Private insurance companies, managed-care programs, employers, and private family members have begun to pay for case management. The result has been a proliferation of models along with the confusion that accompanies growth. The 1990s are likely to see further evolution and clarity of the role of care coordination.

Care coordination is a process (73–75) the components of which are assessment, care planning, arrangement of services, monitoring, and reassessment. Assessment is usually done by a multidisciplinary team that includes a nurse, a social worker, a physician, and other professionals as indicated by the condition of the particular client. Whenever possible, assessment includes evaluation of the home environment and family situation. Based on the results of this assessment, the team concurs on a specific plan of action and recommends an array of appropriate services.

The ongoing care coordinator may be a nurse, social worker, or health care professional trained specifically as a case manager. The care coordinator is responsible for arranging the services ordered by the team and maintaining contact with the client and the service providers to confirm that services are being delivered and are meeting the client's needs. Reassessment of the client's status occurs either according to a regularly scheduled checkup with the clinicians or when the care coordinator detects a change that warrants reevaluation.

The authority of the care coordinator to arrange service use varies. Three basic models exist: broker, service management, and managed care (76). Under the broker model, care coordinators identify needed services and make referrals, but have no authority over service delivery. With service management, the care coordinator has authority over payment but usually has a capitated or predetermined cap limiting how much can be spent. Managed care places the provider at risk, and thus the care coordinator has no set cap but clear financial incentives to use resources carefully and wisely.

A care coordinator can handle 20 to 80 active clients, depending on the breadth and intensity of the program, the dependence level of the clients, and the organizational resources supporting the care coordination operations.

The fee for care coordination is $50–$150 for an initial assessment, then a smaller fee for ongoing monthly service or follow-up consultation. Medicare does not pay for care coordination except in home health. A care coordination program may be paid for entirely or partially by certain state government programs, such as Medicaid, Title XX, mental health or Older Americans Act funds; demonstration grants; private monies, such as grants, foundations, donations; a select group of insurance companies who now cover this as a benefit, or directly by clients or families.

The role of the care coordinator is still evolving and only recently has it received recognition as a separate and distinct role. New variations include care coordinators based in hospitals, HMOs, private insurance companies, employers, and managed-care companies. Meanwhile, traditional care coordinator brokers continue in social services agencies and government programs. Four dimensions characterize care coordination and provide a framework for classifying the myriad models. The four program components are funding/reimbursement, targeting, gatekeeping, and organizational auspices (77).

During the past decade, the providers and payors of health care have recognized the need to develop a cost-effective means of dealing with the complexity of patients' ongoing needs for comprehensive, continuing care, as also discussed in Chapter 12. Care coordination has the potential to coordinate an array of resources, both within a given organization and externally in other community agencies, and to make astute use of a variety of financial resources to maximize the care affordable by the client. The trend to recognize the distinct role of a case manager/care coordinator is further enhanced by the expansion of health care organizations into continuums of care, with more than a single type of service available within the same organization and with a pool of funds for health and social support services that can be spent at the discretion of the provider.

Care coordination/case management is likely to become more prevalent in the future. As part of this expansion, its cost-effectiveness will continue to be examined, and refinement and streamlining of the models is likely to occur.

Integrated Financing

Comprehensive, flexible, and adequate financing are the goals of the ideal continuum. This is the single component of the continuum of care most critical and most challenging in the 1990s. As with many other areas of health care, delivery system changes will be driven by financial incentives. The problems of fragmented and underfunded financing are discussed below under Policy Issues. For a continuum to achieve the access to the full spectrum of long-term care services desired, financial barriers must not dominate placement and

resource allocation decisions. Several trends and demonstrations offer hope that the financing of long-term care is moving in the direction required for the continuum.

The number of seniors enrolled in HMOs continues to increase. In 1990, 2,138,000 people, or approximately 6.7 percent of seniors, were enrolled in HMOs (78). Many people under age 65 with chronic illnesses are also enrolled in HMOs, and the enrollment of younger adults also continues to increase.

Several variations of Medicare HMOs have been formulated by the Health Care Financing Administration (HCFA). All offer a package of services that include acute care with some preventive and long-term services. By having consumers pay for care on a capitated basis, HMOs overcome the access barriers of fragmented funding from the consumer's perspective for at least those services that comprise the service package. Providers may or may not be paid on a capitated basis. Risk sharing, which is now the predominant Medicare HMO model, has financial incentives for providers to be efficient in getting patients the services they need. Risk sharing also has the incentives and the flexibility to match services to a patient's needs rather than according to constrained payment policies.

As currently structured, HMOs are not specifically required to offer a comprehensive continuum of care, nor to provide ongoing services for chronic problems. Nor do they coordinate care or monitor use as ideally as they might. However, many offer a fairly broad array of services. And, as evidenced by the experience of the S/HMOs described below, their structure can be expanded into an integrated continuum when market and financial incentives are right.

Long-term care insurance emerged during the late 1980s as another way to fund long-term care. By 1990, 134 companies offered some type of long-term care product (79). The number of people who had purchased policies grew from 815,000 in 1987 to more than 1.65 million in June, 1990 (80). Although most who purchase it are older, efforts are being made to sell long-term care insurance to younger adults as part of employer-sponsored benefit packages (81). The number of people purchasing long-term care insurance through an employer mushroomed from 20,000 in 1989 to 80,000 by the end of 1990 (82). Long-term care insurance aids the development of comprehensive financing for a continuum of services. For those who have Medicare Part A and Part B or indemnity insurance to cover acute services, long-term care insurance offers complimentary coverage for long-term, ongoing services.

When long-term care insurance policies began to be sold in the early 1980s, they reflected acute-care health insurance by paying based on diagnosis and use of limited services, specifically either nursing homes or home health. By the early 1990s, the policies were based on functional disability and paid on a per-diem basis. Payout of such policies is based on functional disability, not on having a specific disease. The funds are awarded on the basis of a fixed amount per day. The recipient can then spend them to pay for whatever services they use, including nursing homes, home health, home-makers, assisted living, or other formal or informal home support services.

The current generation of long-term care policies remains relatively expensive. In 1991, a policy with $80-per-day nursing home benefit for four years, with a 20-day deductible and no inflation feature would cost a 50-year-old $480 per year and a 79-year-old $3,840 (83). However, the policy is still less than the $25,000–$35,000 annual cost of nursing home care, should such care be needed. The price means that the insurance market is the middle and upper class, and one would not expect those with lower incomes to purchase private insurance. However, as employers add to this benefit packages, and insurance companies incorporate it as a feature of life insurance, the market will broaden. Other ways to expand the private long-term care market are also being examined (84). Related aspects of these insurance issues are also discussed in Chapter 12.

Social HMOs, or S/HMOs, are demonstration projects begun in 1985 by the Health Care Financing Administration (85). The original four sponsors were Kaiser Permanente in Portland, Oregon; Group Health in Minneapolis-St. Paul, Minnesota; Metropolitan Jewish Geriatric Center in Brooklyn, New York; and Senior Health Action Network (SCAN) in Long Beach, California. The demonstration has been extended to 1995 and has been authorized to add up to four sites.

The purpose of the S/HMO is to examine the use and relative cost-effectiveness of a capitated payment system that includes chronic and extended benefits as well as medical services. The Health Care Financing Administration describes the model as follows (86):

The S/HMO model includes four basic organizational and financing features. First, a single organizational structure provides a full range of acute and long term care services to voluntarily enrolled Medicare beneficiaries. Beneficiaries pay a monthly premium for services. In addition to the basic Medicare benefits, services include nursing home, home health, homemaker, transportation, drugs and others. Second, a coordinated case management system is used to authorize long term care services for those members who meet specific disability criteria, within a fixed limit of about $6,000–$12,000 per year. Third, the S/HMOs are designed to serve a cross-section of the elderly population, including both the functionally impaired and unimpaired elderly. Fourth, financing is accomplished through prepaid capitation by pooling funds from Medicare, Medicaid and member premiums. The initial financial risk was shared by the S/HMOs and HCFA. After 30 months of the demonstration, the S/HMO sites assume full financial risk for service costs.

S/HMOs were slower to get started than had originally been expected (87,88). In 1990, the four S/HMOs had 17,869 enrollees and had refined their benefit packages and operations (88). Their long-term financial viability remains in question (89).

The Program of All-Inclusive Care for the Elderly (PACE) is another demonstration of the early 1990s funded by HCFA to test a variation of a capitated payment program linked with a service system for the chronically ill. [PACE replicates On-Lok, a program serving the Chinese community of San Francisco that centers around adult day care. On-Lok and its replicated sites organize a continuum of care for an extremely frail elderly population at considerably less than the cost of care for a comparably ill population not part of an organized system of care (90). The Health Care Financing Administration describes the model as (91):

(It) includes as core services the provision of adult day health care and multidisciplinary team case management through which access to and allocation of all health and long term care services are arranged. Physician, therapeutic, ancillary and social support services are provided on site at the adult day health center whenever possible. Hospital, nursing home, home health and other specialized services are provided extramurally. Transportation is also provided to all enrolled members who require it. Financing is accomplished through prospective capitation of both Medicare and Medicaid payments to the provider.

The PACE project differs from the S/HMO in that it focuses only on frail elderly people who are eligible for nursing home placement, while the S/HMO attempts to get a representative population over which to spread the risk of service use. The PACE projects serve 120–325 people, compared to the 2,500–5,000 served by each S/HMO. The provider network of PACE is smaller, more tightly controlled, and focuses around adult day care. Finally, the financial arrangements are different. PACE receives a capitated amount from Medicare and Medicaid for a frail, high-use population, and may also charge private pay clients on a sliding-scale basis. S/HMOs function more like HMOs, charging enrollees premiums and negotiating with Medicare and Medicaid for capitated payments based on a healthy population.

Both S/HMOs and PACE are efforts to combine acute care and long-term care funding into an integrated system that enables a care manager to allocate resources according to need, rather than be stymied by the constraints of fragmented financing. While only reaching a very small number of people, demonstrations and trends in private insurance and HMOs portent positively for future

financial flexibility that will enable a continuum of care to integrate services according to client need rather than categorical funding.

Policy Issues

The public policy issues pertaining to long-term care are complex, reflecting the diversity and breadth of the field. A comprehensive description would cover the policy issues pertaining to each service and integrating mechanism at federal, state, local, institutional, and societal levels. This section highlights the major policy issues that should be considered by those involved in creating or managing a continuum of care.

Even in the early 1990s, the direction of public policy for all health care is unclear. "National health care reform" is a compelling political issue. Yet, the practical challenges to implementing major change may override the outcries for reform. Public policy for long-term care will be affected by changes in the organization and financing of health care at the broader level.

The discussions of reform have brought the concept of the continuum to the forefront. Proposals for change include organization according to "networks" or "integrating systems," capitated or bundled financing, provider risk for select long-term as well as acute services.

Thus the resolution of the issues identified below may take place gradually, and great impetus for change may await the explosion of demand that will accompany the graying of the Baby Boom generation. As an alternative, a radical change in national health care organization may alter the long-term care continuum by the mid- to late 1990s. In either case, managers must be aware that legislation and regulations may appear in any or all of the following areas.

Financing

Financing is one of the primary problems inhibiting provision and organization of long-term care on a coordinated, continuing basis. The definition of a continuum of care assumes: 1) adequate financing available to provide clients with an array of needed health, mental health, and social services, and 2) access to such financing. At national and local levels, the current mechanisms of financing inhibit the operation of a continuum of care. Under existing financing:

- The federal government does not have a national policy or program that funds long-term care.
- The financing streams for long-term care are highly fragmented (table 7-14).
- The various payors have different eligibility criteria, service coverage, reporting and operating requirements, and payment policies.
- Most providers do not have control over all the pertinent financing streams, thus limiting their ability to pool funds and allocate resources from an internal process to match a client's needs with appropriate care.
- The majority of long-term care is paid for by individuals. In effect, the national policy on long-term care is left to individuals and families, with states, through Medicaid, as a backup.
- The total amount of money expended by the nation may not be sufficient to meet the need, thus resulting in rationing.
- The cost of a universal long-term care program paid for by government funds may prohibit a national policy from being developed in the immediate future.

To understand the challenges of changing long-term care financing from the existing situation to the financing required for the ideal continuum, knowledge of current and projected financing is useful. In 1990, the United States spent $585 billion on personal health care expenditures (92). (This excludes expenditures for administration, research, and the like.) Of the total, $256 billion, or nearly half, was spent on hospital care. About 18 percent was spent on physician services. The amount spent for nursing home care was $53.1 billion, or 9 percent. Home health care accounted for $6.9 billion or 1 percent of total spending. Thus, the proportion of funds spent on acute care dwarfs the amount spent on long-term care. Political attention to revamping the health care delivery system focuses on hospitals and physicians; less attention is given to long-term care.

As noted earlier, two-thirds of those requiring long-term care are age 65 or older. Medicare is the federal insurance program for people age 65 and older; however, Medicare pays primarily for acute care services. In 1990, Medicare accounted for $109 billion of the $585 billion personal health care expenditures, or nearly one-sixth of the nation's health care funds for one-twelfth of its population. Sixty-three percent of Medicare benefits were for hospital care, and an additional 28 percent were for physician services. Medicare spent only $2.9 billion on home health care and $2.5 billion on skilled nursing home care in 1990.

The payment for long-term care is primarily from individuals and states. In contrast to Medicare's allocation of expenditures, federal Medicaid paid $13.7 billion in 1990 for nursing home care, five and one-half times the amount paid by Medicare. This was matched by the amount paid by states, for a total of about $27 billion. Nursing home care is the largest single expenditure of the Medicaid budget in many states. Individuals paid $24 billion, or 47 percent of the costs of nursing home care in 1990, nearly 10 times as much as Medicare. Of the $6.9 billion expenditures for formal home health care, Medicare paid 42 percent, and Medicaid paid 31 percent. Private individuals paid $800 million, or about 12 percent. However, a vast amount of home care is provided by families and friends or paid for privately and thus is not tallied as part of the nation's personal health expenditures.

During the latter part of the 1980s and the early 1990s, state budgets began to tighten, and as a result, Medicaid programs were constrained. Since Medicaid is a major payor for long-term care, these budget cuts affected long-term care. States began to consider how to afford long-term care for their residents (93) and rationing was considered. The state of Oregon implemented a rationing program to limit Medicaid services to the ones proven to be

TABLE 7-14. Major Federal Programs Supporting Long-Term Care Services: Services Covered, Eligibility, and Administering Agency

Program	Services Covered	Eligibility	Administering Agency	
			Federal	State
Medicaid/Title XIX of the Social Security Act	Skilled nursing facility[a] Intermediate care facility[b] Home health[c] Adult day care[b]	Aged, blind, disabled persons receiving cash assistance under SSI; others receiving cash assistance under AFDC; at state option, persons whose income exceeds standards for cash assistance under SSI/AFDC (i.e., the "medically needy")	Health Care Financing Administration/HHS	State medical agency
	2176 "waiver" services (e.g., case management, homemaker, personal care, adult day care, habilitation, respite, and other services at state option)[d]	Aged, blind, disabled, or mentally ill Medicaid eligibles (including children) living in the community who would require nursing-home-level care; at state option, persons living in the community with higher income than normally allowed under a state Medicaid plan		In some case the 2176 "waiver" program may be administered by another agency (e.g., state agency on aging)
Medicare/Title XVII of Social Security Act	100 days of skilled nursing facility care; home health; hospice	Generally Social Security status; persons 65 years and over; persons under 65 years entitled to federal disability benefits; and certain persons with terminal renal disease	Health Care Financing Administration/HHS	Not applicable

Program	Services/benefits	Eligibility	Federal agency	State agency
Title XX of Social Security Act	Various social services as defined by the state, including homemaker, home health aide, personal care, home-delivered meals	No federal requirements; states may require means tests	Office of Human Development Services/HHS	State social services/human resources agency; in some cases other state agencies may administer a portion of Title XX fund for certain groups (e.g., state agency on aging)
Older Americans Act/Title III	Variety of social services as determined by state and area agencies on aging, with priority on in-home services; also case management, day care, protective services; separate appropriation for home-delivered meals	Persons ≥60 years; no means tests, but services are to be targeted on those with social or economic need	Administration on Aging/Office of Human Development Services/HHS	State agency on aging
Supplemental Security Income/Title XVI of Social Security Act	Federal income support; supplemental payment for nonmedical housing and/or in-home services, as determined by state	Aged, blind, disabled persons who meet federally established income and resources requirements; states may make payments to other state-defined eligibility groups	Social Security Administration/HHS	State supplemental payment program may be state or federally administered

^aRequired for individuals over age 21.

^bAt option of the state.

^cRequired for individuals entitled to skilled nursing home care

^dMay be offered under a waiver of Medicaid State plan requirements, if requested by the state and approved by HHS. May include waiver of Medicaid eligibility requirements and stipulation that services be offered on a statewide basis.

source: O'Shaughnessy, C., Price, R., & Griffith, J. (1985, October 17). *Financing and delivery of long-term services for the elderly* (Library of Congress Publication No. 85-1033 EPW). Washington, DC: Congressional Research Service, Library of Congress.

most cost-effective. Should reduced budgets at state levels and rationing at state and federal levels expand, long-term care services are likely to suffer. Their availability will not keep up with the projected growth in demand.

Payment for long-term care is further complicated in that each state has its own payment system. Nursing homes are the largest expenditure and thus have received the most attention. A variety of payment systems for nursing homes have been tried over the years to minimize cost, maximize quality, and provide desired incentives to providers. The most progressive systems base payment on acuity level of patients or intensity of care provided. Similarly, home care, adult day care, and other social support services are paid for primarily by multiple state and local programs. Within a given state, payment may vary by locality.

The private sector recognized that a large share of long-term care funding falls on individual and families. The long-term care insurance market has grown, as described above. Further expansion of private coverage for long-term care could be enhanced by tax incentives (94). Greater understanding of what is covered and protection for the consumer are aspects of long-term care insurance that are the subject of public policy and regulation (95), particularly at the state level.

Expenditures for long-term care will rise dramatically in the near future. Projections for the cost of nursing home care and home care are shown in table 7-15. Because much long-term care supports activities of daily living rather than acute illness, payors are hesitant to authorize funding for fear of unlimited demand. The public policy question then is how all this care will be funded.

Medicare is exploring the possibilities of paying nursing homes and home health agencies on something other than a fee-for-service basis. Demonstrations such as the PACE and S/HMO are being tried, and bundling of specific services is being considered. Incremental changes in Medicare funding are likely to occur during the 1990s. States may or may not adopt the federal system; hence, less federal/state/private-paying variations may continue for some time.

In outlining the considerations for a national health policy that would cover long-term care, the Federal Pepper Commission, which examined the needs of the elderly, estimated the cost at $43 billion (96). This is about half of the total amount spent by Medicare in 1990 and 10 times the amount Medicare spent on nursing home and home care. This was viewed as prohibitively expensive for a nationwide program. The Medicare Catastrophic Care Act of 1988 approached the long-term care arena by incrementally expanding selected Medicare benefits. Funding relied on taxing the older population. Opposition by seniors was so great that the law was quickly repealed. Thus in the early 1990s, the cost of long-term care remains the responsibility of states and individuals, with an

TABLE 7-15. Nursing Home and Home Care Expenditures and Projections

	Nursing Home Expenditures In Billions			Home Care Expenditures In Billions		
	1986–90	2016–20	Change	1986–90	2016–20	Change
Medicaid	$14.1	$46.2	227%	$1.2	$ 2.4	100%
Medicare	.6	1.6	167%	3.1	7.7	148%
Patient	18.3	50.6	176%	2.7	7.2	166%
Other				1.6	4.6	187%
TOTAL	$33.0	98.4	198%	8.6	21.9	154%

Estimates by the Brookings Institution of current spending projected to 2016–20, using 1987 dollars, assuming delivery patterns remain unchanged.

SOURCE: National Association of Home Care.

impending expansion of costs and no consensus on a national approach to payment.

Fragmentation

As is evident from the discussion of services, the continuum of care consists of many different services provided by many organizations, each governed by several different public and/or private sources. To provide any type of comprehensive, continuous care requires achieving cohesion. At the same time, flexibility must be maintained in order to tailor the program to unique individual needs. Individual service providers and agencies must cooperate and share common goals. Although this is readily acknowledged, establishing the mechanisms to do so requires overcoming history and learned preference; state, local, and federal regulations; as well as operational barriers.

Funding for long-term care services comes from health, mental health, social service, public welfare, social security, and housing programs, to mention only the major public programs. Individuals, families, employers, and a variety of insurers and managed care companies represent the private side. Each payor, whether private or public, has distinct requirements. Administration of long-term care services, particularly those that are paid for by public sources, reflects the financing fragmentation. For example, four or five different state agencies may be involved in the payment of home health services. Fragmentation of delivery is likely to continue as long as the funding streams remain separate. The intent of the continuum of care is to be able to pool funding streams in order to provide the specific services required by an individual. Putting in place the mechanisms to accomplish this is the leading challenge of the 1990s.

Availability and Accessibility

For years the cry in the community-based long-term care arena was that services were simply not available. During the 1980s, the nation made great progress in this area. As can be noted from the earlier section on individual services, the number of programs grew: home health agencies doubled, adult day-care centers grew in profusion, hospices became a common and integral component of the system, and hospitals added services specifically for the elderly and chronically ill. In general, most urban areas now have a wide array of community-based services for those requiring long-term care. Trends toward capitation financing are encouraging.

Nonetheless, not all services are available to everyone when they are needed. Affordable homemaker and unskilled home support remains one of the services for which demand exceeds supply. Nursing home beds are in short supply in some areas because the state, in an attempt to limit Medicaid spending, has not allowed construction of new beds. State Medicaid waivers may eliminate financial barriers to community-based services for those who qualify as low-income, but do nothing to minimize costs for those who are just above poverty-level income. Rural areas continue to suffer a lack of many services, not just health care. The operation of a continuum of care assumes the availability and accessibility of key services. To the extent that public policy and funding limit service access or availability, the continuum of care will be abbreviated and patient flow inhibited accordingly.

Quality of Care

Quality has become one of the nation's major concerns about health care. The 1980s saw the initiation of major initiatives to measure and provide quality care for acute and chronic conditions. Long-term care and care for the elderly have also been the focus of initiatives in the public and private sectors.

Stringent regulations are imposed by Medicare and Medicaid, as well as by state licensing and certification programs, to ensure a minimum level of quality. In previous years, the lack of quality in nursing homes was infamous (97). Many of the most egregious problems have been corrected; others remain (98). The growth during the 1980s in the number of organizations providing care for the elderly or chronically disabled has been accompanied both by more visible problems and a large enough nucleus of providers to warrant and fund the development of standards. As the population ages and the general public becomes more aware of long-term care, consumers have added to the cry for high standards.

In the past few years, considerable attention has been given to improving Medicare. The Omnibus Budget Reconciliation Act of 1986 (OBRA 1986) called for a study to "design a strategy for quality review and assurance in Medicare." The recommendations from this study, conducted by the Institute of Medicine, are still working their way into the Medicare system (99).

Professional organizations and consumer groups are also active in establishing criteria and programs to enhance the quality of long-term care (100,101). The Joint Commission on the Accreditation of Hospitals changed its name during the 1980s to the Joint Commission on the Accreditation of Healthcare Organizations. It accredits several major components of the long-term continuum of care: nursing homes, hospital-based step-down units, home health agencies, and hospices. In all of these public and private endeavors, the emphasis has shifted from measuring process to focusing on patient care and outcomes.

The single most significant recent event affecting the quality of long-term care was the passage of the Nursing Home Reform Act of 1987, which was incorporated in the Omnibus Budget Reconciliation Act of 1987 and is thus referred to as "OBRA 1987" (102). This legislation, a series of amendments to the federal budget, created a number of changes affecting nursing homes, home health agencies, and hospitals, as well as other aspects of health care. The emphasis of regulations was changed from process evaluation to outcomes. Increased training was required of aides, essential staff members in nursing homes and home care. Decreased use of restraints was required in hospitals as well as in nursing homes. Medicare eliminated the distinction between skilled

nursing facilities and intermediate care, requiring instead that all facilities meet the requirements for skilled level nursing care. OBRA required more structured patient assessments and care plans, and thus prompted computerization of clinical records and nursing homes. The implementation of OBRA '87 was phased in over a period of years. Health care organizations are still adapting to the changes in the early 1990s.

The issues of quality in long-term care are closely related to the limitations of financing. With minimum financing, long-term care services simply cannot afford the physical or technological luxuries that acute-care services or families can offer. Quality must be balanced with the amount of demand and resource allocation. These become issues for society, as well as for individual patients and organizations.

Consumer Rights and Responsibilities

Quality of life is closely intertwined with quality of care. Only when individuals have dealt with the first issue can society come to consensus on the second. This nation is becoming increasingly aware of the rights and responsibilities of people with chronic and terminal problems. This is reflected in public policy, and in turn, helps to shape it.

The Patient Self-Determination Act of 1990 was landmark legislation. It requires that health care providers explain to patients their options for treatment and gives patients an opportunity to express their desire for extensive or limited use of high technology to maintain their life. The significance is that it forces individuals—health care providers, patients, and families—to determine the quality they desire in their own lives and the potentials and limitations of the health care system. Those with multiple, chronic illnesses and severe functional disabilities must decide to what extent they wish to employ available technologies to prolong their normal course of life. It is the health care providers, however, who must assist the consumer in understanding and making these personal choices.

Living wills and durable powers of attorney for health care are becoming common in the 1990s. The awareness of the need for such documents preceded the passage of the 1990 Patient Self-Determination Act and, in fact, helped to promote its passage. As the population ages, the number of people who are functionally disabled and require guardians or conservators increases. Laws have been implemented, primarily at the state level, to regulate the power one individual can have over another's life and assets. Consumers are increasingly persuaded to consider how they would want their affairs run if they were to become disabled due to physical or mental health problems, to discuss this with family and physicians, and to articulate their choices prior to the advent of problems.

The Americans with Disabilities Act of 1990 further recognized that institutions must assist those with functional disabilities. While the emphasis of this legislation is nondiscrimination for employment and physical access to facilities, the law also affects access to health care. Such legislation offers but a few examples of how the nation is becoming aware of the challenges of meeting the needs of the chronically ill and disabled while using scarce resources wisely.

Staffing and Expertise

The majority of staff in formal organizations providing long-term care have few skills. They receive low pay and their tasks are physically and emotionally demanding. A high proportion are recent immigrants whose native languages and customs differ from those of the majority of frail people for whom they care. Turnover rate is high, reaching as much as 100 percent annually in some nursing homes and home health agencies. Aides are particularly difficult to find and keep. OBRA '87 increased the training required of aides, but did not affect the salary levels nor increase payment to providers to meet the expense of implementing the new requirements. Long-term care providers face a major challenge in trying to provide quality care when they do not have the resources to attract and retain quality staff.

A shortage also exists of experts in chronic care, geriatrics, and rehabilitation. Physicians, nurses, social workers, and rehabilitation therapists who specialize in the care of the elderly or chronically ill are in great demand and short supply. For example, in 1991, physicians certified with a subspecialty in geriatrics number fewer than 5,000. Those with formal academic training in geriatrics number fewer than 2,000. This is not adequate to meet even the assessment needs of the nation's 32 million seniors.

Payment discourages many health care professionals from going into long-term care. Pay scales are lower than in acute settings. Physicians do not get reimbursed adequately for the time it takes them to go to a nursing home or make a home visit, compared to what they get paid for seeing patients in their office.

Attitudes are also an obstacle to attracting and keeping both skilled and unskilled providers in long-term care. Our society is one that values youth. Despite attempts to change the image of older adults, many young people still have a negative stereotype of older people. Health professionals, who are trained to "cure," find it difficult to accept chronic illness and an orientation toward maintaining functional independence rather than recovery.

Federal, state, and private organizations have addressed the issues of long-term care personnel shortages. Educators as well as providers have sought to change attitudes through more knowledge of the aged and the aging process. Many health care provider organizations now conduct aging sensitivity training as part of their orientation and ongoing inservice education.

The Long-Term Continuum of the Future

Do continuums of long-term care exist? Is it possible to overcome the problems of fragmentation, financing, and access to create an effective, efficient, consumer-oriented, high-quality system of care? Few, if any complete continuums of long-term care are now in operation; however, the success of components of a complete continuum of care has been ably demonstrated (31,33,103,104). Select programs throughout the nation provide encouragement for the future. In contrast to Mr. Jackson's experience, how do existing continuums provide long-term care? The following scenario already occurs in exemplary organizations:

Mrs. Smith is an 80-year-old widow who lives alone. She slips in the bathtub and breaks her hip. She uses her voice-activated emergency response system necklace to call for help. The call recipient automatically asks what the problem is, then calls for both a neighbor and emergency assistance. The neighbor comes over to be with Mrs. Smith, having agreed in advance to help in times of emergency.

The paramedics also arrive within minutes, stabilize Mrs. Smith, and take her to the hospital. Mrs. Smith belongs to the hospital-sponsored senior membership program, Silver Services, which was notified automatically via computer when the call came in. A laminated bar-coded ID card from Silver Services gives the paramedics and the doctors in the emergency room all the administrative and clinical information they need to initiate treatment.

While in the hospital, a care coordinator, with whom Mrs. Smith talked when she enrolled in Silver Services, visits her and reassures her that whatever services she needs will be arranged. When Mrs. Smith has recovered enough to be discharged from the acute service, she is transferred to a rehabilitation-oriented skilled nursing facility operated by the hospital. Mrs. Smith never liked the idea of being in a "nursing home," but she does not feel negative about this one because the ambience is positive, the staff are pleasant and encouraging, and she is confident that her physician and care coordinator will arrange for her transfer home.

Indeed, two weeks later Mrs. Smith goes home with home health nursing and rehabilitation. Meals on Wheels brings a hot meal daily, and a homemaker comes in twice a week to help with personal care, shopping, mail, and housekeeping. The emergency response system gives Mrs. Smith the security to remain alone at night, and she knows that she can call the Senior Services number at any time if she has questions or needs nonemergency assistance. Mrs. Smith also knows that her physician is regularly informed of what is happening to her. In another couple of weeks, Mrs. Smith is steady enough to leave her second-story apartment for addi-

tional outpatient therapy. The therapists have automated and immediate access to all of her records and know exactly what exercises the home health staff have recommended she continue.

Mrs. Smith's total spell of illness cost her very little out of pocket. The health care services she used were all participants in the Medicare HMO in which she was enrolled. She made her regular monthly payments somewhat above those required for Medicare Part B, and she acknowledged the HMO as her Medicare Part A and B provider. The care coordinator explained to Mrs. Smith that as long as she did not exceed the lifetime allowance and used the providers within the HMO network, she could use whatever levels of institutional or community-based services her physician and care coordinator felt necessary. Mrs. Smith also had the peace of mind of knowing that she had organized her legal and financial affairs well in advance—just in case anything serious happened. A social worker from Silver Services had helped her prepare a will, designate a sibling to assume durable power of attorney for health care, and express her preferences to her physician about the use of life-sustaining measures.

Long-term care in the United States has undergone major changes in the last 30 years. It has evolved from an insular, isolated potpourri of services bifurcated among nursing homes and social service agencies to a broader, more extensive network of many services available at many locations throughout the community. Its financing sources, coordinating mechanisms, and general outlook have changed greatly as public awareness of its importance increased. Long-term care will continue to change as demand grows. The 1990s will see the basic structure of the long-term care delivery system shift from one of fragmented services to comprehensive continuums of care. The future for the continuum of care, while challenged by the forces facing health care in general, is impressive and exciting.

References

1. General Accounting Office. (1988). *Long-term care for the elderly* (p. 2). Report to the Chairman, Subcommittee on Health and Long-Term Care, Se-

lect Committee on Aging, U.S. House of Representatives, Washington, DC.

2. Young, A. (1985). *Long-term care: An industry composite* (p. 3). New York: Arthur Young International.

3. Weissert, W. (1978). *Long-term care: An overview, health, United States, 1978* (p. 93) (DHEW Publication No. 78-1232). Washington DC: U.S. Government Printing Office.

4. Brody, E. (1977). *The long-term care of older people* (p. 14). New York: Human Services Press.

5. Kane, R., & Kane, R. (1982). *Values and long-term care* (p. 2). Lexington, MA: Lexington Books.

6. Pollack, W. (1979). *Expanding health benefits for the elderly* (Vol. I, *Long-term care*) (p. 2). Washington, DC: The Urban Institute.

7. Brody, S. (1984). Goals of geriatric care. In S. Brody & N. Persily. *Hospitals and the aged: The new old market* (p. 53). Rockville, MD: Aspen Systems Corporation.

8. Katz, S., Ford, A. B., Moskowitz, R. W., et al. (1985). Studies of illness in the aged. The index of ADL: A standardized measure of biological and psychosocial function. *Journal of the American Medical Association. 185.* 94.

9. Lawton, P., & Brody, E. (1969). Assessment of older people, self-maintaining and instrumental activities of daily life. *The Gerontologist. 9.* 179–186.

10. Special Committee on the Aging, U.S. Senate. (1991). *Long-term care: Projected needs of the aging baby boom generation* (p. 2) (GAO/HRD Publication No. 91-86). Washington, DC: Government Accounting Office.

11. U.S. Commission on Aging. (1989, January). Based on middle series projections from U.S. Bureau of the Census, Current Population Reports (Series P-25, No. 1018). *Projections of the population of the United States, by age, sex, and race: 1988 to 2080.*

12. Advisory Panel on Alzheimer's Disease. (1991). *Second report of the Advisory Panel on Alzheimer's Disease, 1990* (p. xi) (DHHS Publication No. [ADM] 91-1791). Washington, DC: U.S. Government Printing Office.

13. U.S. Department of Veterans Affairs. (1989, September). *Annual report, 1988.* Washington, DC.

14. American Association of Retired Persons. (1989). *Veterans and the demand for long-term care* (p. 1). Washington DC: Author, Public Policy Institute.

15. General Accounting Office. (1987, November). *VA health care: Assuring quality care for veterans in community and state nursing homes* (Publication No. GAO/HRD-88-18). Washington, DC: Author.

16. Keenan, M. (1989). *Veterans and the demand for long-term care* (p. 1). Washington, DC: American Association of Retired Persons.

17. National Society to Prevent Blindness. (1988). *Facts on blindness and prevention.* Schaumburg, IL: Author.

18. AIDS Hotline, direct communication. Los Angeles, 1992.

19. U.S. Bipartisan Commission on Comprehensive Health Care (the Pepper Commission). (1990, September). *A call for action, executive summary* (p. 11). Washington DC: U.S. Government Printing Office.

20. Older Women's League, cited 1989.

21. National Center for Health Services Research. (1984). *Caregivers of the frail elderly: A national profile* (p. 4). Washington, DC: U.S. Department of Health and Human Services.

22. The daughter track. (1990, July 16). *Newsweek.* 53.

23. Elder care. (1990, May 20). *Los Angeles Times.* 18.

24. Doty, P. Liu, K., & Wiener, J. (1985). An overview of long-term care. *Health Care Financing Review.* 6.

25. Evashwick, C. (1987). Definition of the continuum of care. In C. Evashwick & L. Weiss (Eds.). *Managing the continuum of care: A practical guide to organization and operations* (p. 23). Rockville, MD: Aspen Publishers.

26. American Hospital Association. (1991). *AHA hospital statistics 1991–92 edition.* Chicago: Author.

27. Evashwick, C., Rundall, T., & Goldiamond, B. (1985). Hospital services for older adults: Results of a national survey. *The Gerontologist.* 631–637. Vol 25 No. 6.

28. Hospital Research and Educational Trust. (1986). *Emerging trends in aging & long-term care services.* Chicago: Author.

29. Evashwick, C. (1982). Long-term care becomes major new role for hospitals. *Hospitals.* Vol 56, No. 13 pp. 50–5.

30. Hospital Research and Educational Trust. (1982). *The hospital's role in caring for the elderly: Leadership issues.* Chicago: Author.

31. Brody, S., & Persily, N. (1984). *Hospitals and the aged: The new old market.* Rockville, MD: Aspen Publishers.

32. Evashwick, C. (1989). *Hospitals and older adults: Meeting the challenge.* Chicago: American Hospital Association.

33. Persily, N. (1991). *Eldercare: Positioning your hospital for the future.* Chicago: American Hospital Association.

34. American Hospital Association. (1991). *AHA hospital statistics 1991–92 edition* (table 12A). Chicago: Author..

35. American Hospital Association. (1991). *AHA hospital statistics 1991–92 edition* (table 4C). Chicago: Author.

36. U.S. Department of Veterans Affairs. (1986, May). *VA in brief* (VA Pamphlet No. 06-83-1). Washington, DC: Author.

37. Veterans Administration. (1984, May). *Caring for the older veteran.* Washington, DC: Superintendent of Documents.

38. General Accounting Office. (1987, November). *VA health care: Assuring quality care for veterans in community and state nursing homes* (Publication No. GAO/HRD-88-18). Washington, DC: Author.

39. American Hospital Association, National Panel Survey. Chicago, December 1991.

40. Coile, R. (1991, March). The second "core business" of hospitals in the 1990s. *Health Strategy Report. 3*(5). 1

41. National Chronic Care Consortium.

42. Hing, E., Sekscenski, E., & Strahan, G. (1989). The National Nursing Home Survey: 1985 summary for the United States. *Vital Health Statistics. 13.* 97.

43. Hing, E. (1989, October). Nursing home utilization by current residents; United States, 1985. *Vital Health Statistics. 13.* 102.

44. U.S. Bipartisan Commission on Comprehensive Health Care (the Pepper Commission). (1990). *A call for action, final report 1990* (p. 93). Washington, DC: U.S. Government Printing Office.

45. Coleman, B. (1991). *The Nursing Home Reform Act of 1987: Provisions, policy, prospects.* Boston: University of Massachusetts.

46. Kemper, P., & Murtaugh, C. (1991). Lifetime use of nursing home care. *New England Journal of Medicine. 324.* 595–600.

47. Kemper, P., & Murtaugh, C. (1991). Lifetime use of nursing home care. *New England Journal of Medicine. 324.* pp. 595–600, Table 2.

48, Hing, E. (1989, October). Nursing home utilization by current residents; United States, 1985. *Vital Health Statistics. 13.* 102 (table F).

49. Hing, E. (1989, October). Nursing home utilization by current residents; United States, 1985. *Vital Health Statistics. 13.* 102 (table M).

50. Levit, K., Lazenby, H., Cowan, C., & Letsch, S. (1991, Fall). National health expenditures, 1990. *Health Care Financing Review. 13*(1). 29.

51. Sonnefeld, S., Walso, D., Lemieux, J., & McKusick, D. (1991, Fall). Projections of national health expenditures through the year 2000. *Health Care Financing Review. 13*(1). 10.

52. National Association for Home Care (1991). *Basic statistics about home care—1991.* Washington, DC: Author.

53. Facts about home care: The numbers. (1986, March 26). *Homecare.*

54. Rice, D., & Wick, A. (1986). *Impact of an aging population on health care needs: State projections* (p. III-7, table 3.6). San Francisco: University of California Institute for Health & Aging.

55. National Association for Home Care. (1991). Special Report.

56. National Association for Home Care. (1991). *Basic statistics* (p. 3). Washington, DC: Author.

57. Lutz. (1991, November 4). Safe harbor rules create infusion. *Modern Healthcare. 21*(44). 32.

58. FIND/SVP: Home Care Services. New York, 1989.

59. Marion Laboratories. (1989). *Marion long term care digest, home health care edition, 1989* (p. 11). Kansas City, MO: Author.

60. Lack, S. A. (1978). *The first American hospice—Three years of home care.* New Haven, CT: The Connecticut Hospice.

61. U.S. Department of Health and Human Services. (1991). *Medicare hospice benefits* (Publication No. HCFA 02154). Washington, DC: U.S. Government Printing Office.

62. Von Behren, R. (1986, October). *Adult day care in America: Summary of a national survey.* Washington, DC: National Institute on Adult Daycare, National Institute on the Aging.

63. Zawadski, R., & Von Behren, R. (1990, June). *The national adult day center census—'89.* San Francisco: University of California Institute for Health & Aging.

64. *Program for day care and respite.* (1992). Princeton, NJ: Robert Wood Johnson Foundation.

65. Health Care Financing Administration, Health Qual-

ity and Standards Bureau. (1980). *Directory of adult day care centers.* Washington, DC: U.S. Government Printing Office.

66. American Hospital Association. (1991, November 22). *Economic discipline and payment reform: Refining the AHA's national health reform strategy.* Chicago: Author.

67. CHA seeks input on systematic reform proposal. (1991, December). *Health Progress.* 12–24.

68. Evashwick, C., & Terrill, T. (1987). Organization and structure. In C. Evashwick & L. Weiss (Eds.). *Managing the continuum of care: A practical guide to organization and operations* (pp. 95–119). Rockville, MD: Aspen Publishers.

69. Evashwick, C., & Weiss, L. (Eds.) (1987). *Managing the continuum of care: A practical guide to organization and operations* (pp. 293–394). Rockville, MD: Aspen Publishers.

70. Bringewatt, R. (1991). *Geriatric care networks* (working paper). Bloomington, MN: National Chronic Care Consortium.

71. Mercy Health Systems. (1989). *Community health care systems concept, strategic plan.* Farmington Hills, MI: Author.

72. Kreger, M., & Weiss, L. (1987). Computer applications with the continuum of care. In C. Evashwick & L. Weiss (Eds.). *Managing the continuum of care: A practical guide to organization and operations.* Rockville, MD: Aspen Publishers.

73. Applebaum, R., & Austin, C. (1990). *Long-term case management* (p. 7). New York: Springer Publishing Company.

74. Steinberg, R., & Carter, G. (1983). *Case management and the elderly.* Lexington, MA: DC Heath & Co., Lexington Books.

75. White, M., Maddox, G., et al. (1987). Case management. *The encyclopedia of aging* (pp. 92–96). New York: Springer Publishing Company.

76. Applebaum, R., & Austin, C. (1990). *Long-term case management* (p. 11). New York: Springer Publishing Company.

77. Austin, C., Roberts, L., & Low, J. (1985). *Case management: A critical review.* Seattle: University of Washington Institute on Aging.

78. Office of Prepaid Health Care Operations and Oversight. (1991, December). *Monthly report Medicare prepaid health plans.* Internal report, Division of Contract Administration. Rockville, MD: Health Care Financing Administration.

79. Health Insurance Association of America. (1991). *The consumer's guide to long-term care insurance* (p. 5). Washington, DC: Author.

80. Van Gelder, S., & Johnson, D. (1991, January). *Long-term care insurance: A market update* (research bulletin) (pp. 4–5). Washington, DC: Health Insurance Association of America.

81. Van Gelder, S., & Johnson, D. (1991, January). *Long-term care insurance: A market update* (research bulletin) (p. 4). Washington, DC: Health Insurance Association of America.

82. Health Insurance Association of America. (1991). *The consumer's guide to long-term care insurance* (p. 6). Washington, DC: Author.

83. Van Gelder, S., & Johnson, D. (1991, January). *Long-term care insurance: A market update* (research bulletin) (p. 7). Washington, DC: Author.

84. Wiener, J., & Hanley, R. (1989, November 8). *Assessing the potential role of private long-term care insurance.* Testimony presented at a hearing on private long-term care insurance. U.S. Bipartisan Commission on Comprehensive Health Care (the Pepper Commission), Washington, DC.

85. Harrington, C., & Newcomer, R. (1990, Spring). Social health maintenance organizations as innovative models to control costs. *Generations.* 49–54.

86. Health Care Financing Administration. (1991, August). *Social health maintenance organization demonstration* (program description). Office of Demonstrations and Evaluation, HCFA, Baltimore, MD.

87. Newcomer, R., Harrington, C., & Friedlob, A. (1991). Awareness and enrollment in the social/HMO. *The Gerontologist. 30*(1). 86–93.

88. Harrington, C., & Newcomer, R. (1991, Spring). Social health maintenance organization's service use and costs. *Health Care Financing Review. 12*(3). 37–52.

89. Harrington, C., & Newcomer, R. (1990, Spring). Social health maintenance organizations as innovative models to control costs. *Generations.* 52.

90. On-Lok, Inc. (n.d.). *PACE* (program brochure). San Francisco: Author.

91. Health Care Financing Administration. (1991, November). *Program of all-inclusive care for the elderly (PACE)* (program description). Office of Demonstrations and Evaluation, HCFA, Baltimore, MD.

92. Levit, K., Lazenby, H., Cowan, C., & Letsch, S. (1991,

Fall). National health expenditures. *Health Care Financing Review. 13*(1). 29–55.

93. Liebig, P., & Lammers, W. (1990). *California policy choices for long-term care.* Los Angeles: University of Southern California, Ethel Percy Andrus Gerontology Center.

94. Wiener, J., & Hanley R. (1991, June 6). *Long-term care and social insurance: Issues and prospects.* Testimony presented at a hearing on health care cost and access. Committee on the Budget, U.S. House of Representatives, Washington, DC.

95. Wiener, J., & Harris, K. (1991, May). Regulation of private long-term care insurance. *CARING Magazine.* 36–42.

96. U.S. Bipartisan Commission on Comprehensive Health Care (the Pepper Commission). (1991, September). *A call for action, executive summary.* Washington, DC: U.S. Government Printing Office.

97. Vladeck, B. (1980). *Unloving care: The nursing home tragedy.* New York: Basic Books.

98. Institute of Medicine. (1986). *Improving the quality of care in nursing homes.* Washington, DC: National Academy Press.

99. Lohr, K. (Ed.). (1986). *Medicare: A strategy for quality assurance* (Vols. I and II). Washington, DC: National Academy Press.

100. Task Force on Long-Term Care Policy. (1988). *A time to be old: A time to flourish: The special needs of the elderly-at-risk.* St. Louis, MO: Catholic Health Association of the U.S.

101. National Citizens' Coalition for Nursing Home Reform, Washington, DC.

102. Coleman, B. (1991, November). *The Nursing Home Reform Act of 1987: Provisions, policy, prospects.* Boston: University of Massachusetts Gerontology Institute.

103. Zawadski, R. (1983). *Community-based systems of long-term care.* New York: The Haworth Press.

104. Miller, J. A. (1991). *Community-based long-term care: Innovative models.* Newbury Park, CA: Sage Publications.

Chapter 8

Mental Health Services

Mary Richardson

Mental health services have experienced considerable growth and change over the last several decades. Who is treated, and the problems they are treated for, have altered with changing definitions of mental illness, changing viewpoints about the appropriate response to mental health problems, and increasing social recognition and acceptance of mental health services as a treatment rather than a custodial function. This chapter describes the development of mental health services in this country, the users and reasons for use, the organization and financing of services, recent trends, and the problems of providing care. Although related issues of utilization and financing are discussed in other chapters, the unique nature of mental health services is presented in detail in this chapter.

Historical Perspectives on Definitions of Mental Illness

Societies have always defined and classified human behavior in ways that differentiated between what was acceptable and what was not. Description of the more subtle maladaptations of human beings to society involves attention to social and cultural values; as value systems change, so do conceptions of deviant behavior. Societal tolerance of deviant behavior partially determines what constitutes mental illness. In more recent times, psychiatric or emotional disability has been defined within biologic, sociologic, and cultural frameworks. However, scientific definitions have philosophical roots in a history that predates much current scientific thought.

During the Middle Ages, aberrant behavior was attributed to demonic influences, evil spirits, and the like. In an agrarian feudal society, deviance relates to the ability to work and sustain oneself. People regarded as "mad" were allowed to wander about if they were not too troublesome (1). Communities were able to offer them some basic support; if they became troublesome, they were driven away.

With the rise of a mercantile society in Europe and a breakdown of feudal estates, major social and political upheavals occurred. Many people were left homeless, with no means of support. Groups of unemployed people and disbanded soldiers drifted around the countryside. People who had previously been defined as mad or insane were classified together with those who were poor or homeless. They were grouped together in a much larger category of people considered to be socially destitute. Small communities quickly lost the ability to offer even minimal support to these people.

In England, the Elizabethan Poor Laws of 1601 heralded a recognition of the responsibility of government, and society as a whole, in addressing the problems of the destitute and the ill. In each community parish, overseers were assigned to provide care for these sick and disaffected members of society. Later, lunatic hospitals were opened throughout England. These hospitals existed more to protect the citizenry by isolating social misfits than to provide even a minimum of care. Conditions in these institutions were generally abominable. Inmates were often chained and provided only the barest essentials of survival.

In 1656 the French Parliament authorized the construction of the Hôpital Generale. The poor, the sick, and the insane were confined in circumstances much like those of the English lunatic hospitals. However, with the 18th century came the Age of Enlightenment and a revolution in scientific thought. In France, Philippe Pinel introduced the idea of mental illness with a medical framework (2). Pinel was initially the physician of the Infirmaries at the Hospice de Bicêtre in Paris. Although he was historically given credit for unchaining the inmates and introducing humanistic treatment, writings discovered more recently reveal that it was actually Jean-Baptiste Pussin, the governor of mental patients, who actually began this more humane treatment (2). The ideas of both Pinel and Pussin, who had once been a patient at Bicêtre, spread throughout Europe and later to the United States.

In the late 1800s, Kraepelin, a German physician, outlined a concise system of classification estab-lishing mental illness as a separate and distinct disease entity subject to the rules that applied to physical or somatic diseases. His work legitimized psychiatry as a branch of medicine. Kraepelin described in detail the symptoms, course of the disease, and prognosis of dementia praecox and manic-depressive psychoses. Sigmund Freud, the father of psychoanalysis, described neuroses in a deterministic fashion by proposing that all events could be traced to a specific origin. He described mental illness as related to disturbances and distortions from unconscious developmental difficulties in psychic growth and maturation and traumatic experiences and conflicts over sexual and self-destructive instincts. Although psychotherapy came to be regarded as a medical and psychiatric specialty. Freud established the psychological viewpoint.

Continuing biomedical research in the 20th century produced evidence that supported the concept of organic causations for mental illness. The discovery of the spirochete that causes syphilis and general paresis and discoveries of chromosomal aberrations in mental retardation were cited as such evidence. Studies of schizophrenia, defined as a diagnosis by Bleuler in the early 1900s (replacing dementia praecox) and manic-depressive syndromes have suggested possible familial tendencies. For example, 10 percent of siblings and children of schizophrenic patients are also diagnosed as schizophrenic, possibly indicating a biogenetic basis for this illness. Transcultural studies of mental illness have demonstrated remarkably uniform prevalence rates for schizophrenia in different countries and cultures. However, modern techniques for the study of chromosomal aberrations do not isolate genetic differences, and even with clinical evidence suggesting a biologic component, critics would argue that a diagnosis of schizophrenia is highly subjective, and that the perception of behavior as being schizophrenic is relative to the environmental context. Studies of other illnesses such as neurotic or drug abuse syndromes have so far been unable to identify biogenetic factors.

Social Psychiatric and Behavioral Definitions

During the 20th century there has been increasing acceptance of pluralistic determinants of mental illness, including biologic, sociologic, and social factors. Harry Sullivan was the first American psychiatrist to develop a theory stressing the importance of interpersonal relations in disease etiology. Concurrent with the development of social psychiatric definitions were new psychological and behavioral concepts of mental illness. Carl Jung broke away from the Freudian approach and formed the field of analytic psychology. Erich Fromme, a psychoanalyst never trained in medicine, and others applied anthropologic and sociologic concepts to Freud's theories. Later, John B. Watson discarded Freudian theory and developed behaviorism, which recognized only observable behavior as critical to the diagnosis of mental illness. He believed that all behavior was predictable on the basis of environmental stimuli. Psychologists introduced classic conditioning and learning theory to psychiatrists and other psychopathologists.

Social psychiatric and behavioral definitions of mental health reduced reliance on the disease concept of mental illness as internally manifested by the client; rather, social and cultural relativity and personality development were emphasized as significant factors in mental health. The development of humanistic psychology also had origins in the behavioral movements. The Freudian approach was considered too pessimistic and the behavioral approaches too mechanistic. Carl Rogers developed the technique of client-centered therapy, which recognized the clients' roles in affecting their own rehabilitation. According to this approach, client behavior is compared to expected behavior for the culture or environment of the patient. Differences between adaptive and maladaptive functioning vary from culture to culture and are more or less acceptable according to one's economic or social status. The validity of these broader environmentally based approaches is supported by transcultural psychiatric research that documents mental illness in all cultures and sug-gests that outward manifestations of these illnesses are shaped by the childrearing practices, indoctrinations, sanctions, encouragements, and discouragements of each culture.

Definitions of mental illness may also be predicated on the social and cultural values of the care provider and may be in conflict with the accepted norms of the recipient. This problem can be difficult if care providers are representative of the majority group within a population and the potential recipient is a member of a minority group. Behavior that is tolerated, accepted, or even encouraged within the minority group may be seen as deviant or sick behavior by the majority group. For example, an epidemiologic study of psychiatric disorders in a Pacific Northwest coastal Indian village revealed differing symptom patterns in men and women (3). Women, suffering more from psychoneuroses, were viewed as ill within this society, whereas men, generally suffering from alcoholism, not only did not seek treatment but were not even considered ill by their community. Hence treatment for women was accepted and even encouraged, whereas treatment of men was not. Finally, defining the overlap between social problems and mental illness is difficult. Are deviations such as delinquency or criminal behavior a mental health problem? What about poverty, discrimination, and unemployment? Mental health professionals must determine the extent of their roles as caregivers and as agents of social change.

Extent of Mental Disorders

The American Psychiatric Association classifies mental illness within three general categories: impairment of brain tissue, mental deficiency, and disorders without a clearly defined clinical cause. Most disorders treated by mental health professionals fall in the third category, but diagnosis of these problems is subjective in actual clinical practice. The *Diagnostic and Statistical Manual* (DSM III), published by the American Psychiatric Association, contains this classification system, which is used extensively in diagnosing mental illness (4).

These classifications are generally used in studies of incidence and prevalence of mental disorder.

The National Institute for Mental Health (NIMH) sponsored a multisite epidemiologic and health services research study, entitled "Epidemiologic Catchment Area (ECA) Program," that assesses mental disorder prevalence, incidence, and service use rates in about 20,000 community and institutional residents (5). An interview schedule, Diagnostic Interview Schedule (DIS), was developed for use by lay interviewers to assess the presence, duration, and severity of symptoms in study participants according to DSM III diagnostic criteria. Interviews were subsequently scored by computer according to diagnostic algorithms specified by DSM III and other diagnostic systems.

Incidence and Prevalence of Mental Illness

An estimated 29.4 million Americans suffer from mental illness (6). An Epidemiologic Catchment Area study of the six-month prevalence of 15 mental disorders in the United States revealed between 16.4 and 23.1 percent of the population to have diagnosable mental disorders (6). Phobias were found to be the most common mental disorder, affecting from 5.1 to 12.5 percent of those surveyed. Substance abuse disorders, including alcohol abuse/dependence, is the second most common category, found in 4.8 to 7.5 percent of Americans. Affective disorders, including major depression, were found in 4.1 to 6.6 percent of those surveyed. Schizophrenia was reported for 0.6–1.2 percent of Americans.

Prevalence rates vary for men and women and according to age. The most frequent diagnosis for men aged 18–64 is alcohol abuse/dependence, with severe cognitive impairment becoming the most prominent diagnosis for men ages 65 and over. Phobias are the most common diagnosis reported for women of all ages. Drug abuse/dependence is cited as the second most prevalent mental health problem for women ages 18 to 24, while major depression is more often cited by women ages 25 to 44.

The rates of mental disorders, except for cognitive impairment, dropped after age 45 for both men and women. Among substance abuse disorders, alcohol-related disorders were two to three times as prevalent as drug-related disorders.

Development of Mental Health Services in the United States

Early Mental Health System

The development of American psychiatry in the 19th century was strongly influenced by Dr. Benjamin Rush, long considered the father of American psychiatry, who was also a pioneer in hospital reform. Before the 19th century, formal treatment centers were nonexistent. Private physician services were available to those with money. The rest faced imprisonment or hospitalization, with one not much different from the other. Ths hospital reform spearheaded by Pinel in the late 1700s in France was paralleled in this country by Rush's activities. The American Psychiatric Association was started through the efforts of affiliated hospital superintendents who, like Rush, were concerned with hospital conditions. Even into the early 20th century, treatment of mental illness based on medical/clinical approaches occurred in state-supported hospitals, which were often located in remote areas and functioned as large human warehouses.

The disease concept of mental illness implies that the patient can become "well" and generally assumes that the therapist, historically a psychiatrist, will diagnose the illness and define subsequent treatment. The Freudian model has led to long-term and intensive psychotherapy and to therapeutic and personal requirements that are beyond the resources available to the state hospitals. Mental illness was also highly stigmatized and subject to funding limitations by state legislatures, with the primary purpose of providing public protection from "crazy people," rather than providing a public good for people with psychiatric problems.

The National Mental Health Act of 1946 (PL79-487) signified an increased federal interest in the plight of the mentally ill. The law created the National Institute of Mental Health and increased appropriations for therapy and research. In addition, recognition of the psychological problems of soldiers during World War II motivated Veterans Administration (VA) hospitals to provide expanded mental health services.

Deinstitutionalization and the Growth of Outpatient Services

The development of psychopharmacology in the 1950s had a profound impact on the field of mental health. Psychotropic drugs led to dramatic breakthroughs in the treatment of mental illness and enabled thousands of patients previously considered incurable to be effectively treated on an outpatient basis. The use of these drugs also created a climate that encouraged the development of various innovative therapeutic approaches.

Before World War II, few outpatient mental health facilities existed. With growing federal interest, the number of outpatient facilities increased. At the same time, the prognosis for the thousands of patients in mental hospitals—many of whom suffered from schizophrenia, depression, and mania—remained dismal. However, the use of antipsychotic medications for schizophrenia, antidepressants for depression, and more recently, lithium in the treatment of mania, rapidly improved the prognosis for these patients. With the development of psychotropic medications, medical/clinical models of treatment continued to be the major influence on hospital treatment of mental illness. Psychotropic drugs also led to a radical decline in hospital lengths of stay for patients with psychiatric diagnoses. Patients now could control their behavior through the use of these drugs and, it was hoped, function within the community. Thus, a mental health system previously based primarily on inpatient facilities had to develop new approaches to serving patients who no longer needed to be hospitalized.

Although mental health professionals continued to expand their understanding of mental and emotional disorders, the general public was still distrustful of, and misinformed about, the nature of mental illness, and there was little advocacy for improvement except from the mental health community. Nevertheless, there was a dramatic increase in outpatient clinics from 400 before World War II to 1,234 by 1954 (7).

Finally, in 1955 the National Mental Health Study Act (PL 84-182) was passed, which authorized $750,000 for a three-year study of the entire mental health system. The result was the *Action for Mental Health Report,* published in 1961. Although this report covered many issues in the provision of mental health services, the primary emphasis of the legislation that followed, during the Kennedy administration, was on outpatient services. Concern was increasingly focused on providing comprehensive mental health services to people not requiring hospitalization as well as to those not previously having access to mental health services. The Mental Retardation Facilities and Community Mental Health Centers Construction Act of 1964 (PL 88-164) provided construction monies for community mental health centers that were to serve designated catchment areas of 74,000–200,000 people. The five basic services that the centers were required to provide included inpatient, outpatient, emergency, day treatment, and consultation and education services. Significantly, the legislation mandated that services be provided regardless of the patient's ability to pay.

Many centers were built with the newly available funding for construction, but money for staffing and operations continued to be scarce. Finally, in 1967, an amendment to the legislation provided the necessary operations money on a matching basis, with funding for each center declining over an eight-year period. This was the "seed money" concept, and it was hoped that the construction and development of a community mental health center would encourage the community to gradually assume financial responsibility for services. Since catchment areas varied in their ability to provide matching funds, the subsidy for services in different areas also varied considerably. And although there was an allowance for poorer communities, the capability to readily obtain local matching funds was a distinct advantage for some centers.

In retrospect, the whole notion of matching local funds ignored the inability of some communities to assume the associated financial burden, especially in areas of greatest need. Since many centers faced closure or significant reduction in services, additional legislation (PL 94-63) was passed in 1975. This law included provision for a one-year distress grant at the end of the eight years of operational support if alternate funding was not obtained. This legislation was designed to overhaul the community mental health center network and also to increase the original five required services to 12, including care for drug abuse problems, children, and the aged, as well as screening, follow-up, and community living services. Planning and evaluation of local community mental health services was mandated; 2 percent of each center's budget was to be used for these purposes.

Community mental health centers are also required to operate under the authority of a board of directors that represents the local community. These boards, however, are often composed of well-educated, upper-middle-income people who are frequently health care providers, despite the location of many mental health centers in lower-income communities.

Concern for the inadequacies of the mental health system led President Jimmy Carter to establish the President's Commission on Mental Health in 1977. The President's wife, Rosalynn, served as honorary chairperson, indicating her active interest in mental health services in Georgia during Carter's tenure as governor. The report produced by the commission went on to influence policy formation and in many ways became the heart of the Carter administration's Mental Health Systems Act, passed by Congress in 1980 (PL 96-398) (1). Although the act authorized continuation of provision to establish additional Community Mental Health Centers and authorized spending for many new initiatives,

it was never implemented. Under the conservative administrations of Ronald Reagan and George Bush, monies authorized were never appropriated.

Although the Systems Act was never implemented, the national plan, also called for by the President's Commission on Mental Health, was produced and underwent limited distribution (8). Titled "Toward a National Plan for the Chronically Mentally Ill" (9), the plan focused on federal mainstream resources, especially those available under the Social Security Act.

Although mental health policy underwent fiscal conservatism, mental health advocates, linked to a doctrine of increased state responsibility, went into action. The National Institute of Mental Health's Community Support Program (CSP), a demonstration program for the care of people with severe mental illness, survived the decade despite repeated attempts by the Reagan administration to eliminate it. In 1986, the State Comprehensive Mental Health Services Plan Act of 1986 (PL 99-660) built on the CSP system by calling on each state to work with the Medicaid agency and prepare a detailed plan for the care of individuals with serious mental illness.

As categorical mental health funds were organized into state block grants, advocates went to work to improve funding in mainstream resources. The four programs upon which these efforts were focused included Supplemental Security Income, Social Security Disability Insurance, Medicaid, and Medicare. The national plan became the blueprint for incremental change. Structural changes were made in each of the four programs that expanded benefits to individuals with mental illness, although full benefit of these changes has yet to be realized.

Mental health policy in the 1990s will be shaped by continuing efforts to expand entitlement programs as well as categorical programs to benefit the mentally ill. In addition, as federal policy makers move to address the pressing problems of the 1990s through consideration of national health care access bills and long-term care proposals, advocates will need to maintain their vigilance in order to ensure appropriate coverage of mental illnesses. One new theme of the policy focus will be set by the passage in 1990 of the Americans with Disabilities Act (PL 101-336), a civil rights bill that ensures the rights of individuals to employment without fear of discrimination and access to all public facilities—whether for transportation, recreation, or other similar activities.

Organization and Use of Mental Health Services

Mental Health Service Settings

Between 1970 and 1986 the number of mental health organizations in the United States increased steadily from 3,005 to 4,747 (10). The number of organizations with inpatient services rose from 1,734 in 1970 to 2,526 in 1980, dropping slightly in 1982—to 2,305—and rising to 3,039 in 1986. The number providing outpatient services rose consistently from 2,156 in 1970 to 2,946 in 1986. Likewise, the number providing partial care services rose rapidly, with a total of 1,947 programs in 1986, nearly triple the 778 in 1970.

The number of patient care episodes increased between 1971 and 1986 from 4.2 million to 7.9 million (10). However, the distribution of episodes by type of service remained fairly constant with inpatient care episodes comprising approximately 26 percent, outpatient care episodes 70 percent, and partial care episodes, 4 percent. This is a reverse of the distribution of patient care episodes in 1955, when 77 percent inpatients or residents, compared to 23 percent who received services in outpatient programs.

The dramatic reduction in episodes of inpatient treatment since 1955 is a direct result of a national philosophy toward deinstitutionalization. Between 1955 and 1980 the resident census of state and county mental hospitals declined from 559,000 to 138,000, or to one quarter of the previous census (11). By 1986, 285 state mental hospitals remained in operation, of which 30 were exclusively for chil-

dren, 12 were security hospitals for the criminally insane, and nine were teaching hospitals. The remaining facilities were not limited to a special program goal or specific clientele.

Although the number of state and county mental hospital beds decreased, VA medical centers, private psychiatric hospitals, and residential treatment centers (RTCs) for emotionally disturbed children increased the number of psychiatric beds between 1984 and 1986 (12). The growth of private psychiatric hospitals and RTCs is believed to be due, in part, to expanded psychiatric hospitalization benefits by a number of insurance carriers.

State and county mental hospitals, however, still accounted for 45 percent of psychiatric beds in 1986 (12). Nationally, the separate psychiatric inpatient services of general hospitals ranked second in number of beds with 17 percent of the total, followed by private psychiatric hospitals, with 11 percent, VA medical centers with 10 percent, RTCs with 9 percent, and multiservice mental health organizations with 8 percent.

Psychiatric outpatient services constitute a large part of the total mental health services delivery system in the United States, accounting for 5.6 million of the 8.1 million patient care episodes (69 percent) (13). The majority (42 percent) are multiservice mental health organizations, 26 percent are freestanding psychiatric outpatient clinics, and 17 percent are psychiatric units of nonfederal general hospitals. The remainder are VA psychiatric organizations, private psychiatric hospitals, and state mental hospitals.

A significant trend in the organization of mental health services has been the rapid growth of the private sector. The private psychiatric hospital is generally categorized as either nonprofit or for-profit. Few, if any, nonprofit hospitals have been founded in decades. Their financing comes from a variety of sources, including fees, endowments, grants, government contracts, and private donations. However, between 1984 and 1986 private psychiatric beds accounted for 41 percent of the growth in psychiatric beds overall (12). Of the for-profit hospitals, approximately 90 percent are owned by corporations (14). The for-profit groups have been characterized by the development of corporate chains.

Another trend affecting mental health services has been the growth of managed-care arrangements as a means of controlling the rate of increase in health and mental health care costs nationwide. Managed care is defined as a set of techniques used by or on behalf of purchasers of health care benefits to manage health care costs by influencing patient care decision making through case-by-case assessments of the appropriateness of care prior to its provision (15). The implementation of managed care strategies follows a series of other cost control measures including insurance benefit limitations and exclusions, prepaid health plans, prospective payment systems, and fee schedules.

Some see managed mental health care as a means of moving to more sophisticated outcomes measurement and management of quality of care (16). With an enrolled population researchers can more accurately measure incidence and prevalence of behavioral health care problems as well as measure the use and outcomes of treatment in a more precise fashion. Critics argue that managed care increases bureaucratization of services, will lead to rationing of services, and does not necessarily reduce the cost of care (17,18). Further, they argue that managed care negatively affects quality of care.

Deinstitutionalization and Chronic Mental Illness

Despite vigorous efforts at deinstitutionalization, state and county mental hospitals continue to be a locus of care for a wide variety of patient populations. In many respects, they serve as the "floor" of the mental health service system. Often they are the "source of last resort" and provide acute inpatient care to patients who have been unresponsive to treatment in other settings or who have exhausted their financial or other resources.

A study of the changes in one state hospital's clientele between 1972 and 1980 showed a 50 percent reduction in long-stay patients and a 27 percent increase in admissions (19). In addition, the authors report a new long-stay population. Over an eight-year period, the hospital has shifted from serving a largely homogeneous population of long-stay schizophrenics plus a smaller short-stay group of patients with similar characteristics to serving a smaller proportion of the original clientele plus larger numbers of patients with differing characteristics. While the old long-stay patients are predominantly middle-aged and elderly schizophrenics, the new patients fall into several categories, including young male schizophrenics, female schizophrenics distributed more evenly across age groups, and elderly female patients with organic brain syndromes.

Deinstitutionalization was to have shifted patient care from long-term care hospitals to short-stay hospitals and/or community mental health centers. Community mental health centers were launched with a philosophy that included responsibility to a total population, as defined within a catchment area, and a mission to serve as the base of community care for people leaving mental hospitals. They were also designed to bring mental health services to previously unserved or underserved populations. Problems beset the community mental health movement as some found fertile ground in some areas of the country and inhospitable ground in others. The availability of community-based services stimulated an increase in utilization of mental health services by many people who had never previously sought services, while the major segment of the targeted population, chronically mentally ill individuals, did not always find their way to the mental health center doorstep.

Of all the organized health care settings, only the nursing home (Chapter 7) can be demonstrated clearly to have become a substitute for the long-term custodial care function of the state and county mental hospital (11). Of slightly more than 1.5 million people over the age of 18 living in nursing homes or personal care homes, approximately 60 percent have some type of mental disorder (20). Approximately 29 percent have dementia only, including chronic or organic brain syndrome, and 13.7 percent have dementia in combination with one or more mental disorders. The remainder had a mental disorder but no dementia.

Concern over the numbers of mentally ill and mentally retarded individuals living in nursing homes was the basis for the Congressional passage of new laws governing nursing homes as part of the Omnibus Budget Reconciliation Act of 1987 (OBRA 1987). Under these provisions, nursing homes must screen all residents to determine their mental status. If placement in the nursing home is related only to mental status and not justified by the level of nursing care required, the individual is to be moved into a more appropriate treatment setting. In the event an individual is mentally ill and his or her nursing care needs require nursing home placement, the nursing home is required to provide treatment appropriate to the mental needs of that patient in addition to the nursing care provided. Great controversy has surrounded enactment of the law, and regulations implementing it have been very slow in coming. Thus, implementation has been hampered and there remains considerable confusion about the ultimate impact.

Deinstitutionalization is undergoing a second-generation effort (21). During this second phase court decisions focus on institutions where deinstitutionalization efforts may have already taken place. It is likely more difficult to sustain remaining patients in the community, even when adequate services are available. Age, specifically age over 60, appears significantly related to longer community tenure and a lower likelihood of readmission. The other most consistently significant predictor is prior hospitalization history. Geller and associates found that many people who have displayed a tendency toward frequent hospitalization will persist in that pattern even in the presence of community-based resources.

More recent studies of long-stay patients raise the question of whether further reductions in insti-

tutional populations are feasible (22). Community mental health centers, intended to form the backbone of community services for the chronically mentally ill, have experienced a shift in policy as federal funds disappeared and centers sought funding from states and other sources. As they changed from federal to state authority, centers have undergone substantial changes in staffing, array of services, and sources of revenue. Thus, program mission has changed substantially, often becoming quite different from that of programs established under the original federal mandates.

The Homeless Mentally Ill Person

The prospect of further deinstitutionalization is daunting. Critics cite many difficulties in implementing deinstitutionalization policies, including inadequate funding, the failure to develop needed community services, and difficulties in maintaining continuity of care after hospital discharge (21). In addition, the numbers of chronically mentally ill young adult patients are growing (23), and deinstitutionalization seems to contribute to the creation of substantial numbers of homeless mentally ill (24).

Mentally ill individuals make up a substantial percentage of the homeless population of the United States, with estimates ranging from 20 to 40 percent of the total (24). The incidence of homelessness in the United States is difficult to quantify; however estimates in recent years place the number of homeless people in a range from a quarter-million to 5 million. Consensus has settled on a survey conducted by the Urban Institute in March 1987 over a one-week period, which resulted in an estimate of 496,000 to 600,000 homeless people in the United States. The Urban Institute further estimated that if 600,000 people were homeless during one week, more than 1 million were homeless at some time during the entire year.

Recent studies estimate that 20 to 40 percent of the homeless population suffers from such serious mental illnesses as schizophrenia, manic-depressive illness, or severe depression. The Urban Institute study indicates that mental illness is most prevalent among single homeless adults, male or female, and is less evident among the typical homeless family of a woman with children, although the prevalence of mental illness among such homeless families is above the average for the general U.S. adult population (25).

The annual report of the Interagency Council on the Homeless notes that the higher prevalence of mental illness in the homeless population and, conversely, the rate of homelessness among those who are mentally ill, is not surprising. Noninstitutionalized mentally ill people are less likely to find employment, housing, or other benefits, or assistance to help keep them from becoming homeless than are those who are not mentally ill. Mentally ill people in the community not only are less likely to be able to function or work, but they are also less aware of the services available to them and less willing to seek help. They face frequent discrimination from employers and landlords and they often face shortages of treatment facilities and housing opportunities in their communities as well.

Abuse of alcohol and other drugs has also been a constant problem among the homeless population, often among the same individuals who suffer from mental illness. The National Institute on Alcohol Abuse and Alcoholism (NIAAA) estimates that 35 to 40 percent of the homeless population suffers from chronic alcohol problems (24). The same agency, in conjunction with the National Institute on Drug Abuse (NIDA) and others, estimates that approximately 10 to 20 percent of the homeless population has chronic problems with drugs other than alcohol. Data from the Urban Institute study indicates that almost half of all severely mentally ill homeless people also have problems with alcohol and other drugs.

There has been quite a bit of talk, but little definitive action on behalf of the homeless mentally ill (25). In 1984 the American Psychiatric Association published the results of a Task Force on the Homeless Mentally Ill, and described homelessness as but one symptom of the problems faced by chronically mentally ill people in the United States.

The APA Task Force called for a comprehensive and integrated system of care for chronically mentally ill people in order to address the underlying problems that cause homelessness. The task force's recommendations called for an adequate number and range of supervised, supportive housing settings; a well-functioning system of case management; adequate, comprehensive, and accessible crisis intervention in the community and in hospitals; less restrictive laws on involuntary treatment; and ongoing treatment and rehabilitative services, combined with assertive outreach programs when necessary.

With few exceptions, these recommendations have not been implemented. In addition to funding problems, a fundamental civil rights issue is being debated. Do the homeless mentally ill have a basic right, irrespective of their mental status and lack of competence, to refuse treatment and appropriate housing, and live on the streets instead? Or does this "right to choice" translate into a life characterized by dysphoria and deprivation, victimization by predators, and the development of life-threatening health care problems—a cruel interpretation of the basic principles of civil rights (26).

Utilization of Mental Health Services

Mental health services are utilized at differing rates depending on such factors as race, age, and sex. The concepts of utilization variables and data assessment presented in Chapter 3 are relevant to understanding and interpreting mental health data; specific aspects of use of mental health services are presented in this section. A diverse group of people were treated in various mental health settings. Overall, approximately 1.7 million people were under care and another 3.9 million were admitted during 1986 to inpatient, outpatient, and partial care programs. In general, outpatient programs served a greater number of people by a wide margin, while partial care programs served far fewer (figure 8-1) (10). Differences in the relative sizes of the under-care and admission populations in inpatient programs is due to the small

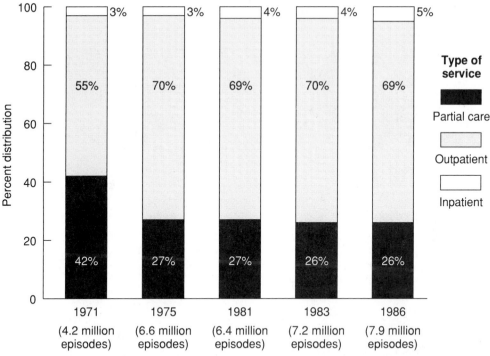

Figure 8-1. Percent distribution of patient care episodes in mental health organizations by type of service: United States, 1971, 1975, 1981, 1983, and 1986 (SOURCE: Manderscheid, R. W., & Sonnenschein, M. A. (Eds.). (1990). *Mental health United States, 1990* (DHHS Publication No. [ADM] 90-1708). Washington, DC: U.S. Government Printing Office.)

proportion of patients who become part of the long-term caseload. In contrast, the number of admissions in outpatient programs was only about one and a half times the number of clients under care.

Individuals from minority races tend to comprise larger percentages of state and county mental hospital populations than they do of other organization types (10). More males were treated in inpatient and partial care services than females, whereas men and women were fairly equally represented in outpatient care. The 24–44 age group comprised the largest percentage (52 percent) of inpatient admissions, while 7 percent were children and youth under the age of 18. Children and youth comprise a rather large percentage of the undercare caseload of private psychiatric hospital inpatient programs. Outpatient program admissions, centered largely in the 25–44 age group, ac-

counted for 45 percent of all clients admitted. Among admissions, however, children and youth represented a higher percentage than they did among those under care (26 percent vs 16 percent) and were the most frequently admitted age group.

Overall, the most frequently occurring diagnostic grouping among admissions to inpatient psychiatric services was affective disorders (31 percent), followed by schizophrenia (23 percent) and alcohol related disorders (15 percent). Schizophrenia was the most frequent primary diagnosis for admission to state and county mental hospitals. It was the second most frequent diagnosis for admission to VA medical centers, nonpublic nonfederal general hospitals, and private psychiatric hospitals (figure 8-2). Affective disorders were the primary diagnosis for only 14 and 13 percent of admissions to VA medical centers and state and county mental hos-

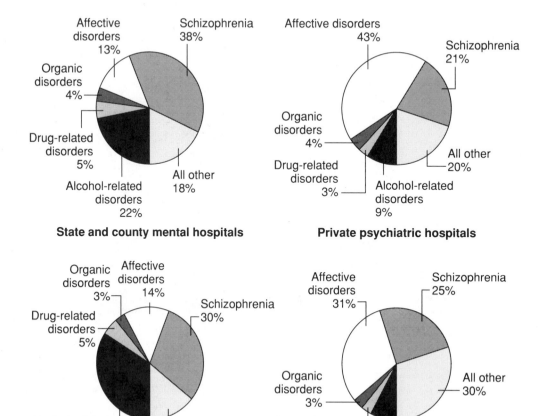

Figure 8-2. Percent distribution of admissions, by selected primary diagnosis and type of inpatient psychiatric service, United States, 1980. (SOURCE: Taube, C. A., & Barrett, S. A. (Eds.). (1985). *Mental health, United States, 1985* (DHHS Publication No. [ADM] 85-1378). Washington, DC: U.S. Government Printing Office.)

pitals, respectively. These data are consistent with the fact that chronically and severely mentally ill persons are more likely to be dependent on the public system of care. However, private settings do serve this population as well.

The percentage of admissions with primary diagnosis of alcohol-related disorders varied considerably by type of inpatient psychiatric service. They represented the most frequent primary diagnoses among admissions to VA medical centers and a significant number of admissions to state and county mental hospitals. Less than 10 percent of admis-

sions to remaining types of inpatient psychiatric service had a primary diagnosis of alcohol-related admissions. More recent trends signify a change in regard to alcohol and drug abuse. Society, and especially employers, have begun to fully understand the major role alcohol and drug abuse/dependence plays in a wide range of physical and mental illnesses. The potential for successful early intervention in mediating the effects of abuse has been the cause for increased efforts to restructure reimbursement mechanisms and allow for improved coverage of drug- and alcohol-related problems. As a result, there has been a significant increase in the number of alcohol and drug treatment programs in a variety of organizational types.

Comparisons among the inpatient psychiatric services show considerable variation in length of stay by type of diagnosis (6). State and county mental hospital admissions with organic disorders had the longest inpatient stay, followed by admissions related to schizophrenia. Length of stay is also affected by principal source of payment. State and county mental hospitals had the longest median inpatient stays for each expected principal source of payment, with the exception of commercial insurance. Admissions expected to use commercial insurance had the longest median stay (21 days) in private psychiatric hospitals. These data support the notion that restructuring of mental health benefits by third-party resources has had a profound impact on the increase of private psychiatric hospitals.

Mental Health Personnel

There are many different types of professionals providing mental health services. They involve a number of interesting and complex issues, mostly unique to the mental health field and discussed in this chapter, but often also similar to other personnel issues discussed in Chapter 1.

The number of full-time-equivalent (FTE) staff employed in specialty mental health organizations in the United States rose from 440,925 in 1984 to 494,591 in 1986 (27). This increase can be attributed in large part to the increase in the number of mental health organizations during this same period. With the exception of freestanding psychiatric outpatient clinics, all of the other types of mental health organizations experienced increases in the number of FTE staff between 1984 and 1986, with the largest numerical increases occurring in private psychiatric hospitals, RTCs, and multiservice mental health organizations.

Of the staff employed by speciality mental health organizations in 1986, 37 percent were employed in state mental hospitals, 20 percent in multiservice

mental health organizations, and 14 percent in separate psychiatric services of nonfederal general hospitals, and 12 percent in private psychiatric hospitals. Each of the organizational types comprised 7 percent or less of the total.

Staff patterns varied among the different mental health organizations, due to such factors as differences in types of service programs offered, caseload mix, budgetary factors, and differentials in the supply and accessibility of specific types of staff. For example, in 1986, 35 percent of the FTE staff in state mental hospitals were classified as "other mental health workers" (holding less than a B.A.); by contrast, in other mental health organizations, the proportion of FTE staff in this category ranged downward, from 22 percent in RTCs to 2 percent for freestanding psychiatric outpatient clinics. Conversely, state mental hospitals had the smallest percentage of FTE professional patient care staff (30 percent). Figure 8-3 denotes the distribution of staff in all mental health organizations for the period 1972–1986.

Psychiatrists

Psychiatry is the medical speciality dealing with mental disorders. Traditional psychiatry offers medical/clinical definitions of mental illness. Social psychiatry, in contrast, is concerned with the environmental and societal phenomena involved in mental and emotional disorders and the use of social forces in the treatment of such disorders. Much of the scientific work of social psychiatry has been in the area of epidemiology, particularly estimation of the incidence and prevalence of mental illness in community and hospital settings. Growing concern for the environment in large mental hospitals during and after World War II also added impetus to the social psychiatric movement, and as early as 1946, the American Psychiatric Association adopted a rigid set of standards for mental hospitals and appointed a Central Inspection Board for enforcement of these standards. Social psychiatry, in an effort to transform these large institutions from custodial care to treatment centers,

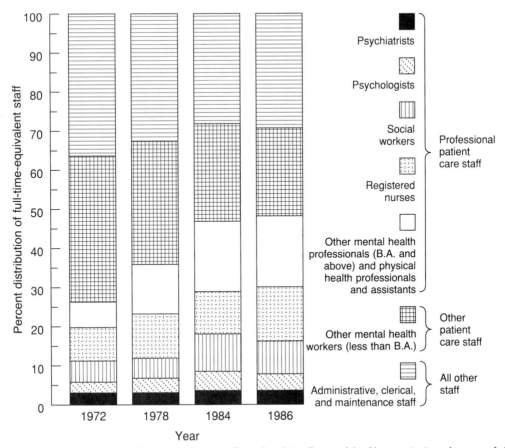

Figure 8-3. Percent distribution of full-time-equivalent staff employed in all mental health organizations, by type of discipline: United States, 1972, 1978, 1984, and 1986 (SOURCE: Manderscheid, R. W., & Sonnenschein, M. A. (Eds.). *Mental health, United States, 1990* (DHHS Publication No. [ADM] 90-1708). Washington, DC: U.S. Government Printing Office.)

developed the concept of the therapeutic community, the fundamental tenet of which is that patients can assist in their own rehabilitation as well as in the rehabilitation of other patients.

Social psychiatry also includes transcultural and community psychiatry. Transcultural psychiatry studies the incidence and prevalence of mental disease across societies and delineates the social forces that affect the manifestations of these illnesses. Community psychiatry has been described as "social psychiatry in action" (28) and is involved in the development, planning, and organization of community mental health programs and consultation to local agencies.

The number of psychiatrists in the United States increased from approximately 7,000 in 1950 to more than 32,000 by 1985, including those working primarily in administration (29). Slightly more than eight out of 10 U.S. psychiatrists in 1982 were men (10). The median age of active psychiatrists in 1982 was 48 years.

Blacks and Native Americans are underrepresented in psychiatry, compared to their proportions of the U.S. population. To address the underrepresentation of racial and ethnic minorities among psychiatrists, the American Psychiatric Association has promoted high school, college, and medical school programs to encourage recruitment.

Psychologists

Psychology, which struggled to create its own professional identity in the early years of this century, has emphasized scientific research in academic settings. Beginning as a philosophy, psychology has become firmly established as a social science, and psychologists have promoted and conducted research on the functioning of the human mind, especially through development of scientific testing instruments. Beginning in the early 20th century, psychological testing began to be used in conjunction with psychiatric treatment. Research by psychologists in classic conditioning and behavior theory also aided psychiatrists, who still provided most therapeutic care.

During World War II, psychologists began to be seen in an increased role in clinical practice. With the expansion of mental health services in VA hospitals, the training of clinical psychologists began in earnest. In 1946 the Veterans Administration, in conjunction with the American Psychological Association, began the Veterans Administration Psychology Training Program, which is still a major source of training for clinical and counseling psychologists. The professional application of psychology received further endorsement at the American Psychological Association Vail Conference of 1973, which emphasized the continued training of clinicians and scientists in psychology.

Psychologists are licensed or certified in all states and the District of Columbia. In almost all states, the training required for licensure is a doctoral degree, although a few states allow limited licensure for graduates of master's degree programs; however, independent private practice is prohibited. Licensure is not required for practice in some settings, however, and unlicensed psychologists most often practice in school or community mental health facilities. The American Psychological Association reports a 1986 membership of 63,000; there may, in fact, be over 70,000 master's- and doctorate-level psychologists (30).

The pool of clinically trained women psychologists, for the most part, tends to be younger and more diverse in terms of racial and ethnic minority representation. In fact, participation by women in psychology has increased in many ways. Within the practice-oriented subfields, women account for 57 percent of all new 1989 Ph.D.s, compared to 21 percent in 1965. Over the next decade, this situation is unlikely to change, given that 62 percent of all full-time students in doctoral clinical, counseling, and school psychology programs are women (10).

Although the proportion of ethnic minority psychologists has remained relatively low compared to their representation in the U.S. population, the number of doctorates awarded to blacks, Asians, and Hispanics has inched upward since the early 1970s (10). In 1975, 42 blacks, 14 Hispanics, and six Asian Americans were earning Ph.D.s in practice subfields. By 1989 these numbers had increased to 63, 63, and 29, respectively. Despite psychology's progress in attracting ethnic minorities to its ranks, minorities are still woefully underrepresented in the field.

Psychiatric Nurses

The professional training of nurses in this country began in the 1860s and consisted primarily of apprenticeships. The first training program that prepared nurses to care for the mentally ill was started in 1882 at McLean Hospital, a private psychiatric facility in Waverly, Massachusetts. Although there was a growing appreciation of nurses who received this type of training, poorly funded psychiatric hospitals continued to employ lesser-trained aides at very low pay. Whatever nursing care did exist in these hospitals consisted mainly of custodial care focusing on the physical needs of the patient, and the nurse continued to practice in a dependent relationship with a physician.

The development in the 1930s of somatic treatments for mental illness, such as insulin shock therapy, psychosurgery, and electroshock therapy, required the services of highly skilled nurses and established a more significant role for nurses in psychiatric treatment. The advent of the therapeutic community in psychiatric hospitals broadened the role of the nurse even further. As the 24-hour care necessary for developing and maintaining the therapeutic milieu was recognized, the nurse became a valuable member of the therapeutic team. The involvement of nurses in group psychotherapy after World War II resulted in federal appropriations for training nurses. However, despite the recognition of psychiatric nursing as a legitimate nursing role, the exact function of the nurse in mental health care remained only vaguely delineated.

Nursing education has become much more academically based over the past 20 years as the need for college-level training programs and nursing research was recognized. Graduates of nursing schools obtained an increasingly strong professional and academic education, often training side by side with psychiatrists, psychologists, and social workers. Nurses who earned advanced degrees were often recruited for teaching, however, and the two-year associate degree and diploma nurses were more prevalent in clinical practice. As nurses began to move into the role of psychotherapists, partially in response to the shortage of psychiatrists in most hospitals, interprofessional conflicts developed. But the exploding demand for psychotherapists further legitimated the nurse's role in therapy, and, by the late 1960s, the clinical specialty of psychiatric nursing was firmly established. The first organization to certify clinical specialists in psychiatric nursing, in 1972, was the New Jersey State Nurses Association.

Nursing education includes training in psychiatric nursing at all academic levels. The associate degree nurse with two years of training in an academic program and the diploma nurse trained in a hospital program most often provide clinical services. Baccalaureate- and master's-level nurses often work in supervisory positions or in teaching, and doctorate-level nurses usually teach rather than provide clinical services.

In 1984, approximately 10,034 master's-prepared psychiatric nurses were working in nursing positions (10). In addition, 2,070 master's-prepared psychiatric nurses were either not working in nursing or not working at all. This is significant in light of projected nursing shortages nationally. Further, a declining number of nurses are entering psychiatric nursing relative to other specialties such as pediatrics and medical surgical nursing.

Ninety-six percent of master's-prepared psychiatric nurses are female. As with all mental health professions, psychiatric nursing reflects serious underrepresentation of minorities in its membership. Approximately 96 percent of all female master's-prepared psychiatric nurses are white, only about 2 percent each are black and Hispanic, and less than 1 percent are Asian, Pacific Islander, or Native American.

Social Workers

The history of social work dates back to the late 19th century and the volunteer mothers who provided disadvantaged persons with charitable aid through the Charity Organization Societies. Social work began to develop as a profession during the early 20th century. Reform-minded women struggling for equality became social workers and began working in medical and psychiatric settings, schools, and correctional institutions. The development of social psychiatry also prompted the formation of a professional identity for social workers. Adopting the Freudian psychoanalytic model of many psychiatrists, social workers struggled for increasing responsibility in the treatment of mental and emotional disorders. The practice of psychotherapy expanded the social worker's domain from providing charitable assistance to the poor to providing a therapy that was viewed as legitimate by the middle and upper classes. Since psychoanalysis and psychotherapy remained medical specialties, social workers were not too successful in developing a separate professional identity, and their practice continued in the shadow of psychiatry.

Training includes two-year associate degree programs graduating human service workers, baccalaureate programs in social work currently recognized as the beginning professional level, master's-level degrees in social work, and doctoral programs. In addition to the basic training of the discipline, social work education offers specialized training in mental health and in human services administration. The National Association of Social Workers lists about 129,092 members (10). Of this total, 81,737 were master's- or doctoral-level social workers. Eighty-one percent are in full-time practice. Social workers are predominantly female (72 percent). Social workers are found in the public sector, including health and mental health services, public welfare, and child welfare, and in the private sector, including employee assistance programs and private practice.

Other Mental Health Personnel Concerns

Professionals with expertise in mental health concerns are practicing an increasingly wide range of disciplines. Schools of education are training counseling and guidance personnel as well as special education teachers who work in schools and other settings. The special needs of people recovering from mental and emotional disabilities have been recognized by such professional groups as occupational and recreational therapists and vocational counselors. Practitioners in marriage counseling, art, music, dance therapy, and religion provide counseling and therapy in many mental health settings. Training for these allied professionals varies tremendously. These personnel serve as mental health workers, alcohol and drug abuse counselors, day-care workers, board and homecare providers, foster parents, patient advocates, and hospital psychiatric aides. In some mental health centers, half of the positions are filled by these individuals.

Indigenous healers are rarely recognized by traditional mental health service providers but they do have an important role in caring for physical and emotional disturbances in many minority cultures. Community volunteers are also an important component of the mental health work force. Thousands of people offer their time and services, performing tasks ranging from assisting with clerical needs to working directly with patients.

Financing Mental Health Care

Most Americans do not pay for all of their own health care. They are covered under some type of third-party reimbursement, whether it is publicly funded—such as Medicaid and Medicare—or by insurance companies. Mental health services have historically been financed through the public sector.

Psychiatric insurance under other forms of insurance is inconsistent. Coverage for mental illness has been characterized by limitations in the form of caps on total coverage available and higher coinsurance and deductibles than for general medical coverage. However, since the 1970s major U.S. employers have become increasingly aware of the need to give greater priority to emotional problems (31). Mental health benefits are experiencing new definitions, designs, and structures for corporate programs. The image of the American worker as being able to cope with any problem is being drowned in a sea of alcoholism, drug abuse, and legal, marital, and financial problems (31). Simultaneously, insurance is focusing more on prevention as a means of increasing efforts to reduce absenteeism and to increase worker productivity.

Total expenditures by mental health organizations increased from $3.3 billion in 1969 to $18.5 billion in 1986 (10). However if adjustments are made for inflation, the total only rose from $3.3 billion to $4.8 billion (figure 8-4). The distribution of expenditures for inpatient mental health care (1986) and ambulatory mental health care (1980) are detailed in figure 8-5.

In the 1950s state psychiatric hospitals accounted for 80 to 90 percent of expenditures for mental illness care. By the 1970s and 1980s the introduction of Medicare and Medicaid, coupled with changing federal policy vis-à-vis the community mental health care system, broadened the funding base. Medicare and Medicaid, however, paralleled the principles and coverage typical of health insurance and only covered acute psychiatric inpatient care in general hospitals in the same

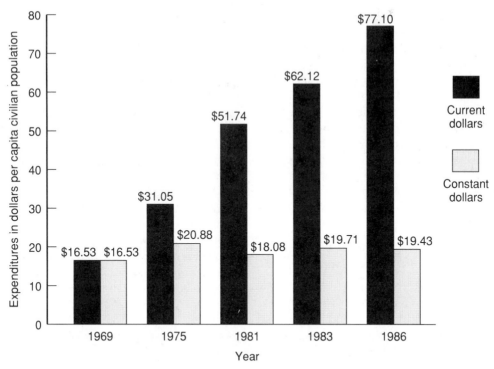

Figure 8-4. Expenditures per capita in current and constant (1969 = 100) dollars, all mental health organizations: United States, selected years 1969–86 (SOURCE: Manderscheid, R. W., & Sonnenschein, M. A. (Eds.). (1990). *Mental health, United States, 1990* (DHHS Publication No. [ADM] 90-1708). Washington, DC: U.S. Government Printing Office.)

manner as medical conditions, limiting care in public or private psychiatric hospitals. Outpatient coverage was severely restricted.

The greater availability of inpatient coverage skewed the growth of mental health services such that general hospital psychiatric services increased during the period 1960–1980, leaving the financing of state mental hospital systems to state governments. Congress felt that states should continue their responsibility for care of the chronically mentally ill and not shift this cost to the federal government.

In the 1980s federal dollars accounted for 19 percent of expenditures for both office-based care and that in organized settings as compared to 29 percent in the health sector. The difference has been absorbed by state and local government, which funded 33 percent of the total, about three

times the corresponding percentage in the health sector (10). Private insurance and direct patient payments accounted for 52 percent of mental health expenditures.

The federal share of the mental health bill was divided primarily between Medicare and Medicaid. Medicaid payments were more than triple those made through Medicare (10). In 1986, estimated Medicare mental illness payments were $1.7 billion; about 63 percent of this total was paid to general hospitals and 19 percent to psychiatric hospitals, for a total of 82 percent in hospital inpatient settings (10). In 1983 Medicaid paid $3.4 billion for mental illness care, with approximately 30 percent going toward hospital inpatient care, 51 percent toward intermediate care/skilled nursing facilities, and the remainder to outpatient services (10).

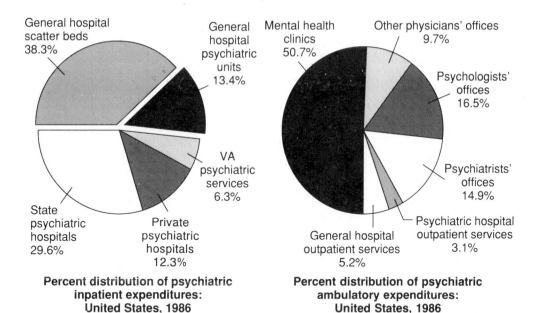

Figure 8-5. Percent distribution of psychiatric inpatient and ambulatory expenditures: United States, 1986 (SOURCE: Manderscheid, R. W., & Sonnenschein, M. A. (Eds.). (1990). *Mental health, United States, 1990* (DHHS Publication No. [ADM] 90-1708). Washington, DC: U.S. Government Printing Office.)

Trends in Financing

America has experienced explosive growth in the costs of health care, and the federal government has responded by legislating an end to the cost-reimbursement system for Medicare providers predominant in the 1960s and 1970s. Rather, the federal payment for health care is now based on payor-determined prices. To date, psychiatry has been excluded from the capitated reimbursement plan under Medicare—diagnosis-related groups (DRGs), which was phased in starting in 1983 (Chapter 11). Hospitals defined as rehabilitation, long-term, pediatric, or psychiatric continue to be paid under a cost-based reimbursement system with limits on rate of growth. The exemptions were based on uncertainty about how well a DRG-based payment system would work for specialized facilities and units.

Current initiatives to contain national health care costs will also affect physicians providing mental health services. The new resource-based relative value scale (RBRVS) Medicare fee schedule, to be phased in over a five-year period beginning in 1992, is likely to have a modest impact initially. Under the RBRVS as proposed, fees for family practitioners, internists, and psychiatrists will rise. A panel convened by the American Psychiatric Association and Harvard University is now working on a reevaluation of fees for psychiatrists under the RBRVS schedule (32).

One organizational type to emerge in response to economic pressures and need for greater integration of the differing parts of the health care system has been HMOs. Insurers and employers have also collaborated with fee-for-service practitioners and hospitals to create PPOs and exclusive provider organizations (EPOs) intended to offer care at a discounted rate. Comprehensive prospective payment systems such as these will play an increasingly important role in the future of psychiatric services. Psychiatric practice in HMOs, concurrently the most common model of prospective payment, has been shown to be cost-effective, and differing models of mental health service delivery have emerged. Psychiatric services are often included in other alternative provider organizations as well. However, they are likely to have modest coinsurance payments and strict limits on the duration of services. Employee assistance programs, originally focused on alcohol treatment, are expanding in scope, and corporate mental health programs are moving in-house through the employment of staff psychiatrists, psychologists, and social workers.

Universal access to health care is a subject of growing public debate as record numbers of Americans find themselves with no access to insurance mechanisms. A number of health care system reform proposals that are designed to improve access while containing costs are being offered by Congressional and state legislators. It remains to be seen what sort of priority mental health services will be given in this national debate.

Legal and Ethical Issues

Policy regarding mental health issues has been affected profoundly by case law in previous years. Three areas of legal change have had major effects on the chronically mentally ill. They include substantive and procedural alterations in civil commitment laws, the limited implementation of a constitutionally based right to treatment, and the partial recognition of a right to refuse treatment (33).

Deinstitutionalization and the way it was implemented was a significant factor in the development of civil commitment laws. The influx of previously hospitalized mentally ill people into the community and the lack of consistent residential and treatment services created a large group of people whose life-styles varied significantly from those of the general population. Philosophical debates raged as to the right of an individual to choose this "alternative life-style," and the responsibility of society to ensure that individuals who appeared unable to care for themselves had protection under the law. Civil commitment laws, initially general in definition, became more definitive and embodied criteria

specifying dangerousness or the incapacity to care for self with the presence of mental illness as a requisite for commitment. Laws also became specific as to the duration of commitment, and the length of time was generally brief. Finally, individuals committed under these laws had rapid access to courts, public defenders, and other elements of the judicial system which ensured due process.

Implementation of laws in most states became quite literal, and dangerousness often became the deciding criterion. Yet, findings suggest that irrespective of commitment criteria, 85 percent of those committed are not dangerous. This emphasis may significantly reduce the number of people who could be helped by commitment and, some would argue, contribute to the increase of urban homeless people (33).

The right to treatment was first addressed in 1952 in civil commitment cases relating to sexual psychopaths. *Rouse v. Cameron* in 1966, based on arguments of cruel and unusual treatment and the right to due process, found that people judged criminally insane had the right to treatment (34). Since the early cases did not define criteria for treatment, but merely stated that some effort was required, there was little immediate impact. A decision by Judge Frank Johnson of Alabama in 1972, based on a class action suit *(Wyatt v. Stickney)* related to conditions in state hospitals, required that right to treatment be enforced and implemented (35). Various courts have subsequently specified minimum standards for treatment. In 1975 the Supreme Court cast significant doubt on a constitutionally derived right to treatment by deciding the case of *Donaldson v. O'Connor* (36) on the narrowest possible grounds. Donaldson, a patient in a Florida hospital for 14 years, sued for damages and demanded his release. The narrowness of the ruling limited the potential impact of the right-to-treatment litigation on increased support for the chronically mentally ill (33).

The right to refuse treatment raises often conflicting interests among society, therapist, and patient. The implications of behavior control through the use of behavior therapies, drug therapy, and psychosurgery create problems that have been addressed by the judicial system and by mental health professionals. The first of two right-to-refuse cases considered by the court was *Mills v.Rogers* (37), a class action suit brought by patients at Boston State Hospital. In the years since, clinicians have been confronted with a bewildering set of pronouncements from the courts (38). Evidence suggests that the right to refuse treatment has significantly increased both use of seclusion and transfers to maximum-security hospitals (33) for chronically mentally ill individuals. In *Stensvad v. Reivitz* (39), the court ruled that the purpose of commitment is custody, care, and treatment, and that such treatment reasonably includes psychotropic medication.

Confidentiality has long been central to the role of mental health care providers. Over the last decade exceptions to confidentiality rules have been developed when the life of a third party is endangered by a patient (40). Most recently, the American Psychiatric Association has proposed a model statute limiting psychiatrist's liability for their patient's violent acts and, at the same time, suggesting that confidentiality may be breached in the context of treating an individual who is infected with the human immunodeficiency virus (HIV) (40).

Advocacy for individual rights is a growing movement in the mental health field. Most recently, the federal government has passed legislation requiring states that accept federal funds for mental health services to create programs for protecting and advocating the rights of the mentally ill. This legislation is patterned after similar legislation in the field of developmental disabilities. Protection and advocacy agencies for developmentally disabled individuals are mandated in each state and funded through federal appropriation. Although meeting mixed enthusiasm among professionals and others in the field of developmental disabilities, advocates for the developmentally disabled have generally been regarded as the pioneers in advocacy movements. They remain a significant and powerful force. Legislation establishing similar advocacy organizations within mental health builds on the developmental disabilities programs by overlaying the new system on the existing one. On the basis of the success of protection and advocacy systems for the developmentally disabled, there is considerable opportunity for mental health advocates and professionals to work together for the betterment of the service system.

Our society is slowly working toward a better understanding of the nature of mental health. Much of what is currently known and believed is predicated on a mixture of fact and untested theory. The mental health system is working vigorously to catch up with current knowledge and philosophy, but its efforts are warped by a confusing mixture of economic and political constraints. Previous philosophy that heralded the ability of all people to live in the community has not been realized. Many people who need mental health services and have no financial or social resources find only limited, or possibly, no services. Mental health services for those who do have resources have expanded and changed considerably, leaving even greater evidence of a two-tiered system of care.

Despite the many problems that remain in the system, mental health professionals, citizen advocates, and consumers continue to labor toward greater access to financial resources, more and improved services, and less stigma for mental illness. Custodial treatment still exists, but we are learning how to better use all of our treatment resources. Many people do go unserved or inappropriately treated, but the problems of the mentally ill continue to receive attention and concern. In short, the mental health system continues to gain credence and legitimacy as a significant and important part of health care.

References

1. Levine, M. (1981). *The history and politics of community mental health.* Oxford, U.K.: Oxford University Press.
2. Weiner, D. B. (1979). The apprenticeship of Philippe Pinel: A new document, "Observations of Citizen Pussin on the Insane." *Psychiatry. 136.* 1128–1134.
3. Shore, J. H., Kinzie, J. D., & Hampson, J. D., et al. (1973). Psychiatric epidemiology of an Indian village. *Psychiatry. 36.* 70–81.

4. *Diagnostic and statistics manual.* (1981). Washington, DC: American Psychiatric Association.

5. Regier, D., Myers, J., Kramer, M., et al. (1984). The NIMH epidemiological catchment area (ECA) program: Historical context, major objectives and study population characteristics. *Archives of General Psychiatry. 41. 934–941.*

6. *Facts and figures from the Alcohol, Drug Abuse and Mental Health Administration* (no. 4). (1986, July). Washington, DC: U.S. Department of Health and Human Services.

7. Rumer, R. (1978). Community mental health centers: Politics and therapy. *Journal of Health Politics, Policy and Law. 3.* 531–558.

8. Koyanagi, C., & Goldman, H. H. (1991). The quiet success of the national plan for the chronically mental ill. *Hospital and Community Psychiatry. 42*(9). 899–905.

9. U.S. Department of Health and Human Services Steering Committee on the Chronically Mentally Ill. (1980). *Toward a national plan for the chronically mentally ill.* Washington, DC: U.S. Public Health Service.

10. Manderscheid, R. W., & Sonnenschein, M. A. (Eds.). (1990). *Mental health, United States, 1990* (DHHS Publication No. [ADM] 90–1708). Washington, DC: U.S. Government Printing Office.

11. Goldman, H., Adams, N., & Taube, C. (1983). Deinstitutionalization: The data demythologicalized. *Hospital and Community Psychiatry. 34.* 129–134.

12. Redick, R., Witkin, M., Atay, J., & Manderscheid, R. W. (1991, March). *Availability and distribution of psychiatric beds, United States and each state, 1986* (Mental Health Statistical Note No. 195). Washington, DC: U.S. Department of Health and Human Services, National Institute of Mental Health.

13. Sunshine, J. H., Witkin, M. J., Atay, J. E., & Manderscheid, R. W. (1991, January). *Psychiatric outpatient care services in mental health organizations, United States, 1986* (Mental Health Statistical Note No. 194). Washington, DC: U.S. Department of Health and Human Services, National Institute of Mental Health.

14. Bittker, T. (1985). The industrialization of American psychiatry. *American Journal of Psychiatry. 142.* 149–154.

15. Gray, G. H., & Field, M. J. (Eds.). (1989). *Institute of Medicine Committee on Utilization Management by Third Parties: Controlling costs or changing patient care? The role of utilization management.* Washington, DC: National Academy Press.

16. Patterson, D. Y. (1990). An approach to rational psychiatric treatment. *Hospital and Community Psychiatry. 41*(10). 1092–1095.

17. Borenstein, D. B. (1990). Managed care: A means of rationing psychiatric treatment. *Hospital and Community Psychiatry. 41*(10). 1095–1099.

18. Dorwart, R. A. (1990). Managed mental health care: Myths and realities in the 1990s. *Hospital and Community Psychiatry. 41*(10). 1087–1091.

19. Craig, T., & Laska, E. (1983). Deinstitutionalization and the survival of the state hospital. *Hospital and Community Psychiatry. 34.* 616–622.

20. Lair, T., & Lefkowitz, D. (1990, September). Mental health and functional states of residents of nursing and personal care homes. In Agency for Health Care Policy and Research. *National Medical Expenditure Survey research findings 7* (DHHS Publication No. [PHS] 90–3470). Washington, DC: U.S. Government Printing Office.

21. Geller, J. L., Fisher, W. H., Wirth-Cauchon, J. L., & Simon, L. J. (1990, August). Second-generation deinstitutionalization, I: The impact of Brewster versus Dukakis on state hospital casemix. *American Journal of Psychiatry. 147*(8). 982–987.

22. Gottheil, E., Winkelmayer, R., Smoyer, P. & Exline, R. (1991, July). Characteristics of patients who are resistant to deinstitutionalization. *Hospital and Community Psychiatry. 42*(7). 745–748.

23. Holcomb, W. R., & Ahr, P. R. (1987). Who really treats the severely impaired young adult patient? A comparison of treatment settings. *Hospital and Community Psychiatry. 38.* 625–631.

24. Klebe, E. R. (1991, April 12). Homeless mentally ill persons: Problems and programs. *CRS Report for Congress* (Publication No. 91–344). Washington, DC: Library of Congress.

25. Interagency Council on the Homeless. (1991). *The 1990 annual report of the Interagency Council on the Homeless.* Washington, DC: Author.

26. Lamb, H. R. (1990, May). Will we save the homeless mentally ill? *American Journal of Psychiatry. 147*(5). 649–651.

27. Redick, R. W., Witkin, M. J., Atay, M. A., & Manderscheid, R. W. (1991, April). *Staffing of mental health organizations, United States, 1986* (Mental Health Statistical Note No. 196). Washington, DC: U.S.

Department of Health and Human Services, National Institute of Mental Health.

28. Lipton, F., Sabatini, A., & Katz, S. (1983). Down and out in the city: The homeless mentally ill. *Hospital and Community Psychiatry. 43.* 817–821.

29. Telephone communication, American Medical Association, 1987.

30. President's Commission on Mental Health. (1978). *Final report, Vol. II, Task panel reports.* Washington, DC: U.S. Government Printing Office.

31. Goldbeck, W. (1983). Psychiatry and industry: A business view. *Psychiatry Hospital. 13.* 11–14.

32. Weil, T. P. (1991, July) Mental health services under a U.S. national insurance plan. *Hospital and Community Psychiatry. 42*(7). 695–700.

33. Lamb, H., & Mills, M. (1986). Needed changes in law and procedure for the chronically mental ill. *Hospital and Community Psychiatry. 37.* 475–480.

34. *Rouse v. Cameron,* 373 F2d 451 (DC Cir. 1966).

35. *Wyatt v. Stickney,* 344 F. Supp. 383 (MD Ala. 1972).

36. *Donaldson v. O'Connor,* 493 F2d 507 (Stu Cir. 1974).

37. *Mills v. Rogers,* 50 USLW 4676 (June 18, 1982).

38. Applebaum, P. (1983). Refusing treatment: The uncertainty continues. *Hospital and Community Psychiatry. 34.* 11–12.

39. *Stensvad R. Reivitz, et al.,* No. 84-C-383-S (W. D. Wis., January 10, 1985).

40. Eth, S. (1990, April). Psychiatric ethics: Entering the 1990s. *Hospital and Community Psychiatry. 41* (4). 384–386.

PART FOUR

Nonfinancial Resources for Health Services

Chapter 9

Medical Technology and Its Assessment

Bryan R. Luce

Technology is credited with the benefits of American medicine as well as what ails it. It is the hope for a long, productive life for millions of people, a primary reason for the spiraling costs of care, and the source of many social and ethical dilemmas such as the rationing of health care and the harvesting of human organs for transplants. It has even given rise to new definitions of death. At different times and places and by different policy makers and analysts it has been accused of not being accessible to all members of the population, being overused, misused, and misunderstood. It has been said to have diffused too rapidly without adequate assessment or regulation, yet today some express a concern that innovation is being stifled, capital is unavailable for technology acquisition, and reimbursement is inadequate.

This chapter is intended to shed light on many of these issues. It will attempt to explain how medical technology fits into the American health care system, what the public policy issues are, and how these issues are being addressed by different elements of society.

The chapter discusses two major issues: medical technology and medical technology assessment. The development and innovation process of medical technology that demonstrates how innovations build on prior knowledge and the amount of investment that is required in terms of both money and time. Next, the reader is provided with a picture of the process of diffusion of medical technologies from an innovative idea to widespread use to obsolescence. The relevance of any particular technology is often related to the stage of its life cycle. Later, it will be seen that the assessment process is also related to the life-cycle stage. Then, the appropriate use of medical technologies, presently the subject of a raging controversy within both the medical and health policy communities, is discussed. As will be clear, it is not possible to discuss medical technology fully without addressing the appropriate practice of medicine. Although the section on appropriateness ends the first part it is a fitting way to introduce the discussion of medical technology assessment, since the assessment process largely involves determination of the appropriate application of medical technology.

The second part of the chapter concerns assessment by first describing the many organizations, public and private, which conduct technology assessments. They include the Food and Drug Administration (FDA), the Congressional Office of Technology Assessment (OTA), and other Department of Health and Human Services (DHHS) activities. Within the private sector many organizations, such as the American Medical Association, the American Hospital Association, and the American College of Physicians, are also active in formal assessment activities.

An overview of some of the more widely used and important methods of assessment—randomized clinical trials, case studies, group judgment methods, quality-of-life measurement, and finally, cost-benefit and cost-effectiveness analyses—is then presented. The chapter concludes with some thoughts about the future of technology and its assessment.

The concept of technology is a very broad one: the application of organized knowledge to practical ends (1). Thus technology connotes much more than either a widget or a machine. Similarly, medical technology is a broader concept than might otherwise be assumed. A comprehensive definition of medical technology in common use today is techniques, drugs, equipment, and procedures used by health care professionals in delivering medical care to individuals, and the systems within which care is delivered (1). From a practice standpoint, however, the discussion in this chapter generally centers on drugs, medical devices, and medical and surgical procedures: that is, the practice of clinical medicine and its tools.

Innovation, Development, and Diffusion

In many ways, the history of medicine is intricately tied to the history of advances in medical technology. Much of modern medical practice can be traced to the origins of the stethoscope in the early 19th century, the thermometer and roentgen rays

in the late 19th century, and the sphygmomanometer and the electrocardiogram (ECG) recorders in the early 20th century, all of which allowed the physician to better understand the internal workings of the human body. Twentieth-century anesthesia permitted surgery to blossom, and the miracle of antibiotics did not occur until well into the 20th century.

Not only is the practice of medicine highly influenced by technological advances; so is the location of that practice. As technology became more sophisticated, complicated, and expensive, it served as a catalyst for centralizing medical care in the hospital. Major surgery such as coronary artery bypass graft (CABG) requires a sophisticated team approach; major diagnostic machines such as the computerized tomography (CT) scanner and the magnetic resonance imaging (MRI) machine require large capital outlays; intensive care units require sophisticated monitoring equipment as well as highly trained integrated staff.

In contrast, today, because of a number of technological innovations as well as financial pressures, technology is allowing patients to be cared for and treated in outpatient settings and at home. Much of ophthalmologic surgery is now being performed in outpatient settings, as are many other surgical procedures and diagnostic testing prior to entering hospitals. Technology permits handicapped people to see, hear, speak, and move. Monitoring devices can permit cardiac implants to transmit vital information over telephone lines; respirators maintain breathing in the home; kidney dialyzers are commonly used at home as is parenteral nutrition, an intravenous technology for patients who cannot swallow or digest food. In fact, technology is a prime reason that home health care expenditures are one of the fastest growing sectors in American health care today. In 1990 expenditures for home health care were $8.5 billion, an increase of 22.5 percent over the previous year, almost as fast as the 24.9 percent growth in 1989 (2).

Technology also profoundly influences who practices medicine. No longer does the general practitioner do everything. The extreme speciali-

underinvested

zation in medicine has been due not only to the increasing volume of medical knowledge but also to sophisticated technological advances, many of which are controlled by specializing subgroups of physicians. For instance, as technological advances occurred in obstetrics, including cesarean section, electronic fetal monitoring, and neonatal intensive care, encouraging births to be located in hospitals, physicians replaced midwives and obstetricians replaced general practitioners. Advances in surgical techniques such as microsurgery, organ implantation, and coronary artery bypass procedures have had similar effects on both general practitioners and general surgeons. Thus technology has helped to transform medicine from primarily an art to a blend of art and science and, in turn, required that physicians become more technologically trained scientists.

The following section discusses the nation's investment in biomedical research and development that has served as the fuel for these technological advancements.

Funding Biomedical Research and Development

Biomedical research and development is funded by both the federal government and the private sector. In 1989 health research and development accounted for 3.5 percent of national health expenditures, down from 3.9 percent in 1972, a 10 percent drop (3). From 1981 to 1991, funding has grown steadily from $8.7 billion to $24.5 billion (figure 9-1). During this time, however, there has been a shift in relative support, with industry increasing its share and government decreasing its share. The U.S. pharmaceutical industry itself reports that it has been increasing its investment in developing new drugs, from 11.7 percent of sales in 1980 to 15.9 percent of sales in 1990 (4). Nevertheless, health research and development spending as a percentage of total national health expenditures has decreased substantially over the past 15 years. Although that proportion is a little higher than the average for all industry in the

United States, it is relatively low for technologically dependent industries (5). Thus, since health care is technologically sophisticated, yet highly labor-dependent, the present level of investment may be unreasonable if the downward trend continues. However, serious concern is being expressed today that changing reimbursement patterns and budgetary pressures due to cost-containment initiatives will significantly dampen industry's investment in new product development (6).

The Diffusion of Technologies

The spread of a technology into society once it is developed is known as *diffusion*. It includes entry, adoption, widespread use, and final obsolescence of an innovation—the life cycle of a technology.

Diffusion is an important concept to study because it is both affected by and, in turn, affects many important socioeconomic processes. Industry is interested in the demand for its products, and that demand is affected by the relative costs and benefits of the innovation, regulatory constraints, reimbursement rules, pricing, and medical acceptance. Whereas the public is concerned with having access to new beneficial procedures, devices, and drugs such as heart transplants and cyclosporin (a drug that inhibits the body's natural rejection mechanisms), payors—including private insurers and federal and state governments—are concerned with adoption of a technology before it has been adequately assessed. Figure 9-2, depicts the life cycle of a technology from basic research to obsolescence. Included in this diagram are some of the many environmental factors such as regulation, evaluation, and reimbursement policies that affect the diffusion process.

The diffusion curve of an innovation is typically described as an S shape (figure 9-3), with an initial slow introduction, and a take-off phase characterized by an increasing rate of adoption that slowly levels off as it matures and, perhaps, decreases as it approaches obsolescence. Several empirical studies have plotted such a course (7,8). For instance, in a 1981 publication the Congressional

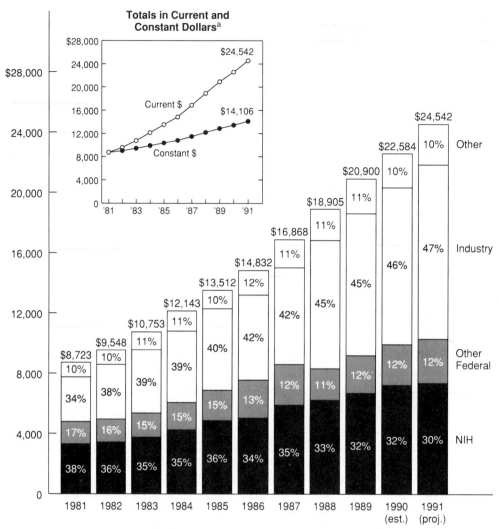

Figure 9-1. National support for health R&D by source, 1981–1991. (dollars in millions). (SOURCE: National Institutes of Health. *NIH Data Book.* (1991.)
[a]*FY 1981 = 100. Constant dollars based on Biomedical R&D Price Index.*

Office of Technology Assessment (OTA) plotted the course of adoption of the CT scanner in the United States (figure 9-4). The CT scanner was introduced into the United States in the early 1970s. In 1974 there were 45 scanners in operation. Within two years there were 475 operational scanners or a tenfold increase. By 1977, scanners were being bought and installed at a rate of about 40 per month. Although total volume continued to increase, a year later the rate of increase was cut in half and continued to decline. During this time, there was a great deal of public debate over control of capital expenditures in health care. Congress enacted the Health Planning and Resources

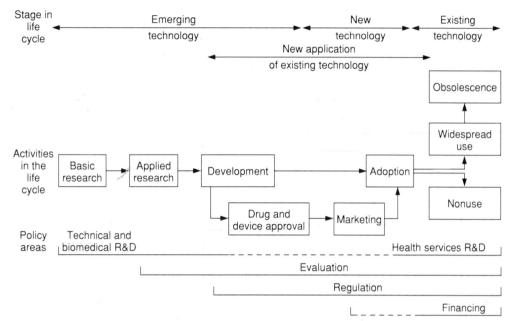

Figure 9-2. Life cycle of a medical technology. (SOURCE: Office of Technology Assessment.)

Development Act of 1974 (PL 93–641), which covered the nation with a system of local health planning agencies. If any single technology was specially targeted for regulatory control with the intentions of creating a more orderly process of diffusion, it was the CT scanner. Later in that decade (1978), the National Guidelines for Health Planning were issued, which attempted to establish

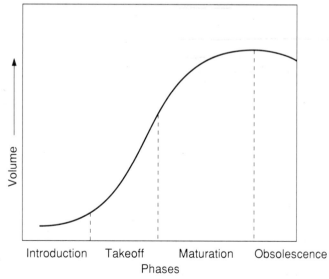

Figure 9-3. Diffusion curve of an innovation.

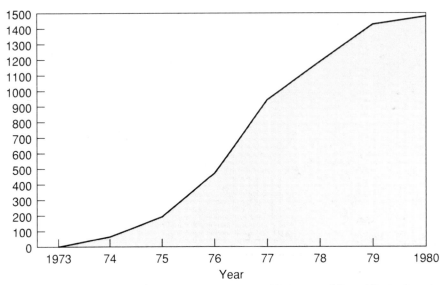

Figure 9-4. Cumulative number of CT Scanners installed (1973–1980). (SOURCE: Office of Technology Assessment.)

utilization guidelines and standards that planning agencies could use for 11 technologies, including the CT scanner. Nevertheless, as figure 9-4 suggests, these and other efforts had little or no effect on diffusion of CT scanning into the U.S. health care system. This widespread diffusion occurred before there was hard evidence of efficacy or cost-effectiveness from well-designed studies (9).

Later, researchers were witnessing diffusion of a similar expensive and dramatic diagnostic technology, magnetic resonance imaging (MRI). By 1985 it was reported to be in its take-off phase of diffusion. But despite the weakening of planning and certificate-of-need (CON) regulations in the 1980s, these regulatory programs are reported to have retarded diffusion in the United States (10). In addition, reimbursement policies such as the Medicare prospective payment system may also have contributed to delaying its diffusion. As with the CT scanner, there is similar concern that adequate testing of the technology's relative value was not systematic prior to widening adoption of the machine.

CABG, an open heart surgical procedure to cor-

rect coronary artery vessel blockage, has diffused very rapidly in this country at great expense but with generally inadequate scientific evidence of safety, efficacy, and cost-effectiveness. In 1972, 2,600 patients had such an operation; by 1981, that figure had grown to almost 53,000 patients, at a total cost of about $500 million (11). In 1989, 368,000 patients had CABG and an additional 259,000 patients had balloon angioplasty (12).

The CT scanner and coronary artery bypass surgery are good examples of technologies that have influenced public health policy development. From the mid–1960s to the end of the 1970s, debate raged over increasing costs due to rapid acceptance of untested and overused technologies. Rising from this debate were health planning and hospital utilization review legislation and increased calls for technology assessment. Because of its perceived ineffectiveness by the 1980s, the regulatory approach began to give way to a more market-oriented approach for controlling diffusion. Payment policies were being changed from cost-based policies to policies being set prospectively, placing the purchaser at increased financial risk for adoption and use of technology. Today, for instance, Medicare pays a set amount of money per hospital admission (i.e., per diagnosis-related group [DRG]), rather than guaranteeing cost recovery. Concern by some immediately shifted from that of overadoption to one of underadoption (5), although a significant shift in diffusion rates has yet to be demonstrated. Nevertheless, there is evidence that new, expensive technologies may not be adequately reimbursed. For instance, a survey of hospitals that have purchased the extracorporeal shock wave lithotripter (ESWL), an imaginative, but expensive, noninvasive method for crushing kidney stones through shock waves, reveals that Medicare's DRG prospective payment system paid only 57 to 82 percent of the costs of the therapy. Since the DRG payment in this case is based on the patient's condition rather than the procedure performed, hospitals are paid the same amount regardless of whether the hospitals have ESWL or whether it is used. Thus, ironically, in 1987, hospitals without ESWL stood to gain an estimated $4.5 to $8.8 million in Medicare payments. Similarly, hospitals with MRIs had a total reported Medicare loss of $31 million (13).

The ultimate effect of these reimbursement policies on technology diffusion—that is, the providers' willingness and ability to purchase technology—is yet to be determined. But little doubt remains that technology continues to spread before adequate assessment is conducted.

The Appropriate Use of Technologies

Studies have shown that there is enormous variation in medical practice, contrary to the general belief of the public (14,15,16,17). Where one lives, who one's practitioner is, and in which setting or hospital that physician practices often determine how one will be treated. This may seem counterintuitive since medical education in this country—indeed, in most of the Western world—has been nearly standardized since the early days of this century, state medical and nursing licensure standards are similar across the states, hospitals conform to standards of the Joint Commission on Accreditation of Health Care Organizations (JCAHO), and nationally read professional medical journals disseminate state-of-the-art knowledge of medical practice. Much of this knowledge stems from the many millions of dollars of clinical research findings funded by the National Institute of Health (NIH) and the private sector as well as results of medical technology assessments to be discussed in a later section of this chapter. Yet large variations in medical practice persist.

In 1978 the Congressional Office of Technology Assessment (OTA) estimated that only 10 to 20 percent of all procedures currently used in medical practice had been shown to be efficacious by controlled (clinical) trial. OTA concluded that "Given . . . examples of technologies that entered widespread use and were shown later to be inefficacious or unsafe, and the large numbers of inadequately assessed current and emerging technologies, improvements are critically needed in the information base regarding safety and efficacy and the processes for its generation" (18).

The concerns expressed in 1978 persist and have been argued to represent a threat to the autonomy of the medical profession. In 1983 the National Academy of Sciences' Institute of Medicine convened a conference on the subject of variations in medical practice. Participants generally agreed that unless the medical profession came to grips to resolve this issue, it risks a future where external pressures from government, insurers, and the public will dictate priorities in the practice of medicine (19).

John Wennberg, in a landmark study in the area of medical practice variation, demonstrated that one's chance of having a major surgical procedure varies dramatically according to where one lives (figure 9-5 demonstrates this point quite clearly). In 1975, within three New England states (Rhode Island, Maine, Vermont), an individual was six times more likely to undergo a tonsillectomy in one location over another and four times more likely

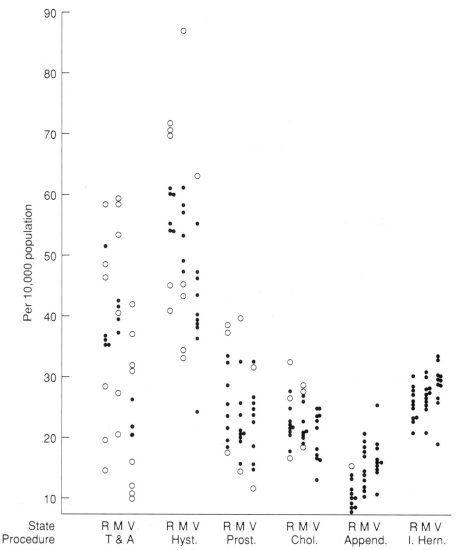

Figure 9-5. Age-adjusted rate of procedure for six common surgical procedures (tonsillectomy-adenoidectomy, hysterectomy, prostatectomy, cholecystectomy, appendectomy, and inguinal hernia) in Rhode Island (R), Maine (M), and Vermont (V) (1975). Rates of surgical procedures vary greatly among hospital areas. The rates shown are for the six most common surgical procedures for the repair or removal of an organ in the 11 most populous hospital areas of Maine, Rhode Island, and Vermont (1975). The rate of tonsillectomy varies about sixfold among the 33 arreas; the rates of hysterectomy and prostatectomy vary about fourfold. Moreover, many of the extreme rates for these procedures differ from the average rate for the state by an amount that is statistically significant (open circles). There is much disagreement among physicians on the value of the high-variation procedures. Similar patterns of variation for these procedures have been observed in Iowa, England, and Norway. (SOURCE: Wennberg JE: Dealing with medical practice variations: A proposal for action. *Health Affairs. 3.* 6–32.)

to have a hysterectomy and prostatectomy (14). He observed in Maine, for instance, that a woman's chance of having a hysterectomy by the time she reached age 70 was 20 percent in one area and 70 percent in another.

These differences cannot be attributed to characteristics of patients, access to service, or insurance protection. Rather, the variation seems to be related primarily to practice styles of physicians. Wennberg's and others' studies indicate that such variation is found throughout the Western world. Disturbingly, the variation is not linked to patient outcomes. Wennberg's explanation of these findings is that scientific evidence of the value of much of medical practice is lacking, ambiguous, or unheeded.

Public policy concern ranges from inefficiencies, to trauma to patients and unnecessary surgical risk, to matters of pure economics. For instance, more than 2,500 "extra" hysterectomies were performed in one Maine market area over another, resulting in a potential avoidable cost in excess of $10 million (15). Nationwide implications of this are staggering. Another study by the Rand Corporation has shown that large and significant variations of medical and surgical procedures persist across large areas in the United States. Of 123 procedures, 67 showed at least threefold differences between sites (16). Both Wennberg and Robert Brook of Rand have estimated that if physicians in high-practice style areas changed their styles to those of their colleagues in low-practice style areas, national health expenditures could be reduced by up to 30 to 40 percent (17). This potential for saving money has recently captured the political attention of both Congress and the Department of Health and Human Services. In 1989 Congress established the Agency for Health Care Policy and Research (AHCPR), directing it to establish a major initiative in outcomes research, including medical effectiveness and medical practice guidelines.

Not only medical and surgical procedures are misused. In 950 B.C., Homer is reported to have stated "many [drugs] were excellent and when mingled, many fatal." A study by the American Hospital Association has estimated that 7 percent of all hospital admissions are related to the misuse of prescribed pharmaceuticals, and in 1983, such drug-induced illnesses led to an estimated 2.7 million admissions costing up to $5 billion (20).

There is similar evidence of the widespread diffusion of medical devices without adequate evidence of efficacy. CT and MRI have already been mentioned. A case study commonly cited in the literature is that of gastric freezing to cure ulcers (21). This medical device was introduced in 1962. Before it was tested for safety and efficacy, 2,500 machines were sold in the United States and an estimated 25,000 operations were performed, causing patients considerable harm. All of this was due to erroneous results of a few uncontrolled case studies that were purported to show dramatic benefit in curing ulcers without medication or surgery. Several years later, gastric freezing was shown by controlled randomized trials to have no benefit whatsoever (21,22).

Gastric freezing is an extreme example of the diffusion of a worthless technology. Mostly, the Food and Drug Administration (FDA) ensures that prescription drugs and certain medical devices are safe and efficacious when applied under prescribed conditions. However, no agency ensures that medical or surgical procedures pass an initial safety and efficacy test prior to diffusion into the general population.

Once any technology is available, whether it is a drug, a device, or a medical or surgical procedure, physicians are constrained in their use solely by their training, ethics, economic considerations, estimate of patient benefit, and the threat of malpractice suits. Thus the appropriate use of all available medical technologies is in the main, left to physician and patient discretion. Testing for appropriateness is a principal purpose of medical technology assessment and is presented in the following section.

Organizing for Technology Assessment

Today a number of organizations in government and the private sector have assumed responsibilities for assessing medical technologies. These organizations attempt to address many of the issues and concerns discussed earlier in this chapter. As a rule, these organizations have been created over time as a response to the perceived needs of society.

Regulation: A Historical Overview

In 1906 the Food, Drug and Cosmetic Act established the new Food and Drug Administration (FDA) to regulate the marketing of drugs and foods for safety. It was passed in response to unsafe and falsely advertised products, primarily of the home remedy or "patent medicine" type. In 1938 an amendment requiring safety of drugs to be demonstrated through more rigorous and sophisticated testing was enacted, largely as a result of public catastrophes such as the elixir of sulfanilamide deaths (23). In 1962 further drug amendments extended regulatory authority of the FDA to require that drugs be tested for efficacy as well as safety prior to marketing. Passage of this legislation was due, in large part, to the thalidomide tragedy (24).

FDA authority over the marketing of medical devices has lagged behind that of drugs. The 1938 amendments sought truth in labeling and provided some marketing control, but only if devices were "adulterated" or "misbranded." By the 1970s, adverse affects of unsafe medical devices had been documented (25), leading to further amendments to the Food, Drug and Cosmetic Act in 1976 empowering the FDA to regulate the marketing of medical devices for safety and efficacy.

In the period following the 1965 Medicare and Medicaid amendments to the Social Security Act, a number of other legislative attempts arose to regulate the adoption and use of medical technologies due mainly to concerns about the ever-increasing cost of medical care. In the late 1960s health planning legislation was passed that helped to spur state-CON legislation around the country. These laws were intended to guide the diffusion of capital-intensive technologies (as well as to guide hospital bed capacity). In 1974 the federal planning legislation was greatly strengthened. (See the earlier discussions of the diffusion of the CT scanner.)

Other legislative routes were followed to regulate hospital utilization, such as the requirement of Medicare that hospitals have utilization review committees and the enactment of the national professional standards review organizations (PSRO) program.

Also during this period, Congress created the Office of Technology Assessment (OTA) to guide itself in the increasingly technological world in which it was operating. OTA's Health Program issued its first major report in 1976 outlining opportunities and needs for assessing medical technologies (26). Two years later, Congress established the National Center for Health Care Technology (NCHCT), whose mission was to "set priorities for technology assessment, and encourage, conduct, and support assessments research demonstrations, and evaluations concerning health care technology" (27). NCHCT was also to advise the Health Care Financing Administration (HCFA) on Medicare-specific coverage policy issues. Before the center could mature, it was defunded in 1981, largely as a result of the medical professions' and the medical device and pharmaceutical industries' belief that its technology assessment activities unduly threatened the innovation process.

Today, there continues to be concern that technologies are not adequately and fully assessed prior to their diffusion and use in medical practice as discussed earlier in this chapter. The more prominent organizations whose missions include the control or assessment of medical technologies are discussed below. Figure 9-6 shows the relationships of the principal organizations engaged in technology assessment in the United States.

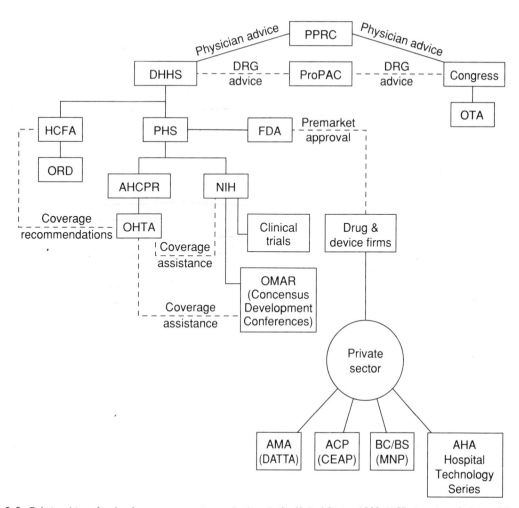

Figure 9-6. Relationships of technology assessment organizations in the United States, 1992. (ACP, American College of Physicians; AHA, American Hospital Association; AHCPR, Agency for Health Care Policy and Research; AMA, American Medical Association; BC/BS, Blue Cross and Blue Shield; CEAP, Clinical Efficacy Assessment Project; DATTA, Diagnostic and Therapeutic Technology Assessment; DHHS, Department of Health and Human Services; FDA, Food and Drug Administration; HCFA, Health Care Financing Administration; IOM, Institute of Medicine; MNP, Medical Necessity Program; NIH, National Institutes of Health; OHTA, Office of Health Technology Assessment; OMAR, Office of Medical Applications of Research; ORD, Office of Research and Demonstrations; OTA, Office of Technology Assessment; PHS, Public Health Service; ProPAC, Prospective Payment Assessment Commission.)

The Food and Drug Administration

The FDA can be considered the backbone of the government's medical technology assessment activities. It regulates entry into the U.S. market of all drugs and relevant medical devices, requiring manufacturing firms to demonstrate that their products are safe and efficacious. Thus FDA *requires* rather than *conducts* assessments. Specifically, it develops product standards, regulates testing, develops and/or approves clinical protocols, evaluates technical and clinical evidence provided to it by manufacturers, and carefully regulates product labeling. It does no clinical testing itself.

FDA generally requires that companies demonstrate safety and efficacy only as claimed in their labeling, not relative to other products or procedures. Thus, testing is usually done compared to a placebo.

Drug Regulation

In order for drugs to enter the U.S. market, the manufacturer must proceed through two major steps established by the FDA: 1) the investigational new drug (IND) application process and 2) the new drug application (NDA) process (28). The IND process normally precedes testing in humans in the United States. The firm describes the proposed clinical studies, the qualifications of the investigators, the chemical properties of the drugs, and the results of all pharmacologic and toxicity testing gained from laboratory animals as well as results from any available human studies, usually from other countries. If FDA approves the IND application, the firm may proceed with the NDA step, normally a three-phase clinical testing program in humans, culminating in relatively large (usually 700–3,000 patients), multisite, randomized, controlled trials. The results of these studies are then presented to FDA for market approval. In some instances, additional "phase 4" postmarketing surveillance studies are required.

The entire drug development process leading to FDA approval reportedly takes as long as seven to 10 years and is extremely expensive. When one includes the development costs of unsuccessful efforts, as much as $231 million is needed for each new chemical entity that reaches the U.S. market (29).

Device Regulation

The 1976 Medical Device Amendments to the Food, Drug and Cosmetic Act require that all medical devices be classified into one of three groups: Class I, general controls; Class II, performance standards; and Class III, premarket approval.

In general, the approval process for medical devices is less onerous than that for drugs. Class I devices (e.g., medical and surgical supplies) essentially require only FDA notification of intention to market and are not closely regulated; Class II devices (e.g., noninvasive diagnostic test equipment) must pass general performance standards; however, Class III devices (e.g., pacemakers, total hip prostheses) are regulated for safety and efficacy and must pass through a clinical testing phase more similar to that mandated for drugs (although much less demanding).

A manufacturer of a Class III device is required to file an investigational device exemption (IDE) application (which is similar to the IND drug process). The IDE permits the firm to test the device in controlled settings on humans in order to establish its safety and efficacy. The resulting evidence is then submitted to the FDA in the form of a premarket approval application (PMAA).

The National Institutes of Health

The National Institutes of Health (NIH) contribute to medical technology assessment by sponsoring clinical trials and by conducting consensus development conferences on specific medical practice issues.

NIH's principal mission is to support basic and applied biomedical research in the United States. Although only 8 percent of its total budget is spent on clinical trials, this amounted to nearly $610 million in 1990. The National Cancer Institute is the largest sponsor of such research, accounting for 40 percent of all NIH monies spent on clinical trials, down from 59 percent in 1985. The decrease is due to additional funding for AIDS research ($146 million, or 24 percent) (3). While funded by NIH, most trials are investigator-initiated by research clinicians at medical centers all over the United States.

The Office of Medical Applications of Research

Another major technology assessment activity of NIH is the consensus development program organized by the Office of Medical Application of Research (OMAR). Whereas NIH-sponsored clinical trials are typically conducted on medical and surgical procedures in a very early phase of development, consensus development conferences generally concern medical practice that is in a much more advanced stage of diffusion. Some topics (e.g., magnetic resonance imaging) are chosen because they are important or controversial new technologies; others (e.g., screening for cervical cancer) are chosen because they involve widespread yet unresolved issues.

These conferences are meetings of experts to arrive at consensus regarding the appropriate use of a given medical technology. The experts are brought together in an open forum to review evidence of safety and efficacy/effectiveness of the technology under study. (*Efficacy* generally refers to the assessment of a technology under ideal conditions of use; *effectiveness,* under average conditions of use.) The panel then secludes itself for a short period of time to reach consensus on a statement of what is known about the application of the technology and what they agree is appropriate state-of-the-art practice.

NIH's objective in sponsoring these conferences is to transfer knowledge to the medical community rather than to create knowledge. The latter is the purpose of the clinical trials. Thus special attention is paid to disseminating the results of the conferences, first by holding a news conference, then by publishing the results in the *Journal of the American Medical Association* and by wide distribution of booklets summarizing the findings.

As of the end of 1991, 87 conferences had been held. Table 9-1 contains a selection of topics chosen to emphasize the diversity of subjects addressed.

The Office of Technology Assessment

The Office of Technology Assessment (OTA) is Congress's technology research and advisory body. Established by Congress in the early 1970s to assist it in better understanding complex techno-

TABLE 9-1. NIH Consensus Development Conferences: Selected Topics

Date	Conference Title
1977	Breast cancer screening
1979	Intraocular lens implantation
	Removal of third molars
1981	CT scan of the brain
1983	Critical care medicine
	Liver transplantation
1984	Lowering blood cholesterol to prevent heart disease
1986	Smokeless tobacco
	Magnetic resonance imaging
1991	Treatment of panic disorder

SOURCE: National Institute of Health, Office of Medical Applications of Research, 1992.

logical issues, OTA is divided into a number of programs, including the Health Program within the Health and Life Sciences Division.

The main purpose of the OTA Health Program is to assist Congress in developing policies concerning medical technologies and their assessment. Its reports tend to be general in nature, drawing conclusions from evidence and expert opinion rather than specific assessments of individual technologies. For instance, OTA was instrumental in educating Congress and the country concerning the lack of safety, efficacy, and cost-effectiveness information of medical technologies.

Although general in scope, OTA's reports are often accompanied by one or many case studies of individual technologies. Even these case studies, however, are often syntheses of information rather than evaluations of primary data. Many assessments include not only cost, efficacy/effectiveness, and cost-effectiveness, but legal and ethical implications as well. By 1991, the OTA Health Program had generated 33 main reports of technology assessment issues plus more than 60 case studies and other background papers and technical memoranda (30). Its 1992 budget is approximately $2 million.

Following a specific request by a Congressional Committee, OTA typically conducts its studies by forming an advisory panel for each major topic, gathering evidence from the literature and expert opinion, writing a report on its findings, and circulating drafts of the report to a wide audience for criticism. It then releases its published report to the requesting committee.

OTA is credited with having guided Congress in a number of major technology issues, including legislation establishing the National Center for Health Care Technology in 1978 (which was defunded in 1981). OTA appoints both the Prospective Payment Assessment Commission (ProPAC) and the Physician Payment Review Commission (PPRC) and was instrumental in passage of the law establishing the Institute of Medicine's Council on Health Care Technology (no longer in existence).

The Health Care Financing Administration

The Health Care Financing Administration (HCFA) is responsible for administering Medicare and the federal aspect of state Medicaid programs. Its medical technology activities are mainly associated with coverage and reimbursement policies and, to a lesser extent, research and demonstrations.

New procedures are evaluated for coverage determination at as local a level as possible and generally must pass a rather loosely defined test to determine whether they are reasonable and necessary (31). When coverage cannot be resolved at the local or regional level, HCFA's central office initiates a more formal process, first by referring the issue to its internal physician panel and then, if still unresolved, referring it to the Office of Health Technology Assessment (OHTA) within the Public Health Service (PHS) for assessment and recommendation. A more structured coverage process which includes the assessment of cost-effectiveness is presently being proposed by HCFA (32).

The HCFA Office of Research and Demonstrations (ORD) conducts and sponsors some studies associated with medical technology and its assessment, but these studies are generally aimed at more general delivery and reimbursement of services than at individual technologies. An exception

was the National Heart Transplant study in which HCFA sponsored a study to help to determine its coverage policy. ORD devotes a relatively small portion of its $35.6 million research and development budget to technology assessment. A selection of previous ORD topics includes heart transplant, kidney dialysis and transplantation, cyclosporin, magnetic resonance imaging, and implantable devices (33).

Agency for Health Care Policy and Research

The Agency for Health Care Policy and Research (AHCPR) both sponsors extramural research for the study of technologies and their assessment and conducts assessments intramurally, mainly through its Office of Health Technology Assessment (OHTA) in support of HCFA coverage policy.

The extramural program consists of investigator-initiated research across all areas of health services research, including especially medical outcomes research as well as topics in health services financing, organization, quality, and utilization; health information systems; the role of market forces in health care delivery; and health promotion and disease prevention as well as research related more directly to medical technology issues. AHCPR's budget in 1992 was $120.2 million.

Office of Health Technology Assessment

Located within the National Center, OHTA is primarily responsible for advising HCFA on coverage policy, assuming this role from the now defunct National Center for Health Care Technology (NCHCT). The Public Health Service (PHS) had previously assisted the Medicare program in guiding coverage policy; however, when NCHCT was created, that process became more formalized. In 1981, when NCHCT was deactivated, the then-National Center for Health Services Research (NCHSR)—now called the Agency for Health Care Policy and Research—created OHTA to continue that coverage advisory function for HCFA.

As stated earlier, when HCFA cannot resolve a coverage issue within its own system, it formally requests the Public Health Service to advise it. PHS refers that request to OHTA, which then publishes a notice to that affect in the *Federal Register,* requesting information and advice from interested and knowledgeable parties.

Traditionally, OHTA assessments have been concerned with safety and efficacy/effectiveness, not cost-effectiveness, and generally have addressed the acceptability and appropriateness of a procedure. In the past, PHS advice was to either cover or not cover a procedure, without explicitly providing guidance as to the appropriate conditions of recommended use. More recently, however, OHTA is addressing the conditions under which a technology should be covered. For instance, in 1986, OHTA recommended to HCFA that heart transplants be covered, but only for persons age 55 and under and only when performed in facilities meeting certain criteria (e.g., high volume, high success rate). In addition, HCFA has proposed coverage rules which include the assessment of cost-effectiveness of new technologies. Presumably, OHTA will have a role in assessing cost-effectiveness.

OHTA reviews and synthesizes existing data, literature, clinical trial evidence, and expert opinion rather than collecting primary data. It also relies heavily on consultation with the relevant medical specialty societies and federal agencies such as FDA and NIH. Between 1981 and 1991, OHTA prepared in excess of 160 coverage recommendations, nearly all of which were accepted by HCFA in its coverage policy determinations.

OHTA technology assessment efforts are guided by its National Advisory Council on Health Care Technology Assessment.

Prospective Payment Assessment Commission

As part of the 1983 Amendments to the Social Security Act, Congress established the Prospective Payment Assessment Commission (ProPAC) to ad-

vise and assist both Congress and the Secretary of DHHS in maintaining and updating Medicare's Prospective Payment System (PPS). Appointed by OTA, ProPAC has two primary responsibilities: (1) recommending to the secretary the annual economic update factor for the entire system that includes an adjustment for changes in technology and (2) recommending changes in the relative weights to the DRGs. The latter responsibility requires ProPAC to study individual technologies as they apply to hospital inpatient care.

When a new technology begins to diffuse into the hospital environment, it must fit within some DRG that has been calibrated based on previous methods of practice. If the new technology either decreases or raises costs of providing care, the DRG may no longer reflect the relative resource intensity of providing care and thus may inappropriately compensate the hospital for that case. ProPAC's responsibility is to assist in determining when a DRG needs to be created or recalibrated and what that change should be. Two examples illustrate the issues involved and the potential impact of the diffusion of important new technologies.

Magnetic resonance imaging was introduced in the 1980s. MRI is an expensive technology that can apply to a growing number of types of hospitalized cases (i.e., DRGs). The question becomes whether—and, if so, how—the Medicare prospective payment system (PPS) should be modified to reflect the additional costs of providing care. If no change is made, hospitals that adopt MRI will likely lose money on such cases (11). If all relevant DRGs are increased to reflect the additional costs to the entire system, hospitals that are slow to adopt MRI will be overcompensated and hospitals that adopt MRI will be undercompensated (since the additional payment is spread across all cases). If an additional DRG "add-on" is made for only those hospitals that adopt MRI or for only those cases where MRI is used, payment may be more equitable on a case-by-case basis. However, such a method begins to resemble the previous inflationary cost-based system that PPS was designed to reform. ProPAC's recommendation was to pay an add-on to the DRG for each scan. However, HCFA has been reluctant to adopt such a policy.

Extracorporeal shock wave lithotripsy (ESWL) provides another example of the new technology– existing DRG dilemma. Prior to the lithotripsy technology, the treatment of kidney stones in a hospital could be managed either medically or surgically, depending on clinical indications, with the surgical DRGs being roughly three times more expensive than the medical DRGs. Although the lithotripster is an expensive machine to buy and install, it crushes kidney stones noninvasively and thus tends to be more expensive per case than medical management but considerably less expensive than surgery. Fitting the lithotripsy into either category could either under- or overpay a hospital for adopting the technology. After studying hospital cost data, ProPAC recommended that HCFA temporarily use the higher of the two medical DRGs that it calculated would just cover costs if the machine were used efficiently. HCFA decided to simply pay ESWL within the existing medical DRGs (34).

Both MRI and ESWL are examples of the importance of ProPAC's role and the potential far-reaching effects of reimbursement policies on the adoption, diffusion, and, ultimately, innovation and development of new technologies.

Other Government Activities

A number of other governmental agencies conduct activities related to medical technology assessment. For instance, the Physician Payment Review Commission (PRPC) has a similar charter to ProPAC in terms of physician payment issues as well as technology-related concerns such as the development of practice guidelines. The new Medicare resource-based relative value scale (RBRVS) fee schedule is designed in part to lower procedure-based services relative to cognitive-based services. This will result in lowering financial incentives for physicians to provide technologically based services. PPRC advises on this new fee schedule system. The National Center for Health Statistics of the Public Health Service collects and disseminates information on health services utilization and health status of the U.S. population and sponsors some relevant methodologic work such as the measurement of health status versus quality of life. The Veterans Administration (VA) funds clinical and health services research, much of it related to technology, throughout its system. The Centers for Disease Control (CDC) support assessments of technologies related to clinical laboratories and disease prevention and health promotion. The Department of Defense conducts some clinical trials, but most of its other medical technology assessment activities are limited to military applications.

Private Sector Technology Assessment Activities

Although public policies and agencies tend to dominate discussion of medical technology assessment issues, the private sector is also very active in this area by contributing funding and generating information.

Pharmaceutical and Device Industries

The pharmaceutical industry devotes enormous resources to the assessment of its products, as mentioned earlier in the discussion of FDA's job in regulating drug entry into the marketplace. The industry reports that 15.9 percent ($6.8 billion) of its 1990 sales was devoted to research and development (4). As noted earlier, each new chemical entity requires seven to 10 years and an average investment of $231 million (29,35). This investment includes all the preclinical and clinical trial research required for FDA premarket approval.

The medical device industry also spends large amounts of money on assessments of its products, although on a much smaller scale than the pharmaceutical industry. A very rough estimate is that 6 percent of sales in the major firms is devoted to research and development, which total almost $2 billion annually (36). In addition, the medical device industry probably devotes only about 4 percent of its research and development (R&D) expenditures to clinical trials (30), in part because it takes less time to bring devices to the market and the necessary FDA evidence of performance standards, safety, and efficacy is usually less rigorous than that required for drugs.

Recently, due to increased pressures from the more competitive marketplace exhibiting greater price sensitivity to costly new technologies, drug and device firms are increasingly investing in cost-effectiveness analysis (CEA) of their products (37). In some cases, firms are integrating economic analysis into premarket clinical trials as well as to sponsor retrospective CEAs using existing literature and data sources such as claims files. These cost-effectiveness studies also differ from more traditional clinical studies by being comparative studies. That is, rather than being compared to placebo, the technologies are being examined for cost-effectiveness compared to competing choices of therapy: for example, coronary artery bypass surgery compared to percutaneous transluminal coronary arteriography (PTCA), a procedure that uses a balloon catheter to open restricted coronary arteries.

Insurers, Medical Associations, and Providers

Most of the remaining technology assessment activities sponsored by private sector organizations rely on synthesizing existing information in order to assist technology policy making. Very seldom are new data collected. In addition, most of these activities assess safety and efficacy issues rather than broader socioeconomic concerns such as cost-effectiveness and legal and ethical implications. Sponsoring such activities are several of the more prominent health care organizations, including the Blue Cross and Blue Shield Association, the American Hospital Association, the American Medical Association, and the American College of Physicians.

All insurers must have some system to determine their coverage policy, just as Medicare must, although private insurers often take a "follow the leader" approach. The leader may be HCFA (for Medicare), or possibly the Blue Cross and Blue Shield Association. In other cases, such as in organ transplantation issues, HCFA has been slower than commercial insurers in making coverage decision. Just as HCFA relies on the Public Health Service, many insurers rely on the appropriate medical societies for guidance as well as having their own internal medical advisory panels.

A prominent and well-defined private insurer assessment activity is the Blue Cross and Blue Shield Association's Medical Necessity Programs (MNP). Established in 1977, MNP attempts to assist in formulating coverage policy by selectively reviewing existing technologies in order to eliminate or reduce coverage for outmoded, ineffectual, and/or misused medical and surgical procedures. By 1985, the program had identified over 90 procedures that were classified as outmoded, had called for the elimination of routine laboratory and X-ray testing, and developed guidelines for respiratory therapy. MNP uses BC/BS's Medical Advisory Panel and requests the cooperation from such medical societies as the American College of Physicians and American College of Radiology to guide its assessments. Commercial insurers are also sponsoring assessment activities to assist in coverage determination.

The American College of Physicians (ACP) sponsors the Clinical Efficacy Assessment Project (CEAP), an expansion of MNP. This program relies on literature review and expert opinion from among its membership to review the appropriate application of established technologies used in the practice of internal medicine.

The American Medical Association (AMA) sponsors the Diagnostic and Therapeutic Technology Assessment (DATTA) program, which is similarly designed to educate its memberships about the value and appropriate use of technologies. DATTA tends to concentrate more on new and emerging diagnostic and therapeutic technologies. For each topic, the DATTA program reviews existing evidence, formulates relevant questions, and surveys a panel of experts within AMA's membership ranks.

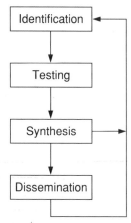

Figure 9-7. Process of assessing medical technologies. (SOURCE: Office of Technology Assessment. (1982). *Strategies for medical technology assessment.* Washington, DC: Author.)

The American Hospital Association's (AHA) Hospital Technology Series is a program that focuses on hospital devices and equipment from the hospital administrator's point of view. The evaluations are concerned primarily with the cost and service implications of technologies that are entering clinical practice. Evaluations are based on synthesis of technical reports and the professional literature as well as selected and focused interviews with technical and hospital experts.

Conclusions

As this overview of several of the major organizations included in medical technology assessment in the United States indicates, the predominant activity is that of assessing existing information. The principal exceptions are the pharmaceutical and medical device firms which must generate primary data for FDA premarket approval, clinical trials sponsored by NIH, and to a much lesser degree other federal agencies.

As was indicated earlier in this chapter, little is known concerning the appropriate use of many technologies. The final section of this chapter addresses some of the methodological issues of assessing medical technologies.

Methods for Assessment

A number of different techniques and methodologies are used in the assessment of medical technologies. Some of the more common ones have already been mentioned: randomized clinical trials (RCT), group judgment methods, and cost-effectiveness analysis.

A helpful way to discuss the methods for evaluating technologies is to use a four-step framework for assessment: identification, testing, synthesis, and dissemination (figure 9-7). This process is applicable even to later stages in the life cycle of a technology due to several factors: technologies may diffuse prematurely without adequate assessment; they are often used for new indications or for different groups of patients; and their relative efficacy may change as new competing technologies are developed.

Identification

It is difficult to determine which technologies should be assessed. Of course, by law, drugs and medical devices can be marketed only with FDA approval, so the industry systematically identifies these technologies for assessment early in their life cycle. Later, these same technologies may face a market test due to price sensitivity of the insurer, the hospital, the health maintenance organization (HMO) or even the physician or the consumer. In such a case, the market itself is identifying the technology—requesting, in effect, that cost-effectiveness be assessed. However, there is nothing systematic concerning this so-called market test.

The previous section discussed the substantial role of the insurer (HCFA, Blue Cross, etc.) in identifying technologies for assessment during the coverage policy determination of a new technology. In other cases, such as with OTA, a technology is chosen for assessment as a case study either for the purpose of illustrating a policy issue or because it has assumed national significance, such as the CT scanner. Other bodies such as the old National Center for Health Care Technology (NCHCT) or BC/BS's Medical Necessity Program rely on advisory councils to develop priorities for assessment using criteria such as high per unit cost, high volume, potential safety issues, and uncertainty concerning efficacy and appropriate use.

Testing

Safety and Efficacy

Testing refers to primary data being generated systematically for analysis. The gold standard for testing technologies is the *randomized clinical trial* (RCT) since it provides the most valid and reliable information. Human subjects are randomly assigned to the experimental and comparison and/or control groups, blinded, if possible, as to which group they are in and followed over time to determine efficacy, safety, and, possibly, cost-effectiveness. When possible, even the clinicians and evaluators are blinded as to which subjects are in which group. Randomization and blinding helps to minimize any bias in the findings.

Many times, blinding or random assignment are impractical or even impossible. For instance, one cannot blind surgeons and patients when testing surgical techniques; sham surgery is unethical. Similarly, once a treatment is thought to be efficacious, it may be unethical to withhold it as would be necessary in random assignment.

Various observation methods are used when randomization cannot be done. For instance, a matched control study attempts to match pairs of patients in both groups on all-important variables that could have an impact on therapeutic outcome such as age, sex, symptoms, and severity of disease.

A very common method found in the medical literature is the *case study*. In fact, individual clinicians develop their own particular practice style based in large part on observations of their own

cases. Although the case study method has its place in informing medical practice, its role may be better served as a method of identifying when a formal assessment is warranted rather than serving as evidence that a technology is or is not efficacious.

Another useful method of study is the *clinical data bank or registry approach*. These types of historical files are set up to follow patients who have certain medical conditions (e.g., cancer) or have undergone a certain procedure (e.g., cardiac catherization). They can be helpful in studying long-term epidemiologic trends and clinical outcomes. Cancer registries are the oldest and most common example of this method. Thus, in themselves, the clinical data bank and registry is not a method of assessment, but rather a way to organize and gather data for assessment.

Cost-Effectiveness Analysis (CEA)

Although most of the technology assessment methods are primarily used for testing safety and efficacy, CEA is becoming increasingly popular since it is clear that when technology decisions are made there are economic constraints that require trade-offs (38). Unlike *cost-benefit analysis* (CBA), which values all outcomes in terms of dollars, thus necessitating the explicit valuing of life, limb, pain, and suffering, CEA is used to calculate the net cost of acquiring some health outcome. A convenient way to conceptualize the cost-benefit and cost-effectiveness approach is shown in figure 9-8.

The medical or health treatment (see box A in figure 9-8) can lead to changes in both health services resource use (e.g., open heart surgery—B) and health status (e.g., years of life saved—C). Changes in health status (C) in turn, can lead to a change in productive output (D) as well as changes in health services (B). Box E depicts the intrinsic economic value that can be placed on that health status change. A cost-benefit analysis calculates the net economic value in boxes B, C, D, and E. Cost-effectiveness analysis generally compares the

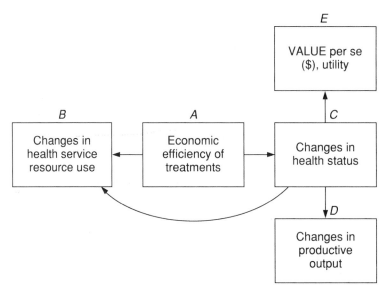

Figure 9-8. Measuring efficiency in health care. (SOURCE: Drummond M. F. (1980). *Principles of economic appraisal in health care.* Oxford, UK: Oxford University Press.)

net economic changes in health resource use *(B)* with the net change in health status *(C)*. Table 9-2 provides comparisons of the cost per year of life saved (or cost per quality-adjusted year of life saved) as reported in a number of cost-effectiveness studies in the literature.

Lately cost-effectiveness analysis has sometimes been added to clinical and observational studies. Typically, patients in the study are followed for standard safety and efficacy evaluation but also monitored for economic outcomes, such as health care utilization patterns and work loss. In addition, special patient survey questionnaires that assess overall health status change are sometimes used. For example, HCFA funded the National Heart Transplant Study, which followed a series of heart transplant patients, assessing effectiveness, quality of life, and direct and indirect economic costs, as well as other social and legal issues (39).

Synthesis

The third component of the process of assessment is the synthesis of information, a practice that is widely used and perhaps overly relied on. Many technology assessments found in the literature today are developed using a technique falling under the general heading of synthesis. The most common and simple method of synthesis is the standard literature review. One person surveys what is written about a procedure, discards that which is deemed unimportant, and draws conclusions regarding the value of the procedure. The quality of a literature review depends on the ability and diligence of the reviewer, that individual's personal biases, and the quality and consistency of the evidence found in the literature. This last point can be a particularly difficult problem because multiple independent clinical studies of a given technology often reveal conflicting results, partially because they are conducted at different times, with different patients using different methods of design and different techniques of analysis.

Today, formal quantitative synthesis techniques, collectively termed *meta analysis,* have been devised to assist in resolving many of these difficulties. Meta analysis permits a reviewer to consolidate the results of multiple, unrelated studies on a given

TABLE 9-2. Costs per Year of Life Saved for Some Health Investments

Investment	Cost per Year of Life Saved (1986 U.S. $) [a]
Neonatal intensive care, 1000–1499 g	$ 5,500
Coronary artery bypass surgery (three-vessel)	$ 7,200*
T4 (thyroid screening)	$ 7,700
Treatment of severe hypertension (diastolic >105 mmHg) in males age 40	$11,400
Treatment of mild hypertension (diastolic 95–104 mmHg) in males age 40	$23,200
Heart transplantation	$26,854*
Estrogen therapy for postmenopausal symptoms in women without a prior hysterectomy	$32,900
Neonatal intensive care, 500–999 g	$38,800
Coronary artery bypass surgery for single-vessel disease with moderately severe angina	$44,200
School tuberculin testing program	$53,100
Continuous ambulatory peritoneal dialysis	$57,300
Hospital hemodialysis	$65,600

[a] Each figure, except for those marked with an asterisk (*), refers to cost per quality-adjusted life year saved.

SOURCE: Adapted from Drummond, M. F. (In press). Economic evaluation and the rational diffusion and use of health technology. Health Policy.

issue, differentially weighting studies depending on the rigor of research design, sample size, and so forth. Thus, an RCT may be weighted more heavily than an observational study; a large trial more heavily than a small one.

A less quantitative but particularly popular method for synthesizing information is a family of techniques termed "group judgment" or "consensus" methods (40). The Consensus Development format used by the NIH was described earlier. There are other variations such as the Delphi and Nominal Group Process techniques, which are more structured methods of eliciting group judgments. The AMA's DATTA program and the American College of Physicians' CEAP, both of which were briefly described in the previous section, are examples of less structured group judgment methods. For instance, DATTA is more of a poll than a group judgment method. Some techniques systematically combine clinical trial evidence with the group judgment (41,42); other techniques assume

that the experts being polled already are aware of the existing evidence (Delphi, DATTA).

Dissemination

The dissemination phase of the assessment process is arguably the most underrated of the four phases being discussed here. Relatively little attention has been paid to how information about clinical practice is disseminated, how it is received once the information arrives, and whether—and why—change really takes place (1). Stated differently, we do not understand very well to what and to what degree doctors pay attention. We simply know that there is clearly much misunderstanding of evidence that both does and does not exist concerning the efficacy, safety, cost-effectiveness, and other social, legal, and ethical implications of the use of technologies. Practicing clinicians rely on their own store of knowledge from their training, personal experience, colleagues, the literature, and other educational materials and programs, perhaps roughly in that order of importance.

Many organizations attempt to make technology assessment information available. There are numerous medical journals, often sponsored by medical societies; the National Library of Medicine catalogs and indexes medical and health journals and is presently establishing a means to include technology assessment reports into MEDLINE; and many of the organizations discussed in this chapter sponsor assessment activities specifically for the purposes of disseminating the results to their membership and the medical community at large. Yet little is known of the effectiveness of these efforts.

Challenges for Technology Assessment

The United States is leaving the era of laissez-faire payment policies that pay—seemingly without question—for whatever is ordered by physicians and whatever is charged for their services. These past payment policies have fueled technological innovation, adoption, and use. Since costs were not much of a constraint, high-tech medicine could soar, as could quality of care, to the extent that the two are linked. It is well known that medicine in the United States is the most technologically advanced system in the world, and believed by many to be the best care in the world.

However, there have been many excesses as well, excesses that are certainly not limited to the United States.

The major threat to the wondrous technological innovations that could be ours in the future probably lies in the hands of the politicians who must control the deficit and in the medical and health services communities which will have to convince an increasingly skeptical public that their own house is in order. The threat is not in the hands of the innovators of health care technology and other venture capitalists, both of whom will respond to the signals that society sends them.

This chapter has attempted to describe medical technology—its development, diffusion, adoption, use, and assessment. Although the United States probably has the most sophisticated technology generating and assessment systems in the world, much still needs to be done. The basic tools are available, however. Sufficient capital and innovative capabilities exist in private industry and NIH. Public agencies and private organizations are in place and assessment methods are useful and available. Basic and applied research monies are available. The country does have an effective system to ensure that drugs and devices are not marketed prior to safety and efficacy being established. However, there is no such system for medical and surgical procedures. Nor is there sufficient information about the appropriate use of any of the classes of technologies in the inventory.

Today, we are seeing more organizations launching assessment activities and existing ones being further developed. This is true of the federal government, medical societies, and insurers. Also, assessment programs are coming under greater scrutiny by policy makers. For instance, OHTA is under the microscope of both Congress and the manufacturers' associations. In general, the assessment enterprise gains greater attention as assessment becomes a gateway to payment and marketing success. Manufacturers are looking beyond safety and efficacy of their products to broader implications such as quality of life and cost-effectiveness. They are also sponsoring more comparative studies.

Nevertheless, despite the gains made to date, the challenge of the future is to learn to use the tools we have in order to better understand the technology and its use within the practice of medicine.

References

1. Office of Technology Assessment, U.S. Congress. (1982). *Strategies for medical technology assessment.* Washington, DC: Author.

2. Levitt, K. R., Lazenby, H. C., Cowan, C. A., & Letsch, S. W. (1991, Fall). National health expenditures, 1990. *Health Care Financing Review. 13.* 1.

3. National Institutes of Health. (1991). *NIH data book.* Bethesda, MD: Author.

4. Pharmaceutical Manufacturers Association annual survey, 1991.

5. Institute of Medicine. (1985). *Assessing medical technologies* (p. 37). Washington, DC: National Academy Press.

6. Bessey, E. C. (1987). Innovation in an era of cost containment. In R. M. C. K. Southby, W. Greenberg, & B. R. Luce (Eds.). *Health care technology under financial constraints.* Columbus, OH: Battelle Press.

7. Russell, L. B. (1979). *Technology in hospitals: Medical advances and their diffusion.* Washington, DC: Brookings Institution.

8. Office of Technology Assessment, U.S. Congress. (1981). *Policy implications of the computed tomography (CT) scanner: An update.* Washington, DC: Author.

9. Office of Technology Assessment, U.S. Congress. (1978). *Policy implications of the computed tomography (CT) scanner.* Washington, DC: Author.

10. Steinberg, E. P., Sisk, J. E., & Locke, K. E. (1985). The diffusion of magnetic resonance imagers in the United States and the world. *International Journal of Technology Assessment in Health Care. 1.* 537.

11. Valvona, J., & Sloan, F. (1985). Rising rates of surgery among the elderly. *Health Affairs. 4.* 108–118.

12. Graves, E. J. (1991). Summary: National Hospital Discharge Survey. *Advance data from vital and health statistics* (no. 199). Hyattsville, MD: National Center for Health Statistics.

13. Chu, F., & Cotter, D. (1986). PPS policies should reflect payment adjustments for new technologies. *Business and Health. 4.* 60.

14. Wennberg, J. E. (1984). Dealing with medical practice variations: A proposal for action. *Health Affairs. 3.* 6–32.

15. Wennberg, J. E. (1984). Dealing with medical practice variations: A proposal for action. *Health Affairs. 3.* 15.

16. Chassin, M. R., Brook, R. H., Park, R., et al. (1986). Variations in the use of medical and surgical services by the Medicare population. *New England Journal of Medicine. 314.* 285–309.

17. Wennberg, J. E. & Brook, R. H. (1985). *Addressing medical practice variations: A challenge for pros and private review agencies.* Paper presented to the National Health Policy Forum, Washington, DC.

18. Office of Technology Assessment, U.S. Congress. (1978). *Assessing the safety and efficacy of medical technologies* (p. 7). Washington, DC: Author.

19. Iglehart, J. K. (1984). Editor's note. *Health Affairs. 3.* p. 3–4.

20. Morse, L. M. (1986). Therapeutic drug use review reduces incidence of drug related illness. *Business and Health. 3.* 58.

21. Fineberg, H. V. (1979). Gastric freezing. A study of diffusion of a medical innovation. In *Medical technology and the health care system: A study of the diffusion of equipment-embodied technology* (p. 173). Washington DC: National Academy of Sciences.

22. Hiatt, H. H. (1987). *Health in the balance: Choice or change* (p. 173). New York: Harper & Row.

23. Lambert, E. C. (1978). *Modern medical mistakes.* Bloomington, IN: Indiana University Press.

24. Lawless, E. W. (1977). *Technology and social shock.* New Brunswick, NJ: Rutgers University Press.

25. Banta, D., Brown, S., & Behney, C. (1978). Implications of the 1976 medical devices legislation. *Man and Medicine. 3.* 131–143.

26. Office of Technology Assessment, U.S. Congress. (1976). *Development of medical technologies: Opportunities for assessment.* Washington, DC: Author.

27. U.S. Department of Health, Education and Welfare, Office of the Assistant Secretary. (n.d.). *NCHCT fact sheet.*

28. Food and Drug Administration, U.S. Department of Health and Human Services. (1977). *General considerations for the clinical evaluation of drugs.* Washington, DC: U.S. Government Printing Office.

29. DiMasi, J. A., et al. (1991, July). Cost of innovation in the pharmaceutical industry. *Journal of Health Economics. 10.* 107.

30. U.S. Congress, Office of Technology Assessment, personal communication, 1992.

31. Lewin & Associates. (1986). *A forward plan for Medicare coverage and technology assessment* (Contract No. 282-45-0062). Prepared for the Assistant Secretary for Planning and Evaluation, U.S.

Department of Health and Human Services, Washington, DC.

32. Medicare program: Criteria and procedures for making medical services coverage decisions that relate to health care technology. (1989, January 30). *Federal Register. 54*(18). 4302–4318.

33. Health Care Financing Administration. Unpublished data, 1986.

34. Office of Technology Assessment, U.S. Congress. (1986, May). *Health technology care study 36: Effects of federal policies on extracorporeal shock wave lithotripsy.* Washington, DC: Author.

35. Pharmaceutical Manufacturers Association. (1987). *PMA statistical fact book.* Washington, DC: Author.

36. Health Industry Manufacturers Association, personal communication, 1992.

37. Elixhauser, A., Luce, B. R., & Taylor. (1990, April). *Standards for socio-economic evaluation of health care products and services.* Berlin, Germany: Springer-Verlag.

38. Warner, K. E., & Luce, B. R. (1982). *Cost-benefit and cost-effectiveness analysis in health care: Principles, practice and potential.* Ann Arbor, MI: Health Administration Press.

39. Health Care Financing Administration, Office of Research and Demonstration. (1985). *National Heart Transplant Study* (Vols. I–VII), Battelle Fund Final Report.

40. Fink, A., Kosecoff, J., Chassis, M., et al. (1984). Consensus methods: Characteristics and guidelines for use. *American Journal of Public Health. 74.* 979.

41. Park, R. E., Fink, A., Brook, R. H., et al. (1986). Physician ratings of appropriate indications for six medical and surgical procedures. *American Journal of Public Health. 76.* 766.

42. Jacoby, I. (1985). The consensus development program of the National Institutes of Health: Current practices and historical perspectives. *International Journal of Technology Assessment in Health Care. 1.* 420.

Chapter 10

Health Care Professionals

Stephen S. Mick
Ira Moscovice

Health care professionals play a key role in the provision of services to meet the health needs and demands of the population. This chapter highlights health care professional trends and discusses issues of provider supply, education and training, distribution, and specialization, and the role of the public sector in the production of health care professionals.

Employment Trends in the Health Care Sector

The 20th century has witnessed a dramatic growth in the number and types of personnel employed in the health care sector. Table 10-1 shows the rapid gains in health sector employment in the United States, starting with a pool of fewer than 500,000 employed persons in 1910 and growing to more than 7 million by 1988. These figures include primarily those people with training and skills unique to the health care sector and exclude clerical staff, artisans, laborers, and others who have supporting roles in the delivery of health services. It has been estimated that almost one-third of all those employed in the health sector fall into this supporting category (1). Although these approximately 1.5 million nonclinical workers are not discussed in this chapter, they are very important because they evidence the role the health care sector has provided for new employment opportunities.

The health care sector has maintained a steadily increasing proportion of all persons employed, and currently includes about 6.2 percent of the U.S. labor force. Thus, growth in employment in the health sector (1,391 percent increase between 1910 and 1988) has outpaced growth in overall employment in the economy (201 percent increase) as well as total population growth (167 percent increase). This growth is underscored by the fivefold increase in the rate of health care personnel per 100,000 population, from a low of 518 in 1910 to a high of 2,872 in 1988 (table 10-1).

More extraordinary than the increased supply of health care personnel has been the emergence of

TABLE 10-1. The Health Sector as a Proportion of All Employed Persons, by Decade: 1910–1980, 1988

	1910	1920	1930	1940	1950	1960	1970	1980	1988
Employment in health sector (thousands)[a]	479	624	859	972	1,394	1,966	3,130	5,030	7,144
Total number of persons employed (thousands)[b]	38,167	41,614	48,829	44,888	56,225	64,639	78,627	97,270	114,968
Health sector as a proportion of all occupations	1.3%	1.5%	1.8%	2.2%	2.5%	3.0%	4.0%	5.2%	6.2%
Total U.S. population (millions)	92.4	106.5	123.1	132.6	152.3	180.7	205.1	227.7	246.3
Rate of health personnel per 100,000 population	518	586	698	733	915	1,088	1,428	2,209	2,872

[a] These figures do not include secretarial and office workers, craftsmen, laborers, and other personnel such as cooks, janitors, and so on who work in supporting roles in the health care sector.

[b] Figures for 1980 and 1988 include employed persons 16 years of age and over; figures from 1940 to 1970 include employed persons 14 years of age and over; earlier data are based on persons 10 years of age and over.

SOURCES: Adapted from Mick, S. (1978). Understanding the persistence of human resource problems in health. *Milbank Memorial Fund Quarterly.* 56. 463–499, table 3; U.S. Bureau of the Census. (1990). *Statistical abstract of the United States: 1990* (110th ed.). Washington, DC: U.S. Government Printing Office.

a wide variety of new categories of personnel, including physicians' assistants (PAs), nurse practitioners (NPs), dental hygienists, laboratory technicians, nursing aides, orderlies and attendants, home health aides, occupational and physical therapists, medical records personnel, X-ray technicians, dieticians and nutritionists, social workers, and the like. The Department of Labor currently recognizes almost 400 different job titles in the health sector (2). Some of the most rapid growth in the supply of health care personnel has occurred in these recently developed categories.

The traditional health care occupations of physician, dentist, and pharmacist have generally experienced declines, some dramatic, in their relative proportion of all health care personnel. For example, physicians (including osteopaths) constituted 30 percent of all persons in health occupations in 1910, but had declined to about 9 percent of the total in 1988. Over the same period, dentists declined from 8 to about 2 percent, and pharmacists 11 to about 3 percent. Registered nurses have

fluctuated up, then down during this nearly 80-year period: 17 percent in 1910 to a high of 36 percent in 1940, then a steady decline to 25 percent in 1988. The group of health care workers that has gained the largest share of the overall number includes allied health technicians, technologists, aides, and assistants: they constituted a mere 1 percent in 1910 but in 1988 they made up over 51 percent. These figures should not mask the fact that *all* groups of health care workers have increased in absolute number from year to year as inspection of any of the tables in this chapter will show. What the data emphasize is the higher growth rate of nontraditional allied health and support personnel, who now constitute more than two-thirds of all personnel employed in the health care sector (3).

The primary reasons for the increased supply and wide variety of health care personnel in the 20th century are the interrelated forces of technological growth, specialization, health insurance coverage, and the emergence of the hospital as

TABLE 10-2. Number of Active Physicians: 1970, 1980, 1990

Health Occupation	1970		1980		1990[a]	
	Number	Personnel per 100,000 Population	Number	Personnel per 100,000 Population	Number	Personnel per 100,000 Population
Physicians	326,200	156.0	457,500	197.0	601,060	240.0
MDs	314,200	150.0	440,400	189.5	543,310	228.9
DOs	12,000	6.0	17,100	7.5	27,750	11.1

[a] Estimated data.

SOURCES: *Fourth report to the President and Congress on the status of health personnel in the United States* (DHHS Publication No. [HRS]-P-0084.4). (1984, May). Washington, DC: U.S. Government Printing Office; *Seventh report to the President and Congress on the status of health personnel in the United States* (DHHS Publication No. [HRS]-P-OD-90-1). (1990, March). Washington, DC: U.S. Government Printing Office.

the central institution of the health care system. The hospital became the setting where new technology could be implemented and where medical, nursing, and other health professional students could be educated. The technological revolution has led to an increased use of hospitals, with the corresponding concentration of health personnel. The rise of private health insurance in the 1940s, plus publicly funded insurance in the mid–1960s (Medicare and Medicaid), fueled hospital growth because reliable payment mechanisms provided hospitals with assured revenues. However, current concerns with escalating health care costs have led to a substantial increase in the use of health care facilities outside the hospital (4). These facilities include urgent care centers, ambulatory surgery centers, hospices, freestanding diagnostic centers, health maintenance organizations (HMOs), and others. Furthermore, the number of people cared for in their own homes has increased, leading to a demand for such personnel as home health aides and inhalation therapists as well as nursing personnel. The hospital sector is no longer likely to be alone as a center for increased employment in the future.

Technological innovation has also lead to increased specialization of health care personnel, primarily during the last 30 years. This specialization has resulted in new categories of health care providers within the traditional professions (e.g., pediatric nephrologists and gastroenterologists in medicine, periodontists in dentistry) and the advent of new types of allied health professions (e.g., occupational and radiological technicians and speech pathologists).

These health care personnel will be discussed in greater detail by focusing on four of the more traditional groups of professions—physicians and osteopaths, dentists, nurses, and pharmacists—and two of the recently developed categories of personnel—PAs and NPs.

The Expanding Supply of Physicians

A Physician Surplus or Shortage?

The number of physicians in the United States has increased rapidly in the last two decades, with an estimated 601,060 active physicians, including osteopaths (described more fully in a later section) practicing in 1990 (table 10-2). Between 1970 and 1990, there was an 84 percent increase in the supply of physicians, resulting in an average of approximately one physician per 414 population. In 1980, the Graduate Medical Education National Advisory Committee (GMENAC) reported to the Secretary of the U.S. Department of Health and Human Services that the surplus of physicians would number 70,000 in 1990 and 145,000 in 2000, underscoring the belief that the nation could substantially reduce its subsidization of medical education (5). This increase in the number of U.S.-

TABLE 10-3. Number of Allopathic Medical Schools, Applicants, Students, Graduates, and Ratio of First-Year Students to Applicants: Selected Academic Years 1965–1966 through 1990–1991

Academic Year	Number of Schools	Number of Applicants	Number of Students		Number of Graduates	Ratio of First-Year Students to Applicants
			Total	First Year		
1965–1966	88	18,703	32,835	8,759	7,574	1:2.4
1970–1971	103	24,987	40,487	11,348	8,974	1:2.2
1975–1976	114	42,303	56,244	15,351	13,561	1:2.8
1980–1981	126	36,100	65,497	17,204	15,667	1:2.0
1985–1986	127	32,893	66,604	16,929	16,125	1:1.9
1990–1991	126	29,243	64,986	16,803	15,499	1:1.7

SOURCES: Undergraduate medical education. (1980). *Journal of the American Medical Association. 243.* 849–866; Jonas, H., Etzel, S., & Barzansky, B. (1991). Educational programs in U.S. medical schools. *Journal of the American Medical Association. 226.* 913–923.

trained physicians was one of two reasons contributing to the overall growth in supply; the other was the immigration of foreign-trained physicians into the United States, particularly between the early 1960s to the late 1970s (6).

Table 10-3 shows the substantial increase in both the number of medical schools and the number of medical students (first-year and total enrolled) over the last 25 years. By 1990–1991, the yearly number of graduates had more than doubled the 1965–1966 number. This increase can be directly attributed to massive federal outlays for training, research, and construction in the 1960s and 1970s. By the early 1970s, 40 to 50 percent of medical school support came from federal sources (7). However, the retreat of the federal government from an active role in the financial support of medical education was initiated in the early 1980s as a result of overall pressures to reduce federal spending and the perception that there was an adequate aggregate supply of physicians in the United States. In 1989, the federal government provided approximately 23 percent of medical school financial support through direct subsidies and research funds. The comparable proportions were 40 percent in 1960, 44 percent in 1970, and 29 percent in 1980 (8).

The reduction of federal funds is just one of several factors that have helped to produce a lev-

eling off in the 1980s of the admission and graduation of U.S. medical graduates. The most intriguing factor is the large decline in people applying to medical schools. Since the high point in the mid–1970s (42,303 in 1975), medical school applicants dropped to 26,721 in 1988, a 37 percent decrease, although the numbers have begun to move back up (table 10-3). This decline has been caused by the reduced number of reapplicants, the number of accepted applicants electing to attend other graduate training programs, and the soaring costs of medical school tuition. The cost of attending medical school has increased to the point that the average debt of a graduating medical student was about $46,000 in 1990, an increase of 77 percent from 1980, after adjustment for inflation (9).

Other factors influencing the decline include changes in the practice of medicine such as restrictive reimbursement policies by public and private insurers, vulnerability to allegations and claims of malpractice, perceived loss of professional autonomy by hospital utilization and quality review units and by external governmental agencies, and the expansion of so-called managed care schemes—e.g., health maintenance organizations and preferred provider organizations. Some feel that the practice of medicine is not as attractive as it once was. Surveys of physicians have revealed a

TABLE 10-4. Foreign Medical Graduates (FMGs) in Residency Positions: Selected Years 1980 through 1990

	1980	1982	1984	1986	1988	1990
Total FMGs	12,259	13,123	13,525	12,207	12,433	14,914
Percentage of total residents	19.9	18.6	18.0	15.7	15.3	17.9
U.S.-citizen FMGs	4,814	6,388	7,386	5,845	5,131	5,026
U.S.-citizen FMGs as a percentage of all FMGs	39.3	48.7	54.6	47.9	41.3	33.7

SOURCES: Crowley, A. (1985). Graduate medical education in the United States, 1984–1985. *Journal of the American Medical Association.* 254. 1585–1593; Etzel, S., Egan, R., Shevrin, M., & Rowley, B. (1989). Graduate medical education in the United States. *Journal of the American Medical Association.* 262. 1029–1037; Rowley, B., Baldwin, D., McGuire, M., Etzel, S., & O'Leary, C. (1990). Graduate medical education in the United States. *Journal of the American Medical Association.* 264. 822–832; Jonas, H., Etzel, S., & Barzansky, B. (1991). Education programs in U.S. medical schools. *Journal of the American Medical Association.* 226. 913–923.

surprising amount of discontent among practicing physicians: in 1990, 38 percent of a random sample of physicians said they would not recommend medicine as a career choice to a high school or college student (10). Thus, many people who would have applied to medical school in the past have elected to apply to and enroll in business, engineering, and other areas.

The decline in interest in medical education has not been translated into much decrease in entering class sizes or numbers graduating annually (table 10-3). Thus one can conclude that the flow of new U.S.-trained physicians will hold constant for the near future.

The second important factor in the increased supply of physicians has been the influx of foreign medical graduates (FMGs) into the United States. By the mid–1960s, favorable immigration policies for physicians had encouraged this movement; there was in addition an unceasing demand for interns and residents in U.S. hospitals as measured by the existence each year of unfilled house officer positions (11). By the early 1970s, FMGs accounted for more than 40 percent of new physician licentiates, 30 percent of filled residency positions, and 20 percent of the active physicians in the United States. One-third of the growth of the physician supply in the 1970s was due to increases in the number of physicians trained outside the United States (12).

The vast majority of the increase in FMG supply occurred before 1976, and that year marked the

passage of PL 94-484 (the Health Professions Education Assistance Act of 1976), which stated, "there is no further need for affording preference to alien physicians and surgeons in admission to the United States under the Immigration and Nationality Act." The enactment of PL 94-484 noticeably limited the immigration of FMGs to the United States. The number of FMGs filling residency positions decreased from 18,395 in 1972–1973 to 12,259 in 1980–1981. This figure stabilized at between 12,000 and 13,000 during most of the 1980s (table 10-4).

Another interesting facet of the FMG phenomenon has been the growing numbers of U.S. citizen FMGs, men and women who went abroad to receive a medical education and then returned to the United States. Virtually nonexistent before 1970s, U.S. citizen FMGs grew in number throughout the 1980s, and by the mid–1980s, they actually surpassed the number of foreign national FMGs (54.6 percent of all FMGs in 1984). However, the U.S.-citizen FMG has since declined in numbers, to about 33.7 percent of all FMGs in 1990. Recent research has also shown that many of these U.S.-citizen FMGs were and are actually naturalized U.S. citizens who were not born in the United States and who did not gain U.S. citizenship until they entered medical school or until they arrived in the United States to begin residency training. The majority of these people are Spanish-speaking and were educated in Mexico, Spain, and the Dominican Republic (13).

By 1989, the number of FMGs again began to grow and registered a marked increase to 14,914 residents in 1990, a level not seen since the late 1970s. The new upturn may not portend a trend of the magnitude of the late 1960s and early 1970s FMG migration, but it does underscore the continuing importance of FMGs in the United States because there are more than 130,000 FMGs (21 percent of all licensed physicians) in the United States (14). The new upturn, coupled with a once-again increasing number of unfilled residency positions, also provides evidence that the surplus of physicians predicted throughout the 1980s, and discussed below, may have been overstated.

In summary, there was a marked increase in the supply of U.S. physicians in the 1970s and 1980s due to an increased number of U.S. medical schools and the number of U.S. medical school graduates. The immigration of FMGs supplemented this increase during the 1970s, but contributed to an increasingly smaller proportion of this increase during the 1980s. However, very recent data suggest that the number of FMGs, especially foreign-national FMGs, may once again be increasing, simultaneous with a leveling-off trend of U.S. medical graduates. The obvious question related to the dramatic increase in physicians is why it was necessary to use a dual strategy of increasing the supply. The answer is twofold: first, before the 1970s, policy makers and medical experts strongly believed that there was serious shortage of physicians in the United States, with several studies estimating the shortage in 1975 to be in the range of 10,000 and 50,000 (15). Second, our nation has not had a coordinated physician personnel policy, as has, for example, Canada; undergraduate and graduate medical education systems have operated independently of each other (16). Thus, the policy of increasing the number of U.S. medical schools and U.S. medical graduates has not been closely connected to the graduate training system, with the result that students graduating from U.S. medical schools have filled a smaller proportion of available residency positions, often leaving the less desirable positions (both for residencies and per-

manent employment) for FMGs. FMGs have helped staff U.S. hospitals and have been more willing than U.S. medical graduates to practice in relatively less popular geographic, specialty, and institutional areas and settings (13,17).

As the physician shortage was perceived to turn into a surplus, the number and proportion of FMGs fell to lower levels. Specialties once heavily populated by FMGs gained appreciable numbers of U.S. medical graduates, and the number of unfilled residency positions almost disappeared. Most observers believed that FMGs were less able to compete against U.S. medical graduates for scarcer residency slots. However, our nation is now witnessing a reversal of earlier thinking that a surplus exists (18,19). Mounting skepticism of a physician surplus now coincides with an increasing number and proportion of unfilled residency training positions as well as an increase in the number and proportion of FMGs beginning their graduate medical education in the United States. Although few would predict that the FMG phenomenon will return to the magnitude that it assumed in the early 1970s, some observers note that international physician migration appears to be following a cyclical pattern.

Trends in Specialty Distribution

Whether or not a surplus exists, there has been a significant increase in the supply of physicians, which has led to major concerns about their specialty and geographic distribution. Simply increasing the supply of physicians has not guaranteed that necessary medical services would be readily available to the general population. Of particular interest was the availability of primary care—the entry level into the health care system where basic medical services are provided. Primary care includes diagnosis and treatment of common illness and diseases, preventive services, home care services, and uncomplicated minor surgery and emergency care.

The increased supply of physicians has not resulted in major changes in the proportion of physicians in primary care specialties—general practice, family practice, general internal medicine, and general pediatrics (table 10-5). There has been substantial growth of primary care specialties between 1970 and 1990 (90 percent increase), but the growth of other specialty groupings has been greater, 470 percent, 92 percent, and 116 percent, respectively. Efforts to increase support for primary care residencies appeared to have helped increase their proportion of all active physicians only slightly to a little more than 38 percent in 1980. Since then, however, the proportion in primary care fell to 35 percent in 1986 and is estimated to drop to 33 percent by 2000. This decline is a major concern in view of the amount of public and private funding that has occurred during the last two decades to increase the number and proportion of primary care physicians.

The Graduate Medical Education National Advisory Committee (GMENAC) ranked most medical specialties by the degree to which each would or would not meet the estimated needs of the U.S. population. Most of the primary care specialties, e.g., family practice, general internal medicine, and general pediatrics, as well as osteopathic general practice, ranked as "near balance" specialties—i.e., those in which an adequate number of physicians was available for the estimated need. By contrast, specialties that GMENAC predicted to be in the surplus range included most surgical specialties and many medical subspecialties. In view of the ongoing proportionate decrease and increase of primary care specialties and medical subspecialties, respectively, the potential shortages in primary care predicted by GMENAC will continue unless specific efforts are made to reverse the trend.

The real goal of any physician supply policy should be to provide appropriate medical services that are readily accessible to the general population. Knowledge of the physician specialty distribution does not provide information on physician productivity, practice case mix, or the scope of services provided. The controversy over the extent of primary care provided by specialists and specialty care provided by primary care physicians highlights this point (20,21). Future demand for physicians cannot be based solely on the number and types of physicians in our country.

Geographic Distribution of Physicians

One of the assumptions underlying federal health personnel policy in the 1960s and early 1970s was that a significant increase in the overall supply of physicians would both resolve the problem of a serious shortage and improve the geographic distribution of physicians. But although there is now debate between the surplus and shortage hypotheses, there is less debate about the persistent chronic shortages in rural and inner-city areas (22,23,24).

With the output of physicians from medical schools outpacing the growth of the U.S. population, the population/physician ratio declined from one physician per 840 people in 1960 to one per 513 people in 1980 and to one per 415 people in 1990. From 1960 to 1970, the vast majority of these physicians located in urban areas. However, the supply of physicians increased in both metropolitan statistical areas (MSAs) and non-MSAs after 1970. Among the total population living in both MSAs and in non-MSAs, there was a 28 percent decrease in the population/physician ratio during the period 1970–1983. Thus, there was some evidence in favor of the market "diffusion" theory that argued that an abundance of physicians in urban areas would cause movement in these crowded areas to less densely populated rural areas provided that demand for medical services was present (25).

Policy makers have traditionally assumed that physicians, particularly specialists, would not locate in nonurban areas. But these views have been challenged by research that concluded that economic or market forces have caused some change in the distribution of those specialists who are certified by one of 23 specialty boards—i.e., med-

TABLE 10-5. Number of Active Physicians (MDS): And Percentage Distribution by Specialty Groups: Selected Years 1970, 1975, 1980, 1986, 2000

Specialty	1970		1975		1980		1986		2000[b]	
	Number	Percent	Number	Percent	Number	Percent	Number	Percent	Number	Percent
All Specialties	310,845	100.0	340,280	100.0	414,916	100.0	521,780	100.0	681,880	100.0
Primary care specialties[a]	117,761	37.9	130,634	38.4	159,922	38.5	182,110	34.9	223,920	32.8
Other medical specialties	17,401	5.6	19,010	5.6	25,882	6.2	60,700	11.6	99,170	14.5
Surgical specialties	86,042	27.7	96,015	28.2	110,778	26.7	134,440	25.8	165,550	24.3
All other specialties	89,641	28.8	94,621	27.8	118,334	28.5	144,530	27.7	193,240	28.3

[a]Includes general practice, family practice, general internal medicine, and general pediatrics.
[b]Projected.

SOURCES: *Fifth report to the President and Congress on the status of health personnel in the United States.* (DHHS Publication No. [HRS]-P-OD-86-1). (1986, March). Washington, DC: U.S. Government Printing Office; *Seventh report to the President and Congress on the status of health personnel in the United States.* (DHHS Publication No. [HRS]-P-OD-90-1). (1990, March). Washington, DC: U.S. Government Printing Office.

ical societies that confirm via a number of procedures that a physician is especially qualified to engage in his or her specialty (26). By the late 1970s, locales with populations of more than 20,000 often had at least one board-certified physician in each of a variety of specialties. But, communities with populations of fewer than 20,000 were not as likely to have physicians such as these, and in view of the propensity of board-certified physicians to move to non-MSA areas in which regional centers exist with a preexisting group of specialists (27), counties with smaller populations still have difficulty in attracting physicians of any kind, be they board-certified or not. Rural counties with the smallest populations have gained few new physicians during this period, and in some states, the number of counties without a primary care physician has actually increased (28).

The impact of specialization on the geographic distribution of physicians is not surprising. Until recently, general practitioners were the majority of physicians in rural areas. The supply of general practitioners has since almost disappeared, to be replaced in the late 1970s and 1980s by recently trained family practitioners and other specialists. Graduates of family practice residency programs have located in non-MSA areas more frequently than have other specialists, with, for example, 27 percent of family practice residents who graduated in 1991 locating in towns of 25,000 people or fewer that are not within 25 miles of a large city. When one adds those graduating family practice residents in the same size towns but within 25 miles of a large city, the proportion jumps to 42 percent (29). Family practitioners appear to have become the new core of rural physician supply, particularly in smaller towns.

Physicians have been reluctant to locate in rural areas for such reasons as lack of adequate medical facilities; professional isolation; limited support services; inadequate organizational settings, including lack of group practices; excessive workloads and time demands; limits on earnings; lack of social, cultural, and educational influence; and spouse's influence (30). Efforts to improve the distribution

of physicians have tried to address some of these factors.

Federal efforts to improve the distribution of physicians have included loan forgiveness, the National Health Service Corps, Area Health Education Centers, and extensive support for the development of family practice training programs (31,32). However, these programs were largely dismantled during the Reagan administration's attempt to stem the rise of health care costs.

Other efforts to improve physician distribution include the attempts of Offices of Rural Health in states like North Carolina, North Dakota, and Nevada to increase the recruitment and retention of health care providers in rural areas, and cooperative ventures of consortia of states to decentralize medical education programs and coordinate the placement of graduates (30). Examples of cooperative programs include the WAMI program (Washington, Alaska, Montana, and Idaho) and WICHE (Western Interstate Commission for Higher Education). In addition, the development of rural hospital consortia and networks of cooperatives has had a positive impact on improving physician distribution. Examples include the Northern Lakes Health Care Consortium and the Wisconsin Rural Health Care Cooperative.

Despite the variety of approaches used to alter the urban/rural location of physicians, unequal distribution persists. Market forces have altered to varying degrees the distribution of physicians, but many rural communities still find it difficult to recruit and retain physicians. The same is true for many inner-city locations. Often those locales with the greatest need continue to have the biggest problems attracting physicians.

Developing policies to alter physician distribution has turned out to be a difficult undertaking. The task requires not only knowledge of which areas are underserved, but also an explanation of why this is so and the amount and type of resources needed to address equalizing the distribution (33). The limited impact of previous attempts suggests that broader policy options should be considered. The possibilities include changing reimbursement systems to provide a financial reward for physicians practicing in underserved areas. The 1992 adoption by the U.S. Department of Health and Human Services of a resource-based relative value system (RBRVS) for physician services to Medicare patients may be a step in this direction. RBRVS will reimburse physicians in so-called cognitive specialties—e.g., internal medicine and family practice—at a higher rate than they have been historically and will reimburse physicians in procedural specialties—e.g., surgical specialties—at lower than historical rates. A possible effect of this system is that more physicians may choose to practice in the former group of specialties and that more of them may practice in underserved areas since the majority of physicians in such areas are in primary care specialties like family medicine. This is an open question at this time, however.

Another remedy might be to modify medical school admissions to place emphasis on applicants interested in primary care practice, or to change the undergraduate and graduate medical education systems to ensure that the curriculum, counseling, clinical setting, and role models presented are better related to health needs of the underserved.

Physician maldistribution persists in the United States despite the much larger numbers of physicians who have been educated over the last two decades. Inefficient and ineffectual policies that continue to produce excesses of specialists in return for a diminishing proportion of primary care physicians need to be examined. With the distinct possibility that the surpluses of recent times may turn out to be smaller than predicted or even nonexistent in some cases, this issue should increase in importance over the next decade. Future policies that influence the training and reimbursement of physicians should be compatible with goals for improved physician distribution.

Changes in Medical Education

The past 20-year period has been one of change for both undergraduate and graduate medical ed-

ucation. The stereotype of the typical medical student—a white urban male who will eventually practice a medical or surgical specialty in a large urban setting—has changed.

On the undergraduate level, from 1970–1971 to the current time, the first-year medical school class size increased by more than 48 percent, with the 1990–1991 entering class totaling 16,803. First-year enrollments have hovered in the 17,000 range throughout the 1980s and into the 1990s (34). Compared to the early 1970s figures, there is no question that U.S. medical schools responded to the call—enabled by massive federal and state funding of medical education—to increase the supply of physicians. But, with the concern that the nation may have trained too many physicians, the number of undergraduate medical students has leveled off, as noted earlier.

The undergraduate medical curriculum remains broad-based, with the first two years consisting of lectures and laboratory work in the basic sciences, followed by two years of work in the clinical sciences through seminars and work in hospital wards and clinics. The role models and values in most medical schools continue to emphasize acute care for hospitalized patients (34). However, the recent increase in ambulatory and noninstitutional services due to hospital cost containment pressures could lead to the development of medical role models outside the hospital. The professional socialization of the medical student shows signs of changing, with increased emphasis on preceptorships in primary care settings and shifts in the focus of a growing number of medical school faculty from research to the provision of patient care. The latter has occurred due to recent changes in the distribution of medical school funding that have resulted in a deemphasis of federal support and greater reliance on state and local support as well as revenues from faculty practice plans (8).

Another important issue affecting the system of medical education has been the number of women and minority students in medical schools. Concerted efforts to increase their enrollment have borne fruit: over the past 20-year period, the first-

TABLE 10-6. Students in Allopathic Medical Schools, by Gender: Selected Academic Years 1970–1971, 1980–1981, and 1990–1991

Academic Year	All First-Year Students	Female Students	Percent Female of First-Year Students	Total Students Enrolled	Total Female Students	Percent Female of Total Students
1970–1971	11,348	1,256	11.1	40,487	3,894	9.6
1980–1981	17,204	4,970	28.9	65,497	17,373	26.5
1990–1991	16,803	6,499	38.7	64,986	24,164	37.2

SOURCES: Crowley, A., Etzel, S., Petersen, E., et al. (1985). Undergraduate medical education. *Journal of the American Medical Association. 254.* 1565–1572; Jonas, H., Etzel, S., & Barzansky, B. (1991). Educational programs in U.S. medical schools. *Journal of the American Medical Association. 226.* 913–923.

year enrollment has increased from 11 to 38 percent for female first-year medical students; total female enrollment increased from 10 to 37 percent (table 10-6). A more modest, but still significant, increase in minority students has been registered: from 1970–71 to 1988–89, the percentage of minority students in allopathic medical schools increased from about 9 percent to nearly 26 percent of all first-year students (table 10-7). The greatest increase in minority students has been among Asian Americans, Hispanic Americans, Native Americans, and African Americans, in that order. For example, although African Americans increased their numbers by 74 percent over the nearly two-decade period just noted, Asian Americans increased over tenfold.

The graduate medical education "pipeline" has also undergone major changes in the past two decades. The total number of residency positions increased significantly, from 65,615 in 1971 to 89,566 in 1991 (35,36). The percentage of positions filled had increased until 1985 when only 1,696 posts, or 2 percent of the total, remained vacant. Since 1986, however, there has been a steadily increasing percentage of unfilled posts (to 5 percent in 1989), a somewhat unexpected phenomenon. And, as noted earlier, the proportion of FMGs in residency slots has reversed itself and is now on the rise again. Between 1986 and 1990, the percentage of FMGs in U.S. residency positions increased from 16 percent to 18 percent.

Graduate medical education specialty distributions changed during the 1970s in favor of primary care specialties, so that by 1980 nearly 45 percent of all residents were in the primary care specialties of family practice, internal medicine, and pediatrics. However, a serious erosion of the primary care movement has occurred, with a decline to 38 percent of all residents in these primary care specialties in 1990 (36). Thus, the stabilization of primary care training in the mid–1970s and the demise of federal and state policies to stimulate further growth have led to actual declines, and the negative impact has been greater than what some had predicted (37).

In summary, undergraduate and graduate medical education has changed in the past 20 years. Even under the shock of the feared surplus of physicians, some of the recommendations of the final report of the GMENAC, such as a decrease in the size of medical school classes by 10 percent by 1984, were largely ignored. In 1987, for example, 19 medical schools had reduced their first-year classes by five or more students, with an average reduction of only 8.2 (38). Other recommendations, such as no longer using capitation payments to influence specialty choice, were effected. The decline in interest among U.S. college graduates in medical careers cannot be denied, and the shrinking availability of federal grants and loans probably contributed to this indifference. There remain imbalances across specialties and geo-

TABLE 10-7. Minority Students in the First Year of Allopathic Medical School: Selected Academic Years 1970–71 through 1988–89

Academic Year	All First-Year Students	Racial/Ethnic Category						Percent Minority of First Year Students
		African American	Native American	Hispanic American	Asian American	Other Minority[a]	Total Minority	
1970–1971	11,348	697	11	100	190	—	998	8.8
1975–1976	15,295	1,036	60	461	282	73	1,912	12.5
1980–1981	17,186	1,128	67	818	572	—	2,585	15.0
1985–1986	16,929	1,030	61	953	1,164	—	3,208	18.9
1988–1989	16,868	1,210	76	949	2,100	—	4,335	25.7

[a]Data were not provided for the category "Other Minority" for certain years. Where data were provided, they include a number of persons now counted under "Hispanic American."

SOURCE: *Minorities & women in the health fields, 1990 edition* (DHHS Publication No. [HRSA]-P-DV 90-3). (1990). Washington, DC: U.S. Government Printing Office.

graphic locations, with rural areas hit particularly hard. And, oddly, there is a renewal of concern that the physician surplus predicted a decade ago has not materialized to the degree thought. Federal and state decision makers must continue their efforts to develop effective policies that influence physician training despite these changing trends.

Osteopathy

Often neglected in discussions of medical personnel is the small but significant number of osteopaths in the United States. Osteopathy differs from allopathic medicine in that osteopaths traditionally emphasize treatments that involve corrections of the position of the joints or tissues and they stress diet or environment as factors that might destroy natural resistance. Allopathic medicine views the physician as an active interventionist attempting to neutralize effects of a disease by using treatments that produce a counteracting effect. Despite this difference, osteopaths are licensed to practice medicine and perform surgery in all states, are eligible for graduate medical education in either osteopathic or allopathic residencies, and are reimbursed by both Medicare and Medicaid, the two major federal financing programs.

The growth in osteopaths has been great, but this is partially due to the small base number to begin with; in 1970, there were 12,000 osteopaths; in 1990, there were an estimated 27,750, an increase of 131 percent. The ratio of osteopaths to population was 11 per 100,000 in 1990 (table 10-2). However, this figure is deceptive because osteopaths are extremely unevenly distributed around the country. Four of five osteopaths were located in just 16 states, led by Michigan, Pennsylvania, Ohio, Florida, Texas, and New Jersey, in descending order. Hence, in states like these, osteopaths make a contribution to health care disproportionate to their overall numbers. Finally, although there were only five doctors of osteopathy per 100,000 population in metropolitan areas in 1986, the rate in rural areas was six times as great or 30 per 100,000 in nonmetropolitan areas (23). This is, of

course, the opposite of allopathic physicians, whose ratio is larger in metropolitan than nonmetropolitan areas.

There are 15 schools of osteopathy and they are located, not surprisingly, in the states with the largest number of osteopaths. From 1975 to 1985, there was an increase in first-year class size of about two-thirds, but like allopathic first-year classes, there has been a slight decline since then (table 10-8). There has been an increasing proportion of first-year female students—14 percent in 1975 to 29 percent in 1987—as well as an increase in minority first-year students—5 percent to 13 percent over the same period. In 1987, there were actually more osteopaths in allopathic residency programs than in osteopathic programs (2,025 v. 1,292, respectively), underlining the narrow difference between osteopaths and allopathic physicians (39). Nearly 40 percent of osteopaths train in the primary care specialties of general internal medicine and general practice, which, combined with their concentration in specific states and regions, underscores their importance to health care delivery of primary care medicine.

In short, osteopathic medicine is a small but important form of health care delivery that shares the burden of medical care with allopathic physicians. It has experienced the same changes—e.g., increasing proportion of women and minorities, decreasing applicant pool, as its larger cousin has undergone.

Dentistry: A Profession in Transition

By 1988, there were approximately 146,800 active dentists practicing in the United States. Although the supply of dentists has been increasing during the past decade, the ratio of active dentists to population fluctuated from a high of 51.5 per 100,000 population in 1950 to a low of 49.4 per 100,000 population in 1960, and remained level until 1975, when it barely surpassed the 1950 level with 51.6 per 100,000. Since then, the ratio has climbed to 59.4 dentists per 100,000 population in 1988 (table 10-9). As in medicine, the increases

TABLE 10-8. First-Year Students by Gender and Minority Status, Graduates of Osteopathic Medical Schools, Selected Academic Years, 1975–1976, 1980–1981, 1985–1986, and 1987–1988

Academic Year	First-Year Students Enrolled	First-Year Female Students	Percent Female of First-Year Students	First-Year Minority Students[a]	Percent Minority of First-Year Students	Total Number of Graduates
1975–1976	1,038	140	13.5	55	5.3	809
1980–1981	1,496	329	22.0	99	6.6	1,151
1985–1986	1,737	489	28.2	185	10.7	1,560
1987–1988	1,692	490	29.0	213	12.6	1,564

SOURCE: *Minorities & women in the health fields, 1990 edition* (DHHS Publication No. [HRSA]-P-DV 90-3). (1990). Washington, DC: U.S. Government Printing Office.

[a] Includes African, Hispanic, Native, and Asian Americans.

that occurred can be attributed to federal legislation passed in the early 1960s and early 1970s that directly attempted to remedy the perceived shortage. This legislation resulted in increases in the number of dental schools from 47 to 60 in the period 1960 to 1980 and an increase in the number of first-year dental students from 3,600 to more than 6,000 in the same period (table 10-10). However, since 1980, the total number of dental students and the first-year class has continued to drop, so much so that the number of first-year dental students is now below the number enrolled in 1970. The 1980 to 1988 decline in first-year class size was 31 percent.

Some of the recent trends that are descriptive of medical schools are also descriptive of dental schools. The percentage of female first-year students has soared from a low of 2 percent in 1970 to 33 percent in 1988 (table 10-10). The proportion of minority first-year dental school students has also increased dramatically: from 3 percent in 1970 to 26 percent in 1988. Dental schools have started to deemphasize their support from federal sources and have increased their state support, dental clinic revenues, and fees from tuition. Also as with medicine, there has been a sizable decrease in the number of applicants to dental schools, although the decline has been steeper for dentistry. Since 1975, when dental school applications peaked at 15,734, there has been a steady decline—in

1988, only 5,017 people applied, less than one-third the 1975 number (39). The declining applications, smaller class sizes, and increased costs have forced at least three dental schools to announce their closing during the early 1980s.

Unlike their physician counterparts, dentists typically work in solo private general dental practices. However, the current economic pressures on the dental profession have initiated changes in the delivery of dental services. During the 1980s, a variety of nontraditional practice settings have emerged for dentists, including HMOs and retail locations in malls, stores, and plazas. Although only a small proportion of dental services is currently provided in these settings, this innovation is an indication of the more competitive environment in denistry in the 1980s and early 1990s.

The vast majority of dentists are in general practice. Only about one-seventh of all dentists are specialists, and the proportion of specialists has remained relatively stable throughout the 1980s. Orthodontists comprise one-third of all dental specialists, with oral surgeons totaling almost another one-fourth of the specialist population (table 10-11).

There is significant variation in the distribution of dentists across regions of the United States and metropolitan vs. nonmetropolitan areas. This variation is caused by the same factors that have led to physician maldistribution, as well as by the lack

TABLE 10-9. Total and Active Dentists and Dentist/Population Ratios: Selected Years, 1950 through 1988

Year	Number of Dentists[a]		Total Population (Thousands)	Dentists per 100,000 Population		Active Civilian Dentists[b]	Civilian Population (Thousands)	Active Civilian Dentists per 100,000 Civilian Population
	Total	Active		Total	Active			
1950	89,730	79,190	153,622	58.4	51.5	75,310	151,238	49.8
1960	105,200	90,120	182,287	57.7	49.4	84,500	179,742	47.0
1970	116,250	102,220	206,466	56.3	49.5	95,680	203,499	47.0
1975	126,590	112,020	217,095	58.3	51.6	106,740	214,957	49.7
1980	147,280	126,240	228,831	61.7	55.2	121,240	226,715	53.5
1988	na	146,800	247,284	na	59.4	142,200	245,172	58.0

[a]Includes dentists in federal service.
[b]Dentists in the Veterans Administration and U.S. Public Health Service are counted as civilian dentists.

SOURCES: *Fourth report to the President and Congress on the status of health personnel in the United States* (DHHS Publication No. [HRS]-P-0084.4). (1984, May). Washington, DC: U.S. Government Printing Office; *Seventh report to the President and Congress on the status of health personnel in the United States* (DHHS Publication No. [HRS]-P-OD-90-1). (1990, March). Washington, DC: U.S. Government Printing Office.

TABLE 10-10. Number of Dental Schools, Students, and Graduates: Selected Academic Years 1960–1961 through 1990–1991

| Academic Year | Number of Schools | Number of Students[b] | | First-Year Female Students | Percent Female of First-Year Students | Total Minority Students[a] | Percent Minority of Total Students | Total Number of Graduates[b] |
		Total	First Year					
1960–1961	47	13,580	3,616	—	—	—	—	3,290
1970–1971	53	16,553	4,565	94	2.1	552[c]	3.3	3,775
1980–1981	60	22,842	6,030	1,194	19.8	2,453	10.7	5,550
1988–1989	—	17,094	4,148	1,368	33.0	4,411	25.8	4,519

[a]Includes African, Hispanic, Native, Asian Americans, and, for 1970, "Other Minorities."
[b]Excludes graduates of the University of Puerto Rico.
[c]Estimated minority enrollment.

SOURCE: *Minorities and women in the health fields, 1990 edition* (DHHS Publication No. [HRSA]-P-DV 90-3). (1990). Washington, DC: U.S. Government Printing Office.

of reciprocity in the licensing of dentists across states. More than half of all dentists practice in the state in which they were trained, yet 18 states have no school of dentistry (12). The northeastern and western portions of the country have the highest dentist/population ratios, and the south, with its larger rural areas, has the lowest ratio (table 10-12). In 1980, metropolitan areas had 60 dentists per 100,000 population compared to 37 per 100,000 in nonmetropolitan areas. These figures do not reveal the even larger supply of dentists practicing in the biggest metropolitan areas and nonmetropolitan areas with large cities. Thus, the smallest, poorest rural communities continue to have the greatest undersupply of dentists and probably the greatest need. For example, in 1987, there were 758 federally designated dental shortage areas approximately three-quarters of which were in nonmetropolitan areas (39). The likelihood of improving this situation in the near future is not good, as previous efforts to broaden the distribution of dentists have generally been ineffective (30).

Auxiliary Personnel

The practice of dentistry has undergone major technological and organizational changes in the past several decades. Of particular importance has been the increased use of dental auxiliary personnel. The three major types of dental auxiliaries are dental hygienists, dental assistants, and dental laboratory technicians. Dental hygienists provide oral prophylaxis services and dental health education and comprise the only group of dental auxiliaries that is licensed. Dental assistants have generally supported the dentist at chairside and have had the opportunity in some states to perform expanded functions under the dentist's supervision. Dental laboratory technicians make oral appliances following the written prescription of a dentist. In 1988, there were an estimated 70,000 full- and part-time active dental hygienists, 197,000 dental assistants, and 67,00 dental laboratory technicians (39).

TABLE 10-11. Number of Active Dental Specialists by Specialty: 1986

Type of Specialist	All Dental Specialists	
	Number[a]	Percent Distribution
Orthodontists	7,150	33.6
Oral Surgeons	4,730	22.2
Periodontists	3,030	14.2
Pedodontists	2,600	12.2
Endodontists	1,900	8.9
Prosthodontists	1,560	7.3
Public Health Dentists	170	0.8
Oral Pathologists	160	0.8
Total All Specialists	21,300	100.0

[a] Includes dentists in federal service.

SOURCE: Sixth report to the President and Congress on the status of health personnel in the United States (DHHS Publication No. [HRS]-P-OD-88-1). (1988, June). Washington, DC: U.S. Government Printing Office.

In 1988, nearly all dentists employed some dental auxiliary personnel on a full- or part-time basis, and over one-half employed at least one dental hygienist (39). The government has supported the training of expanded-function dental auxiliaries (dental hygienists or dental assistants who receive additional education and training that enables them to perform a broader array of clinical functions), as well as the training of dental students to help improve their administrative and organizational skills in managing multiple auxiliary team practices (40). Support for the auxiliary concept has been due largely to an increase in the productivity of dental practices that employ auxiliaries.

The dental profession is in transition. There has been a relative increase in the supply of dental services in recent years, resulting in a potential surplus of dentists in the future, but there has also been a significant decrease in dental school enrollments, which will counteract any surplus. The role of the expanded-function dental auxiliary is still unclear, given this potential surplus, and much depends on the state of the economy. The demand for dental care is very sensitive to economic con-

TABLE 10-12. Dentist/Population Ratios According to Geographic Region, United States, 1970, 1980, 1986

Geographic Area	1970 Number of Active Civilian Dentists per 100,000 Civilian Population	1980 Number of Active Civilian Dentists per 100,000 Civilian Population	1986 Number of Active Civilian Dentists per 100,000 Civilian Population
United States	47.0	53.5	57.3
Northeast	58.9	66.2	68.5
New England	51.9	66.1	69.0
Middle Atlantic	61.1	66.2	68.3
North Central	46.3	52.7	59.9
East North Central	45.9	52.4	59.7
West North Central	47.4	53.4	60.5
South	35.3	42.6	46.5
South Atlantic	35.8	45.0	48.2
East South Central	32.6	40.3	47.4
West South Central	36.2	40.2	43.4
West	54.9	59.2	61.2
Mountain	45.5	52.3	55.1
Pacific	57.9	61.7	63.4

SOURCE: *Sixth report to the President and Congress on the status of health personnel in the United States* (DHHS Publication No. [HRS]-P-OD-88-1). (1988, June). Washington, DC: U.S. Government Printing Office.

ditions and can decrease during recessionary periods, despite the significant growth in third-party payment for dental services—in 1986, more than one-third of dental expenditures were paid by dental insurance, covering two-fifths of the population (41). Under ordinary economic circumstances, the projection until the year 2000 is that there will be relatively faster growth in demand for dental services than in the ability of dentists and their auxiliaries to supply these services (39).

Thus, aspects of the dental situation resemble the medical one: a renewal of demand that may outstrip supply at the same time as the number of new entrants into the profession is declining or remaining constant. Substantial gains made in the prevention of dental disease through community water supply fluoridation will tend to reduce the demand for some dental services, while the aging of the population will increase demand for others.

In addition, any further extension of dental insurance will fuel additional demand for services. How these many factors combine to affect the future of dentistry should be watched closely.

Nursing: Shortages and Future Role Changes

The Paradox of Increased Supply But Continued Shortage

Registered nurses are the largest group of licensed health care professionals in the United States. The active supply of registered nurses (RNs) grew more than twofold, from 750,000 in 1970 to 1,627,035 in 1988, an increase that resulted in a change from 366 RNs per 100,000 population to 560 RNs per 100,000 population. The annual number of nursing graduates has increased accordingly: 35,000 in 1966, 74,000 in 1982, and 94,594 in 1987 (39,42).

Table 10-13 presents a profile of the registered nurse supply from a survey in 1980 that was sponsored by the federal Bureau of Health Professions. Where possible the information was updated to 1988. The first important thing to note is that the number of nurses actually in nursing is about 80 percent of all nurses. Put another way, one-fifth of all trained nurses were not employed in nursing in 1988. It can also be seen that most nurses were women, almost seven of ten were married, and only 8 percent were from minority groups. About half of RNs were diploma school graduates, usually from hospital-based programs, and almost one-fourth were baccalaureate or advanced-degree graduates. The shifting educational pattern of RNs, with increased emphasis on a four-year baccalaureate degree and continued significant reductions in diploma school graduates, is discussed in greater detail below.

The percentage of nurses employed in nursing has increased throughout the decade: it was 77 percent in 1980, 79 percent in 1984, and 80 percent in 1988, as already noted. However, despite the overall absolute increase in the number of nurses and the increasing proportion of nurses employed in nursing, there has been and continues to be a shortage of nurses relative to demand (43). Understanding the causes of the imbalance between the supply and demand is not easy. Some have pointed to the large number of inactive nurses—despite the reduction over time in this statistic—as the main reason for the perceived shortage. Although a 20 percent inactive rate may seem high, the labor force participation of nurses is similar to that of women in comparable professions. Personal characteristics and the role of women in society appear to be as important as job characteristics in influencing nurses to work (27). Only 8 percent of unemployed nurses are actively seeking nursing employment; the vast majority of unemployed nurses are over 50 years of age or are married with children at home (44). One job characteristic that appears to influence the nurse employment rate is salary (45). Nurses are not paid well relative to their training and responsibilities, and thus, the nurse shortage has been termed a shortage due to lagging salaries (46).

Approximately one-third of employed nurses work part-time (43), and the majority of these are married with children at home. Although concern has also been focused on nursing attrition due to burnout or poor working conditions, or both, surveys indicate only a small increase in the number of nurses working in other professions (43). Thus, the possible shortage of nurses cannot be attributed to increases in the number of part-time workers or attrition from the profession.

The reason for the perceived shortage of nurses is unclear. The most likely explanation appears to be an increased demand for nursing services from several sectors of the health care system—acute, hospital-based care; long-term care for the growing number of chronically ill people; home health care; and preventive care. Two-thirds of all nurses are estimated to have worked in hospitals in 1990 (39), and that proportion has not decreased since 1985 (47). Thus a proportionate shift away from hospital-based employment to ambulatory care employment has not yet materialized. This may be because patients admitted to hospitals are increasingly sicker and may require more, not less, intensive nursing care. Nevertheless, because of the burgeoning growth in ambulatory care settings, the proportion of nurses in hospitals may eventually decline.

The demand for nursing services should continue to grow, and the federal government's predictions are that requirements for nursing personnel will continue to outstrip the supply well into the next century. This is due not only to the factors already mentioned but also to the trend—beginning in the mid–1980s—of a decline in annual admissions to nursing programs; in 1984, admissions were over 120,000; in 1988, they were well under 100,000. More alarming in this regard are the graduation statistics: in 1985, there were slightly over 80,000 nursing graduates; in 1988, there were about 65,000 (39). This trend is expected to con-

TABLE 10-13. Statistical Profile of Registered Nurses, 1980 and 1988

Characteristics	Total Registered Nurses	Total Employed in Nursing	Total Not Employed in Nursing
Total Number, 1988	2,033,032	1,627,035	405,997
Median Age, 1988	39.0	—	—
Percentage Male, 1988	—	3.3	—
Percentage Minority, 1988	8.3	8.5	—
Percentage Married, 1980	70.8	68.1	79.8
Percentage Married with children at home, 1980	47.5	46.3	51.6
Percentage whose basic nursing education in 1988 was:			
Diploma	48.7	—	—
Associate degree	28.3	—	—
Baccalaureate or higher degree	22.3	—	—
Other	0.7	—	—

SOURCES: Levine, E., & Moses, E. (1982, p. 480). Registered nurses today: A statistical profile. In L. Aiken (Ed.). *Nursing in the 1980's: Crises, opportunities, challenges.* Philadelphia: Lippincott; *Seventh report to the President and Congress on the status of health personnel in the United States* (DHHS Publication No. [HRS]-P-OD-90-1). (1990, March). Washington, DC: U.S. Government Printing Office; *Minorities & women in the health fields, 1990 edition* (DHHS Publication No. [HRSA]-p-dv 90-3). (1990). Washington, DC: U.S. Government Printing Office.

tinue (48). Like other health professional groups, during the 1980s, there has been a somewhat unexpected diminution of interest and decline in enrollment in training programs. To move toward a balance between supply and demand, institutional and other employers must become more sensitive to the special needs of working women.

Like many other health care professionals, nurses are not distributed evenly throughout the United States. The maldistribution appears to be due to the geographic immobility of women who are married and second wage earners in a family, as well as the inability of rural and inner-city hospitals to offer an adequate range of incentives (e.g., flexible working hours, increased salaries, and fringe benefits) to attract nurses (27).

Rural institutions have found that urban-based education and training programs are often not relevant to rural needs. Rural hospitals must frequently hire recent nursing graduates with limited skills and often resort to depending on pool nurses from temporary employment agencies (27). This problem is of particular concern because of the increased responsibilities and range of skills of rural nurses. In the near future, rural providers are not likely to improve their chances of attracting well-trained nurses with a broad range of skills.

Nursing Education and Role Changes

The federal government provided almost $2.0 billion for nursing education during the period 1965–1985. This support, as well as market forces, helped to increase the number of nursing graduates entering the profession. Table 10-14 shows the more than twofold increase in the number of admissions to RN programs during the period 1960–1980. However, the 1987 information reveals the overall declining admissions picture already mentioned. Despite this decline, of particular interest is the switch that has occurred in the control of nursing education from the hospital to nursing educators in colleges and universities.

Three forms of training lead to licensure as an RN: three-year diploma programs that are hospital-based, two-year associate degree programs that are generally community college-based, and four-year baccalaureate nursing programs in universi-

TABLE 10-14. Admissions to Schools Offering Initial Programs in Registered Nursing by Type of Program, 1960–1961, 1970–1971, 1980–1981, and 1987–1988

Academic Year	Baccalaureate[a]	Diploma	Associate Degree	Total
1960–1961	8,674	38,460	2,085	49,219
1970–1971	20,299	28,792	29,433	78,524
1980–1981	35,808	17,494	56,899	110,201
1987–1988	28,732	8,389	57,473	94,594

[a]Includes students in a few generic programs leading to a master's or doctoral degree.

SOURCES: *Fourth report to the President and Congress on the status of health personnel in the United States* (DHHS Publication No. [HRS]-P-0084.4). (1984, May). Washington, DC: U.S. Government Printing Office; *Seventh report to the President and Congress on the status of health personnel in the United States* (DHHS Publication No. [HRS]-P-OD-90-1). (1990, March). Washington, DC: U.S. Government Printing Office.

ties or four-year colleges. As table 10-15 indicates, in 1987, only 9 percent of new nursing students were enrolled in diploma programs; in 1960 78 percent were.

The nursing profession is attempting to change its role in the health care system. The leaders of the profession have called for an expansion of the independent role of the nurse within the hospital and the creation of new professional roles outside the hospital. Nurses are seeking to clarify their relationship to physicians, particularly within the context of clinical decision making in the hospital (45). They have developed new delivery modes, such as primary nursing, in which the nurse assumes direct responsibility for comprehensive care for a group of patients over a given time period.

A variety of new roles has emerged for the RN. Included are such positions as clinical nurse specialist, nurse practitioner, nurse anesthetist, and nurse clinician. These positions involve employment in new ambulatory care settings (e.g., HMOs, ambulatory surgery centers), nursing homes, and home care programs providing care for the elderly and others with chronic illness, as well as positions in hospitals. Nurses are also finding significant opportunities in statewide, regional, and hospital-level utilization and quality review roles in which they participate in close inspection of clinical records describing patient care.

Nursing professionals want to control their future. They are trying to shed the traditional stereotype of the nurse as an underpaid female hospital laborer. In the process, considerable controversy has been created both inside and outside the profession. This is often most visible when labor collective bargaining groups attempt to unionize nurses, forcing to the surface the ambivalence many nurses feel between being a highly skilled professional delivering personalized services versus an underpaid employee in a bureaucratic health care organization. Associate degree and diploma graduates want to continue to function in viable roles within the nursing profession. Institutions want to employ combinations of nursing personnel suitable for their particular environments. These forces, as well as the current restrictive interpretation of state nurse practice acts, suggest that there will be no easy solutions to changing and, one hopes strengthening the future relationships among nurses, physicians, and health care institutions.

Pharmacists

As is the case for all of the health professional groups discussed, pharmacists are also undergoing extensive change. Until recently, pharmacists performed the traditional role of preparing drug products and filling prescriptions. In the 1980s and

TABLE 10-15. Number of Active Pharmacists and Number of Pharmacy Students, by Gender and Minority Status, Selected Years 1970, 1980, 1988

Academic Year	Total Active Pharmacists	First-Year Students[a]	First-Year Female Students[a]	Percent Female of First-Year Students[a]	First-Year Minority Students[a]	Percent Minority of First-Year Students[a]
1970	112,600	5,694	1,349	23.7	na	na
1980	142,400	7,551	3,655	48.4	891	11.8
1988	157,800	7,867	4,655	59.2	1,361	17.3

[a]Includes students in the first year of the three years of pharmacy education, excluding any students in prepharmacy years.

SOURCES: *Seventh report to the President and Congress on the status of health personnel in the United States* (DHHS Publication No. [HRS]-P-OD-90-1). (1990, March). Washington, DC: U.S. Government Printing Office; *Minorities and women in the health field, 1990 edition* (DHHS Publication No. [HRSA]-p-dv-90-3). (1990). Washington, DC: U.S. Government Printing Office.

1990s, the pharmacist has expanded that role to include drug product education and acting as an expert for clients and patients about the effects of specific drugs, drug interaction, and generic drug substitutions for brand-name drugs. The role has even expanded to include selecting, monitoring, and evaluating appropriate drug regimens and providing information not only to the patient but also to other health care professionals. Finally, in their roles as businesspeople, pharmacists have had to learn more about the managerial and financial aspects of working in a retail trade.

There has been steady growth in the number of pharmacists in the United States during the last quarter-century, although the percentage growth has not been as great as in other health care professions (table 10-15). From 1970 to 1988, there was a 40 percent increase in the overall numbers. First-year enrollment in pharmacy schools leveled off during the 1980s, although there was a major increase in the proportion of female first-year students, from about 24 percent in 1970 to about 59 percent in 1988. The growth of minorities in pharmacy, although not as great, has been steady, increasing from about 12 percent in 1980 to 17 percent in 1988. Another phenomenon of note is the popularity of doctorate in pharmacy programs, which lead not only to research and teaching positions but also to levels of higher administrative responsibility, often in health care organizations.

Pharmacists are employed in a number of settings, but the growth of chain drugstores has been notable. In 1988, about 40 percent of all pharmacists were employed by chains. From 1979 to 1987 the proportion of new pharmacy graduates hired by chains rose from 27 percent to 42 percent (39). The remainder of the 1987 graduates worked in hospitals (22 percent) and independent pharmacies (18 percent), with the rest divided among manufacturers, government, graduate studies, and other areas.

Making projections about the future supply of pharmacists in relation to future need or demand is difficult because of rapidly changing employment circumstances in the field. Further, the aging of the American population would suggest that more medication prescriptions will be written and more work for pharmacists will result. At the same time, because pharmacists are expanding their role to include nontraditional activities, as mentioned, the amount of time an individual pharmacist might spend in traditional "druggist" activities will decline. However, with computerized information processing systems, assistance from pharmacy technicians, and mail order approaches that pharmacists will be using in increasing numbers, one would expect a positive gain in productivity. In short, a number of factors make predicting the future balance of supply and demand difficult, and given the importance of drug therapies for modern medical care, policy makers should watch this important health profession closely.

Physician Assistants (PAs) and Nurse Practitioners (NPs)

The perceived shortage of physicians in the mid–1960s led to the development of two new types of health care providers—PAs and NPs. About 30 years ago, the first PA training program was established at Duke University; the initial NP program was started at the University of Colorado.

PAs are qualified by academic and practical training to provide patient services under the direction and supervision of a licensed physician who is responsible for the performance of the PA (49). PAs are able to diagnose, manage, and treat common illness; provide preventive services; and respond appropriately to common emergency situations. The typical PA training program consists of two years of didactic study followed by clinical training. However, programs vary widely in terms of admission requirements, curriculum, and site of educational training. There were 51 accredited PA programs in 1989 (39). In 1988, about 55 percent of PAs were in primary care specialties, and the remaining 45 percent were in nonprimary care specialties such as surgery, psychiatry, and emergency and industrial medicine. In 1989, there were an estimated 20,000 PAs in the United States, with programs graduating about 1,200 new PAs a year.

NPs are registered nurses who have completed formal programs of study preparing them for expanded roles and responsibilities (50). These expanded roles include obtaining comprehensive health histories, assessing health status, performing physical examinations, formulating and managing a care regimen for acute and chronically ill patients, teaching, and counseling (51). There are a range of training programs for NPs, including pediatric, nurse-midwife, family, adult, psychiatric,

and geriatric programs. Slightly more than half of the more than 200 NP training programs are certificate programs that generally last for eight to 12 months; the remainder are master's programs lasting from one to two years. GMENAC has estimated that approximately 16,000 NPs had graduated by 1980, and that around 2,000 new NPs were expected to graduate each year after that (50).

About 32 percent of PAs work in hospitals, another 31 percent in physicians' offices, and 12 percent in HMOs (39). The remainder are employed in clinics, health centers, correctional institutions, and the like. In the mid–1980s, almost one-third of PAs were working in rural or small towns with fewer than 25,000 inhabitants (39). NPs have been more likely than PAs to locate in urban areas, but research suggests that the structure and location of NP training programs affects the geographic distributions of NPs and PAs (50).

There are important differences in the perceptions of the roles of PAs and NPs (52). PAs are viewed by the medical profession as physician "extenders" who can perform many of the usual functions completed by physicians. Nurses view NPs as registered nurses in an expanded role. The expanded role includes greater supervision of and responsibility for primary patient care, with extra emphasis on the traditional nursing values of prevention and counseling. Despite these perceptual differences, as well as differences in education and training, many of the performance characteristics of PAs and NPs appear to be similar.

Issues in PA and NP Use

Among the issues that need to be resolved before PAs and NPs can be used fully are legal restrictions concerning practice, reimbursement policies, and relationships with physicians. The legal status of PAs and NPs is uncertain and varies considerably across states. Some states permit considerable delegation of tasks and responsibilities to the PA, including prescribing drugs when a physician countersigns within 24 hours. State legislation expanding medical delegation has been unduly restrictive with respect to the scope of practice of qualified nonphysicians (53).

Laws and regulations governing the expanded role of the nurse are changing rapidly but inconsistently. Although the majority of states have altered their nurse practice acts to facilitate expanded roles, the constraints on the scope of NP practice vary from state to state. The restrictions appear to be fewer for NPs than for PAs, but changes in legal authority must take place before NPs will be able to practice independently. The nonphysician health care provider technical panel of GMENAC had recommended that state laws and regulations should not require physician supervision of NPs and PAs beyond that needed to assure quality of care (50).

Third-party reimbursement imposes another constraint on the use of PAs and NPs. Current policies generally link their reimbursement directly to the employing physician or institution. Most insurers do not recognize PAs and NPs as legitimate providers of medical care. Private fee-for-service physician practices or other ambulatory settings have had difficulties in securing reimbursement for nonphysician services. Reimbursement problems may be even greater than legal restrictions. Some significant progress has been made in certain ways, however. For example, if a hospital or clinic is located in a federally designated "health manpower shortage area" or a "medically underserved area," NPs and PAs can be employed, within the constraints of state law, and the hospital can be reimbursed by Medicare under a more liberal cost-based scheme, as opposed to the prospective payment system (PPS). Although by 1988 many rural hospitals had not taken advantage of this—because of the third problem discussed below—clinics located in rural areas have responded to this economic incentive and have employed NPs and PAs (54). This new reimbursement policy is very promising and should help mid-level health professionals gain an important role in patient care.

The third area of concern is current and future PA and NP relationships with physicians. In the

past, physicians were reasonably accepting of these personnel (55). Yet, about the time these mid-level practitioners were becoming popular among those seeking a lower-cost substitute for physician services, the physician surplus was discovered, and physicians were wary of employing personnel who might take away their work. Further, there was, as noted earlier in this chapter, a tendency for some physicians to move into previously medically underserved areas. Despite certain recommendations by GMENAC in favor of NPs and PAs, there were also recommendations calling for more research on these personnel and for a stabilization, not an increase, in the numbers in training (5).

Now that there is a growing concern that the surplus GMENAC predicted may have been overstated, the future of NPs and PAs is uncertain. There are still many roles that these personnel can fill: providing primary care to underserved areas and populations, like the elderly and the mentally ill, providing preventive care, and providing specialty services in hospitals in lieu of house staff. New practice settings for NPs and PAs include schools, industrial settings, prisons, nursing homes, HMOs, and managed care settings generally. If the physician surplus actually does begin to disappear, then the original impetus for these mid-level practitioners will once again emerge and will complement the above list of employment opportunities. However, there still remain the problems of legal restrictions and reimbursement policies to be resolved before the potential productivity gains and improved access to services can be realized (55).

The Changing Nature of the Health Professionals

This chapter has summarized trends in the supply of health professionals. From the 1960s through the early 1980s, federal and state support resulted in large increases in the number of graduates in most health professional occupations. Simultaneously, women and minorities have greatly benefited from this overall growth. With the disappearance of large federal subsidies for the training of health professionals, the nation has witnessed a decline in the number of applicants, first-year students, total student enrollments, and graduates in most health care fields discussed here. Some declines have been dramatic, as in the cases of nursing and dental education. Other declines have been limited to the number of applicants but not to the number of first-year students, total enrollments, and graduates, as is the case in medicine. But, overall there is strong evidence of a return to the numbers of new health professionals that preceded federal and state governments' generous support of health professional education.

The federal and state investment in health care personnel improved access to health care, and helped schools training in the health professions remain fiscally viable. The reduction of government spending for the health professions has been caused by the reallocation of these funds to other portions of federal and state budgets, and the belief in the existence of a surplus of many types of health professionals added to the logic of reduced spending. Many of the major trends affecting the U.S. health care system, such as restrictive public and private sector reimbursement, growth of alternative delivery systems and managed care, and the general increase of health care costs, portend even further efforts to reduce spending. This will undoubtedly have direct and indirect impact on future employment opportunities available for health professionals (56).

In some instances such as nursing and medicine, the supply of practitioners will increase at a decreasing rate, and in both instances, there is worry that the need for services will outpace the supply. Although this has been a worry for nursing personnel for some time, it is a new concern for medicine, given the enormous publicity of GMENAC's surplus predictions. As noted earlier, increased demand has surprised the experts: total hours that physicians spent in patient care rose 21 percent from 1982 to 1987, whereas physician supply—even though it was increasing faster than population growth—rose by 16 percent (18). Some argue that it is unlikely that future demand for

physician services will be less than the growth in the supply (19). The United States is facing new and renewed dilemmas that were not adequately considered in the late 1970s and early 1980s when perceived surpluses were predicted. The care needed by those with AIDs, the homeless, unemployed, and uninsured, the elderly, and those living in rural areas has added extra burdens to the health care system.

The increasing number of women in all of the health professions also suggests that, on balance, with the rise of single-parent households and the continued disproportionate household and child-rearing responsibilities that married working women bear, women health professionals, particularly physicians, will work fewer weeks per year than men. This adds up to the need for more personnel because overall productivity will be lower. For example, if the proportion of women entering medicine continues at the current pace, the effective full-time-equivalent supply of physician services will decline by about 4 percent between 1986 and 2010, other things being equal (57). On the other hand, the increase in the number of organizational settings, such as HMOs, in which care is delivered increases the overall productivity of health workers and acts to increase the overall full-time-equivalent supply of personnel (58). Such conflicting forces make predicting the balance between need and demand versus supply of health personnel a very difficult enterprise as the lessons of GMENAC demonstrated.

It is still important to develop health care cost containment strategies in concert with health care personnel policies. Given the increasing possibility of personnel shortages within the context of constrained spending, major system changes like competition among health providers and alterations in reimbursement policies can best be implemented if constraints on the flexible use of health personnel are reduced. Alternatives to the existing methods of training, licensing, regulating, and reimbursing health care personnel should be serious considered. It is unlikely that federal and state governments will soon return to the high levels of subsidization of health care professional education we witnessed in the 1960s and 1970s. Therefore, we will need new and creative solutions to health personnel training and deployment, not ones that simply call for expansion in overall numbers. Although there is a high level of uncertainty about what our present and future policies should be, there is also great opportunity to effect positive changes that have been suggested for decades (59).

References

1. Sorkin, A. (1984). *Health economics.* Cambridge, MA: Lexington Books.
2. U.S. Department of Labor. (1977). *Dictionary of occupational titles, fourth edition.* Washington, DC: U.S. Government Printing Office.
3. U.S. Bureau of the Census. (1990). *Statistical abstract of the United States: 1990* (110th ed.). Washington, DC: U.S. Government Printing Office.
4. Blendon, R., & Ginzberg, E. (Eds.). (1985). *Policy choices for the 1990's: An uncertain look into America's future in the U.S. health care system.* Totowa, NJ: Rowman & Allanheld.
5. *Report of the Graduate Medical Education National Advisory Committee to the Secretary, DHHS, Vol. 1; GMENAC summary report* (DHHS Publication No. [HRA] 81-653). (1980). Washington, DC: U.S. Government Printing Office.
6. Mick, S., & Worobey, J. (1984). Foreign medical graduates in the 1980s: Trends in specialization. *American Journal of Public Health. 74.* 698–703.
7. Reinhardt, U. (1975). *Physician productivity and the demand for health manpower.* Cambridge, MA: Ballinger.
8. Jolin, L. D., Jolly, P., Krakower, J. Y., & Beran, R. (1991). US medical school finances. *Journal of the American Medical Association. 226.* 985–990.
9. Hughes, R. G., Barker, D. C., & Reynolds, R. C. (1991). Are we mortgaging the medical profession? *New England Journal of Medicine. 325.* 404–407.
10. Harvey, L. K., & Shubat, S. C. (1990). *Physician opinion on health care issues.* Chicago: American Medical Association.
11. Mick, S. (1975). The foreign medical graduate. *Scientific American. 232.* 14–21.
12. *Third report to the President and the Congress on the status of health professions personnel in the United States* (DHHS Publication No. [HRA] 82-2). (1982). Washington, DC: U.S. Government Printing Office.
13. Mick, S. (1992). *The 1987 career characteristics of foreign and U.S. medical graduates who entered the U.S. medical system between 1969 and 1982.* Report submitted to the Education Commission for Foreign Medical Graduates, Philadelphia, PA.
14. Page, L. (1991, May 13). Dr. Todd condemns unequal licensure policies for FIMGs. *American Medical News.* 2–26.
15. Hanson, W. (1970). An appraisal of physician manpower projections. *Inquiry. 7.* 102–114.
16. Stevens, R. (1975). The muddle over medical manpower. *Prism. 3.* 10–63.
17. Mick, S., & Worobey, J. (1984). Foreign and United States medical graduates in practice: A follow-up. *Medical Care. 22.* 1014–1025.
18. Schwartz, B., & Mendelson, N. (1990). No evidence of an emerging physician surplus: An analysis of change in physician's work load and income. *Journal of the American Medical Association. 263.* 557–560.
19. Schwartz, W. B., Sloan, F. A., & Mendelson, D. N. (1988). Why there will be little or no physician surplus between now and the year 2000. *New England Journal of Medicine. 318.* 892–897.
20. Aiken, L., Lewis, C., et al. (1979). The contribution of specialists to the delivery of primary care. *New England Journal of Medicine. 300.* 1363–1370.
21. Rosenblatt, R., Cherkin, D., & Schneeweiss, R. (1982). The structure and content of family practice: Current status and future trends. *Journal of Family Practice. 15.* 681–723.
22. Fruen, M., & Cantwell, J. (1982). Geographic distribution of physicians: Past trends and future influences. *Inquiry. 19.* 44–50.
23. Hicks, L. (1990). Availability and accessibility of rural health care. *Journal of Rural Health. 6.* 485–505.
24. Kindig, D. A., & Movassaghi, H. (1989). The adequacy of physician supply in small rural communities. *Health Affairs. 8.* 63–76.
25. Newhouse, J. (1990). Geographic access to physician services. *Annual Review of Public Health. 11.* 207–230.
26. Schwartz, W., Newhouse, J., & Bennett, B. (1980).

The changing geographic distribution of board-certified physicians. *New England Journal of Medicine. 303.* 1032–1037.

27. Moscovice, I., & Rosenblatt, R. (1985). A prognosis for the rural hospital part II: Are rural hospitals economically viable? *Journal of Rural Health. 1.* 11–33.

28. Hicks, L. (1984). Social policy implications of physician shortage areas in Missouri. *American Journal of Public Health. 74.* 1316–1321.

29. *Report on survey of 1991 graduating family practice residents.* (1991). Washington, DC: American Academy of Family Physicians.

30. Rosenblatt, R., & Moscovice, I. (1982). *Rural health care.* New York: Wiley.

31. Rosenblatt, R., & Moscovice, I. (1980). The National Health Service Corps: Rapid growth and uncertain future. *Milbank Memorial Fund Quarterly. 58.* 282–309.

32. Gessert, C., & Smith, D. (1981). The national AHEC program: Review of its progress and consideration of the 1980's. *Public Health Reports. 96.* 116–120.

33. Hadley, J. (1979). Alternative methods of evaluating health manpower distribution. *Medical Care. 17.* 1054–1060.

34. *Report of GMENAC to the Secretary, DHHS: Vol. 5: Educational Environmental Technical Panel* (DHHS Publication No. [HRA] 81-655). (1980). Washington, DC: U.S. Government Printing Office.

35. American Medical Association. (1972). Graduate medical education: Annual report on graduate medical education in the United States. *Journal of the American Medical Association. 222.* 991–1016.

36. Rowley, B., Baldwin, D., & McGuire, B. (1991). Selected characteristics of graduate medical education in the United States. *Journal of the American Medical Association. 266.* 922–943.

37. Steinwachs, D., Levine, D., Elzing, J., et al. (1982). Changing patterns of graduate medical education. *New England Journal of Medicine. 306.* 10–14.

38. Clare, F., Spratley, E., Schwab, P., & Iglehart, J. (1987). Trends in health personnel. *Health Affairs. 6.* 90–109.

39. *Seventh report to the President and Congress on the status of health personnel in the United States* (DHHS Publication No. [HRS]-P-OD-91-1). (1990). Washington, DC: U.S. Government Printing Office.

40. Machlin, S. (1981). Dental manpower. In *Health,* *United States, 1981* (DHHS Publication No. [PHS] 82-1232). Washington, DC: U.S. Government Printing Office.

41. Beazoglou, T., Brown, L., & Heffley, D. (1989). *Determinants of dental care expenditures over time.* Paper presented at Eastern Economic Association meeting.

42. *Fourth report to the President and Congress on the status of health personnel in the United States* (DHHS Publication No. [HRS]-P-OD-84-4). (1984). Washington, DC: U.S. Government Printing Office.

43. Levine, E., & Moses, E. (1982). Registered nurses today: A statistical profile. In L. Aiken (Ed.). *Nursing in the 1980's: Crises, opportunities, challenges.* Philadelphia: Lippincott.

44. Moses, E. (1981). *The registered nurse population: An overview* (DHHS Report No. 82-5). Hyattsville, MD: Bureau of Health Professions.

45. Aiken, L. (1982). The impact of federal health policy on nurses. In L. Aiken (Ed.). *Nursing in the 1980's: Crises, opportunities, challenges.* Philadelphia: Lippincott.

46. *The recurrent shortage of registered nurses.* (DHHS Publication No. [HRA] 81-23). (1981). Hyattsville, MD: Bureau of Health Professions.

47. LeRoy, L., & Ellwood, D. (1985). Trends in health manpower. *Health Affairs. 4.* 77–90.

48. Joint Rural Task Force of the National Association of Community Health Centers and the National Rural Health Association. (1989). Health care in rural America: The crisis unfolds. *Journal of Public Health Policy. 10.* 99–116.

49. *Physician assistants: Education, accreditation, and consumer acceptance.* (1975). Chicago: American Medical Association.

50. *Report of GMENAC to the Secretary, DHHS: Vol. 6: Nonphysician Health Care Provider Technical Panel* (DHHS Publication No. [HRA] 81-656). (1980). Washington, DC: U.S. Government Printing Office.

51. Abdellah, F. (1982). The nurse practitioner 17 years later: Present and emerging issues. *Inquiry. 5.* 470–497.

52. Kane, R., & Wilson, W. (1977). The new health practitioner—the past as prologue. *Western Journal of Medicine. 127.* 254–261.

53. Kissam, P. (1975). Physician's assistants and nurse practitioner laws: A study of health law reform. *Kansas Law Review. 24.* 1–65.

54. Mick, S., Morlock, L., Salkever, D., de Lissovoy, G., et al. (1992). *Medical, professional, and other personnel in rural hospitals: Trends from 1983 to 1988*. University of Michigan: Studies in Rural Health Care.

55. Weiner, J. P., Steinwachs, D. M., & Williamson, J. W. (1986). Nurse practitioner and physician assistant practices in three HMOs: Implications for future US health manpower needs. *American Journal of Public Health. 76.* 507–511.

56. Ginzberg, E. (Ed.). (1985). *The U.S. health care system—a look to the 1990's*. Totowa, NJ: Rowman & Allanheld.

57. Kletke, P. R., Marder, W. D., & Silberger, A. B. (1990). The growing proportion of female physicians: Implications for U.S. physician supply. *American Journal of Public Health. 80.* 300–304.

58. Steinwachs, D. M., Weiner, J. P., Shapiro, S., et al. (1986). A comparison of the requirements for primary care physicians in HMOs with projections made by the Graduate Medical Education National Advisory Committee. *New England Journal of Medicine. 314.* 217–222.

59. Mick, S. (1978). Understanding the persistence of human resource problems in health. *Milbank Memorial Fund Quarterly. 56.* 463–499.

PART FIVE

Financial Resources for Health Services

Chapter 11

Financing Health Services

Alma L. Koch

The system for financing health services in the United States reflects the fragmentation of health care as a whole. In view of the large number of Americans who are uninsured or underinsured for health care, one may say that it is not really a system at all; rather, it is a patchwork of loosely connected financing mechanisms varying by provider type and reflective of age, health, and economic status of the specific patient groups that are being served. However, this observation only frustrates the study of the financing apparatus as it now exists. If one looks at the system in light of the role of tradition and the values of the American people, as well as the political philosophy of the times, the organization of health finance in the United States comes into better focus.

This chapter will examine the size and scope of the health care financing system in the United States. Where possible, comparisons will be drawn between the United States and other countries. Special attention will be paid to differences and similarities in the public and private financing components of the system, reimbursement of various provider categories, and trends that we may expect to see by the end of the century. The role of health insurance as a financial conduit will be explored and monetary business objectives will be contrasted with the altruistic goals of health care as a human service.

Health Expenditures

Size of the U.S. Health Care Industry

In dollar volume, the U.S. health care industry is eclipsed only by the U.S. manufacturing sector, ranking third after total durable goods and total nondurable goods. For personal consumption, Americans spend more only on food and housing than they do on medical care. In terms of U.S. general public expenditures, the health care industry ranks third following national defense and education. Furthermore, it is by far the largest service industry in the country (1,2). In 1990, Americans spent $666 billion on health care, comprising 12.2

reasons for the costs ↑

TABLE 11-1. Aggregate and Per Capita National Health Expenditures, United States, Selected Years

Year	Total (Billions)	Per Capita *	GNP (Billions)	Percent of GNP
1940	$ 4.0	$ 30	$ 100	4.0
1950	12.7	82	287	4.4
1960	27.1	147	515	5.3
1970	74.4	346	1,015	7.3
1980	250.1	1,062	2,732	9.2
1990	666.2	2,566	5,465	12.2

SOURCE: Adapted from Sonnefeld, S. T., Waldo, D. R., Lemieux, J. A., & McKusick, D. R. (1991, Fall). Projections of national health expenditures through the year 2000. *Health Care Financing Review. 13*(1). 16.

*Based on July 1 Social Security area population estimates.

percent of the gross national product (GNP) and amounting to $2,566 per capita (3). The United States spends far more on health care than other industrialized democracies. For example, in 1988, the United Kingdom and Japan fell at the lower end of the spectrum, spending 5.9 and 6.7 percent of their respective gross domestic products on health care. Sweden, France, Germany, and Canada came closer to U.S. figures with 9.0, 8.7, 8.6, and 8.5 percent of their respective gross domestic products spent on health, with most other industrialized nations falling in the established range (1).

Growth in Health Expenditures

Since 1940, national health expenditures have grown at a rate substantially outpacing the GNP. Table 11-1 shows that, prior to World War II, only 4 percent of the GNP was devoted to health care, both public and private. By 1990, the proportion of the GNP expended for health care increased by more than eight percentage points. Since the onset of Medicare and Medicaid in mid–1966, national health expenditures have grown particularly rapidly, from about 6.3 percent of the GNP to the present figure. In fact, 1984 was the only year since 1973 where the percentage of GNP devoted to health care actually showed a slight downturn (0.1 percent) from the previous year. Most of this growth is quantitatively explained by economywide infla-

tion, excess medical inflation, increased intensity in the provision of health care services, and other factors. Only a small fraction of growth in health care can be attributed to the growth in the U.S. population (4).

A variety of qualitative factors is believed to have contributed to the disproportionate growth in health care spending relative to the growth in GNP. These include 1) rising expectations about the value of health care services; 2) rapid development and dissemination of medical technology, which expanded the treatment of disease; 3) government financing of health care services; 4) the nature of third-party reimbursement; 5) growth in the proportion of elderly; and 6) lack of competitive forces in the health care system to increase efficiency and productivity in the delivery of services.

Monetary Flow

Payment Sources

Figure 11-1 contrasts the monetary inflow and outflow in the U.S. for total health spending in 1990. Private health insurance finances one-third of all health expenditures; direct patient payment finances another one-fifth. These payment sources, together with other private sources (mostly philanthropy), account for the 58 percent of all health expenditures which is privately financed in the United States. The other 42 percent is financed publicly by federal, state, or local governments. The largest single public program is Medicare (the federal social security health insurance plan for the elderly, disabled, and other groups), followed by Medicaid (the federal/state welfare program for health care) and other government programs (3).

Spending for Medicare and Medicaid has been increasing even more rapidly than total national health expenditures. In 1990, Medicare and Medicaid together comprised 27 percent of the total health care bill; in 1967 the two programs represented only 15 percent of the total health care bill. Out of approximately 260 million people in the United States in 1990, almost one-quarter (60 million) were enrolled in either or both programs. Medicare's role was clearly most substantial for

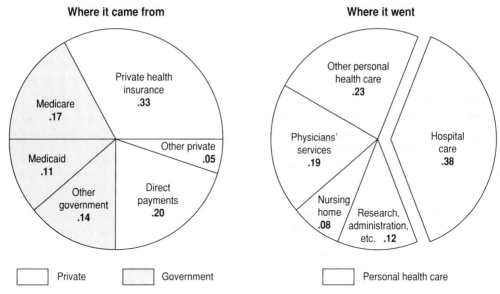

Figure 11-1. The nation's health care dollar, 1990. (SOURCE: Levit, K. R., Lazenby, H. C., Cowan, C. A., & Letsch, S. W. (1991). National health care expenditures, 1990. *Health Care Financing Review. 13.* 1–29.)

hospital care, and Medicaid's role was most prominent for nursing home care; the growth in these two services has certainly been spurred on by the two public programs (3).

Outlays

In terms of outlays, 46 percent of the money spent for health in 1990 was used to purchase hospital and nursing home services, although hospital expenditures, which totaled $256 billion, have dropped slightly as a proportion of health care expenditures in recent years. Another 42 cents was evenly divided among physicians' services and other personal care items (i.e., dentists' services, drugs, eyeglasses and appliances, and other professional services. Research and construction, program administration, and public health activities comprised the final 12 cents of the health care dollar for 1990 (3).

Personal Health Care

Figure 11-2 shows financing trends since 1950 for personal health care expenditures (total health ex-

penditures minus program administration, public health activities, research, and contruction) (3,5,6). Government and private insurance carriers, as funding sources for health care, have grown continuously in the postwar era, and out-of-pocket payments by patients have dropped commensurately. Compared to previous decades, the 1980s manifested considerable stability among payors.

Sources of funding for major providers of personal health care are depicted in figure 11-3. Government funding dominates hospital reimbursement, with about 55 percent financed by Medicare, other government programs, and Medicaid, in that order. Another 35 percent of the national hospital bill is footed by private health insurance. Physician outlays are clearly dominated by the private sector. Private insurance and direct patient payments account for more than 65 percent of physician funding; Medicare, which in recent years has grown as a financier of physicians' services, picks up another 24 percent. Nursing home funding reflects the "rich man, poor man" dichotomy of the long-term care industry, wherein patients must "spend down"

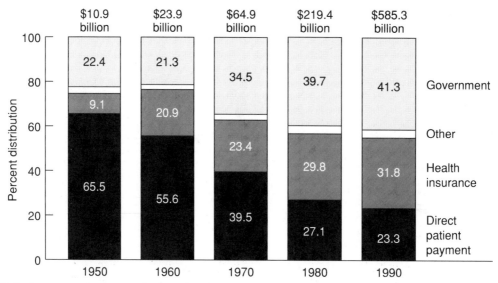

Figure 11-2. Percentage distribution of personal health care expenditures by source of funds, United States, selected years. (SOURCE: Adapted from Leavit, R., Lazenby, H. C., Cowan, C. A., & Letsch, S. W. (1991). National health expenditures, 1990. *Health Care Financing Review. 13.* 1–50.)

their assets in order to qualify for government assistance. Ninety percent of nursing home revenues are evenly divided between direct patient payment and Medicaid (3).

Health Insurance

Origins of Health Insurance

Health insurance originated in Europe in the early 1800s when mutual benefit societies arose to lighten the financial burden for those stricken with illness. The focus was on low-skill, low-income workers who were industrially employed. (Providers in Europe wanted to keep high-skill employees in the private medical market.) The first government health insurance program arose in Germany in 1840, mandating workers below a certain income level to belong to a "sickness fund." The concept of health insurance as linked to employment in the industrial sector persists internationally to this day. The health insurance networks of many nations grew out of this linkage and still reflect an emphasis on nonagricultural employment and coverage of the worker, irrespective of dependents (7,8).

Today in the U.S., the framework of health insurance stems clearly from its European antecedents and breaks down into three categories which, in some sense, reflect employment status. *Voluntary health insurance* (VHI) is private insurance, usually denoting current industrial employment; *social health insurance* (SHI) reflects participation in a government entitlement program linked to previous employment; *public welfare* health care programs connote lack of employment, low-income employment, or the inability to gain employment stemming from a disabling condition.

Distributing Risk

Insurance is a way of pooling or distributing risk, the risk being the probability of incurring a loss. Risk stems from two kinds of occurrences 1) unanticipated events such as fires, car accidents, or airplane crashes, and 2) anticipated events such as death, old age, and sickness. Health or, more correctly, illness is an anticipated event associated with old age and death. Thus, we know that illness is a likely event, but we don't know when it will strike, to whom it will happen, or how severe it will

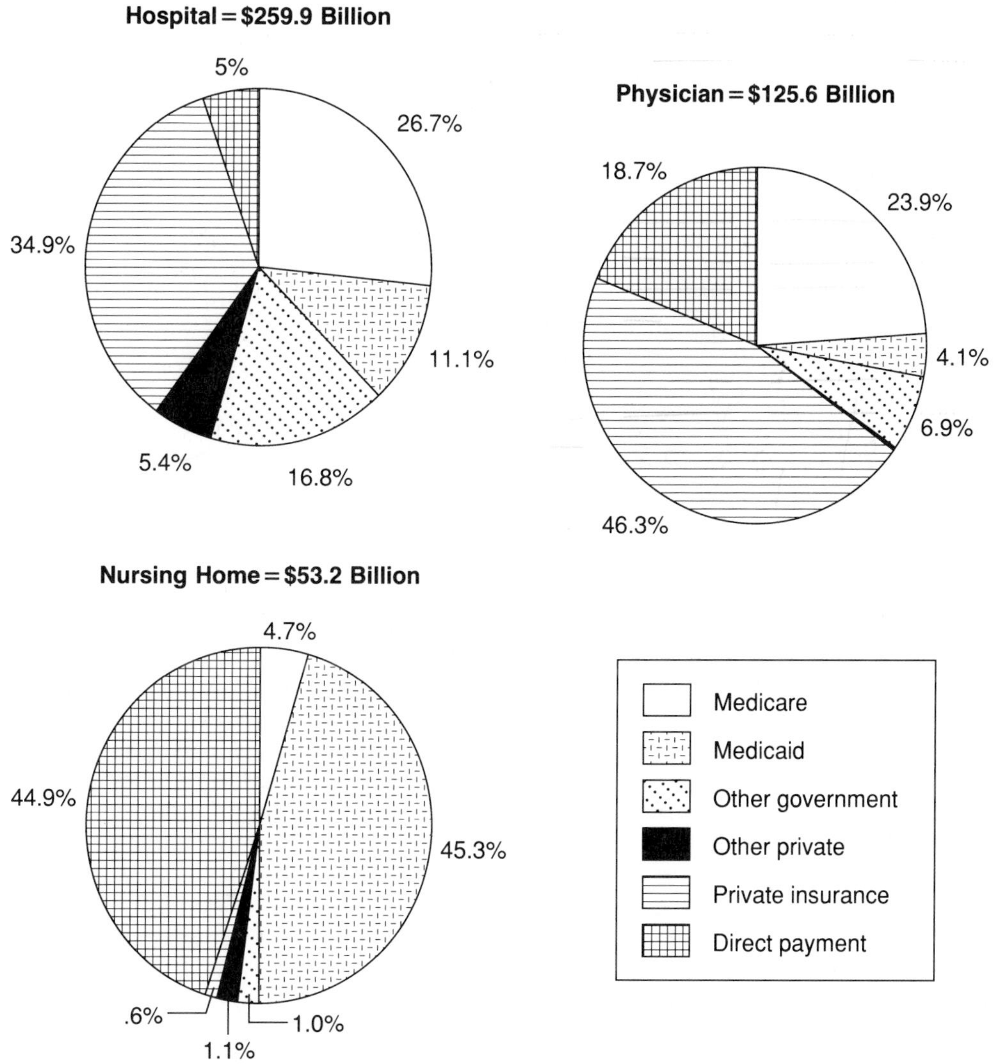

Hospital = $259.9 Billion

5%

26.7%

34.9%

11.1%

5.4%

16.8%

Physician = $125.6 Billion

18.7%

23.9%

4.1%

6.9%

46.3%

Nursing Home = $53.2 Billion

4.7%

44.9%

45.3%

.6%

1.1%

1.0%

Legend:
- ☐ Medicare
- ⊞ Medicaid
- ⋯ Other government
- ■ Other private
- ≡ Private insurance
- ▦ Direct payment

Figure 11-3. Personal health care expenditures for total population, by type of service and source of funds, United States, 1990. (SOURCE: Adapted from Leavit, K. R., Lazenby, H. C., Cowan, C. A., & Letsch, S. W. (1991). National health expenditures, 1990. *Health Care Financing Review. 13.* 52.)

be. Therefore, health is uncertain for the individual but not for a group. Groups are actuarially (statistically) predictable. *Why workplace is a natural risk pool pop.*

Moral Hazard

In all insurance, it is assumed that risks are independent of each other: 1) what befalls one person does not affect another, and 2) that for a single individual, risks are independent. Neither assumptions are true in health insurance because one person's sickness may spread contagiously and illness in one part of the body may weaken another part. These phenomena, together with the *moral hazard* inherent in medical care, make health insurance and health costs, in general, extremely volatile. Moral hazard means that, to the extent that the event insured against can be controlled, a temptation exists to use the insurance. (The classic example of moral hazard is setting fire to a failing business in order to collect the insurance.) Health insurance usage is highly discretionary; doctors and patients can conspire (intentionally or not) to use the insurance. An example is where the privately insured patient is kept in the hospital an extra day because it would be difficult or inconvenient for the family to receive the patient back home on the earliest possible discharge day. In this example, the insured extra day in the hospital, at a cost of $500 or more to the carrier, saves a loss in earnings for the family, and the expense is borne by purchasers of the policy, as reflected in the price of the premium.

Benefit Structure

Because of moral hazard, health insurance usually pays less than the total loss incurred by levying out-of-pocket or direct costs on the patient. In fee-for-service provider reimbursement, paying less takes the form of deductibles and copayments. A *deductible* is a sum of money that must be paid, typically every year, before the insurance policy becomes active. Deductibles have long been criticized in health insurance because they pose an impediment to first-contact care, discouraging the patient from seeking care until the condition becomes severe. Since higher costs may be incurred for more severe illness, deductibles have been seen as contributing to health cost inflation, rather then stimulating parsimonious consumer use. A *copayment* is paid as the beneficiary uses the insurance. For example, in a policy with a traditional *indemnity benefit,* a fixed cash amount is paid to the beneficiary per procedure or per day in the hospital (e.g., $800 for a one-night stay in the hospital following a hernia repair). If the hospital charges $1,100, then the patient must pay a copayment of $300. Thus the patient is liable for any amount in excess of the indemnity payment. An insurance plan with a *service benefit* reimburses on a percentage basis and the patient pays *coinsurance.*

Using the example above, the insurance plan would pay 80 percent or $880 of the surgeon's charges, leaving only $220 in coinsurance to be paid by the patient. Thus, if the percentage rate is high, the reimbursement structure of service benefits usually works to the patient's advantage, compared to indemnity benefits.

Pure types of indemnity or service benefits are becoming increasingly rare. Nowadays, to control health care inflation, there is a growing trend toward hybrid benefit structures, combining both service and indemnity features. A plan may, for example, pay a percentage of charges up to a specified limit, beyond which point the patient becomes responsible for the balance. Preferred provider organizations (PPOs) use this technique, often in concert with low price ceilings, to reimburse nonparticipating providers. Using the example above, the PPO might pay 80 percent up to an $800 limit on charges for a nonparticipating hospital. The plan would pay $640 and the patient would thus incur a $460 copayment. However, if the patient uses a hospital that participates in the PPO, the plan might pay 90 percent of the discounted fee of $1,000, resulting in a copayment of only $100 for the patient.

Premium Determination

Due to the financial implications of choosing one type of health insurance plan over another and because the possibility of moral hazard is a real one in health care use, health insurance plans are particularly vulnerable to the phenomenon of *adverse selection.* Adverse selection may be at work when an insurance policy experiences a higher number of claims due to sickness than would be probable on a random basis. If an employee is offered an alternate choice of plans, for example, a "sicker" person or a potentially higher user of health care services is likely to elect the plan with more generous provisions (i.e., lower deductible and copayments or fewer limitations and exclusions), even if the employee's share of the premium is higher. Therefore, more liberal fee-for-service plans may experience an adverse selection of sicker enrollees compared to a more restrictive managed care plan, such as a PPO or a health maintenance organization (HMO). This may result in ever-spiraling claims for the liberal plan as costlier people join and as healthier individuals defect to the lower-cost alternative plans.

Because of adverse selection, most health insurance plans today are *experience rated*; the premiums are based on demographic characteristics, such as age and sexual composition, of the employer group or on the actual experience of the group in that plan in prior years. *Community rating,* originated by Blue Cross and Blue Shield, bases premiums on the wider use of the defined geographic area (e.g., census tracts, city, county, etc.). Today, most fee-for-service plans are experience rated, even the Blues, which must contend with stiff price competition from commercial carriers. HMOs, on the other hand, use community ratings more widely for their enrolled groups, but even this is fading as HMOs face price competition or enter the for-profit arena.

Voluntary Health Insurance

Voluntary or private health insurance in the United States can be subdivided into three distinct categories: 1) Blue Cross and Blue Shield, 2) private or commercial insurance companies, and 3) health maintenance organizations (HMOs). The respective sponsorships of these types of VHI are providers, third parties or middlemen, and patients or independent carriers.

Growth and Development

Nineteen twenty-nine was a landmark year for VHI. In spite of active opposition from the American Medical Association (AMA) to any type of health insurance from 1920 onward, both Blue Cross and the HMO movement got their start in this last pre-Depression year. Blue Cross was initiated by Baylor teachers in Dallas, Texas, who organized to provide hospital care for three cents a day. Michigan and New Jersey were next in the movement for hospital

insurance. In 1934, the depths of the revenue depression for hospitals, the American Hospital Association (AHA) united these plans into the Blue Cross network. Today Blue Cross has broken away from its original AHA sponsorship, but the hospital-sponsored underpinnings remain strong in many locales (7,8).

In Oklahoma also in 1929, the Farmer's Union started its Cooperative Health Association, the first HMO. Independently, in the same year in Los Angeles, two Canadian physicians founded the Ross-Loos group practice and sold the first doctor-sponsored health insurance plan with prepayment to the Department of Water and Power and Los Angeles City workers.

As these and other plans grew during the 1930s, the AMA reversed its opposition to VHI in response to dwindling physician and hospital incomes and, in 1939, the California Medical Society developed and sponsored a plan known as Blue Shield to pay doctor's bills in a hospitalized environment (7,8).

By 1946, private health insurance plans were experiencing astronomical growth as wage and price restrictions in the post-World War II period spurred the growth of fringe benefits, especially in unionized industries. Insurance companies, already on the inside track in sales and actuarial information in life insurance, barged headlong into the health insurance business in competition with Blue Cross and Blue Shield.

Although voluntary health insurance plans were initiated by consumer cooperatives or employers, followed by provider-sponsored plans in the 1920s and 1930s, and supplemented by commercial insurance companies in the 1940s, the rate of growth in VHI programs has been in the reverse order. Today, most programs in the United States are sponsored by insurance companies, then providers, with consumers lagging far behind. Blue Cross currently administers a network of 61 member plans extending its public service concept internationally. Similarly, Blue Shield administers 65 plans, 53 of which are joined with Blue Cross. About 650 commercial insurance companies offer health insurance plans (2).

Population Coverage

About three-quarters of the U.S. population in 1990 is covered by private health insurance. About 40 percent of this group have health insurance as an employment benefit. These employees, in turn, cover another 38 percent of the population as dependents under their policies. In addition, almost three-quarters of the elderly, who with few exceptions are covered by Medicare, hold private insurance coverage to supplement their Medicare benefits. In 1988, about 77 percent of the population under 65 had some form of VHI and an equal proportion of employees worked for firms where they were eligible for health insurance. Firms that do not offer any health benefits at all tend to be small and nonunionized, hire seasonal workers, and employ relatively large numbers of low-wage employees. The industry groups supporting the highest rates of health insurance coverage are government, mining, manufacturing, and finance/insurance, which offer insurance to over 90 percent of their employees. Retail trade and construction are the least well-insured groups, offering coverage to less than 65 percent of their employees (2).

An unfortunate effect of employment-linked private health insurance is that people who are least able to pay for health care have the least insurance because they are unemployed (or work only part-time). The alternatives for these people are to purchase a nongroup or individual plan, usually a less generous and more expensive option in terms of out-of-pocket premiums, or to accept the risk of doing without any health insurance. Estimates vary, but according to the U.S. Census Bureau, about 13 percent of the total U.S. population in 1988 (31.5 million people) had no health insurance coverage at all, either public or private (2).

Benefits

Private health insurance coverage varies widely in terms of benefits provided, the extent of reimbursement for covered services, and exclusions or limitations. Based on the most recently available survey data, figure 11-4 depicts the most commonly covered services for the privately insured. *Basic*

insurance plans are designed to provide limited protection for the most expensive services and usually cover inpatient hospital and physician services, and outpatient hospital services, including laboratory procedures. Limits may apply to a group of related services such as those provided during the course of a hospitalization.

Major medical insurance extends basic benefits to such services as physician office visits, outpatient mental health care, prescribed medicines, durable equipment and supplies, ambulance services, and the like. Thus, this type of insurance is designed to protect against large medical bills as well as many expenses associated with routine types of medical care. For a traditional indemnity claim, the insurer typically pays a specified share of total covered expenses (e.g., 80 to 90 percent) in excess of a deductible (usually $100 to $200 per year for an individual), with a high maximum allowance. The beneficiary pays the deductible and coinsurance, which comprise the share of the incremental expenses not covered by the plan, subject to a limited amount known as the *out-of-pocket limit* or *stop-loss provision*. A limit of this kind may range from $1,500 to $2,500. Many major medical plans limit deductibles for family members to a specified amount (typically $300 to $500 per family) or waive the deductible for the rest of the family once two or three members have met their deductibles (9).

Comprehensive plans

Combine the features of both basic insurance and major medical plans. The deductible and other provisions apply to all expenses for all covered services. In contrast, "Medigap" plans are designed to reimburse only the deductibles and coinsurance associated with Medicare-covered services (9).

Two other types of private insurance coverage are noteworthy: hospital indemnity plans and HMOs. Hospital indemnity plans offer specified cash payments (e.g., $100 per day) for each day of inpatient hospitalization, regardless of the expenses actually incurred. Thus, it is not linked to the amount or type of medical services provided, but rather to

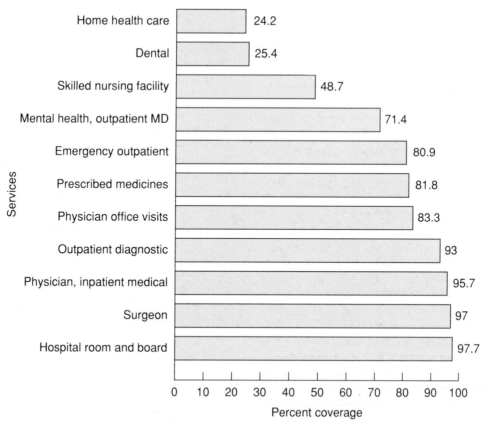

Figure 11-4. Coverage of the U.S. population: percent of privately insured persons under 65, by selected services. (SOURCE: Adapted from Farley P. J. (1986). In National Center for Health Services Research and Health Care Technology Assessment. *Private health insurance in the United States.* Data preview 23, National Medical Care Expenditure Survey (DHHS Publication No. [PHS] 86-3406, p. 19). Washington, DC: U.S. Government Printing Office.)

length of the hospital stay, and the payment is not generous in relation to the actual hospital expenses. This type of coverage is held by less than 8 percent of the privately insured (2,9).

Prepaid Plans

HMOs and other similar plans provide fairly comprehensive coverage in return for a prepaid fee, usually without deductibles and coinsurance for most services, and therefore offer coverage against the risk of large health care financial losses. Prepaid health plans are a rapidly growing segment of the private health insurance market. Today, there are about 590 HMOs in the United States, com-

pared to about 50 in 1973, prior to the passage of the HMO Act (2). This act requires employers with more than 25 employees to offer a dual choice of health plans, including an HMO if one is available locally.

It was anticipated that the HMO concept would foster incentives toward prevention and cost-consciousness on the part of physicians who are encouraged to be frugal in the use of secondary services, particularly hospitalization. However, because the prepayment of premium does not necessarily translate into capitated provider reimbursement and tight prospective budgeting, cost-containment experience is mixed. Due to legislative and economic incentives, almost 35 million Americans belonged to HMOs in 1989—a threefold increase since 1983 (2).

Social Health Insurance

The U.S. government sponsors two major mandatory social health insurance programs: 1) Worker's compensation for the costs and pain of suffering job-related accidents, and 2) Medicare for the elderly, disabled, and other special groups. Several states sponsor social insurance programs in the areas of temporary disability (California) or health insurance (Hawaii) (7).

Worker's compensation is offered in all 50 states to some extent. It is usually the first type of social insurance enacted in a nation and the vast majority of nations worldwide have some form of industrial accident insurance. The first worker's compensation law in the U.S. was passed by New York State in 1914 in response to the tragic Triangle Shirt Factory fire in which 146 women lost their lives. In 1950, Mississippi became the last state to enact worker's compensation. In recent years, over 80 percent of the U.S. workforce has been covered to some extent by worker's compensation, leaving the remaining workers, many of whom are agricultural, casual, and domestic workers, without coverage. Unfortunately, it is often these same people who are not covered by any type of health insurance (7).

Worker's compensation provides two basic benefits: 1) cash replacement of a portion of wages lost due to disability, and 2) payment for all or part of the medical care necessary. Worker's compensation may be underwritten by a private insurance company, a state government insurance fund, or a corporate contingency fund. Premiums are usually determined by experience rating. In 1988, Worker's compensation paid out about $10 billion in hospital and medical expense claims.

Medicare In 1935, national health insurance almost became a reality as part of the Social Security Act. Due to strong opposition from the AMA and conservative members of Congress, national health insurance was scrapped from the act by President Roosevelt, who did not want to risk passage by Congress. In 1939, and every two years for several Congresses thereafter, the Wagner, Murray, Dingell national health insurance bill was proposed in Congress. The timing of this bill coincided with the growth curve of private health insurance enrollment, which precluded a pressing interest in national health insurance. However, private health insurance was largely sponsored by employers and thus did not serve the nonworking population, particularly the aged. Nonetheless, about 50 percent of the elderly enrolled in voluntary health insurance programs during the 1957–64 pre-Medicare period (7).

In 1957, Representative Forand of Rhode Island introduced the bill that was the precursor of Medicare (Title XVIII of the Social Security Act). On July 30, 1965, Medicare became the first entry of the federal government into the provision of social health insurance rather than medical assistance (public welfare medicine) such as offered by the Kerr-Mills Act of 1960—"Medical Assistance for the Aged."

Strictly speaking, only Medicare Part A—Hospital Insurance (HI)—is social health insurance (figure 11-5). Part B—Supplementary Medical Insurance (SMI)—is neither compulsory nor funded by a trust fund. Seventy-two percent of the funds for SMI comes from the general treasury and the other 28 percent comes from Medicare Part A recipients who elect that Part B premiums be deducted from their monthly Social Security check (3).

Medicare uses an *indirect pattern* of finance and delivery, wherein the Health Care Financing Administration (HCFA), a branch of the U.S. Department of Health and Human Services, contracts with independent providers. Medicare recipients also access providers independently. HCFA sees to it that the provider is paid, but the providers are neither owned nor hired by the government, as in SHI systems using the *direct pattern* of delivery. Generally speaking, if the private medical market is strong at the time when SHI is enacted, an indirect pattern of delivery emerges. If the market is weak, a direct financing route emerges.

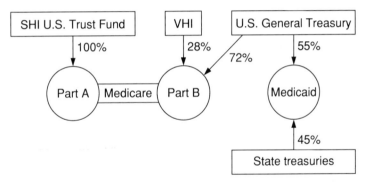

Figure 11-5. Flow of federal and state financing for Medicare and Medicaid.

Welfare Medicine

Public assistance of welfare medicine is sponsored by a plethora of federal, state, and local government programs, but the most far-reaching program is Medicaid (Title XIX of the Social Security Act). Administered at the federal level by HCFA, Medicaid is financed by an average federal contribution from the general treasury of 55 percent and from state treasuries at an average contribution of 45 percent (figure 11-5). Federal matching varies from 50 to 77.5 percent, depending on the income of the individual state (5). General treasury funds are generated from personal income tax, corporate income tax, and various excise taxes. To the extent that these taxes are borne by higher-income individuals and organizations, Medicaid represents a type of transfer payment to the poor.

The distinction between welfare medicine and social health insurance, both of which are public programs, is an important one and rests on the philosophical difference between a transfer payment and entitlement. Medicaid is a *transfer payment* "in kind," meaning that medical services are provided as a welfare benefit in lieu of cash. Welfare recipients also receive cash subsidies to pay for their living expenses, but medical benefits are paid directly to the provider so that the recipients will not be tempted to spend the money on expense items other than health care. (Food stamps are another "in kind" benefit, providing vouchers solely for the purpose of purchasing food and other

groceries.) Thus the transfer payment is a type of "relief" that government bestows upon the poor.

Social health insurance is an *entitlement* program, not charity. It is a right earned by individuals in the course of their employment. The funds for SHI programs are contributed by a payroll tax (for 1990, 2.9 percent for the first $51,300 of wages), which in the case of Social Security, is divided equally between the worker and the employer. Worker's compensation too is financed, at least in part, by worker contributions. When the worker retires or suffers a temporary or sustaining injury related to employment, SHI becomes an advocate for the worker and dependents. The fundamental aim of a compulsory, government-provided or -supervised SHI program is social adequacy—to provide members of society with protection against hazards so widespread as to be considered risks that individuals cannot afford to deal with themselves. Eligibility in SHI is derived from contributions having been made in the program and benefits are a statutory right not based on need. Recipients are thus entitled to the benefits of SHI. About half the countries in the world have an SHI system for financing health care (7).

Medicare

Medicare, the principal SHI program in the United States, provides a variety of hospital, physician, and other medical services for 1) persons 65 and over, 2) disabled individuals who are entitled to Social Security benefits, and 3) end-stage renal disease victims. In 1990, Medicare financed $111.2 billion in health services, comprising 41.4 percent of all publicly financed health expenditures and 18.6 percent of personal health care expenditures. Medicare reimbursed 26.7 percent of all hospital expenditures, and 23.9 percent of all physician expenditures in 1990 (3).

Hospital Insurance

Ninety-five percent of the aged population of the United States is enrolled in Part A of Medicare, Hospital Insurance (HI). Part A finances four basic benefits for the covered population:

1. Ninety days of inpatient care in a "benefit period." (A benefit period is a spell of illness beginning with hospitalization and ending when a beneficiary has not been an inpatient in a hospital or skilled nursing facility for 60 continuous days. There is no limit to the number of benefit periods a beneficiary can use.)
2. A lifetime reserve of 60 days of inpatient care, once the 90 days are exhausted.
3. One hundred days of posthospitalization care in a skilled nursing facility.
4. Home health agency visits.

Since the inception of the Medicare program, hospital insurance has required the beneficiary to participate in cost sharing. The patient is required to pay an inpatient hospital deductible in each benefit period which approximates the cost of one day of hospital care ($652 in 1992). Coinsurance based on the inpatient hospital deductible is required for the 61st–90th day of inpatient hospitalization and is always equal to one-fourth of the deductible ($163 in 1992). For the 21st–100th day of skilled nursing facility (SNF) care, the coinsurance equals one-eighth of the deductible ($81.50), and for the 60 lifetime reserve days, the patient pays one-half of the deductible ($326) for each day of inpatient hospitalization. Nearly 70 percent of Medicare enrollees have private "Medigap" policies, which primarily cover some or all of the deductibles and coinsurance under Medicare. About 15 percent of the aged and 21 percent of the disabled have Medicaid coverage also (a group known as "crossovers"), and Medicaid usually as-

sumes responsibility for the cost-sharing under Medicare (5).

While hospital expenditures have grown at a rapid rate since the inception of Medicare, skilled nursing facility, home health agency, and outpatient benefits have all shifted significantly as a percent of total Medicare benefit payments. Skilled nursing facility payments have dropped from 6.5 percent of payments in 1967 to only 2.2 percent in 1990. Home health agency payments rose from 1.0 percent to 2.6 percent and outpatient outlays. Currently the fastest growing component of Medicare, home health agency payments are slated for reduction in the near future (5).

Catastrophic Coverage

In 1988, amendments to Medicare were enacted to shield Medicare beneficiaries from catastrophic hospital and doctors' bills related to acute illnesses. While the bill provided no new benefits for long-term care, it did provide for the first broad coverage of outpatient prescription drugs. Due to pressure from organized groups of elderly who objected to the additional income taxes and substantial premium increases targeted at them, Congress repealed the bill in 1989. Only a few minor provisions in the amendment were subsequently incorporated into the regular Medicare benefit structure.

Supplementary Medical Insurance

Ninety-seven percent of Part A beneficiaries are enrolled in Part B—Supplementary Medical Insurance (SMI). Part B is the third largest federal domestic program, exceeded only by the social security cash benefit program and Medicare's Part A program. SMI was designed to complement the HI program. It provides payments for physicians, physician-ordered supplies and services, outpatient hospital services, rural health clinic visits, and home health visits for persons without Part A.

SMI requires the beneficiary to meet a deductible (currently $100) each year, in addition to paying a monthly premium ($31.80 in 1992). Under "buy-in" agreements, most state Medicaid programs pay the premiums for Medicaid enrollees who qualify to participate in SMI (5).

Drugs on an outpatient basis, dental care, routine eye examinations and eyeglasses, preventive services, and long-term institutional services are not covered by either part of Medicare. Hospice benefits, however, became available for terminally ill persons in 1983. Enrollees in Medicare can elect the hospice benefit for two 90–day periods and one 30–day period, with a subsequent extension period during the individual's lifetime.

From 1967 to 1988, Part B of Medicare grew faster than Part A—at a compound growth rate of about 20 percent, compared to 15 percent. Therefore, although Part B represents less than 40 percent of Medicare expenditures, Part B has almost doubled as a proportion of Medicare expenditures since 1967 and Part A has shrunk commensurately (2). To constrain SMI inflation, the Deficit Reduction Act of 1984 placed a freeze on Medicare maximum payment levels (originally slated for 15 months beginning July 1, 1984, but continuing for several years) and introduced the concept of "participating physicians," who are those who accept assignments for all services. Incentives to participate were introduced and resulted in substantial increases in assignment.

Provider Reimbursement

Medicare has operated primarily on a fee-for-service basis for physicians and related services and, until 1983, on a cost-based retrospective basis for hospital services. Hospitals were reimbursed for any reasonable costs incurred in the provision of covered care to Medicare patients. Commencing in 1983, payment rates were prospectively determined on a case basis. The Medicare hospital prospective payment system (PPS), discussed in detail later in this chapter, uses diagnosis-related groups (DRGs) to classify cases for payment. All providers must bill Medicare directly in order to qualify for reimbursement.

Under Medicare Part B, physicians may elect one of two reimbursement strategies. The first is to accept the Medicare fee determination as pay-

ment in full, billing Medicare directly, and receiving 80 percent payment from the Medicare intermediary—a practice called "accepting the assignment." The beneficiaries are liable for the remaining 20 percent coinsurance. On unassigned claims, the beneficiary is additionally liable for the difference between the physician's charge and the Medicare-allowed charge.

The Deficit Reduction Act of 1984 created two classes of physicians: "participating" and "nonparticipating." A participating physician must accept assignment of all claims for all Medicare patients. Several incentives of a pecuniary and marketing nature, have been employed by Medicare to entice physicians to participate. A nonparticipating physician can continue to treat Medicare patients, accepting assignments or not on a claim-by-claim basis, but Medicare will reimburse only 95 percent of the Medicare fee schedule amount (10).

Claims are processed by *intermediaries* or fiscal agents, such as Blue Cross or a commercial insurance company, contracted by the Medicare program to review and pay the bills. Enrollees can also join HMOs, and similar forms of prepaid health care and special reimbursement provisions apply to these organizations. The Tax Equity and Fiscal Responsibility Act of 1982 (TEFRA) included major revisions to the Medicare law to encourage growth in the number of HMOs and other comprehensive medical plans enrolling Medicare beneficiaries. TEFRA also set limits on Medicare reimbursements for hospital costs at the per-case level and also placed a limit on the annual rate of increase for Medicare's reasonable costs per discharge.

Utilization

The average aged Medicare enrollee spent in excess of $2,500 in 1988. As in any insurance program, however, use is uneven. A study of 1983 data showed that two-thirds of the enrolled population had small claims of $500 or less or none at all. The highest 9.6 percent of users had reimbursements of $5,000 or more and these enrollees consumed 72.2 percent of program payments (5). Other studies have demonstrated that high Medicare reimbursements are related to terminal illness. Lubitz and Prihoda (11) found that reimbursements for decedents averaged $4,527 for the last year of life, whereas reimbursements averaged $729 for a comparison group who survived the period under study. Fuchs (12) showed that the greatest proportion of medical care costs are incurred in the year prior to death, regardless of the age of natural death. For Medicare enrollees in 1976, the average reimbursement for those in their last year of life was 6.6 times as large as for those who survived at least two years. Thus, one may surmise that the principal reason why health expenditures rise with age is that the proportion of people near death increases with age. Other studies have found a great deal of consistency over time in the use of health expenditures by the highest users, the top 1 percent accounting for 20 or more percent of health care dollars (5).

Medicaid

Program Structure

Medicaid was enacted into law on July 30, 1965, as Title XIX of the Social Security Act, and became part of the existing federal-state welfare structure to assist the poor. Until 1956, there had been no federal participation in health care for the poor. This public obligation was delegated to the states as part of their police powers. Prior to Medicaid, many doctors donated their services or used a sliding scale of fees in treating the poor and, as a rule, hospitals admitted charity cases. However, under the purview of the states, health care for the poor varied widely from state to state and manifested all the forms of discrimination tolerated in each locale. The Kerr-Mills Act of 1960—Medical Assistance for the Aged—was the forerunner of the Medicaid model and was later subsumed under Title XIX.

Eligibility

Supported by federal grants and administered by the states, Medicaid is limited to specific groups of low-income individuals and families (figure 11-6). Medicaid is welfare medicine and thus has no entitlement features. Recipients must prove their eligibility according to their income and, prior to 1976, states were permitted to put a lien on a recipient's home or other personal property.

The program was designed to cover those groups who are eligible to receive cash payments under one of the two existing welfare programs established under Social Security—Aid to Families with Dependent Children (AFDC) and Supplemental Security Income (SSI). In most instances, receipt of a welfare payment under one of these programs means automatic eligibility for Medicaid. The mandatory "categorical" assistance groups covered by Medicaid include adults who receive AFDC, and other low-income parents: children in AFDC families, other low-income children, and low-income pregnant women; aged, blind, and disabled individuals who receive SSI: and certain other specifically defined groups. Figure 11-6 compares the distribution of Medicaid recipients to that of expenditures by eligibility category. AFDC families were the largest group of recipients (68.2 percent) in 1989, but accounted for a relatively small part of the Medicaid budget (25.4 percent), which is a reflection of the relatively good health of most Medicaid children. Due largely to high use of nursing home services, 34.1 percent of total Medicaid outlays was attributable to the aged, who comprise only 13.3 percent of the Medicaid population. Similarly, outlays for the disabled totaled 38.3 percent of Medicaid expenditures, compared to 15.3 percent of recipients, largely reflecting the high rate of expenditures for the 142,000 individuals in intermediate-care facilities for the mentally retarded (13).

States also hold the option of providing Medicaid to "categorically needy" groups. Most of these optional groups share characteristics of the mandatory groups (parents and children, aged, blind, and disabled), but the income eligibility ceilings are higher (e.g., 1.85 times the federal poverty level). "Medically needy" persons comprise another optional group—those who spend down their

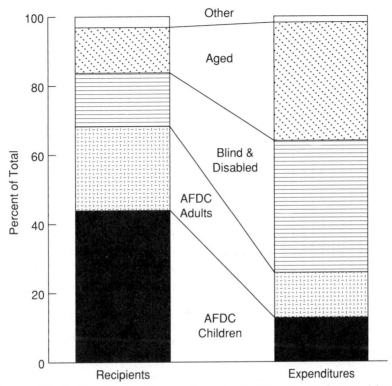

Figure 11-6. Distribution of Medicaid recipients and expenditures, by eligibility category. (SOURCE: Adapted from Reilly, T. W., Clausen, S. B., & Baugh, D. K. (1990). Trends in Medicaid payments and utilization, 1975–89. *Health Care Financing Review*. *12(Annual Supplement)*. 15–33.)

income and wealth, due to medical bills, to the medically needy standard. Under federal guidelines, states set income and asset levels for cash assistance and medical eligibility. Because there is considerable variation in the coverage of optional groups by the states and in income standards across Medicaid jurisdictions, the degree to which programs cover the poverty population varies considerably.

Benefits Provided

Services

Title XIX of the Social Security Act mandates that every state Medicaid program provide specific basic health services:

- Hospital inpatient care
- Hospital outpatient services
- Prenatal care
- Laboratory and X-ray services
- SNF services for those age 21 and older
- Home health services for those eligible for SNF services
- Physicians' services
- Family planning services and supplies
- Rural health clinic services
- Early and periodic screening, diagnosis, and treatment for children under 21 years of age
- Nurse-midwife services
- Certain federally qualified ambulatory and health center services

States may determine the scope of services offered (e.g., limit the days of hospital care or the number of physician visits covered) and provide a number of other elective services. The most commonly covered optional services include:

- Clinic services
- Intermediate care facility services (ICF) for the aged, blind, disabled, and mentally retarded
- Optometrist services and eyeglasses
- Prescribed drugs
- Prosthetic devices
- Dental care

Administration

Medicaid operates primarily as a vendor payment program. Payments are made directly to providers of service for care rendered to eligible individuals. With certain exceptions, a state must allow Medicaid recipients freedom of choice among participating providers of health care.

Methods for reimbursing physicians and hospitals vary widely among the states, but providers must accept the Medicaid reimbursement level as payment in full. Payment rates must be sufficient to enlist enough providers so that comparable care and services are available to the Medicaid population as are available to the general population in the area. Notwithstanding, Medicaid physician reimbursement rates are usually less generous than those of Medicare.

In long-term care facilities, individuals are required to turn over income in excess of their personal needs and maintenance needs of their spouses (the monetary level being determined by the state) to help pay for their care. States may require cost sharing by Medicaid recipients, but they may not require the categorically eligible to share costs for mandatory services. As noted previously, most state Medicaid programs have buy-in agreements with Medicare in which Medicaid assumes the responsibility for the Medicare cost sharing for people covered under both programs (5,14).

States participate in the Medicaid program at their option. All states (except Arizona, which has a demonstration project of capitated health delivery that excludes long-term care services) currently have Medicaid programs. The District of Columbia, Puerto Rico, Guam, the Northern Marianas, and the Virgin Islands also provide Medicaid coverage.

The states administer their Medicaid programs within broad federal requirements and guidelines. These requirements allow states considerable discretion in determining not only eligibility, but covered benefits and provider payment mechanisms as well. Some states also include in the Medicaid program persons known as "state-only" enrollees, who do not meet federal requirements and hence do not qualify for federal matching funds. As a result of state options and policy decisions, the characteristics of Medicaid programs vary considerable from state to state. In the Omnibus Budget Reconciliation Act of 1981, the states were given even more flexibility in the administration of their programs as well as additional options, including the introduction of home- and community-based service programs as alternatives to institutionalization.

Medicaid expenditures vary widely across the states. In 1984, four states had per capita Medicaid expenditures of less than $70, whereas four states had more than $190. Similarly, seven states had Medicaid expenditures per person in poverty of less than $500, and eight states had expenditures of $1,500 or more (5).

Growth of Medicaid

Providers

From 1980 to 1990, growth in Medicaid expenditures (287 percent) rivaled that of Medicare, which grew by 352 percent over the same period. Hospital care (inpatient, outpatient, drugs, and hospital-based home health and physician services) accounted for a much smaller proportion of 1990 Medicaid expenditures (40 percent) than Medicare personal care outlays (63 percent in 1990). Nursing home care, including SNFs, ICFs, and intermediate care facilities for the mentally retarded (ICF/MR), is the second largest component of the Medicaid budget, accounting for more than one-third of all outlays for personal care (3,13).

Medicaid continues to be the largest third-party

payer of long-term care services, financing 45.4 percent of nursing home care in 1990. Although growth in spending for SNFs and ICFs has slowed considerably in recent years Medicaid has funded about 90 percent of all public spending for nursing home care since the early 1970s. Compared with the other services Medicaid provides, Medicaid payments for long-term care are also the most costly per user. A 1984 study showed that the average Medicaid payment for SNF services was $8,594; for ICF services, the payment was $7,377; and for ICF/MR, the payment averaged a whopping $29,995. In 1989, the fastest-growing services in the Medicaid budget were ICF/MR care and home health care, with annual compound rates of growth of 22 and 26 percent, respectively (3,5,13).

Growth

Medicaid is the fastest-growing component of aggregate state spending. In 1990, Medicaid spent $71.3 billion of combined federal and state funds for personal health care. Growth in program spending for about 25 million Medicaid recipients accelerated from 13.6 percent in 1989 to 20.6 percent in 1990, the fastest annual rate of growth in Medicaid spending since 1975. As a result Medicaid's share of personal health care expenditures grew from 11.2 percent in 1989 to 12.2 percent in 1990 (3).

In order to curtail Medicaid growth, cost-containment initiatives were instituted in the early 1980s. During this time important experiments were launched in prepaid managed health care; utilization review; case management; reimbursement via diagnosis-related group (DRGs); and new services for the elderly, disabled, and persons with AIDS. In the mid–1980s, as state economies improved, Congress moved to careful and selective expansion of Medicaid coverage, particularly for low-income women and children. Currently, the focus is on shifting Medicaid funding from the federal coffers to state budgets and encouraging states to model their systems on HMOs (15).

Physician Reimbursement

Paying the doctor traditionally calls upon one of three reimbursement mechanisms: fee for service, prepayment, or salary. Health insurance plans, either public or private, may use any or all of these reimbursement types; there is no optimal system. According to the most recent data available on the U.S. population under 65 years of age who are privately insured, more than 80 percent are covered for physician office visits, more than 95 percent are insured for physician inpatient medical care and surgeon's fees, and more than 70 percent are covered for outpatient mental health care (9).

Fee for Service

Fee for service (FFS) is widely used throughout the world for paying the doctor and is typically the physician's preferred mode of payment. In FFS, the unit of remuneration is the medical act, either a service or a procedure. In the days before health insurance for physician reimbursement was widespread, most physicians had a sliding-fee scale wherein poor patients paid lower fees than wealthier ones did. With the advent of health insurance in both the public and private sectors, physician payment became more regulated and physicians adopted one schedule of charges used for all payors, whether they were individuals or third parties.

Among the advantages of fee-for-service reimbursement are that the remuneration adjusts automatically for case complexity, linking the provider's reward closely to the output of services. The billing system, in turn, provides a great deal of "transparency" of the physician's profile of practice. The ease with which patients may change physicians in a fee-for-service system enables them to directly exercise considerable economic clout over practitioners (16).

Indemnity

Insurance policies that reimburse on a fee-for-service basis offer payment either by indemnity or service benefits or by fixed fees. *Indemnity payment* stipulates a certain dollar value per procedure usually according to a "Table of Allowances." The provider can charge anything above the stipulated amount and collect the remainder directly from the patient. Often, the Table of Allowances is based upon a "Relative Value Scale," in which each procedure is rated according to a point system that reflects the relative technical difficulty and time cost of the procedure, and each point is worth so many dollars. This type of system is easy to administer and update for inflation and changing practice patterns, but no provision is made by the insurer to protect the patient from outlandish charges.

Service benefits pay a percentage per procedure, usually 80 percent of "usual, customary, and reasonable" (UCR) fees. In this scheme, the UCR fee schedule protects the carrier from unlimited liability in the wake of high charges and also may give the patient information about reasonable fee norms. UCR means that the fee is "usual" in that doctor's practice, "customary" in that community, and "reasonable" in terms of the distribution of all physician charges for that service in the community. The last is commonly expressed as a percentile (e.g., the policy will pay up to the 75th percentile). Up until 1992, Medicare Part B used a similar standard of "customary, prevailing, and reasonable fees."

Hybrid fee-based systems came into vogue with the advent of PPOs and combined features of both indemnity and service reimbursement for cost containment. In a hybrid system, the intermediary contracts with the participating physician (or hospital) to accept a discounted version of the UCR table of allowances. The plan considers these "allowed amounts" to be the maximum covered expenses. For a participating provider, the PPO will typically pay 90 percent of the allowed amount for most procedures, with the remaining 10 percent paid by the patient as coinsurance. This arrangement protects both the intermediary by effectively capping the reimbursement (as in an indemnity payment)

and the patient by not making him liable for the difference beyond 10 percent of the allowed amount (as in a service benefit).

Fixed Fees

In some reimbursement plans, physicians can only charge, and will only be paid, according to fixed fees. If the provider accepts the plan, then he must accept the fee schedule. This arrangement exists in Medicaid and many private plans also stipulate fixed fees to protect the patient and contain costs.

Prepayment

In prepayment or capitation, the person served, rather than the medical act, is the unit of remuneration. The capitation payment takes care of reimbursement for a stipulated length of time, usually a year. Using capitation as a reimbursement methodology, physicians have formed contracted networks known as independent practice associations (IPAs), usually organized around an HMO. In recent years, IPAs have been gaining in popularity for physicians and consumers, along with the HMO movement. Advantages to prepayment are that it is administratively simple; it facilitates advance global budgeting; and it gives physicians incentive to control the cost of medical treatments. If patients can switch physicians from time to time, they still retain some economic clout over physicians (16).

Salary

Salary is payment to the doctor for his time, irrespective of units of service or number of patients. On a large scale, salaried practice almost always takes in a highly organized network such as the National Health Service in Great Britain. On a smaller scale in the United States, urban public hospitals that serve indigent populations often have large attending salaried staffs. Countries in which salaried practices are common rarely include specialists in this payment mechanism. Instead, general practitioners or primary care providers have a "panel" of patients in the community. Advantages of salaried reimbursement for physicians are that it is administratively simple, the medical treatments selected are not influenced by relative profitability, and it encourages cooperation among physicians. Furthermore, salaries facilitate budgeting for health expenditures *ex ante* (16).

Monitoring   *Incentives*   *FFS vs prepaid vs salaries*

All payment mechanisms have faults and each must be monitored for abuses. In FFS, the incentives are for overwork by the physician and overuse by the patients. FFS fosters unnecessary or duplicative service to the point where the high volume of services may adversely affect the quality of care. Unfortunately, in the United States, malpractice suits have encouraged defensive medicine, wherein overuse and extra fees are simply passed on to the consumer in higher insurance rates. Also, if fees for all procedures do not stand in constant proportion to costs incurred, the choice of treatment may favor more profitable procedures. For these and other reasons that foster inflation, fee-for-service reimbursement is very difficult to budget to in advance (16).

In prepayment, on the other hand, underuse must be monitored because the incentives are to decrease costs and services provided vis-à-vis the capitation payment. In many prepayment schemes, any cost savings realized are distributed to the participating physicians, which may be an inducement to cut costs too far. In HMOs where only the primary care physicians are capitated, there also exists the incentive to refer excessive numbers of patients to specialists. Likewise, capitation gives physicians incentives for "dumping" patients with complex, costly conditions onto other providers. Finally, the administrative system for prepayment yields little insight as to the physician's practice profile (16).

In salaried practice, incentives favor underwork or seeing too few patients. Doctors literally "get paid by the hour," resulting in no inducement to increase volume. According to Reinhardt (16), unless the salary is linked to output and patient

satisfaction, patients lose economic clout over the physician, who, in turn, may render care as an act of noblesse oblige. Like capitation, salaried practice reveals little about the physician's practice profile.

Thurs.

Recent Initiatives in Health Care Finance

Factors in Health Care Inflation

The implementation of Medicare and Medicaid in 1966 heralded a 25-year era of unprecedented health care cost inflation. Gornick et al., succinctly list the multiplicity of factors feeding the inflationary process (5:16):

Several different factors in the health care system have been identified with the continuing increase in costs: the rise in wages and price levels in the health care industry; increases in the number of certain customary services such as laboratory tests; the development of new and costly medical technologies such as open-heart surgery; changes in the organization of care, such as the growth of intensive care units in hospitals and increases in personnel; and the growth of institutions for long-term care.

Factors often cited as giving impetus to these changes include: the increase in demand for more costly health care services, as a result of Medicare, Medicaid, and other third-party payment that removed the individual from direct consequences of the cost of services; the response of health care providers to reimbursement methods that offered financial incentives to increase medical care spending; and the rising expectations in the Nation with regard to health care services.

Cost-Containment Measures

In the 1970s, the federal government experimented with a number of programs and reimbursement methods to contain health care costs. Major programs included 1) the establishment of reasonable cost limits for hospitals; 2) the initiation of state and local networks of health planning agencies along with the "certificate-of-need" procedure for augmenting capital plant and equipment; 3) the establishment of the professional standards review organization (PSRO) program to review care and to eliminate unnecessary hospital days for federally funded patients; and 4) encouragement of the growth of HMOs to promote the use of preventive services and to decrease the use of hospital inpatient care. It can be safely said that the programs of the 1970s were unsuccessful in containing health care costs.

Early in the 1980s, during the Reagan administration, legislative efforts to change the monetary incentive system in health care began in earnest. While the past decade has witnessed considerable flux in health care financing, along with inducements to reduce overuse, cost-containment efforts have not been successful. Furthermore, they have held painful consequences for many groups of people. The balance between reasonable costs and equitable access has not yet been struck, but it is clear that the traditional health care market has no apparatus to reflect social or economic rationing decisions regarding the provision of health care that might help to stem inflation. Managed care, particularly capitated prepaid care, holds better incentives for efficiency, productivity, and management coordination. Yet, even with more closely managed use and seemingly never-ending growth, universal realized access to health services remains illusive.

Procompetition

Early in the 1980s, Enthoven (17) and other health economists exposited strategies of "procompetition," which were meant to restrain health care costs by creating competitive market conditions, via direct incentives for both consumers and employers who purchase group health insurance policies. Among these strategies were the imposition of a "tax cap" on employer income tax deductions for health insurance expenses, raising the threshold for individual income-tax deductions, and employers offering multiple choices of health insurance plans. While the threshold for personal income-tax deductions for medical out-of-pocket expense was raised to 7.5 percent of gross income, the

other strategies, while not formally enacted, had a profound effect on the thinking of health policy makers. The programs of the 1980s reflect this conservative philosophy and, in most cases, the scorecards for their success are mixed, at best.

TEFRA

The Tax Equity and Fiscal Responsibility Act (TEFRA), signed into law in September 30, 1982, and enacted the next day, set limits on Medicare reimbursements on a per-case basis for hospital costs and also placed a limit on the annual rate of increase for Medicare's reasonable costs per discharge. TEFRA was expected to reduce Medicare reimbursement by 4.5 percent in real dollars over the ensuing three years, during which time reimbursement increases, based on projected inflation rates, would be in effect. Due to the fast enactment of the prospective payment system one year later, it was difficult to evaluate the impact of the act. However, TEFRA was the harbinger of prospective payment and a number of features of the latter program were borrowed from it. These features were part of the *Section 223 limits* on hospital costs. They included 1) grouping hospitals by bed size and size of locale, 2) wage adjustments by locality, and 3) an adjustment for case-mix index (18).

Today, most hospitals that are excluded from the Medicare prospective payment system are reimbursed according to TEFRA regulations.

The Section 223 limits were calculated according to a complicated formula whereby the labor-related component for the hospital region, adjusted by a geographic wage index, was added to a regional nonlabor component. The product was then multiplied by a case-mix index specific to each hospital. These figures were all specified by Health Care Financing Administration and published in the *Federal Register*. The formula used to calculate the Section 223 limits was substantially retained for figuring reimbursement rates for the prospective payment system.

HCFA developed institutional-specific case-mix indexes based on a diagnosis-related group (DRG) system designed at Yale University. The DRG classification system sorts patients into uniform, clinically compatible groups that have been categorized on the basis of traditional resource use by patients with similar diagnoses. The original Yale DRGs were modified to reflect variation only in Medicare cases. For each hospital, HCFA used a 20 percent sample of the Medicare billing forms submitted for calendar year 1980. Using the 10,167 ICD-9-CM diagnosis codes from these claims and each hospital's Medicare cost report, HCFA developed the case-mix index. (See table 11-2.) In essence, this case-mix index was intended to compare a particular hospital's case mix with that of all other hospitals in the nation (18).

Target Rates

Another ceiling established by HCFA, concurrent with the Section 223 limits, was the *target rate ceiling*. This target rate limited the allowable amount of growth in Medicare-reimbursable inpatient operating costs limits, based on historical Medicare-allowable operating costs per discharge, increased by an inflation factor. Medicare operating costs were defined as routine operating costs, ancillary service costs, and special care unit costs, excluding capital-related costs, medical education program costs, and medical malpractice insurance costs.

TEFRA reimbursement gave bonuses to hospitals whose inpatient operating costs per discharge were less than the target rate ceiling, providing that the target rate was below the Section 223 limit. Today, while the Section 223 limits have been abandoned, the target rates have been retained. If a hospital's per-discharge costs fall below the target rate, the hospital is given 50 percent of the difference. On the other hand, if a hospital's per-discharge costs are above the target, the hospital is reimbursed at the target rate plus 50 percent of

the costs in excess of it, as long as the excess is limited to 10 percent of the target rate. In this way, TEFRA provides an incentive system for hospitals to lower their costs on Medicare discharges rather than incur spiraling excesses year after year (18).

The Prospective Payment System

The prospective payment system (PPS) was enacted on October 1, 1983, two years ahead of schedule. The Social Security Amendments of 1983 (PL 98-21) initiated the Medicare prospective payment system and contained provisions to base payment for hospital inpatient services on predetermined rates per discharge for diagnosis-related groups (DRGs). By the end of the first year of PPS, a total of 5,405 hospitals, which comprised 81 percent of all Medicare-participating hospitals, were operating under PPS. This figure represented virtually all of the short-stay acute care hospitals participating in the Medicare system (19,20).

Under PPS, the majority of U.S. hospitals are no longer reimbursed for inpatient services on the basis of reasonable costs. Excluded from PPS are psychiatric, rehabilitation, alcohol/drug, and children's hospitals; long-term care hospitals; and other medical facilities that have an approved waiver. Except for childrens' hospitals, which are still reimbursed according to costs, these facilities remain on TEFRA regulations.

PPS is a major departure from the preceding reimbursement system—cost-based reimbursement—in that payment bears no direct relationship to length of stay, services rendered, or costs of care. For a given discharge, a hospital with actual costs below the designated PPS rate for a given DRG is permitted to keep the difference in payment. If discharge costs exceed the payment level, the hospital is required to absorb the loss. Certain costs, such as capital depreciation and direct medical education costs, are exempt from PPS provisions and have their own payment formulas. Payment for hospital-based physician services (e.g., radiology, anesthesiology, pathology, etc.), which

TABLE 11-2 Calculation of Medicare Case-Mix Index[a]

Hospital	DRG 1	DRG 2	DRG 3	DRG 4	DRG 5	Total (Percent)	DRG Weighted Expected Cost Per Case ($)[b]	Case-Mix Index[c]
A	2.5	27.3	10.5	41.5	18.2	100	1660.40	0.8900
B	21.0	.9	30.1	2.0	46.0	100	2401.30	1.2872
C	40.6	5.0	2.3	47.2	4.9	100	1346.30	0.7227
D	5.1	18.4	62.5	10.0	4.0	100	2990.70	1.6031
E	30.4	65.0	1.0	1.6	2.0	100	929.00	0.4980
Average proportion for all hospitals	19.92	23.32	21.28	20.46	15.02	100	1865.54	—
DRG cost weight	$1000	$800	$4100	$1500	$2000	—	—	—

[a]Adjusted to make these 5 DRGs hypothetically represent all 356 Medicare DRGs.
[b]For hospital A, calculated as follows:

$$0.025(1000) + 0.273(800) + 0.105(4100) + 0.415(1500) + 0.182(2000) = \$1660.40$$

[c]For hospital A, calculated as $1660.40 divided by $1865.54 = 0.8900.

SOURCE: Deloitte Haskins & Sells. (1982). *Tax Equity and Fiscal Responsibility Act of 1982: Management strategies for health care providers.* New York: Author.

previous to enactment of PPS were reimbursed on the basis of reasonable costs under Medicare Part A, are included in the hospital's PPS rate. As a result, many such physicians have defected to Part B of Medicare, billing patients directly for their services.

Standardized Payment Amount

PPS pays a standardized amount for each DRG. Standardized amounts are issued each year by HCFA according region of the country (e.g., New England, Middle Atlantic, etc.) and by urbanization of the area (large urban, other urban, and rural). This amount is further divided into two components—a labor-related amount and a nonlabor-related amount. To compute the payment amount for a DRG of 1.0000, the labor-related amount is multiplied by a wage index, specific to each locality, and the product is added to the nonlabor-related amount. In 1992, for example, a hospital in San Diego is subject to a large urban labor-related amount of $2,374.81, multiplied by a wage index of 1.1945, plus a nonlabor-related amount of $1,155.02. Thus, the DRG payment for a hospital in San Diego is $3,991.76.

DRG Weights

The DRG weight classifications used in TEFRA were updated for use in PPS using a stratified sample of 400,000 medical records drawn from patient discharges in 332 hospitals during the last half of 1979 (19). To date, 492 DRGs have been developed, expanding on the original 468 principal diagnoses. A contracted fiscal intermediary, such as Blue Cross or a commercial insurer, assigns a DRG from a bill submitted by the hospital for each case. Using classifications and terminology consistent with the ICD-9-CM and the Uniform Hospital Discharge Data Set (UHDDS), the intermediary assigns the DRG using the Grouper Program (an automated classification algorithm), which compares information contained in the bill with appropriate DRG criteria. Criteria include the patient's age, sex, principal and secondary diagnoses, pro-

cedures performed, and discharge status (21). (Figure 11-7 presents a schematic diagram of the Grouper Program.) For all but a few DRGs, which require clarification by the hospital before the payment amount is determined, the intermediary determines the payment amount and pays the hospital.

Outliers

Bills for "outliers," which result in extra payment for the hospital above the standard DRG rate, require special consideration. About 5 percent of the pool of total PPS payments is reserved for outliers. Length-of-stay or day outliers are identified by the intermediary and, after appropriate review, payment is made to the hospital. Cost outliers, however, are not identified by the intermediary. The hospital must identify cost outliers and request payment. (It is important to note that the classification of DRGs depends largely on the principal diagnosis, which may not be the diagnosis consuming the most resources.)

For a discharge to be considered as an outlier, the rules are very stringent. In 1992, the threshhold for a day outlier expanded to 34 days beyond the geometric mean length of stay for a specific DRG or three standard deviations above the mean, whichever is less. A simple appendectomy (DRG 167) with a mean length of stay of four days, for example, would not be considered an outlier until the inpatient episode reached 15 days. Cost outliers must exceed two times the DRG rate of payment or $44,000.

Quality Indicators

A clear incentive in the PPS system is for hospitals to expand services still qualifying for cost-based Medicare reimbursement. Opportunities for marketing expansion include specific ambulatory programs; satellite clinics; health-related services such as family planning, chemical dependency treatment, and laboratory; or other ancillary services used by physicians. Hospital-sponsored skilled nursing, rehabilitation, home health services, and

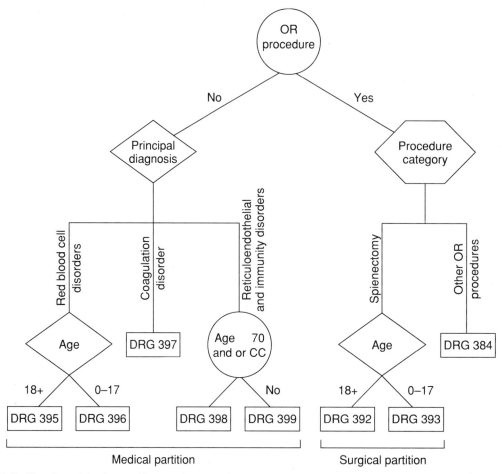

Figure 11-7. Flowchart of the Grouper Program for major diagnostic category 16: Disease and Disorders of the Blood and Blood-Forming Organs and Immunological Disorders. (OR, operating room; CC, comorbidity and/or complication.) (SOURCE: American Medical Association. (1984). *Diagnosis-related groups (DRGs).* Chicago: Author.)

other services that may facilitate earlier discharge of patients and provide additional sources of revenue for hospitals have experienced marked growth since the inception of PPS. Many of these programs may be accomplished by conversion of acute care beds, replacing services eliminated by PPS-induced financial considerations or making use of excess capacity.

The major deleterious incentives anticipated in the enactment of PPS included: 1) multiple, unnecessary admissions of the same patient for a set of related procedures resulting in more discreet DRG payments, a practice known as *"churning;"* 2) *"skimming"* more profitable, less severely ill patients in each DRG, or *"dumping"* high-cost patients; and 3) reducing length of stay, tests, and procedures per admission to dangerously low levels, thereby increasing mortality and morbidity.

Empirical findings as to the validity of these assertions have shown few ill effects of PPS or are inconclusive due to the rapidly changing nature of the health care sector (20,22,23). Prior to PPS, hospital admissions had been falling for all payors for a number of years and once PPS was enacted, Medicare admissions went down as well. The figures for fiscal year 1984 indicated an 11.3 percent decrease in admissions, resulting in a per-Medicare enrollee decline of 15.9 percent, which was counter to the steady rise in Medicare admissions during the 1978–84 period (20,22). While anecdotal evidence of skimming and dumping did surface, widespread use of these practices by hospitals had largely been documented for the uninsured and, in some states in particular, for Medicaid patients, rather than for Medicare patients.

Length of stay has been falling for Medicare since the inception of the act. Under the PPS system, an even steeper decline in average length of stay (down 17 percent for the first three years of PPS), combined with reduced admissions, has resulted in declining patient volumes. This reduced length of stay has been achieved through shorter stays across the board, rather than efforts aimed specifically at patients who have the longest stays (i.e., the most severely ill). This phenomenon indicates that PPS has been effective in encouraging hospitals to improve efficiency in the provision of inpatient care (22).

The Medicare Case-Mix Index increased sharply and the percentage of hospital days spent in special care units increased in the first three years after the implementation of PPS, possibly due to more judicious selections of candidates for inpatient hospitalization. Other studies of severity of illness at admission and discharge also show increases in the post-PPS period. The discharge of patients "quicker and sicker" has fostered rapid growth in the use of SNF and home health agency services by Medicare enrollees. Research indicates a tendency under PPS to increase the care provided to patients in other than inpatient settings (20). A survey of 200 physicians in five states shows that under prospective payment, hospitals encourage physicians to reduce ancillary services, shorten hospital stays, and increase outpatient testing (23). Hospital mortality rates for the Medicare

population have increased under PPS, but studies have explained this movement in terms of changing case mix and heightened severity of illness of patients (22). All in all, there is no systematic evidence that access to needed care has been hampered by PPS (23).

Criticisms of PPS

A number of criticisms have been levied against the incentives inherent in the DRG system. First, speculation exists that DRGs may not be "economically neutral" in that a hospital may be rewarded or penalized for performing an activity. To the extent that individual DRGs reflect procedures actually performed (e.g., types of surgery) as well as diagnosis, the choice of treatment may vary according to the "profitability" of that DRG and treatment decisions may not be made on purely clinical grounds. In a similar vein, physicians, in their clinical notes, and medical records administrators, in abstracting data for the DRG grouper program, might call upon "gaming" strategies to assure "DRG creep" to higher-level, more revenue-enhancing diagnoses (24).

Other criticisms involve the structure and mathematical integrity of DRGs. Several methods for changing PPS to a severity-based, rather than diagnosis-based, case-mix system have been postulated, along with schemes for refining DRG coding to reflect the severity of the condition (24,25,26). Research has demonstrated that the mathematical constructs of the DRGs lend themselves to "compression" in DRG prices; the prices of the truly high-cost DRGs are set low relative to their actual costs, whereas the prices of truly low-cost DRGs are set high relative to their costs (27). Recent research has confirmed the persistence of this phenomenon (28). Compression could create a situation in which hospitals may want to discriminate against providing service to patients in the high-cost DRGs or, on a positive note, it could encourage a few hospitals in competitive markets to specialize in efficiently providing "high-cost" services, such as coronary bypass surgery, at more profitable rates.

Financial Performance

Hospitals have generally fared well financially under PPS, but the distribution of results is uneven. On average, hospitals received Medicare reimbursements that exceeded considerably their corresponding costs. In the first three years of PPS, urban, large, and teaching hospitals experienced wider payment margins than their rural, small, nonteaching counterparts. In terms of overall financial performance, urban and proprietary hospitals, as well as regional referral centers, have manifested large margins, and sole community hospitals are disproportionately represented at the lower end of the range (22). The spate of hospital bankruptcies that were predicted at the inception of PPS have not taken place, but acquisitions and mergers have been rampant in the health care industry in recent years.

PPS appears to have decelerated the rate of increase in Medicare inpatient hospital expenditures. Although outpatient payments, which are excluded from PPS, have mushroomed, total Medicare benefit payments are increasing at a slower rate due to the sharp decline in growth of Part A payments. From fiscal year 1974 (which marked the end of wage and price controls under the Nixon administration) through fiscal year 1982 (the last year prior to enactment of TEFRA), Medicare inpatient hospital benefit payments increased at an annual rate of 10 percent in real terms. Under TEFRA, this rate of increase dropped to 6.8 percent in real terms. For the first three years of PPS, the slowdown was even more dramatic —a real annual rate of increase of 3.5 percent (20,22).

Economic projections have shown that PPS reduced Medicare's hospital costs substantially. Expenditures for hospital insurance would have been $18 billion more in 1990 were it not for PPS, representing a savings of about 20 percent (29).

Medicare Physician Reimbursement

From 1975 to 1990, Medicare's total payments for physician services grew at a faster rate than payments for hospital services. By 1990, physician services reached 27.5 percent of total Medicare spending, up from 21.4 percent in 1975. Over the same period, hospital care dropped as a share of total Medicare expenditures from 74.4 to 62.7 percent. Although the Reagan administration had intended to reform physician reimbursement for Medicare, these plans were postponed due to pressures from private-sector opponents of government regulation. Nonetheless, there was general agreement that physician payment under Medicare needed to be revised (4,30).

Congress directed the administration to study physician payment reform when it established Medicare's DRG-based prospective payment system for hospital care. One of the favored options was to develop a national fee schedule that would set a price for each type of service with adjustments for local wage costs. Another possible reform alternative was to establish physician DRGs. Research into this option, however, disclosed thorny problems in 1) applying DRGs to outpatient care, which is typified by a large number of encounters at a relatively small price per visit; 2) dividing the DRG payment among a number of doctors who may be involved in one illness episode; 3) marked geographic variations in practice patterns; 4) cost variability in DRGs used to reimburse the medical versus the surgical specialties, the latter of which are more homogeneous and lend themselves better to DRG-based payment (31,32).

Resource-Based Relative Values

On January 1, 1992, Medicare initiated a new system for reimbursing physicians using a resource-based relative-value (RBRV) scale, which will be phased in over four years. The new payment method divides resources needed to produce physician services into three components: physician work, practice expenses, and malpractice insurance costs. For each procedure, each of the three components is characterized by a numerical value representing its relative contribution to the expenses incurred in delivering the service (table 11-3). The total units drive the fee, which is derived by multiplying the total units by a conversion factor. The conversion factor is a single national value ($31 in 1992). In addition, as shown in table 11-4, the relative values of the three components are adjusted for geographic cost/price variations. The final fee is thus a geographically weighted summation of the three components of the RBRVs times the conversion factor (33,34,35).

For surgery, the RBRV payment schedule also establishes a uniform definition of "global surgery" to ensure that identical payments are made for the same amount of work and resources expended in furnishing specific surgical services on a nationwide basis. The initial evaluation or consultation by a surgeon is paid separately from the global surgery package. The global fee includes all preoperative visits and all medical and surgical services related to a procedure, covering a 90-day postoperative period for all visits by the primary surgeon (35).

Simulations done by the Harvard University developers of the new reimbursement system (33), show that certain types of physicians will be financial winners and losers under RBRVs in comparison to what they would have earned under the old fee schedule. Pathologists, radiologists, thoracic surgeons, cardiovascular surgeons, and ophthalmologists stand to lose from 25 to 45 percent of their former Medicare fees. Internists, immunologists, and family practitioners, on the other hand, are likely to gain from 35 to 65 percent over their previous Medicare earnings.

Selective Contracting

In 1982, the California legislature cleared the way for the state Medicaid program (Medi-Cal) and private insurers to enable payors to draw up contracts for the delivery of health services to their beneficiaries, selecting only hospitals and physi-cians that agreed to accept a negotiated price for their services. This practice of "selective contracting" was first embraced by the Medi-Cal program to contract hospitals at low per diem rates. The selection rule was uncomplicated: if the price was right and other specified conditions were met, a contract would be secured.

Not all hospitals competing for contracts, including large traditional Medi-Cal providers, gained them and, as a result of these shocks in the health care marketplace, the contracting process was enormously successful, with 67 percent of California hospitals, accounting for 72 percent of the Medi-Cal patients, awarded contracts by the end of the first year of negotiations. Furthermore, during the first two years of selective contracting, there was no evidence of reduced access to health resources for Medi-Cal patients or any change in the quality of care they received. Savings to the state were estimated at $165 million for the first year of the program and $235 million for the second year (36,37).

Cost cutting on an unprecedented scale was reported by hospitals receiving Medi-Cal contracts, demonstrating that competitive bidding shifts the burden of proof in hospital rate setting and encourages an active search for economies of operation. For contract hospitals, total payments (in constant dollars) fell 9.6 percent in the first year of the program; average payments per day fell 18.4 percent and payments per admission fell 19.7 percent. Teaching, nonprofit, and investor-owned hospitals absorbed the largest reductions in average payment per day. Even though the per diem rates held incentives for increasing inpatient stays, length of stay fell 1.5 percent. Hospital financial analyses showed that contractors were, on the whole, not adversely affected by selective contracting in the first two years (38).

Preferred Provider Organizations

The entry of private insurers and firms into selective contracting began in earnest in 1984 and quickly became known as "preferred provider or-

TABLE 11-3 Resource-Based Relative Value Units (RBRVs), Medicare 1992: Selected Procedures

Description	Physician Work	Practice Expense	Malpractice Insurance	Total Units
Repair of inguinal hernia, age 5 years or older	5.12	4.75	0.98	10.85
Cholecystectomy without cholangiography	9.81	8.03	1.70	19.54
Replacement of aortic valve	25.25	32.30	5.66	63.21
Coronary arteries bypass	25.63	38.90	6.81	71.34
Insertion of intraocular lens subsequent to cataract removal	8.39	13.16	0.69	22.24
Repair of retinal detachment, schleral buckling, with or without implant	14.87	22.15	1.16	38.18
Arthroscopy, knee, surgical; with meniscectomy (medial or lateral, including meniscal shaving)	7.93	12.02	1.94	21.89
Interpretation of computerized axial tomography scan of the brain with and without contrast	1.23	0.60	0.09	1.92
Vasectomy, unilateral or bilateral, including post-operative semen examination(s)	3.40	2.74	0.29	6.43
Transurethral resection of prostate, including control of postoperative bleeding, complete	12.23	12.65	1.23	26.11

SOURCE: Adapted from Grimaldi, P. L. (1991). RBRVs: How new physician fee schedule will work. *Healthcare Financial Management. 45*(9). 64.

ganizations" (PPOs). PPOs have become a rapid growth area in health insurance. By 1986, enrollment in PPOs had increased to 6.2 million people, with 28 percent of the nation's patient care physicians contracting with a PPO. With California leading the pack in selective contracting, five of the nation's 10 largest PPOs are in that state. By 1989, 685 PPOs were operational in the United States (2,39).

A PPO is an arrangement or contract between a panel of health care providers, usually hospitals and physicians, and purchasers of health care services. The providers agree to supply services to a defined group of patients on a discounted fee-for-service basis. The exclusive provider organization (EPO) is the extreme form of a PPO, wherein services provided by nonparticipating providers are not reimbursed at all (forcing the patient to pay the entire cost out of pocket unless care is rendered by an affiliated provider). Many PPO plans are sponsored by health insurance companies or self-insured employers (40).

PPOs generally have five key elements: 1) a limited number of physicians and hospitals; 2)

negotiated fee schedules; 3) utilization review; 4) consumer choice of provider with incentives to use PPO participating providers; and 5) expedient settlement of claims (41).

Utilization review is the principal mechanism used by PPOs for controlling costs via reducing inappropriate use of services. Typical methods of utilization review include preadmission certification of hospital stays and mandatory second opinions for surgery. Other mechanisms used by PPOs for cost control are contracting with low-cost providers and establishing a reimbursement system that realizes savings through discounted provider charges or incentives for reduced use. Discounts are generally 10 to 13 percent below usual charges and insurers are reporting premiums 10 to 20 percent below standard indemnity plans (39,40).

Health Care Reform

National Health Insurance

National health insurance (NHI) has been espoused by many for almost 60 years because it

TABLE 11-4. Geographic Practice Cost Indexes Used to Weight Components of RBRVs: Selected Cities, 1992

Locality	Physician Work	Practice Expense	Malpractice Insurance
Birmingham, AL	0.981	0.913	0.824
Los Angeles, CA	1.060	1.196	1.370
San Francisco, CA	1.038	1.303	1.370
Colorado	0.999	0.988	0.683
Washington, DC, area	1.059	1.168	0.947
Miami, FL	1.034	1.025	1.641
Atlanta, GA	0.975	1.022	0.752
Lexington and Louisville, KY	0.984	0.917	0.667
New Orleans, LA	0.994	1.003	1.185
Detroit, MI	1.059	1.091	1.763
St. Paul-Minneapolis, MN	1.014	1.024	0.748
Montana	0.967	0.926	0.718
New York, NY (Manhattan)	1.059	1.255	1.647
Dallas, TX	0.996	0.971	0.504
Vermont	0.942	0.941	0.533
Urban Massachusetts	1.002	1.131	0.855
Chicago, IL	1.004	1.114	1.773
North central Iowa	0.971	0.916	0.666

SOURCE: Adapted from Grimaldi, P. L. (1991). RBRVs: How new physician fee schedule will work. *Healthcare Financial Management. 45*(9). 66.

contains health care costs and provides universal access for the population. NHI came close to becoming part of the Social Security Act of 1935 and numerous bills, representing a spectrum of schemes, have been introduced and seriously debated by congressional session ever since. In the mid–1970s the NHI issue became so heated that both political parties introduced bills that were strikingly similar. NHI bills ran the gamut from expanding Medicare to new population groups (e.g., children under five years of age) to a national health service (NHS) concept like that of Sweden or Great Britain where the government owns the hospitals and the doctors are paid on the basis of capitation or salary by the NHS.

When Carter was elected to the presidency in 1976, many in the health arena assumed that NHI would be an eventuality. But early on it was evident that Carter took little interest in health issues. In the 1980s and early 1990s, the Reagan and Bush administrations were active in introducing cost-containment measures, such as PPS and RBRVs, for Medicare, but no serious consideration was given to sweeping reform of the entire system.

Heath care reform has been touted to be the domestic political "issue of the 1990s." Pressures for such reform have come from a wide variety of groups including providers, the elderly and disabled, labor unions, state and local governments, and insiders within the Washington establishment. Even health insurers and managed-care organizations are calling for change. The two main targets of discontent are 1) the growing numbers and financial burden of uninsured and underinsured Americans, and 2) the ever-spiraling costs of health care, which serve to erode American competitiveness in the international marketplace.

The Uninsured

According to estimates from the 1987 National Medical Expenditure Survey (42) one in five Americans (48 million) was uninsured for all or part of the year. About half of those uninsured (more than 24 million) were without coverage for the entire year; this amounts to 10.2 percent of the population. The other half either gained or lost some type of public or private coverage during 1987. On any given day, about 36 million were uninsured.

The majority of the uninsured were poor or hovering close to poverty level. The poor, according to the federal definition of poverty, accounted for about one-third of the uninsured. One-third are children 18 and under and one-third are either black or Hispanic. More than 40 percent live in the South and almost 25 percent live in the West (42).

A variety of estimates indicate that the proportion of uninsured Americans has been creeping up over the last decade. In addition to the growing ranks of poor, anecdotal evidence attests to the transiency of private insurance coverage for all Americans, linked as it is to employment status and subject to fluctuations in the economy. Constantly changing eligibility requirements for Medicaid and other public programs also add to the problem of frictional uninsurance for many of the nation's low-income population.

The plight of the uninsured impinges on the health care of all Americans for several reasons. First, it results in reduced access to care for the uninsured themselves, who are likely to postpone needed care until their medical conditions have escalated in severity. Thus, the heightened intensity of caring for sicker people increases the cost of care. Second, providers must recoup the costs of serving the uninsured from their paying customers—private insurers or the government. Insurance premiums go up commensurately and the taxpayer's burden enlarges. Third, this cost shifting imposes yet another pressure on the efficient production of American goods and services, many of which stand to lose their competitive advantage in the world economy. Finally, in a spiral effect, uninsurance feeds on itself. With health insurance premiums constantly escalating, many businesses, especially small ones, cannot afford to initiate or continue health insurance, thus adding to the problem.

Strategies for Reform

An unprecedented issue of the *Journal of the American Medical Association* appeared in May 1991 (43). The entire issue was devoted to health system reform proposals, a subject traditionally anathema to organized medicine. Thirteen articles, by authors spanning a variety of special interests, detailed a number of strategies for achieving a new system.

Most proposals called for a revised system administered by private insurers with employer/employee premium sharing, supplemented by some form of government financing for nonworking individuals and families. With few exceptions, the proposals called for universal access to health care and for the provision of health insurance to all employees (44). Looking to the political left, it was interesting that no plan advocated a national health service model, where the government owns the facilities and employs the doctors directly. On the right, only one of the plans called for increased privatization and freedom of choice.

In what can only be called a courageous editorial, George D. Lundberg, the editor of the *Journal* summed up the findings (45:2566):

Although there may be consensus that our society must provide basic medical/health care for all of our people, we seem not to be close to a consensus on how to do it. Virtually all comprehensive health care proposals involve major legislation of some sort. Since consensus means "general agreement or unanimity; group solidarity in sentiment or belief," it is unlikely that, either as a society or as a profession, we will ever reach a true consensus on how to proceed, so we must not wait for one. To pass federal legislation requires only a simple majority in both houses of Congress plus presidential approval.

International Comparisons

A great deal of interest of late has been focused on the health care systems of Canada and Germany (46,47,48,49,50). While each has its flaws, both countries have achieved universal access, ostensibly high quality, high-volume care, and significant cost controls. The Canadian system is financed equally by federal and provincial government general revenues in most provinces; Germany relies primarily on social health insurance linked to employment, supplemented by public general revenue funds. In both systems, global budgets are prospectively determined on an annual basis. In both systems, providers are predominantly private, independent contractors with the relevant health ministry acting as third-party payer—the sole purchaser and reimburser of health services. Many assert that it is this monopsony purchasing power that foster coalition building around issues of cost control, negotiated rate setting, and sustained quality of care. It is also argued that a universal reimbursement system promotes efficiencies that vastly reduce administrative costs.

In contrast to the Canadian and German national health insurance systems, the national health service model has been a growing movement in Europe (51). Among 12 nations in the European Community, six now have a national health service model—the United Kingdom, Denmark, Spain, Italy, Greece, and Portugal. France, Germany, Belgium, Luxembourg, Ireland, and the Netherlands remain without an NHS. Increasing regulation of health care is also notable in Western Europe.

Bush Proposal

In 1992, President Bush unveiled his proposal for health care reform. Calling on conservative principles, he advocated a type of voucher system, whereby needy families would be allowed to take up to a $3,750 family tax credit, inversely related to income, for the purchase of private health insurance. With the goal of providing better access to the poor, states would be financially induced to capitate and expand Medicaid programs.

Critics of the proposal noted that the tax credit voucher approach, linked to income taxes, might bypass many nonworking poor. Further, they held that it would take as much as $100 billion in additional government revenues to compensate for taxes lost to the credits, and Mr. Bush gave no indication as to how such funding would be forthcoming. Finally, the plan did not elucidate how cost controls would be achieved in the market-based approach.

Conclusion

Financing health services in the United States includes a plethora of institutions and activities. The growth of employer-based private health insurance discussed in detail in the next chapter, has stimulated unprecedented growth in health expenditures and biomedical advancement for the nation in the postwar era. The advent of Medicare and Medicaid in 1966 heralded a period of even more rapid growth, along with unbridled inflation, that persists to this day.

Inequities in access to health care, thought to have been alleviated by Medicare and Medicaid, and the extensive provision of voluntary health insurance for employed groups, have not been resolved. Universal health coverage has not been realized, and a substantial and growing amount of the U.S. population goes uninsured. State revenues have grown at rates slower than health care costs, inducing across-the-board reductions and more restrictive eligibility requirements for state Medicaid programs. The prospective payment system, the new Medicare physician fee schedule, selective contracting, and prepaid plans hold potential for ameliorating uncontrolled inflation in health care spending. However, effective means for identifying and monitoring the adequacy and appropriateness of health care, in an environment of either over-utilization or underutilization, have not been developed.

The cry for health care reform resounds in all sectors of the U.S. economy. While most policy makers agree on universal access, they are far from agreement on how to finance the system, reimburse the providers, and impose cost controls. Whatever transpires in the future is likely to revolve around the fundamental politic of health finance: private versus public, entitlement versus social welfare, monopsony purchasing versus competitive concessions, fee for service versus prepayment.

This chapter has provided a historical and methodological framework for understanding and analyzing health care finance in the United States today. The principles that have been presented will apply to health finance, no matter how dynamic the future of the health care sector proves to be.

References

1. U.S. Bureau of the Census. (1991). *Statistical abstract of the United States: 1991* (111th ed.). Washington, DC: U.S. Government Printing Office.
2. Health Insurance Association of America. (1991). *Source book of health insurance data, 1990.* Washington, DC: Author.
3. Levit, K. R., Lazenby, H. C., & Letsch, S. W. (1991). National health expenditures, 1990. *Health Care Financing Review. 13*(1). 29–54.
4. Sonnefeld, S. T., Waldo, D. R., Lemieux, J. A. & McKusick, D. R. (1991). Projections of national health expenditures through the year 2000. *Health Care Financing Review. 13*(1). 1–27.
5. Gornick, M., Greenberg, N. J., Eggers, P. W., et al. (1985). Twenty years of Medicare and Medicaid: Covered populations, use of benefits, and program expenditures. *Health Care Financing Review.* (Annual suppl.). 13–59.
6. Gibson, R. M. (1980). National health expenditures, 1979. *Health Care Financing Review. 2.* 1–36.
7. Roemer, M. I. (1978). *Social medicine: The advance of organized health services in America.* New York: Springer.
8. Roemer, M. I. (1977). *Comparative national policies on health care.* New York: Marcel Dekker.
9. Farley, P. J. (1986). *Private health insurance in the United States.* Data preview 23, National Medical Care Expenditure Survey (DHHS Publication No. [PHS] 86-3406, pp. 1–106). Washington, DC: National Center for Health Services Research and Health Care Technology Assessment.
10. American Medical Association. (1984, July 30). *Q&A: New provisions for physician reimbursement under Medicare.* Chicago: Author.
11. Lubitz, J., & Prihoda, R. (1984). Use and costs of Medicare services in the last two years of life. *Health Care Financing Review. 5.* 117–131.
12. Fuchs, V. R. (1984). "Though much is taken": Reflections on aging, health, and medical care. *Milbank Memorial Fund Quarterly. 62.* 143–166.
13. Reilly, T. W., Clausen, S. B., & Baugh, D. K. (1990). Trends in Medicaid payments and utilization. *Health Care Financing Review. 12*(Annual Suppl.). 15–33.
14. Waldo, M. O. (1990). A brief summary of the Medicaid program. *Health Care Financing Review. 12*(Annual Suppl.). 171–172.
15. Altman, D., & Beatrice, D. F. (1990). Perspectives on the Medicaid program. *Health Care Financing Review. 12*(Annual Suppl.) 2–5.
16. Reinhardt, U. E. (1985). The compensation of physicians: Approaches used in foreign countries. *Quality Review Bulletin. 11.* 366–377.
17. Enthoven, A. (1981). The competition strategy; status and prospects. *New England Journal of Medicine. 304.* 109–112.
18. Deloitte Haskins & Sells. (1982). *Tax Equity and Fiscal Responsibility Act of 1982: Management strategies for health care providers.* New York: Author.
19. Deloitte Haskins & Sells. (1982). *Medicare prospective payment system—1983: Strategies for health care providers.* New York: Author.
20. Guterman, S., & Dobson, A. (1986). Impact of the Medicare prospective payment system for hospitals. *Health Care Financing Review. 7.* 97–114.
21. American Medical Association. (1984). *Diagnosis-related groups (DRGs) and the prospective payment system.* Chicago: Author.
22. Guterman, S., Eggers, P. W., Riley, G., Greene, T. F., & Terrell, S. A. (1988). The first three years of Medicare prospective payment: An overview. *Health Care Financing Review. 9*(3). 67–77.
23. DesHarnais, S., Kobrinski, E., Chesney, J., et al. (1987). The early effects of the prospective payment system on inpatient utilization and the quality of care. *Inquiry. 24.* 7–16.

24. Jencks, S. F., Dobson, A., Willis, P., et al. (1984). Evaluating and improving the measurement of hospital case mix. *Health Care Financing Review*. (Annual Suppl.). 1–11.

25. Smits, H. L., Fetter, R. B., & McMahon, L. F., Jr. (1984). Variation in resource use within diagnosis-related groups: The severity issue. *Health Care Financing Review*. (Annual Suppl.). 71–78.

26. Horn, S. D., & Horn, R. A. (1986). Reliability and validity of the Severity of Illness Index. *Medical Care*. 24. 159–178.

27. Lave, J. R. (1985). Is compression occurring in DRG prices? *Inquiry*. 22. 142–147.

28. Keeler, E. B., Kahn, K. L., Draper, D., Sherwood, M. J., et al. (1990). Changes in sickness at admission following the introduction of the prospective payment system. *Journal of the American Medical Association*. 264(15). 1962–1968.

29. Russell, L. B., & Manning, C. L. (1989). The effect of prospective payment on Medicare expenditures. *New England Journal of Medicine*. 320(7). 439–444.

30. Hadley, J. (1984). How should Medicare pay physicians? *Milbank Memorial Fund Quarterly*. 62. 279–299.

31. Mitchell, J. B. (1985). Physician DRGs. *New England Journal of Medicine*. 313. 670–675.

32. Culler, S., & Ehrenfried, D. (1986). On the feasibility of physician DRGs. *Inquiry*. 23. 40–55.

33. Hsiao, W. C., Braun, P., Dunn, D., Becker, E. R., DeNicola, M., & Ketcham, T. R. (1988). Results and policy implications of the resource-based relative-value study. *New England Journal of Medicine*. 319(13). 881–888.

34. Hsiao, W. C., Braun, P., Yntema, D., & Becker, E. R. (1988). Estimating physicians' work for a resource-based relative-value scale. *New England Journal of Medicine*. 319(13). 835–841.

35. Grimaldi, P. L. (1991). RBRVs: How new physician fee schedule will work. *Healthcare Financial Management*. 45(9). 58–75.

36. Johns, L., Derzon, R. A., & Anderson, M. D. (1985). Selective contracting in California: Early effects and policy implications. *Inquiry*. 22. 24–32.

37. Johns, L., Anderson, M. D., & Derzon, R. A. (1985). Selective contracting in California: Experience in the second year. *Inquiry*. 22. 335–347.

38. Mennemayer, S. T., & Olinger, L. (1989). Selective contracting in California: Its effect on hospital finances. *Inquiry*. 26. 442–457.

39. Rice, T., Gabel, J., & de Lissovoy, G. (1989). PPOs: The employer perspective. *Journal of Health Politics*. 14(2). 367–373.

40. Gabel, J., Ermann, D., Rice, T., et al. (1986). The emergence and future of PPOs. *Journal of Health Politics*. 11. 305–322.

41. de Lissovoy, G., Rice, T., Ermann, D., et al. (1986). Preferred providers organizations: Today's models and tomorrow's prospects. *Inquiry*. 23. 7–15.

42. Short, P. F. (1990). *Estimates of the uninsured population, calendar year 1987* (DHHS Publication No. [PHS] 90-3469). National Medical Expenditure Survey Data Summary 2. Rockville, MD: Agency for Health Care Policy and Research.

43. *Journal of the American Medical Association*. (1991). 265(19).

44. Blendon, R. J., & Edwards, J. N. (1991). Caring for the uninsured: Choices for reform. *Journal of the American Medical Association*. 265(19). 2563–2565.

45. Lundberg, G. D. (1991). National health care reform: An aura of inevitability is upon us. *Journal of the American Medical Association*. 265(19). 2566–2567.

46. Iglehart, J. K. (1986). Canada's health care system: Part one. *New England Journal of Medicine*. 315(3). 202–208.

47. Iglehart, J. K. (1986). Canada's health care system: Part two. *New England Journal of Medicine*. 315(12). 778–784.

48. Neuschler, E. (1990). *Canadian health care: The implications of public health insurance*. Washington, DC: Health Insurance Association of America.

49. Reinhardt, U. E. (1990). West Germany's health-care and health-insurance system: Combining universal access with cost control. In the Pepper Commission. *A call for action: Final report of the U.S. Bipartisan Commission on Comprehensive Health Care*. Washington, DC: U.S. Government Printing Office.

50. Hurst, J. W. (1991). Reform of health care in Germany. *Health Care Financing Review*. 12(3). 73–101.

51. Abel-Smith, B. (1985). Who is the odd man out? The experience of western Europe in containing the costs of health care. *Milbank Memorial Fund Quarterly*. 63. 1–7.

Chapter 12

![decorative bar]

Private Health Insurance and Employee Benefits

Gary Whitted

After Medicare, private health insurance is the most prevalent source of financing for the United States health care system. Few other industrialized countries maintain systems of private medical insurance programs that even approximate those established in the United States. Private health insurance coverage is by far the most comprehensive source of medical care financing for Americans, and it continues to play a pivotal role in influencing the direction and structure of the U.S. medical care system.

The term "health insurance" often is employed to mean a wide array of health care financing mechanisms—the "social insurance" of Medicare, the public assistance of Medicaid, the "self-insurance" techniques adopted by large employers, and the managed care programs of health maintenance organizations (HMOs) and preferred provider organizations (PPOs). This chapter is limited in discussion to those variants of "insurance" that do not involve government, since the subjects of Medicare, Medicaid, and other prominent government-sponsored medical care financing programs are covered in Chapter 11. Since health insurance and employee medical benefits are inextricably linked for most American families, this chapter will often look at these two concepts together, even though many medical benefits programs are not "insurance" in the technical or legal sense.

Insurance Concepts

Central to any definition of "insurance" is the notion of "risk." One standard insurance text defines "risk" as "the possibility of an adverse deviation from a desired outcome that is expected or hoped for," or more simply as "a possibility of loss" (1). Insurance is a mechanism for managing or controlling the financial exposure to this risk through two basic principles: 1) transferring or shifting risk from an individual to a group; and 2) sharing losses on some equitable basis by all members of the group (2). Depending on individuals' or employers' preferences about how much risk they want to assume, as well as their various abilities to withstand the economic consequences of the losses, the amount and type of insurance required can vary substantially.

When health insurance began in the United States, conceptually it was similar to most other types of insurance—for example, auto insurance. In both cases, insurance was purchased to protect an individual from an expensive loss—hospital care or a badly damaged automobile. However, as private health insurance evolved to cover more people and a wider variety of medical expenses, it began to assume characteristics very dissimilar from traditional forms of insurance, by violating certain implied rules, such as:

1. A "loss" is supposed to be something out of the ordinary, as well as something to be avoided. However, ill health is not a substantially abnormal event for most people, and in many cases the "loss" being indemnified (e.g., a physician office visit) is not necessarily an event to be dreaded.
2. "Losses" are intended to be fairly independent events. In contrast, the very nature of infectious illness (or in the extreme, an epidemic) implies a great degree of dependency among insureds' losses.
3. The "loss" should be of such financial magnitude that it is realistically unbudgetable for most insureds. The growth of so-called "first-dollar" base/major medical health plans (prominent in the 1970s and early 1980s) directly violated this tenet. Even today, providing insurance coverage for items such as pharmaceuticals or vision care stretches the limits of the "insurance" principle.

Thus, it is not surprising that health insurance has become a fundamentally different product from most all other forms of insurance. And many health care observers have noted that these unique characteristics of health insurance, when added to the economic structures of the medical care marketplace, have made health insurance a chief contributor to the continued rapid growth of health expenditures in the United States. Ironically, the presence and growth of health insurance in the 1950s and 1960s provided a financial foundation for much of medical-industrial complex that now fuels medical expenses. And the presence of health insurance creates a "Catch-22" situation in which

the existence of the insurance mechanism (often distorted to include first-dollar coverage of non-catastrophic expenses) stimulates demand and increases medical care prices, thereby raising the cost of health care and encouraging even greater insistence on more comprehensive coverage.

A Brief History of U.S. Health Insurance

The history of medical expense insurance in the United States, discussed briefly in the previous chapter, goes back to the middle of the 19th century, when in 1850 the Franklin Health Insurance Company of Massachusetts offered coverage for bodily injuries that did not result in death (3). Ten years later, the Travelers Insurance Companies first extended health coverage in a form similar to today's insurance. By 1866, 60 other insurance companies were writing forms of such coverage. At the end of the century, accident and life insurers were writing health insurance policies, primarily to indemnify against loss of income and for certain acute illnesses. However, the real beginning of modern private health insurance took place in 1929, when a group of teachers made a contract with Baylor Hospital in Dallas, Texas, to provide coverage against certain hospital expenses, thereby starting the first "Blue Cross" plan.

During the 1930s and until the wartime period of the 1940s, health insurance coverage grew rather slowly, in terms of both the insured population and the types of coverage offered. In 1940, insurers provided some form of medical expense protection to 12 million people, 9 percent of the total U.S. population (table 12-1). A series of legal and tax developments in the mid–1940s and early 1950s provided nontrivial inducements for both employers and employees to purchase comprehensive health insurance benefits (4–8). In 1942, only 37 insurers wrote group health insurance coverage; by 1951, this number had climbed to 212 (8). By 1950, the number of people covered by the nation's health insurers had climbed to nearly 77 million, 53 percent of the U.S. population. Fueled by the strong union gains of the 1950s and 1960s,

TABLE 12-1. Distribution of Covered Persons, by Type of Private Health Insurance

Year	Net Number of Persons with Private Health Insurance (Millions)	Percentage Distribution		
		Commercial Insurance Companies	Blue Cross/ Blue Shield Plans	HMOs and Self-Funded Plans
1940	12.0	31%	50%	19%
1945	32.0	33%	59%	8%
1950	76.6	46%	48%	5%
1955	101.4	48%	46%	6%
1960	122.5	56%	47%	5%
1965	138.7	52%	44%	5%
1970	158.8	52%	43%	5%
1975	178.2	50%	43%	7%
1980	187.4	47%	38%	15%
1985(e)	181.3	43%	34%	24%
1988(e)	182.3	39%	31%	30%

SOURCE: Health Insurance Association of America. (1991). *Source book of health insurance data, 1990* (p. 23). Washington, DC: Author.

NOTE: Percentages sum to 100 percent, as persons with duplicate coverages are counted multiple times.

(e) = Estimate; 1988 data exclude coverage for hospital indemnity coverage by commercial insurers, which is included for prior years.

collectively bargained employee benefits packages quickly became the norm throughout industrial America.

In 1960, 123 million Americans held some type of health insurance protection, generating about $5 billion in payments and accounting for nearly 21 percent of the financing for personal health care expenditures (see tables 12-1–12-2). During the 1960s, health insurance coverage was expanded to an additional 36 million Americans, while health insurance payments tripled to $15 billion, representing more than 23 percent of total U.S. personal health care expenditures. The inauguration in 1965 of Medicare and Medicaid greatly expanded Americans' protection against catastrophic medical expenses for our most vulnerable citizens, the elderly and indigent. But these two programs also gave substantial impetus to the notion that affordable access to the health care system was as much a right for Americans.

The decade of the 1970s witnessed another 29 million Americans added to the roster of the health-insured population, as the health insurance industry plateaued in terms of the depth of medical coverage, while introducing new forms of health insurance protection (principally dental and prescription drug insurance). By 1980, health insurance paid nearly 30 percent of the nation's personal health care bill, more than $65 billion. Although the 1980s saw proportionately slower growth in the number of Americans with private health insurance protection than in earlier decades, private health insurance expenditures nearly tripled to $191 billion by 1990, even though neither the depth nor breadth of coverage increased nearly as dramatically as in previous eras. In 1990, private health insurance and employee benefit programs are responsible for financing nearly one-third of all personal medical care expenditures (see table 12-2).

Despite an increase from 12 million people protected by private health insurance in 1940 to 185 million in 1985 (about 76 percent of the civilian noninstitutionalized population), political concern escalated in the early 1990s about the number of

TABLE 12-2. Private Health Insurance as a Health Care Financing Vehicle

Year	Private Health Insurance Expenditures (Billions)	Per Capita Health Insurance Expenditures	Private Health Insurance as a Percent of Total Personal Health Care Expenditures
1960	$5.0	$26	20.9%
1965	$8.7	$42	24.2%
1970	$15.2	$71	23.4%
1975	$31.2	$139	26.6%
1980	$65.3	$277	29.8%
1985	$114.0	$461	30.8%
1990	$191.2	$737	32.5%
1995(e)	$302.6	$1,113	31.6%
2000(e)	$444.6	$1,572	30.5%

SOURCES: Waldo, Daniel R., et al. (1986). National health expenditures, 1985. *Health Care Financing Review,* *8*(1), p. 16. Levit, K. R., et al. (1991). National health expenditures, 1990. *Health Care Financing Review.* *13*(1), p. 49. Sonnefield, S. T. (1991). Projections of national health expenditures through the year 2000. *Health Care Financing Review.* *13*(1), p. 18–24.

(e) = Estimate.

individuals without any financial protection for health care expenses. Perhaps the best evidence of concern over the uninsured was demonstrated by the normally staid American Medical Association, which devoted an entire issue of its journal (and subsequent articles in later issues) to this topic (9).

The National Center for Health Statistics estimated that in 1989, 34 million people in the civilian, noninstitutionalized population (nearly 14 percent) lacked health care coverage of any type (private health insurance, Medicare, Medicaid, or military and VA) (10). This substantial number of Americans made vulnerable to the economic consequences of serious medical illness (or for low-income individuals, even relatively routine medical care) has become a potent political cause as the U.S. enters the last decade of the 20th century. Lack of health insurance protection is greatest for the unemployed, minority, younger-age, and low-income/moderate-income segments of the U.S. population (10,11,12).

Yet even among the employed population under age 65, more than 14 percent were without health insurance protection, due principally to lapses of coverage between jobs, the preexisting condition limitation clauses of most employee benefits pro-

TABLE 12-3. Percentage of Companies Offering Group Health Insurance Coverage to Employees, by Size of Firm

Year	Number of Employees in Firm			
	1–24	25–99	100–499	500+
1979	36%	65%	77%	86%
1988	39%	66%	74%	81%

SOURCE: *Wall Street Journal,* November 22, 1991; data are from the U.S. Small Business Administration.

TABLE 12-4. Composition of U.S. Business Establishments, Employees, and Payroll, by Size of Establishment, 1982

Number of Employees	Percentage of Total Establishments	Percentage of Total Employees	Percentage of Total Payroll
1–19	88%	27%	23%
20–99	11%	28%	25%
100–499	2%	24%	24%
500–999	—	7%	9%
1,000+	—	14%	20%

Figures may not sum to 100%, due to rounding.

SOURCE: U.S. Department of Commerce, Bureau of the Census. (1982). *County Business Patterns 1982, United States,* Washington, D.C.—U.S. Government Printing Office, p. xii and p. 3.

grams, and lack of employee benefits for employees in many small businesses and the self-employed. Indeed, two-thirds of the uninsured population are in families of full-year, steadily employed workers, most of whom are employed full-time. Nearly half of uninsured workers are self-employed or are employed in small concerns with fewer than 25 employees (11). Employees working in small establishments are particularly vulnerable to inadequate or nonexistent health insurance coverage (table 12-3). Contrary to popular opinion, most Americans are not employed by *Fortune* 500 corporations, as table 12-4 clearly depicts.

Alternate Health Insurance Taxonomies

Most of what falls into the category "health insurance" is a combination of true insurance and employee benefits. One methodology for gaining an overview of health insurance is to subdivide the general area using different criteria. First, the principal insurance vehicles provide benefits associated with ill health: 1) basic employee benefits (primarily medical, dental, vision, and prescription drug coverage); 2) disability (short- and long-term insurance offered as part of many employee benefits programs, as well as compulsory temporary disability insurance mandated by five states); and 3) workers' compensation. Employers pay for some or all of each category of insurance, with the first

type of insurance reimbursing most of the expenditures attributed to "health insurance."

A second major categorization of health insurance is by the type of organization furnishing the coverage. First and foremost among such organizations are the approximately 800 insurance carriers that comprise the "commercial" health insurance industry (13). Second, there are 73 Blue Cross and Blue Shield plans. While technically offering insurance, the "Blues" historically maintained a different tax status from that of the "commercials." (The Tax Reform Act of 1986, PL 99-514, removed the federal tax exemption for Blue Cross and Blue Shield organizations engaged in providing commercial-type insurance.) Third, health maintenance organizations (HMOs) offer a form of health insurance, although not in the same legal definition as either the Blues or the commercials. HMOs, in addition to retaining different tax and regulatory structures from those of either the Blues or commercials, differ from those two entities in one very fundamental sense: HMOs are not guaranteeing to *reimburse* the insured for medical expenses; rather, their obligation to the insured is more direct—to actually *provide* medical services to them. A fourth major entity in furnishing health insurance is employers (primarily large corporations) that self-fund or partially self-fund employee benefits for workers and their families. Although declining in importance, unions are a fifth type of health insurance sponsor. Finally, corporations and

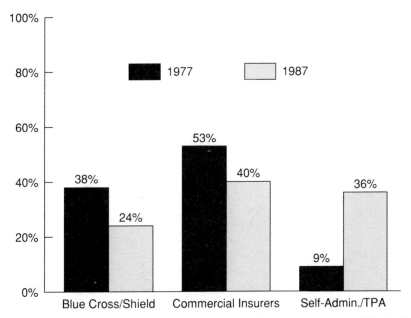

Figure 12-1. Market shares for "Conventional" health insurance, by type of intermediary (SOURCE: DiCarlo, S., & Gabel, J. (1989). Conventional health insurance: A decade later. *Health Care Financing Review. 10*(3). p. 82.) "Conventional" Is Non-HMO & Non-PPO.

unions sometimes jointly sponsor and administer "Taft-Hartley" health and welfare funds.

A third taxonomy of health insurance is by funding mechanism: 1) Fully insured; 2) Partially insured; and 3) self-funded or self-insured. The funding mechanisms of health insurance should not be confused with the three principal administrative intermediaries: 1) insurers; 2) third-party administrators (TPAs); or 3) self-administration. The market shares for these types of intermediaries have changed drastically during the last 15 years (figure 12-1).

What makes these taxonomies confusing is that there is substantial overlap between (and even within) each categorization. The Travelers Insurance Companies is indicative of this complexity. Under the umbrella of Travelers are a number of individually licensed insurance companies, providing an array of traditional health insurance, disability, and workers' compensation products, primarily for employers, unions, and Taft-Hartley plans. Each of these products is offered in fully insured, partially insured, or self-funded capacities. The

Travelers also owns 11 licensed HMOs, administers medical benefits through nearly 60 preferred provider organizations (PPOs) and more than 40 "point-of-service" networks, and operates a nationwide dental PPO network. Finally, The Travelers maintains a subsidiary called Travelers Plan Administrators, a network of 14 TPAs—the third largest such organization in the United States. Other large commercial insurers maintain an analogous series of interlocking products, financing options, and administrative alternatives. Similarly, the Blues offer comprehensive medical insurance products (primarily in an insured capacity) and they operate both HMOs and PPOs.

The Commercial Health Insurance Industry

There are several ways to describe the "commercial" health insurance industry. Perhaps the most fundamental distinction is between "mutual" and "stock" insurers. Mutual insurance companies essentially are owned by their policyholders, in contrast to stock insurance companies, which are owned in the more traditional corporate fashion by stockholders. In 1989, approximately 60 percent of net premiums for accident and health insurance were written by stock companies (14), which include such large insurers as Travelers, CIGNA, and Aetna (well-known mutual health insurers are Prudential, Metropolitan, and Mutual of Omaha). Within each type of insurer are so-called "multiline" carriers and "single-line" insurers. Multiline insurers, such as Travelers, Aetna, and CIGNA, offer life insurance and accident and health insurance, as well as "property/casualty" insurance (e.g., auto, homeowners, workers' compensation, comprehensive general liability, etc.) Many multiline insurers also operate businesses that offer a range of financial products and services, particularly in the pension and investment areas. In contrast, single-line insurers usually offer the majority of their insurance products in the life insurance, property/casualty, or health insurance/employee benefits arena. Examples of single-line insurers are State Farm and Allstate.

Despite the approximately 800 companies that participate in writing health insurance and/or providing employee benefit programs, the commercial health insurance industry is moderately concentrated. As table 12-5 depicts, about one-quarter of the $62 billion in total net accident and health premiums written by accident and health insurers in 1990 was contributed by only five large insurers, with the top 10 insurers maintaining 38 percent of the premium volume and the top 50 insurers responsible for 71 percent of total premiums. In 1990, 11 large commercial accident and health insurers each wrote more than $1 billion in premiums (15). (Use of the word "premium" generally refers only to true "insured" products, not to partially insured or self-funded medical payments that flow through insurance companies via other administrative arrangements. These latter monies often are described as "premium-equivalents," which usually are several times the size of true premiums.) Because most the major U.S. self-funded employee benefits programs are administered by

TABLE 12-5. Market Concentration in the Insurance Industry

	Percent of Total Premiums Written	
	Accident & Health Insurers	Property/ Casualty Insurers
Top 5 Insurers	23%	29%
Top 10 Insurers	38%	40%
Top 50 Insurers	71%	74%
Top 250 Insurers	N/A	94%
Top 300 Insurers	97%	N/A
Total Net Premiums Written (Est.)	$60 Billion	$218 Billion
Number of Insurers With Greater Than $1 Billion in Premiums	11	42

SOURCES: *Best's Review* (Property/Casualty Edition), July 1991 *Best's Review* (Life/Health Edition), December 1991 © A.M. Best Company—Used with permission.

the largest accident and health insurers, the concentration of the total generic health insurance/employee benefits industry is even more pronounced than indicated by accident and health insurance premium volume alone.

Blue Cross and Blue Shield Plans

As noted earlier, Blue Cross plans initiated the modern era of private health insurance in 1929. Throughout the early portion of their history, Blue Cross plans focused attention on medical insurance for hospital costs, and Blue Cross itself was closely affiliated with the hospital industry. Approximately 10 years after its establishment, Blue Shield began offering medical insurance protection for physicians' services. As with Blue Cross, Blue Shield was loosely affiliated with organized medicine because of its focus on insuring physician expenditures.

Since their inceptions, many Blue Cross and Blue Shield plans have merged their activities, becoming essentially a single insurance entity in a state. However, by the 1980s, a number of Blue Cross and Blue Shield plans reversed this posture and divorced themselves from each other, in a few cases becoming bitter rivals. Today, there are 73 Blue Cross and Blue Shield plans throughout the United States. In recent years, the national Blue Cross and Blue Shield Association, which heretofore had provided only a minimal amount of integration among its member constituents, has become more aggressive in attempting to marshal the resources of individual plans (e.g., in the area of centralized claims processing). This cooperation has been necessary in order to compete effectively with large national commercial insurance companies for the business of employers operating in more than one state. The Blue Cross and Blue Shield Association also has developed a national HMO network, for the same reason.

Unlike commercial insurance companies, which are regulated in most states by a state insurance department, Blue Cross and Blue Shield plans are subject to special enabling state legislation. In addition to the historically close affiliations of the Blues with hospital and physician providers, the Blues have differentiated themselves historically from commercial insurers by establishing premium levels using a "community" rating methodology (in contrast to the "experience" rating most often used by commercial insurers).

Another key area of differentiation historically between the Blues and commercial insurers was the former's adoption of "service" benefits (i.e., reimbursement for the total costs of covered benefits), rather than the "indemnity" benefits (i.e., payment of a fixed sum for a covered benefit) of commercial insurers. Today, however, particularly for group insurance, commercial insurers offer service benefits; major exceptions are some individual and supplementary policies, as well as specialty insurance (e.g., cancer insurance).

One final point of distinction for the Blues is their traditional reluctance to underwrite quite as rigidly as commercial carriers, particularly with respect to refusing coverage for entire industry groups or for individuals. In some states, for some populations, the Blues are the only health insurer of any significant size. However, all these historical differences between the Blues and commercial insurers are rapidly disappearing.

Due in part to these unique historical roles and unconventional insurance financial practices, a number of large Blues plans recently have been chronicled as teetering on financial instability (16). Most notably, during 1990 Blue Cross of West Virginia essentially became insolvent, leaving behind $50 million in unpaid medical bills. Its financial obligations and territory were assumed by Blue Cross and Blue Shield of Northern Ohio.

Health Maintenance Organizations *[Managed care]*

Although coining of the term health maintenance organizations (HMO) was attributed to Dr. Paul Ellwood in the early 1970s, these insurance-like organizations have been in existence for over a half-century. In 1929, the Ross-Loos Clinic in Los Angeles was the first generally recognized HMO (or prepaid group practice, to use the pre-Ellwood term); however, one can argue that the true roots of prepaid group practice began at the Mayo Clinic in the late 1800s.

Beginning with Kaiser's coverage of the health needs associated with workers building the Grand Coulee Dam in the 1930, health maintenance organizations grew relatively slowly until the Nixon administration sparked new interest in these providers of predominantly group medical benefits (Chapter 13). Enrollment has been strongest since the mid–1980s (table 12-6), fueled by employers' dissatisfaction with the escalating costs of their employee medical benefits programs and the concomitant published research demonstrating the cost-containment success of many HMOs (particularly large, well-established plans such as Kaiser, Health Insurance Plan of New York, and Group Health Cooperative of Puget Sound). Growth of HMOs was also stimulated by the HMO Act of 1973 (PL 93-222) and its subsequent amendments. These statutes required employers with more than 25 employees to offer an HMO option if a

TABLE 12-6. HMO Growth, 1976–1990

Year	Number of Plans	Enrollment (Millions)
1976	174	6.0
1978	202	7.5
1980	235	9.1
1982	264	10.8
1984	304	15.1
1986	623	25.7
1989	604	31.9
1990	572	33.0

SOURCE: U.S. Department of Health & Human Services, Public Health Service, Center for Disease Control, National Center for Health Statistics. (1991). (DHHS Publication No. PHS 91-1232). Hyattsville, M.D.: U.S. Government Printing Office.

local, federally qualified HMO so "mandated." The legislation also required employers to contribute toward the HMO premium of its employees an amount equal to that contributed toward indemnity plan premiums—the so-called "equal contribution" rule.

At the beginning of 1991, Interstudy data indicated that 34 million Americans were covered by HMOs, about 14 percent of the total U.S. population (17). In 1990, the Group Health Association of America (GHAA) counted 570 HMOs. Data from the GHAA shows that 70 percent of HMO enrollees reside in the 27 largest metropolitan areas, with one-quarter of all HMO members living in either greater Los Angeles or San Francisco (18). In some cities (such as San Francisco or Minneapolis), HMO market penetration is 45 percent. However, in some northeastern metropolitan areas, such as greater New York City, market penetration is only 11 percent. Nine major cities have been served by HMOs for at least 30 years.

In the 1990s, HMO growth has slowed somewhat, due to several factors. First, the emergence of competing "alternative delivery systems," such as preferred provider organizations (and more recently "point-of-service" and "triple choice" managed care options), have provided employers with

cost-effective, middle-of-the-road medical benefit plan options. Principal among the attractions to employers of these non-HMO options is the enhanced employee freedom of choice regarding providers, particularly physicians. Second, the wave of enthusiasm for HMOs regarding their potential cost containment prowess was tempered during the late 1980s, when many HMOs' premium increases reached levels nearly as great as those of indemnity insurers and the Blues (19). In addition, research findings (aided by the "gut" feelings of many large employers) indicted HMOs for "cream skimming" the healthier risks toward the HMO, supposedly leaving the remaining indemnity medical plan options saddled with the "sicker" insured (20,21). Finally, for reasons of administrative ease and fear of the financial and liability consequences of dealing with potentially insolvent HMOs, some employers have trimmed substantially the number of HMOs offered to employees. This trend undoubtedly will continue during the 1990s, particularly beginning in 1995, when the dual-choice "mandating" provision of the 1973 HMO Act will no longer apply to employers, due to legislative amendments enacted in 1988. This same legislation, updated by the Department of Health and Human Services in 1991, also will permit greater employer flexibility in determining their required contributions to HMO premiums (22).

As discussed in detail in Chapter 13, HMOs generally are characterized by their form of organization, according to one of our principal structures: 1) group; 2) staff; 3) independent practice association (IPA); and 4) network (see figure 12-2). In group plans (Kaiser is the most prominent one), a physician medical group contracts with an entity that is financially responsible for covering enrollees. For example, the Kaiser Permanente Medical Care Program actually is a combination of three different groups: 1) The Permanente Medical Groups (providing professional services); 2) Kaiser Foundation Hospitals (providing hospital care); and 3) Kaiser Foundation Health Plans (providing administrative and financial services). In the network model, the HMO contracts with two or more in-

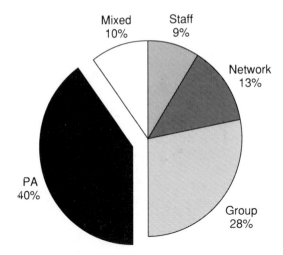

January 1991 Enrollment (34 Million)

Figure 12-2. HMO enrollment, by type of plan (SOURCE: Kenkel, Paul J. (1991). HMOs Choosing IPA Partners with Care. *Modern Healthcare. 21* (49), p. 42.)

dependent group practices. Staff model HMOs (such as Group Health Cooperative of Puget Sound) employ most primary care physicians and major speciality physicians on a full-time, salaried basis. Hospital services and the rarer physician specialities are arranged through separate contracts. IPA-model HMOs forge the same types of hospital arrangements as staff-model HMOs, but physicians' services are established with a relatively large number of generally small or medium-sized group practices, with physicians receiving some type of discounted fee-for-service payment from the HMO, rather than the salaried reimbursement of staff-model HMO physicians.

As stated earlier, HMOs differ fundamentally from the true "insurers" (i.e., commercials and Blue Cross/Blue Shield), because HMOs are not offering reimbursement for health care outlays; rather, HMOs actually guarantee the *provision* of covered health services. Like the historical record of Blue Cross and Blue Shield plans, HMOs generally have relied on community, not experience rating. (Indeed, the HMO Act of 1973 required federally qualified HMOs to price insurance in this manner.) However, due to both competitive pressures and employers' in-

creasing paranoia about perceived cream skimming by HMOs, HMOs are being pressured to engage in experience rating (which has been permitted since 1989 by subsequent amendments to the HMO Act of 1973). Another distinction between HMOs and their pure "insurance" colleagues is that HMOs often are regulated by an entirely different set of statutes and organizations than either commercial insurers or the Blues. In California, for example, there is (state) Insurance Department regulation for commercial insurers, while HMOs are overseen by the Department of Corporations.

HMOs not only can be freestanding organizations (Kaiser is the largest example, with United Health Corporation and U.S. Healthcare Inc. also very large HMO competitors), but the Blues and commercial insurers also own and operate HMOs. As depicted in table 12-7, for example, the Blue Cross and Blue Shield Plan HMOs form an integrated network that is nearly as large as industry leader Kaiser, while CIGNA, Aetna, and Prudential own HMO networks that place these insurers among the 10 largest HMO operators in the United States. Although the earliest large HMOs (such as Kaiser, Health Insurance Plan of New York, and Group Health Cooperative of Puget Sound), as well as some of the newer, well-respected HMOs (such as the Harvard Community Health Plan in Boston), were organized as not-for-profit entities, many of the newer, rapidly expanding HMOs (such as U.S. Healthcare Inc.) and most of the commercial insurance company-sponsored HMOs are for-profit organizations.

Private Health Insurance as a Financing Mechanism

Private health insurance is made up of the three principal entities just described (commercial carriers, the Blues, and HMOs), plus self-funded plans. As indicated in figure 12-3, the importance of private health insurance as a source of financing for personal health care expenditures has increased slowly but steadily. In 1960, private health insurance funded more than one-fifth of these

TABLE 12-7. Top 10 General Service HMOs, June 1991

Health Maintenance Organization	Members (Millions)	Tax Status
Kaiser Permanente Medical Care Program	5.9	Not For Profit
Blue Cross & Blue Shield Plan HMOs	5.2	Varies
CIGNA HealthPlan Inc.	2.2	For Profit
United HealthCare Corporation	1.4	Varies
Aetna Health Plans	1.3	Varies
U.S. Healthcare Inc.	1.2	For Profit
Health Insurance Plan of Greater New York	1.0	Not For Profit
Prudential Health Plans	1.0	For Profit
HealthNet	0.8	Not For Profit
Sanus Corporation Health Systems	0.7	For Profit

SOURCE: Kertesz, Louise. (1991). Clear Goals Necessary to Pick Among Broad Field of Providers. *Business Insurance*, p. 1.

expenses; by 1990, nearly one in every three dollars spent for personal health care was reimbursed by private health insurance (23).

As noted earlier, private health insurance began with coverage principally for hospital and physicians' services. In 1960, virtually all of total net private health insurance payments were devoted to these two types of health care (see figure 12-4).

As figure 12-5 depicts, private health insurance has funded a steady one-third of personal health care expenditures for hospital services since 1960. However, between 1960 and 1990, private health insurance grew in importance as a source of financing for physicians' services, providing 30 percent of the funding in 1960 and 46 percent by 1990. The largest percentage impacts of health insur-

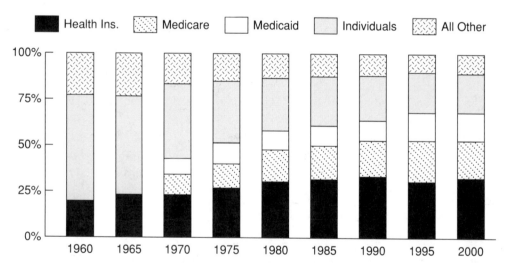

Figure 12-3. Private health insurance as a payor of personal health care expenditures (SOURCES: Waldo, Daniel R., et al. (1986). National health expenditures, 1985. *Health Care Financing Review, 8*(1), p. 16; Levit, K. R., et al. (1991). National health expenditures, 1990. *Health Care Financing Review, 13*(1), p. 50; Sonnefield, S. T. (1991). Projections of national health expenditures through the year 2000. *Health Care Financing Review, 13*(1), p. 18–25.)

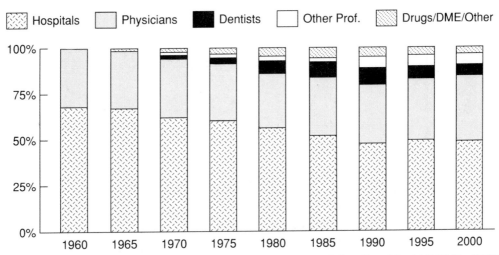

Figure 12-4. Recipients of private health insurance payments (SOURCES: Gibson, Robert M. and Daniel R. Waldo. (1981). National health expenditures, 1980. *Health Care Financing Review, 3*(1), p. 45, 47; Waldo, Daniel R., et al (1986). National health expenditures, 1985. *Health Care Financing Review, 8*(1), p. 20; Levit, K. R., et al. (1991). National health expenditures, 1990. *Health Care Financing Review, 13*(1), p. 51; Sonnefield, S. T. (1991). Projections of national health expenditures through the year 2000. *Health Care Financing Review, 13*(1), p. 18–24.)

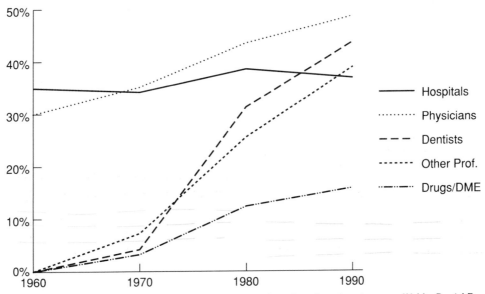

Figure 12-5. Private health insurance as a percent of total payments for selected services (SOURCES: Waldo, Daniel R,, et al (1986). National health expenditures, 1985. *Health Care Financing Review, 8*(1), p. 20; Levit, K. R., et al (1991). National health expenditures, 1990. *Health Care Financing Review, 13*(1), p. 51–52.)

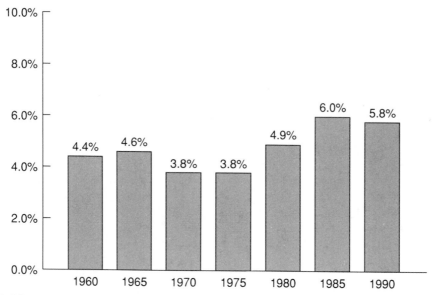

Figure 12-6. Administrative expenses as a percent of total national health expenditures. (Includes net cost of health insurance.) (SOURCES: Sonnefield, S. T. (1991). Projections of national health expenditures through the year 2000. *Health Care Financing Review, 13*(1). p. 17. Levit, K. R., et al. (1991). National health expenditures, 1990. *Health Care Financing Review, 13*(1), p. 47.)

ance financing have occurred in the areas of dental services, nonphysician professional services, and pharmaceuticals. Private health insurance for these expenses was negligible until about 1970, and even at that time, reimbursements from private health insurance were less than 7 percent of total payments in each of the three categories. But by 1990, private health insurance was responsible for 43 percent, 38 percent, and 15 percent of personal expenses for dental services, nonphysician professional services, and pharmaceuticals and durable medical equipment expenses, respectively (figure 12-5). Although in 1990 hospital and physicians' services still commanded about 80 percent of private health insurance payments, almost $39 billion in private health insurance reimbursement was available for other types of medical care services (24).

The most recent projection of health care expenditures by the Health Care Financing Administration (HCFA) forecasts total national health care expenditures of $1.6 trillion by the year 2000, of which $1.46 trillion will represent personal health care (25). Between 1990 and 2000, HCFA estimates that private health insurance expenditures will more than double, from $223 billion to nearly $508 billion. However, the proportion of personal health care expenditures funded by private health insurance is expected to decline slightly during this period, from 32.5 percent to 30.5 percent (see table 12-2), as publicly funded health care programs grow more rapidly than private financing.

As political debates in the United States continue regarding forms of national health insurance, there has been considerable arguing and criticism about the "overhead" generated by the private health insurance mechanism (26,27). In 1990, the total administrative costs of public medical programs, philanthropic organizations, and the net cost of private health insurance amounted to nearly $39 billion, 5.8 percent of total national health expenditures (see figure 12-6). (This estimate excludes the nontrivial administrative costs to providers regarding the filing of claims.) In 1990, Americans

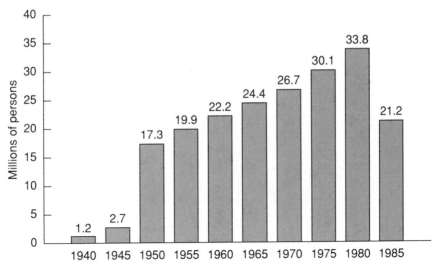

Figure 12-7. Persons covered by commercial insurers' individual health policies (SOURCE: Health Insurance Association of America. (1991). *Source book of health insurance data, 1990* (p. 23). Washington, DC: Author.)

paid $217 billion in health insurance premiums and received $186 billion in benefit payments, resulting in a net cost of private health insurance equaling $31 billion (28). This $31 billion includes insurers' administrative costs, net additions to reserves, rate credits and policyholder dividends, premium taxes, and carriers' profits or losses.

While there is no denying that some government health insurance programs such as Medicare deliver benefits at far less administrative cost per dollar of reimbursement than the private health insurance industry, health insurance *by itself* is not a significantly profitable business for most insurers. This is particularly true at the high end of the market, where self-funded "administrative services only" customers generate profit margins of only 1–2 percent for most group insurers. Indeed, the health insurance industry has suffered a net underwriting loss (the difference between premiums and claims paid) in most of the years since 1976 (29). Health insurance is beneficial for insurers primarily because it serves as a vehicle for selling other, more profitable products (such as life insurance), and because health insurance premiums generate revenues via investment income.

Health-Related Insurance Programs

Individual Coverage

Although a number of insurance entities (mostly commercial carriers and the Blues) offer insurance coverage for individuals, fewer insurers every year are interested in this line of business. Many of the nation's largest commercial accident and health insurers sell few or no individual policies. The number of people covered by commercial insurers' individual policies has decreased steadily since the late 1970s (figure 12-7).

Much of the current individual insurance sold today is "supplementary" in nature—for example, to pick up coverage for the many expenses that Medicare does not cover, or covers only with significant cost sharing. Ordinary individual policies for basic medical (hospital and physician) coverage are extraordinarily expensive, as policy premiums can easily reach several thousand dollars, even for plans with extensive cost-sharing provisions. Underwriting guidelines for individual policies have become increasingly stringent, so many people who might wish to purchase coverage are not able to do so. In some states, the only recourse for such individuals is through high-risk state insurance pools. At the end of 1990, 26 states had enacted broad-based pools for uninsurable individuals.

Demand for individual medical policies has diminished with enactment of PL 99-272, the Consolidated Omnibus Budget Reconciliation Act of 1985 (COBRA). Under this statute, employers with 20 or more employees are required to extend group health care coverage to former employees for up to 18 months after leaving their jobs (voluntarily or not), and for up to 36 months for dependents of employees following events such as death or divorce. Employers can charge a premium not to exceed 102 percent of the average cost of group health insurance for that employer.

Group Coverage

In the United States, employment not only provides the financial means of support for families, but it is the principal source of insurance protection against medical expenses and income loss associated with both on- and off-the-job illness and injury. Through sponsorship by a number of different groups (principally employers, but also unions, employer/union Taft-Hartley plans, multiple-employer-trusts [METs], and multiple-employer welfare arrangements [MEWAs]), Americans receive the preponderance of their health insurance protection. Indeed, according to a study by the Employee Benefit Research Institute, the United States is the only major industrialized country in which voluntary, employment-based health plans are the primary source of health insurance for its citizens (30).

In 1990, 70 percent of the population under age 65 obtained its health insurance through some employment-based group (31). The rapidly accelerating costs associated with medical care, and the tax-exempt nature of employee medical benefits, have stimulated the expansion of group health coverage. The importance of this latter factor is evidenced by calculations of the Congressional Budget Office that, in 1991, employers and em-

ployees were able to exclude $56–$58 billion in taxation from employer-paid employee benefits (31).

As noted earlier, small employers often provide meager health insurance benefits, if they provide them at all. But for workers of medium-size and large employers, medical insurance protection is nearly a universal benefit. For example, in a survey by the U.S. Chamber of Commerce of 957 firms (including 100 firms with fewer than 100 employees), various types of health insurance were provided as follows (32):

Medical: 99%
Long-Term Disability: 65%
Dental: 56%
Short-Term Disability: 41%
Retiree Medical: 33%

A more scientific survey of 1,647 medium-size and large business establishments by the Bureau of Labor Statistics produced these results (33):

Medical: 92%
Dental: 66%
Long-Term Disability: 45%
Sickness and Accident: 43%

Funding Alternatives for Group Health-Related Insurance

As mentioned earlier in this chapter, there are three principal options to funding health-related insurance: 1) fully insured; 2) partially insured; and 3) self-funding. At least for "conventional" health insurance (defined as non-HMO and non-PPO health plans), substantial differences exist in the use of funding alternatives among the Blues, commercial insurers, and self-administered/third-party administrator plans (figure 12-8). For certain health-related benefits, such as accidental death and dismemberment (AD&D), travel accident, long-term care, and long-term disability, funding (even within large corporations) is usually on a fully insured basis. This funding mechanism is employed because premiums are relatively small and stable, and the frequency of loss is so small that the only sound actuarial basis for establishing a premium

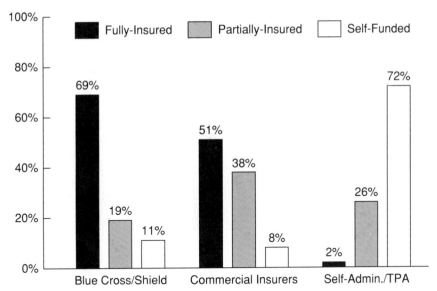

Figure 12-8. Type of funding for conventional health insurance, by type of intermediary, 1987 (SOURCE: DiCarlo, S., & Gabel, J. (1989). Conventional health insurance: A decade later. *Health Care Financing Review. 10*(3), p. 83.) "Conventional" is non-HMO & non-PPO

is to combine exposures from many different employers.

For medical and dental employee benefits, however, all three of the aforementioned funding alternatives are used. Which one makes most sense to an employer is primarily a function of the size of its employee population, and an employer's degree of risk aversion. Clearly for employers with more than several thousand employees, pure self-funding is actuarially viable, because medical expenses are relatively predictable. With 100 percent self-funding, employers basically choose some organization (an insurer or third-party administrator) to administer their medical benefits program and perform claim adjudication. Depending on the self-funding contract, additional services (e.g., actuarial, employee communications, etc.) also may be performed for the employer. Thus, the employer basically pays two types of employee benefits expenses: 1) medical service claim expenses submitted to the administrator for reimbursement by employees; and 2) an administrative fee, usually called "retention." This latter fee can be computed as a per capita charge, a percent of claim payments, or a transaction-related fee.

Self-funding of employee benefits is one of the principal trends in health insurance since the late 1970s (see figure 12-9). There are four principal advantages to self-funding. First, the employer avoids the risk charges paid to the insurer that are inherent whenever any entity purchases insurance. Second, employers may be able to avoid administrative fees for services that are bundled with a normal insurance premium, but which the employer may wish to purchase through alternate channels (e.g., actuarial or loss-prevention services). Third, since self-funding is technically not insurance, employers can avoid the nontrivial premium taxes (usually amounting to several percentage points) assessed by states on insured group health products.

Finally, and perhaps the biggest enhancement of self-funding, the Supreme Court ruled in June 1985 that the 1974 federal Employee Retirement Income and Security Act (ERISA) statute preempted states from regulating self-funded group medical programs (34,35). The most important advantage

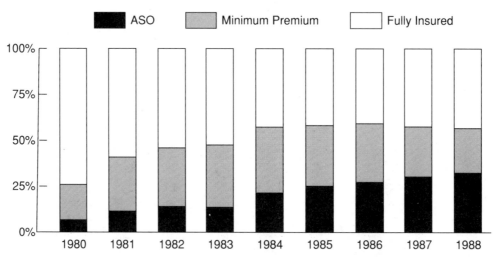

Figure 12-9. Insurance company group health claim payments, by type of funding (SOURCE: Health Insurance Association of America. (1991). *Source book of health insurance data, 1990* (p. 27). Washington, DC: Author.)

of this preemption is the ability of employers to avoid the mandated benefit provisions of states, which require insured benefit plans to cover specific types of benefits. One recent tally places the number of state-mandated health insurance benefits at nearly 1,000 (36). These state mandates originally served as a useful stimulus to encourage appropriate coverage for types of care or for conditions not previously covered by typical group health plans (alcoholism is a notable example). In recent years, however, state legislatures have greatly expanded the scope and specificity of coverage to include personal preferences of powerful state legislators, and for care where cost-effectiveness is unproven.

Some observers blame mandated benefits for increasing the costs of medical benefits, especially for small employers, thereby exacerbating the uninsured problem (37,38). In effect, large employers began to see that their multimillion-dollar employee benefits programs were being crafted by politicians, who bore no responsibility for the financial impact of their decisions. Thus, self-funding not only provides financial savings for large employers, but permits them significantly greater flexibility in designing benefit plans and establish-

ing employee cost-sharing responsibilities. Some states, such as Texas, have become so concerned about the loss of tax revenues that they have attempted (so far, without success) to seek legal rulings that would permit taxation of self-funded employee benefit expenses, which would reverse ERISA preemption (39).

Many employers, particularly those with 500 to 5,000 employees, are reluctant to assume the financial risk of a fully self-funded arrangement. For these employers, there are several forms of "partial" self-funding (the most common of which is usually referred to as a "minimum premium plan"). Generally, these financial options permit the employer to self-fund claim expenses up to a certain predefined maximum amount, after which an "insured" policy assumes financial liability. Another variant of self-funding involves the purchase of "stop-loss" (or "specific and aggregate") insurance. Again, the employer pays directly for all medical claims, except those which, either in the aggregate or individually, exceed a predetermined threshold.

Finally, there is the standard fully insured program, which remains the principal funding mechanism for the millions of small and medium-size businesses that form the foundation of employment for most Americans. For the small employer (in Travelers' case, for employers with fewer than 200 employees), premiums for this coverage are set prospectively (akin to auto insurance premiums, for example). For larger employers, a form of retrospective "experience" rating often is used, so that this year's premium is affected (either positively or negatively) by the previous year's claim expense history for each individual employer.

All three of these standard funding mechanisms are employed by both commercial carriers and the Blues. In contrast, most HMOs price their services prospectively, on a per capita basis. HMOs then are financially responsible for providing all necessary, covered medical services for this capitated premium. (Despite the feeling of some health care observers, there really is not much practical difference between the capitated premiums of HMOs and the group health premiums of fully insured insurance plans.) Historically, these capitation amounts were community-determined, unrelated to the claim experience of individual employers. As stated earlier, however, competitive pressures and amendments to the 1973 HMO Act are now stimulating funding approaches for HMO services that are more similar to the approaches used by the Blues and commercial insurers, particularly in the area of experience rating.

"Core" Medical Employee Benefits

Today's core medical employee benefits consist primarily of medical and dental coverage. In addition, larger employers may offer separate plans for coverage of prescription drug and vision services (although coverage for these expenses can be combined under the general medical plan).

Medical Plans

This coverage is the oldest and most vital form of health insurance, since it protects against those financial expenses that can be truly catastrophic. For most major types of providers (e.g., hospitals, physicians, nonphysician providers, laboratory and radiology, etc.) there is somewhat uniform coverage under indemnity group policies, but with different cost-sharing responsibilities for employees. The most generous plans (but also the type of plan rapidly losing favor with employers) are called "base/major medical" plans. Under these arrangements, there is first-dollar coverage for a few key providers (e.g., hospitals and sometimes physicians); then more limited coverage (e.g., with 20 percent employee coinsurance required) for all other services. Except for so-called "corridor" deductibles that may exist between the "base" and "major medical" expenses, these plans generally contain no up-front employee cost sharing. Perhaps the biggest disadvantage of base/major medical plans is that many do not place any upper limit on the expenses borne by the patient in a calendar year.

In contrast, the most prominent type of medical benefit plan today, the "comprehensive" design, retains little (if any) first-dollar coverage. A comprehensive plan design usually has a relatively small annual deductible (e.g., $200) that pertains to all medical expenses, then it reimburses the patient a fixed percentage (most commonly 80 percent) of all medical claims that exceed the deductible, up to a maximum "out-of-pocket" patient expense (typically $1,000–$2,000 per insured person). When the patient reaches this out-of-pocket maximum, 100 percent of all subsequent expenses are borne by the medical plan. Both base/major medical and comprehensive plans usually place lifetime maximums on the total amount of benefits that will be paid to any individual. A 1989 Bureau of Labor Statistics survey found that while 78 percent of plan participants were so restricted, about half of these limits were set at $1 million or more (40).

In a 1989 Bureau of Labor Statistics survey of medium and large firms, 74 percent of medical insurance participants were covered by a fee-for-service medical plan, with the remainder of participants covered by an HMO (17 percent) or PPO (10 percent) (41). This survey also found that 53 percent of workers had their own coverage wholly financed by the employer, but this percentage was much smaller (34 percent) for dependent coverage (42). Forty-two percent of employees with a medical plan became eligible for coverage on the date of hire, while another 37 percent became eligible within three months of employment (43). Most medical plans today impose at least some managed care requirements on plan participants, the most common programs being utilization review and case management.

The benefit structure of medical plans offered by HMOs is somewhat different from fee-for-service "indemnity" coverages. First, the scope of coverage often is broader in HMO plans than in indemnity programs (although there are notable exceptions, particularly regarding the coverage of psychiatric and substance abuse illnesses). Second, the more generous HMO plans usually have no deductibles. Third, instead of coinsurance, HMOs feature fixed-dollar copayments for selected services, most commonly physician office visits ($5–$15 per visit) and medications ($3–$7 per prescription). Finally, HMOs traditionally have displayed greater attentiveness to fostering health promotion than have indemnity insurers. Therefore, covered expenses in HMO benefit plans often include medical care not covered in indemnity plans, such as immunizations, well child care, and physical examinations.

Dental Plans

Although Continental Casualty Company was the first commercial insurer to issue a comprehensive group dental insurance plan (in 1959), insurance for dental expenses was not generally available until the 1970s. Plan designs for dental insurance generally follow more of a "comprehensive" than a "base/major medical" structure. Usually there are three tiers of benefits. For preventive services (e.g., semiannual prophylaxis and routine dental X rays), coverage often is 100 percent, without a deductible. For the two remaining benefit tiers, there is a small annual deductible ($50–$100 per insured person) the patient must satisfy before any benefits

are paid. Restorative services (e.g., amalgams), oral surgery, endodontics (e.g., root canal), and periodontics then are paid with relatively standard coinsurance (usually 80 percent). Services such as crowns, inlays, and prosthetics are reimbursed only 50 percent by the dental plan. Cosmetic dentistry (e.g., bonding) usually is covered at this lower level, or it may be excluded from coverage entirely. Orthodontic services usually receive a relatively limited lifetime benefit (e.g., $1,000), unless special orthodontic coverage is elected. Plans of dental HMOs (DMOs) and Delta Dental plans are analogous to medical HMO coverages, with slightly broader coverage and fewer cost-sharing requirements for the employee, when compared to indemnity dental plans.

In a 1989 survey by the Bureau of Labor Statistics of medium and large firms, 91 percent of dental insurance participants were covered by a fee-for-service plan, with the remainder covered about equally by dental HMOs and PPOs (41). This survey revealed that individual coverage required no employee contribution for 52 percent of participants, while dependent coverage was free to only 37 percent of participants (42). Unlike medical benefits, dental plans are more restrictive in terms of annual limits on reimbursement. The Bureau of Labor Statistics survey found that 82 percent of dental plan participants were subject to an annual maximum, and for 62 percent of participants this threshold was $1,000 or less (44).

Vision Plans

Expense benefits for vision care were first introduced by private insurers in 1957. Many health care observers believe that vision care is a prime example of what should not be covered by an insurance program, since vision care is relatively inexpensive for most Americans. According to a 1989 Bureau of Labor Statistics survey, approximately 35 percent of medical care plan participants in medium and large organizations retained insurance coverage for vision services (45). For those individuals covered for vision services, nearly all received coverage for examinations, while two-thirds were covered for eyeglasses and contact lenses. Usually there are limits regarding the frequency with which examinations and lenses are reimbursable. With the advent of managed care, vision care may be available as a "carve-out" benefit, sometimes with a separate deductible. These vision care programs usually are offered in conjunction with large, national chains of vision care products, offering employees substantial discounts on these products if they are purchased through the "preferred" providers.

Prescription Drug Plans

This benefit is another example of a specialized employee benefit that increasingly is carved out of the regular medical benefit program, in order to take advantage of managed care features. Generally, coverage assumes one of two forms. In the traditional fashion, prescription drugs simply are a covered expense under the medical benefit plan. There may be individual copayments per prescription, and sometimes these copayments are higher for branded drugs than for generics. (Traditional coinsurance, typically 80 percent, may be substituted for the copayment type of cost sharing.) Nearly all types of prescription drugs are eligible for reimbursement, with the principal exceptions being certain injectibles (except insulin), contraceptives, and experimental drugs. Prescription drugs for acute conditions (e.g., antibiotics) may be covered in part by the regular medical plan, while "maintenance" drugs are available through mail order. Mail-order plans permit employers and employees to take advantage of steep discounts and some drug use review, while offering the convenience of home delivery. Mail-order programs have been particularly well received by older employees and retirees. The latest trend in pharmacy programs, however, is a full "carve-out" program for all prescription drugs, a feature that may or may not include a mail-order companion product.

Long-Term Care Coverage

The most recent option for a number of corporate employee benefits programs is long-term care insurance, which first became available for groups during the last half of the 1980s. In 1990, private health insurance paid only $600 million of the nation's more than $53 billion in nursing home expenditures (46). Much of these benefits was paid by individual long-term care policies and group medical plans (although nursing home coverage usually is quite limited for the latter programs). By December 1989, 118 U.S. insurers had sold about 1.5 million policies (mostly individual) covering long-term care (47). The group policies now available are largely 100 percent employee-funded, as employers are fearful of assuming any additional fiscal liability for insurance protection, even though the long-term actuarial value of this type of insurance is highly uncertain. Unlike the service benefits of most group medical and dental plans, long-term care insurance is largely an indemnity product, offering a fixed daily reimbursement payment for nursing home care and related services. Coverage generally is not allowed for custodial care, nor for chronic organic illnesses such as Alzheimer's disease.

Retiree Medical Coverage

The foregoing description of the principal forms of group health insurance applies to active employees. (Of course, a very small percentage of active employees or their family members may receive primary insurance coverage through Medicare, such as individuals with chronic renal failure who require dialysis). For active employees between the ages of 65 and 70, the Tax Equity and Fiscal Responsibility Act (TEFRA) of 1982 required employers' group health insurance plans to remain the primary payors, with Medicare retaining only secondary coverage. In 1984, the Omnibus Deficit Reduction Act (PL 98-369) extended Medicare as the secondary payer for aged spouses of workers under age 65. (These statutes are just two examples of how the federal government has shifted fiscal responsibility for the financing of some medical care from government to the private sector.)

According to a 1989 Bureau of Labor Statistics survey of medium and small firms, 42 percent of plan participants were enrolled in plans that continued health insurance coverage after retirement (48). For 79 percent of retirees less than age 65 and 72 percent of retirees older than age 65, there was no change in health insurance coverage from their active coverages (49). However, for those retirees with health insurance coverage, 29 percent under age 65 and 26 percent older than age 65 were subject to a minimum company service requirement. Another 26 percent of retirees under age 65 and 30 percent of retirees older than age 65 were required to qualify for the company pension program in order to be eligible for health insurance coverage.

For retirees, there has been a profound reexamination by employers of providing continuing medical expense protection, particularly for early retirees who have not yet reached age 65 (and therefore are ineligible for Medicare) (50). This rethinking of retiree medical coverage has occurred for several reasons. First, the unrelenting growth in employers' medical benefit expenses—acceleration that is two or three times as rapid as the increase in other costs of doing business—has forced most employers to reassess whether they can afford to finance retiree medical expenses as generously as in the past.

Second, as one would expect, early retirees' average annual medical expenses easily can be double or triple those of the active population. For employers with significant numbers of retirees (such as long-standing manufacturing companies like auto and steel producers), early retiree medical costs can significantly raise an employer's overall average financial liability for medical benefits. Third, all employers (even relatively young firms) are faced with the undeniable "aging" of America, so the pressures on employers' total medical benefit expenditures will become more severe over the next several decades.

Finally, regulations proposed by the Financial Accounting Standards Board (referred to as "FASB 106") will take effect at the beginning of 1993 (51). Before 1990, virtually all employers used the pay-as-you-go approach to value the cost of retiree medical benefits on their financial statements. By 1993, employers must accrue retiree health care liabilities as an expense against earnings, from the date an employee is hired until that employee becomes eligible for benefits. In addition, retiree health liabilities that have accumulated as of the date that employers adopt FASB 106 accounting rules must be recognized at once, or be amortized (generally, over 20 years). In 1990 and 1991, a number of prominent corporations decided to take their FASB 106 medicine, with a number of these companies assuming multibillion dollar write-offs. For example, General Motors estimates the value of its FASB 106 obligations at a whopping $16–$24 billion (52).

Since incorporation of these amounts on corporate balance sheets result in only a minimal diminution of actual cash flow (since FASB 106 is merely an accounting acknowledgment of future liabilities), its direct effect on employers' day-to-day operations is minor. However, the enormous financial impact of FASB 106 has jolted senior corporate executives into explicitly acknowledging the increasingly onerous burden of all medical benefits (not just retiree obligations) on employers' overhead expenses, perhaps more than any other single legislative or regulatory rule enacted to date.

As a result of these combined forces, most employers are reexamining how (and even if) they want to provide medical coverage for retirees. Some employers have even attempted to rescind retiree health insurance coverage (51). The courts generally have ruled that employers retain the right to rescind or amend retiree medical benefit programs, as long as this option is clearly stated in employers' benefit documentation (53). For retirees under age 65, benefit protection often is the same as that for active employees. For retirees over age 65, employers' liability is diminished significantly, since the group health insurance plan becomes secondary to Medicare coverage. For both groups, however, employers are reconsidering their funding options.

One approach is to eliminate retiree medical coverage entirely for all new hires, or to link coverage with length-of-service requirements, much as pension plans' "vesting" periods. Another option is to require retirees to contribute much more generously than in the past to their medical coverage. Unfortunately, current tax laws impede the ability of employers to establish tax-exempt trusts to fund retiree medical benefits. There have been some proposals in Congress to make it easier to prefund retiree medical expenses by both employers and employees, for example, via an analog of 401(k) pension plans.

But the most fundamental choice most employers must make these days is whether they will continue to offer medical benefits to retirees under a "defined benefit" concept, or whether (like pensions) retiree medical benefits should be switched to a "defined contribution" program. This latter option generally limits employers' future liabilities by making them much more predictable (like pension benefits), and clearly places most of the concern over the ultimate magnitude of medical care cost escalation squarely on retirees. If defined contribution programs for retiree medical benefits become the norm, retirees will need to be much more concerned about issues of plan design and cost containment than they have in the past. Active employees also will be required to assume significantly more responsibility for funding their retiree medical benefits far ahead of when they will be incurred, just as workers must plan now to ensure that they will retain enough retirement income via pension benefits and 401(k) plans.

Disability Insurance

Serious illness or injury not only creates economic hardship due to the high costs of medical care, but it also inhibits the ability of workers to maintain a wage stream to support the everyday costs of living. Thus, loss-of-income policies are one of the oldest forms of health-related insurance. In contrast to the disability programs available through Social Security for chronic loss of income via disability, private insurance vehicles have focused on the short to medium term. Unlike most health insurance, disability insurance pays indemnity benefits, not medical service benefits. Except for the compulsory temporary disability insurance programs mandated by five states (Rhode Island, 1942; California, 1946; New Jersey, 1948; New York, 1949; and Hawaii, 1969), which combine wage-replacement with medical expense reimbursement for nonoccupational disabling illness or injury, short- and long-term disability programs do not reimburse for expenses associated with medical services.

Short-Term Programs

Coverage for loss of income due to illness can be available to workers through two avenues: 1) sick leave or salary continuation benefits; or 2) short-term disability insurance. A 1989 Bureau of Labor Statistics survey of medium and large firms observed that 89 percent of the working population was covered by one or both of these programs (54). While sick leave benefits usually replace all or most of an ill employee's wages, reimbursement often is limited to no more than a few weeks, at best. Eligibility for sick leave, and the length of sick leave benefits, are usually related to an employee's length of service.

According to the Bureau of Labor Statistics survey, in 1989 approximately 43 percent of workers were eligible for short-term disability insurance (54). Of those workers eligible, 84 percent of their programs were employer-financed. Short-term disability insurance retains several important features, many of which differentiate disability insurance from health insurance. First, there is a short "elimination period" (usually one to seven days) between the onset of disability or illness, and the date when benefits begin to be paid. In the most generous short-term income protection employee benefits, sick leave benefits dovetail with short-term disability insurance, so that the ailing worker has no front-end gaps in coverage.

Second, as their name implies, short-term disability programs protect workers only for relatively brief periods. In the Bureau of Labor Statistics survey, 96 percent of short-term disability plan participants had coverage of six months or less (55). Finally, three-quarters of short-term disability insurance plan participants had a length-of-service requirement before they were eligible for coverage, usually three months or less (56). This period of time to become eligible for coverage is called a "waiting period."

Long-Term Programs

Long-term disability insurance can be perceived in two different lights. In its most generous version, this coverage dovetails with an employer's short-term income maintenance program to create a seamless layer of wage protection for periods of several years. In its more primal role, long-term disability insurance is the disability equivalent to a catastrophic medical benefit plan, because benefits are paid only after the insured has retained a significant amount of loss.

According to the Bureau of Labor Statistics survey, in 1989 45 percent of American workers were protected by long-term disability (LTD) insurance (57). For 78 percent of the workers eligible for coverage, premiums were entirely employer-financed. Like short-term coverage, long-term disability insurance maintains a waiting period before employees are eligible for coverage. Nearly two-thirds of the LTD participants surveyed by the Bureau of Labor Statistics were subject to a length-of-service requirement of generally less than one year (58). In addition, the Bureau of Labor Statistics survey found that nearly half of plan participants had an elimination period (no coverage) of six months (59).

In order to induce workers to return to the job, and because long-term disability payments can be exempt from both state and federal taxation, benefits are paid at rates usually in the range of 50–67 percent of a worker's wages (60), although there are often maximums to these payments. Due to the existence of Social Security disability programs, most long-term disability policies include provisions that permit benefits to be reduced commensurate with the amount of Social Security disability benefits paid. This provision is analogous to the "coordination of benefits" feature common in nearly all medical and dental insurance policies.

Workers' Compensation Insurance

Like Medicare, workers' compensation insurance is a "social insurance" program. Usually, employee benefits professionals do not consider workers' compensation a health insurance program. But changes in the nature of workers' compensation benefits over the years, as well as the way in which these programs are now being affected by new managed care techniques, argue that workers' compensation should be discussed as a vehicle providing nontrivial medical benefits.

Workers' compensation programs really were the first types of broad coverage, health-related insurance in the United States. Beginning with a federal statute in 1908, workers' compensation-type insurance programs were enacted by nine states in 1911, and by 1920, all but six states had inaugurated such a program (61). Today, there are 55 workers' compensation programs in operation—one in each of the 50 states as well as in Puerto Rico, the District of Columbia, and the U.S. Virgin Islands. There are also two special federal workers' compensation programs covering government employees and longshoremen and harbor workers. In addition, there are unique occupational illness and injury programs for coal miners suffering from pneumoconiosis ("black lung" disease) and railroad workers.

Covering nearly 94 million employees, or 87 percent of the nation's work force, workers' compensation insurance is compulsory for most private employment, except in New Jersey, South Carolina, and Texas. This protection provides workers and their families with three types of benefits: 1) indemnity cash benefits to help replace lost wages; 2) medical expense reimbursement; and 3) survivors' death benefits. Despite generally broad-based coverage, many state workers' compensation programs do not cover domestics, agricultural workers, and casual laborers. Many programs also cover public employees, as well as workers in nonprofit and charitable institutions, with varying degrees of comprehensiveness. Initially focusing on workplace injuries, workers' compensation programs increasingly are being pressured financially by the long-term affects of occupational illness (even though nationwide, occupational disease accounts for only about 2 percent of all workers' compensation claims).

In 1988, employers paid $43 billion for workers' compensation insurance, and workers' compensation benefits exceeded $29 billion (62). The large difference between premiums and benefit payments reflects the long payout time frame on workers' compensation claims, so premiums collected in one year must anticipate claims filed for many subsequent years. Employers provide funding for virtually all workers' compensation premiums. About 20 percent of premiums are contributed to state high-risk pools, which provide coverage for high-risk employers that cannot obtain workers' compensation insurance through commercial carriers. Each state establishes its own regulatory mechanisms, eligibility rules, benefit schedules, and funding alternatives.

In 42 states, employers may purchase workers' compensation insurance through private insurers, either property/casualty single-line carriers, or multiline carriers. The nation's largest writer of workers' compensation coverage, Liberty Mutual, is largely unknown to most health insurance professionals. However, in eight jurisdictions, commercial insurance is not permitted. Four of these areas have an exclusive state workers' compensation insurance fund. In four other states, employers can purchase workers' compensation coverage through the state program, or they can self-fund. In 14 states, state

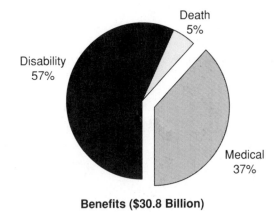

Benefits ($30.8 Billion)

Figure 12-10. Workers' compensation benefit payments, by type of benefit, 1988 (SOURCE: Nelson, W. J. (1991, March). Workers' compensation: Coverage, benefits, and costs, 1988. *Social Security Bulletin. 54*(3). 15.)

funds compete with commercial insurers. Since 1980, there has been a consistent distribution among payors of workers' compensation benefit payments, as commercial insurers have been responsible for about 60 percent of benefits, with state funds and self-funding equally splitting the remainder of payments (63).

One important development in workers' compensation programs over time has been the degree to which they provide reimbursement for medical benefits. In 1988, about 37 percent of all workers' compensation benefits (totaling $11.5 billion) were for medical care, a percentage not reached since 1940 (figure 12-10). As figure 12-11 depicts, this percentage has been increasing slowly but steadily since 1980. This trend is due both to states' restrictions on cash compensation benefit levels, as well as to the higher growth rate for medical care when compared to wages. Nearly all standard employee benefit medical programs contain provisions that exclude coverage for medical care for work-related accidents, in order to avoid duplicate payments by both the medical plan and workers' compensation.

Between 1978 and 1988, Worker's Compensation benefits accelerated at an annual average rate of 12.4 percent, with self-funded programs rising

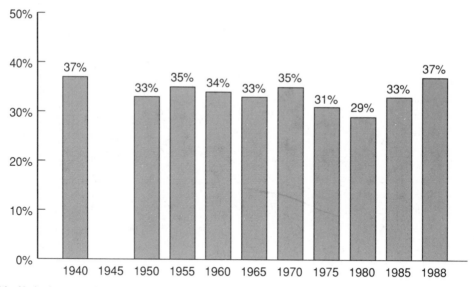

Figure 12-11. Medical care reimbursement as a percent of total workers' compensation payments (SOURCE: Worker's compensation. (1991). *Social Security Bulletin. 54*(9), p. 30.)

even more rapidly at 14.6 percent (64). For this reason, many employers are beginning to observe their increasing workers' compensation expenses as closely as the accelerating costs of medical benefit programs. Thus, it is no surprise that many of the cost-management techniques (particularly managed care) that have been successful in moderating medical benefit plan expenditures are now being modified for workers' compensation programs. These strategies are more workable in some states than in others, however, as states differ in the degree of provider freedom-of-choice that is afforded to the injured worker. In 32 jurisdictions, the employee may seek treatment from any physician, although in some cases this choice is restricted to lists of physicians established by state funds or insurers. Therefore, in these states it may be difficult or impossible to encourage workers to use a "preferred provider" network. Even utilization review may be only marginally effective in such circumstances. It is not surprising that some of the most aggressive transference of managed care techniques from the employee benefits arena to workers' compensation is occurring in those states

which provide employers with unilateral physician selection powers.

Changes Facing the Health Insurance Industry

Private health insurance has been an integral part of the American health care system for so long, it is hard to conceive that forces will be successful in eliminating it from the scene. Health insurance is such an economic commodity that the Chicago Board of Trade (CBOT) planned, then postponed, the trading of health insurance futures on the CBOT commodity exchange during 1991 (65). Yet as we enter the last decade of the 20th century, there is reason to believe that some fundamental changes in the health insurance mechanism will be cast, perhaps by the middle of the decade. Nineteen ninety-one marked a rebirth of interest in rising health costs and the uninsured. These topics have become front-page banners in major periodicals (66,67,68). Corporate America's increasing frustration with the financial impact of employee medical benefits is also becoming more noticeable

(69–71). Spurred by the rumblings of discontent evident during the 1991 elections (72), health care issues could well be the chief domestic polemic of the 1996 presidential election.

With this background, five basic trends in private health insurance seem most probable:

1. *Greater Regulation and More Aggressive Insurance Industry Responses:* On insured health insurance products, states will continue to impose more mandated benefits, and to exert greater control over the way in which managed care is operated. Successful grass-roots outrage over insurance practices, such as California's controversial Proposition 103 limits on automobile insurance, easily could spread to health insurance. The health insurance industry, in an effort to defuse criticism about the uninsured, to sidetrack aggressive attempts in Congress to repeal the Mc-Carren-Ferguson Act (the landmark 1945 legislation that permitted state, not federal, regulation), and to amend key antitrust legislation, is moving forward with its own reforms for small business insurance.

   In particular, insurers are increasingly sensitive about the adverse political impact of the uninsured problem, and they are becoming more aggressive in promoting and implementing plans to ameliorate perceptions surrounding this issue. For example, in Connecticut, home to many large insurers, 1990 legislation 1) guaranteed health insurance to small employers; 2) ensured automatic renewals; 3) limited waiting periods for coverage when a worker changed jobs; 4) placed a ceiling on annual rate increases; and 5) established a reinsurance pool to cover high-risk individuals and very small employers. Similar initiatives have been endorsed more formally by the Health Insurance Association of America, a trade association of 300 private health insurers that covers 95 million Americans (73). With these types of programs, the health insurance industry hopes to avoid more intrusive mandates on health coverage that would render health insurance less profitable or diminish the pool of potential health insurance purchasers.

2. *Continued Consolidation of Major Health Insurers:* The purchase of Equicor's health insurance business by CIGNA in 1990, and the departure of Lincoln National from the group health insurance and managed care market in early 1992, are just two recent examples of insurer consolidation. For health insurance, profitability increasingly demands the economies of scale derived from very large policyholder bases. The significant investments required to deliver today's comprehensive, increasingly sophisticated managed care technologies and provider networks are becoming insurmountable barriers to entry for new insurers (although several large Japanese insurers appear interested in the U.S. marketplace). And if a combination of public and private initiatives are successful at shrinking interest in individual health insurance policies and supplemental Medicare coverage, specialty health insurers will become rarer.

3. *Increasing Use of Managed Care:* The nation's largest insurers now view their roles as not so much fiscal intermediaries, but managed care firms. "Conventional" health insurance is steadily moving in the direction of greater managed care (74). This evolution has not occurred without some miscalculations, however (75). Nevertheless, health insurers are becoming active participants in the growing national debate over definitions of "appropriate" care. At least one well-known health care researcher has noted that as insurers become more directly involved in the actual delivery of medical care (or at least in its concurrent monitoring), there are opportunities for considerable cost savings, thereby freeing funds that could be used to finance improved health care access for uninsureds (76).

   Insurers interested in the high end of the health insurance market simply are unable to gain and retain large customers today without broad, serious managed care capabilities. These skills also are needed increasingly for the middle and smaller health insurance segments, because these employers correctly perceive that their larger corporate siblings are performing their own form of cost shifting, namely from employers with managed care benefit plans to businesses without such programs. Managed care techniques already have migrated to dental products, while specialty programs have been inaugurated with considerable success in mental health/substance abuse and prescription drug arenas. Yet the largest growth of managed care in the mid–1990s is likely to be first in the areas of disability and workers' compensation, and then in select areas of property/casualty coverage such as automobile insurance, where health costs are a key contributor to its significant and steady rate increases.

4. *Greater Merging of Managed Care With Individual Freedom of Choice:* Many medium-size and large employers are likely to continue to be interested in health insurance products that deliver aggressive managed care, yet still permit some measure of provider freedom of choice for patients. In product design, health insurance plans are evolving toward a more common middle ground. So-called open-ended HMOs, which allow some non-HMO use, albeit with nontrivial financial penalties, have been growing far

more rapidly than traditional HMO plans, as enrollment in such programs has accelerated from about 400,000 in 1988 to more than 1 million in 1991 (77). At the indemnity end of the health insurance spectrum, the benefit design receiving the greatest attention today among larger employers is the "point-of-service" medical plan, a hybrid product that combines aspects of both HMOs and PPOs. In total, HMO and commercial insurers' point-of-service plans are estimated to cover 3.3 million enrollees today, up from 600,000 as late as 1989 (78). While employees and their families will retain some freedom of choice, the financial disincentives for not complying with managed care guidelines will become increasingly onerous, unless the liability climate changes drastically.

5. *Continued Self-Funding:* In order for employers to avoid ever-expanding government regulation and taxation, and to maintain greater internal control over employee medical plan details, businesses are not likely to return to an insured basis for their health benefit programs. It is arguable whether the advent of so-called pay-or-play health insurance reforms, advocated by some business giants (79), would really lead to an exodus of major corporations from self-funded employee benefit programs to government-sponsored health care, given the emasculation of employee benefits autonomy that such a movement would engender.

References

1. Vaughn, E. J., & Elliott, C. M. (1978). *Fundamentals of risk and insurance* (p. 7). New York: John Wiley & Sons.
2. Vaughn, E. J., & Elliott, C. M. (1987). *Fundamentals of risk and insurance* (p. 17). New York: John Wiley & Sons.
3. Health Insurance Association of America. (1991). *Source book of health insurance data, 1990* (pp. 1–2, 103–109). Washington, DC: Author.
4. Greenspan, N. T., & Vogel, R. J. (1980). Taxation and its effects upon public and private health insurance and medical demand. *Health Care Financing Review. 1*(4). 39–46.
5. In the future, employee health may tax employer. (1979). *Employer Benefit Plan Review. 34*(3). 38.
6. Feldstein, M., & Friedman, B. (1977). Tax subsidies, the rational demand for insurance and the health care crisis. *Journal of Public Economics. 7*(2). 155–178.
7. Congressional Budget Office, Congress of the United States. (1980). *Tax subsidies for medical care: Current policies and possible alternatives.* Washington, DC: U.S. Government Printing Office.
8. Congressional Budget Office, Congress of the United States. (1991). *Rising health care costs: Causes, implications, and strategies* (pp. 11–14). Washington, DC: U.S. Government Printing Office.
9. *Journal of the American Medical Association.* (1991, May 15). *265*(19).
10. National Center for Health Statistics. (1991, June 18). *Characteristics of persons with and without health care coverage: United States, 1989.* Advance Data #201 (DHHS Publication No. PHS 91-1250). Washington, DC: U.S. Government Printing Office.
11. Health Insurance Association of America. (1991). *Source book of health insurance data, 1990* (pp. 13–14). Washington, DC: Author.
12. Congressional Budget Office, Congress of the United States. (1991). *Rising health care costs: Causes, implications, and strategies* (pp. 67–80). Washington, DC: U.S. Government Printing Office.
13. *National underwriter profiles, 1990, health insurers.* (1991). Cincinnati: National Underwriter.
14. Accident and health premiums, 1989. (1990). *Best's Review (Life/Health Edition). 91*(8). 68–75.
15. Accident and health premiums, 1990. (1991). *Best's Review (Life/Health Edition). 92*(8). 60–66.
16. Blue Cross beset by financial problems. (1991, March 27). *Wall Street Journal.* p. A6.
17. Kenkel, P. J. (1991, December 9). HMOs choosing IPA partners with care. *Modern Healthcare. 42.* p. 42.
18. Locke, A. C. (1991, January 21). HMOs strong in cities. *Business Insurance. 3, 8.*
19. Shellenbarger, S. (1991, February 27). As HMO premiums soar, employers sour on the plans and check out alternatives. *Wall Street Journal.*
20. Scanlon, J., & Austin, N. (1987). Bringing HMOs in line with cost management goals. *Business and Health. 5*(2). 12–17.
21. HMOs: Employers shed casual attitudes, contracts. (1988). *Hospitals. 62*(12). 60–61.
22. Geisel, J. (1991, August 26). Relief for HMO costs. *Business Insurance.* 27.
23. Levit, K. R., et al. (1991). National health expenditures, 1990. *Health Care Financing Review. 13*(1). 29–54.

24. Levit, K. R., et al. (1991). National health expenditures. *Health Care Financing Review. 13*(1). 49.

25. Sonnefeld, S. T. (1991). Projections of national health expenditures through the year 2000. *Health Care Financing Review. 13*(1). 1–27.

26. Woolhandler, S., & Himmelstein, D. (1991). The deteriorating administrative efficiency of the U.S. health care system. *New England Journal of Medicine. 324*(18). 1253–1258.

27. Letters to the editor. (1991). *New England Journal of Medicine. 325*(18). 1316–1319.

28. Levit, K. R., et al. (1991). National health expenditures, 1990. *Health Care Financing Review. 13*(1). 38.

29. Health Insurance Association of America. (1991). *Source book of health insurance data, 1990* (p. 16). Washington, DC: Author.

30. Schachner, M. (1990, October 22). United States has only health care system based on employer plans. *Business Insurance.*

31. Congressional Budget Office, Congress of the United States. (1991). *Rising health care costs: Causes, implications, and strategies* (pp. x, 12). Washington, DC: U.S. Government Printing Office.

32. U.S. Chamber Research Center. (1990). *Employee benefits, 1989* (p. 35). Washington, DC: U.S. Chamber of Commerce.

33. U.S. Department of Labor, Bureau of Labor Statistics. (1990). *Employee benefits in medium and large firms, 1989* (p. 4). Washington, DC: U.S. Government Printing Office.

34. *Metropolitan Life Insurance Company v. Massachusetts.* 84-325 (Supreme Court 1985).

35. Rublee, D. A. (1985). Self-funded health benefit plans. *Journal of the American Medical Association. 255*(6). 787–789.

36. Tally of mandated benefits nears 1000. (1991). *Modern Healthcare. 21*(47). 8.

37. Stipp, D. (1988, December 28). Laws on health benefits raise firms' ire. *Wall Street Journal.* B1.

38. Goodman, J. C. (1991, December 17). Health insurance: States can help. *Wall Street Journal.*

39. Judge strikes down Texas tax on self-funded benefit plans. (1989, March 6). *Business Insurance.* 1, 2.

40. U.S. Department of Labor, Bureau of Labor Statistics. (1990). *Employee benefits in medium and large firms, 1989* (p. 53). Washington, DC: U.S. Government Printing Office.

41. U.S. Department of Labor, Bureau of Labor Statistics. (1990). *Employee benefits in medium and large firms, 1989* (p. 50). Washington, DC: U.S. Government Printing Office.

42. U.S. Department of Labor, Bureau of Labor Statistics. (1990). *Employee benefits in medium and large firms, 1989* (p. 124). Washington, DC: U.S. Government Printing Office.

43. U.S. Department of Labor, Bureau of Labor Statistics. (1990). *Employee benefits in medium and large firms, 1989* (p. 66). Washington, DC: U.S. Government Printing Office.

44. U.S. Department of Labor, Bureau of Labor Statistics. (1990). *Employee benefits in medium and large firms, 1989* (p. 71). Washington, DC: U.S. Government Printing Office.

45. U.S. Department of Labor, Bureau of Labor Statistics. (1990). *Employee benefits in medium and large firms, 1989* (pp. 6, 62). Washington, DC: U.S. Government Printing Office.

46. Levit, K. R., et al. (1991). National health expenditures, 1990. *Health Care Financing Review. 13*(1). 49.

47. Health Insurance Association of America. (1991). *Source book of health insurance data, 1990* (p. 12). Washington, DC: Author.

48. U.S. Department of Labor, Bureau of Labor Statistics. (1990). *Employee benefits in medium and large firms, 1989* (pp. 6, 66). Washington, DC: U.S. Government Printing Office.

49. U.S. Department of Labor, Bureau of Labor Statistics. (1990). *Employee benefits in medium and large firms, 1989* (p. 67). Washington, DC: U.S. Government Printing Office.

50. Solomon, J. (1990, May 17). Retirees, companies head for showdown over moves to reduce health coverage. *Wall Street Journal.* B1.

51. Now that wasn't so bad, was it? (1991, December 2). *Business Week. 3234.* 123–124.

52. Templin, N. (1991, November 11). GM is facing a huge charge up to $24 billion. *Wall Street Journal.* A3.

53. Geisel, J. (1989, January 2). Court says firm can't alter retiree health plan benefits. *Business Insurance.* 2, 7.

54. U.S. Department of Labor, Bureau of Labor Statistics. (1990). *Employee benefits in medium and large firms, 1989* (p. 22). Washington, DC: U.S. Government Printing Office.

55. U.S. Department of Labor, Bureau of Labor Statis-

tics. (1990). *Employee benefits in medium and large firms, 1989* (p. 29). Washington, DC: U.S. Government Printing Office.

56. U.S. Department of Labor, Bureau of Labor Statistics. (1990). *Employee benefits in medium and large firms, 1989* (p. 33). Washington, DC: U.S. Government Printing Office.

57. U.S. Department of Labor, Bureau of Labor Statistics. (1990). *Employee benefits in medium and large firms, 1989* (p. 4). Washington, DC: U.S. Government Printing Office.

58. U.S. Department of Labor, Bureau of Labor Statistics. (1990). *Employee benefits in medium and large firms, 1989* (p. 38). Washington, DC: U.S. Government Printing Office.

59. U.S. Department of Labor, Bureau of Labor Statistics. (1990). *Employee benefits in medium and large firms, 1989* (p. 37). Washington, DC: U.S. Government Printing Office.

60. U.S. Department of Labor, Bureau of Labor Statistics. (1990). *Employee benefits in medium and large firms, 1989* (p. 34). Washington, DC: U.S. Government Printing Office.

61. Workers' compensation. (1991). *Social Security Bulletin. 54*(9). 28–36.

62. Nelson, W. J. (1991). Workers' compensation: Coverage, benefits, and costs, 1988. *Social Security Bulletin. 54*(3). 12–20.

63. Nelson, W. J. (1991). Workers' compensation: Coverage, benefits, and costs. *Social Security Bulletin. 54*(3). 17.

64. Nelson, W. J. (1991). Workers' compensation: Coverage, benefits, and costs. *Social Security Bulletin. 54*(4). 17.

65. Taylor, J. (1991, September 4). CBOT puts insurance futures on hold. *Wall Street Journal.* C1.

66. The health care crisis: A prescription for reform. (1991, October 7). *Business Week. 3234.* 58–66.

67. Castro, J. (1991, November 25). Condition: Critical. *Time.* 34–42.

68. Faltermayer, E. (1990, May 21). How to close the health care gap. *Fortune. 121*(11), p. 121.

69. Business leaders bring their clout to Washington. (1990, April 20). *Hospitals. 64*(8), p. 32.

70. Kenkel, P. J. (1991, July 29). Business-led efforts to control costs. *Modern Healthcare.* p. 48.

71. Winslow, R. (1991, January 29). Medical costs soar, defying firms' cures. *Wall Street Journal.* B1.

72. A roar of discontent: Voters want health care reform—now. (1991, November 25). *Business Week. 3241.* 28–30.

73. Schramm, C. J. (1991). Health care financing for all Americans. *Journal of the American Medical Association. 265*(24). 3296–3299.

74. DiCarlo, S., & Gabel, J. (1989). Conventional health insurance: A decade later. *Health Care Financing Review. 10*(3). 77–88.

75. Whitted, G. S. (1991). Insurers and managed care: No easy solutions. In P. Boland (Ed.). *Making managed healthcare work: A practical guide to strategies and solutions* (pp. 102–103). New York: McGraw-Hill Inc.

76. Brook, R. H. (1991). Health, health insurance, and the uninsured. *Journal of the American Medical Association. 265*(22). 2998–3002.

77. Geisel, J. (1991, September 16). Open-ended HMOs catch on. *Business Insurance.* 1, 97.

78. Kenkel, P. J. (1991). Insurance regulators recommend requiring cash reserves for open-ended plans. *Modern Healthcare. 21*(6). 52.

79. Garland, S. (1991, November 18). Already, big business' health isn't feeling so hot. *Business Week. 3240.* 48.

Chapter 13

Managed Care: Restructuring the System

Stephen J. Williams
Paul R. Torrens

Probably the most dramatic realignment of the nation's health care system in recent years has been the development of managed care plans. *Managed care* is a generic term that has evolved over the past few years to encompass a variety of forms of prepaid and managed fee-for-service health care.

Under managed care programs, the fundamental incentive structure of traditional fee-for-service medicine is dramatically altered to encourage greater control over the use and costs of health care services. The concepts incorporated into managed care programs involve restructuring the delivery system for health care services; providing appropriate incentives and barriers for providers and consumers to contain costs; imposition of an administrative structure with various components related to managing the enrolled population and its use of services; and facilitating the paperwork required on the part of consumers (1).

This chapter discusses the history, promises, and shortcomings of managed care. Since managed care is an evolving concept that, in all likelihood, will continue to change in the future, the emphasis in this chapter is on the structural changes in health care delivery imposed by the managed care approach, and the implications for providers and consumers alike.

Managed care represents a serious challenge to both providers and consumers in their traditional approach to the provision of health care. The underlying concepts of managed care hold promise for allowing more comprehensive services to greater numbers of people while, at the same time, providing significant incentives to contain the use and cost of services. It is essential that the structure and implications of managed care systems be well understood by everyone involved in providing and using health care.

While managed care has evolved over the years, many of the underlying concepts of managed care have become institutionalized within the health care system. These principles are likely to remain in place, in one form or another, regardless of the further evolution of managed care and of the health care system itself.

The Historical Origins of Managed Care

The fundamental concept of managed care, prepayment of services or discounted fee-for-service arrangements for defined, enrolled populations, has a rather extensive history. As discussed in Chapter 5, managed care has actually existed for quite some time. Such long-standing programs as the Kaiser health care system and Group Health Cooperative of Puget Sound in the United States, as well as the British National Health Service, have long exemplified some of the forms of managed care that are recognized today. These providers have been some of the most successful and well-documented "managed care" efforts ever. The rapid proliferation of managed care programs in recent years, however, has reflected the development of many other models for providing health care to enrolled populations.

The Evolution of HMOs

The recent origin of today's managed care programs in the United States can be traced back to the 1970s with the development of health maintenance organizations (HMOs). Health maintenance organizations were written into federal legislation during the Nixon administration as an approach to reorganizing health care services to facilitate cost containment and to control utilization.

The federal HMO program was initiated in 1973 to promote prepayment plans and incorporated both the group practice and IPA models. The concept was originally proposed by the President as a means of promoting private-sector medicine through self-regulation, while at the same time incorporating some incentives for containment of health care costs. The HMO law provided grants and loans for the planning and establishment of HMOs and required that certain services be provided (table 13-1).

TABLE 13-1. Health Services Originally Required under the Health Maintenance Organization Act of 1973

- Physician professional services
- Outpatient services
- Short-term mental health services
- Short-term rehabilitative services
- Certain services for substance abuse
- Laboratory and radiology services
- Home health service
- Family planning services
- Certain social services
- Immunizations and preventive health services
- Health education
- Arrangements for emergency care
- Arrangements for out-of-area coverage

The federal HMO program and prepaid group practices had early success in providing comprehensive and acceptable quality health services at lower total costs than the fee-for-service sector. However, some of these plans had difficulties attaining financial viability. This problem may have been partially the result of program requirements that included offering a full range of services and having a period of open enrollment during which anyone could join.

Some provisions of the federal program, however, helped developing HMOs. These provisions included the dual-choice requirement under which certain employers had to offer an HMO as a health care option to employees. This established the precedent for employer endorsement of these plans. Now many employers are increasingly offering only forms of managed care.

The most successful prepaid groups have generally been the larger, better capitalized plans or those serving populations with high levels of insurance coverage. Poor management and lack of commitment on the part of organizers and providers have been identified as major reasons for the failure of some early HMOs.

The initial form of HMO that fit the federal prototype was the staff model group practice. In this approach, typified by Kaiser, group practices provide prepaid, rather than fee-for-service, health care through intermediaries that enroll consumers and assume responsibility for all covered care. The passage of federal and state HMO legislation formalized these arrangements into law.

When HMOs were originally proposed, consideration was given to also allowing forms of prepaid health care that could be provided by community-based physicians, rather than by just the closed medical staff group practices. A second organizational format, the independent practice plan (IPP) or independent practice association (IPA), was provided for. An early plan that used this approach was the San Joaquin Foundation in California.

IPAs are affiliations of independent practitioners in the community who, in addition to their fee-for-service patients, contract to provide care for prepaid, enrolled individuals. The IPA sells the insurance product as a prepaid program with a set monthly premium for all covered services. The IPA pays participating physicians on either a capitated or fee-for-service basis, depending on the terms of the plan. The IPAs sign up community-based solo and group practitioners, and provide an opportunity for participation in prepaid health care by physicians who are not part of closed panel providers such as Kaiser.

Many of the early independent practice plans reimbursed physicians using an open-ended, fee-for-service fee schedule, while the plan itself collected revenues on a prepaid basis. These IPAs failed to control the use of services by physicians, since the physician's incentive continued to be to increase use. Many of these plans experienced severe financial difficulties, and some became insolvent. This early lesson in managed care has led to many changes in the operation of these programs today.

Even in these early developmental years, HMOs were viewed by both governmental policy makers and employers as an alternative to traditional fee-for-service medicine and one that would help stem the rapid escalation in health care costs. HMOs gained employer political support and consumer credibility. Some HMOs, however, tarnished the image as a result of managerial incompetence or, occasionally, outright fraud.

Physician Reimbursement and Cost Controls

Some health maintenance organizations, such as Kaiser, reimburse physicians predominantly by salary. Other HMOs and managed care programs provide for incentive-oriented reimbursement of providers while at the same time retaining many of the virtues of prepayment. Experimentation in organizing prepaid programs and in providing incentives to providers and consumers has occurred over the years. Today's managed care programs still have not completely succeeded in fine-tuning these incentives in such a manner as to ensure access to high quality care while also containing costs.

Historically, most prepaid plans have achieved their lower costs for health care services through hospitalization rates that were lower than those in the fee-for-service sector. Ambulatory care use has been generally higher in managed care or HMOs as services have been increasingly shifted from inpatient to outpatient settings. The financial incentives to provide care on an outpatient basis, combined with such changes in the practice of medicine as the increasing use of ambulatory surgery facilities, have enhanced this effect.

Prepaid systems have also rationed services by using a number of mechanisms. These include the use of waiting times to obtain appointments, encouragement of self-care, and triaging of patients to provide care first to more seriously ill individuals. The significant reductions in hospitalization achieved in managed care programs are particularly important, since there is little evidence that managed care providers offer any specific service, such an an office visit or a day in the hospital, at substantially lower cost than fee-for-service providers.

The traditional organizational form of HMOs is presented in figure 13-1. This simplified organizational structure of a typical plan incorporates a

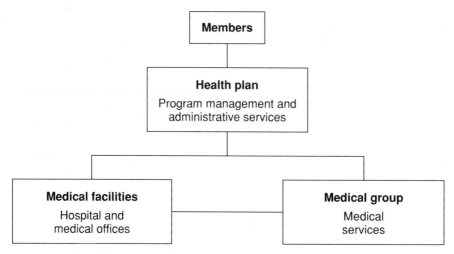

Figure 13-1. Typical Prepaid Health Plan Organizational Relationships.

group practice and affiliated medical facilities, and a health plan or insurance entity that enrolls members and arranges for the provision of care by the provider organizations. Today many other organizational forms are also used.

Under the procompetitive approach of the Reagan and Bush administrations, HMOs and other prepaid plans have had considerable appeal because of their internal incentives for cost containment, and their ability to provide relatively comprehensive services for a predetermined monthly premium. They are also valuable in arranging for care in government entitlement programs, particularly Medicare and, to an extent, Medicaid (2).

Federal subsidies for the development of HMOs have been reduced on the assumption that the appeal of managed care programs will lead to their creation without external government financing. The 1973 legislation has also been amended to reduce restrictions on HMOs in the health care marketplace—for example, decreasing the scope of mandated benefits and allowing premiums to be computed on a more financially sound basis, such as by using experience rather than community rating.

Another important recent trend in managed care programs has been a shift toward for-profit plans.

A large number of older, established plans have converted from not-for-profit to for-profit status or have been assimilated by for-profit entities. For-profit status allows these plans to obtain equity financing and to earn and distribute profits. Public accountability may even be greater in the for-profit sector with public stock ownership.

The Empirical Evidence

The empirical evidence regarding the "first phase" of HMO development, although not entirely consistent throughout all studies, has accumulated over the past few years and suggests distinct advantages for prepaid plans. These advantages were reviewed in a comprehensive and analytical manner by Luft (table 13-2).

The accumulated evidence supports many of the proclaimed advantages of prepayment, although there are also significant disadvantages. Two important concerns are the maintenance of an acceptable level of quality of care and assurance of access to care.

More recently Peter Fox and LuAnn Heinen examined the determinants of HMO success (3). Some of their conclusions are listed in table 13-3.

The role of the medical staff and contracting

TABLE 13-2. Selected Early Empirical Evidence Concerning HMOs

Area of Knowledge	Evidence
Consumer preference	HMOs appeal due to broader benefits. Existing physician relationships are a negative factor. HMOs use hospital services less and ambulatory care more. Adverse selection not a problem.
Health care costs	Prepaid group practice has 10–40% lower costs. IPAs don't achieve the same savings. Out-of-pocket costs are often lower.
Use of services	HMOs have lower hospitalization rates. HMOs have similar lengths of stay and more use of ambulatory care. IPAs have lower surgical rates than other plans, but PGPs do not.
Use of resources	PGPs have higher laboratory and radiology use. HMOs have higher ambulatory and preventive use. HMOs probably provide each unit of service at similar cost. Productivity of physicians is higher in HMOs.
Quality of care and consumer satisfaction	Limited quality comparisons do not clearly favor HMOs. Quality of medical records, appropriateness of care, and health status may be more favorable in HMOs. HMO enrollees tend to be satisfied. Continuity of care may be lower in PGPs. PGP enrollees are less satisfied with physician interaction. Out-of-plan use in PGPs is about 5 to 10%.
Physician satisfaction	Physicians work fewer hours, earn less, have less autonomy, may be less happy with patient relationships in HMOs.

SOURCE: Adapted from H. S. Luft. (1981). *Health maintenance organizations: Dimensions of performance.* New York: John Wiley & Sons, Inc.

physicians, especially in IPAs and networks, is critical. Incentives to control use, to be receptive to patients, and to support the plan are essential (4). In PPOs and similar plans, financial incentives and controls must also encourage containment of total costs (4,5). Hospitals are also assuming an increasingly important role in plan design, operation, and success (6). Hospitals, in turn, succeed in managed care contracting when they have strong medical staff commitment and leadership.

Managed care is successfully being developed for a wider array of services. Mental health and dental services are especially popular, but even other, more highly specialized care is the subject of contract arrangements and even capitation (7). Mental health often is provided less intensively in some managed care settings, especially HMOs (8).

Recent evidence confirms earlier studies that HMOs in particular have lower hospitalization rates,

possibly lower consumer satisfaction for some groups, but probably not lower health outcomes (9). Physician opposition to managed care is a continuing barrier (10). Some physician incentive approaches and HMO organizational arrangements may affect physician clinical practice patterns, and further investigation is needed to determine these effects on the quality of care (11). Designing incentives to control costs and use, while not adversely affecting quality of care and patient and provider satisfaction, is a major challenge in managed care (12,13).

Recent Growth and Evolution of HMOs and Managed Care

The number of HMOs, and the number of consumers enrolled in these plans, have skyrocketed in recent years. Table 13-4 indicates that the number

TABLE 13-3. Some Recent Evidence on HMO Performance

External Success Factors
- Early entry into the marketplace
- Solid provider structure
- Commitment to the marketplace
- Targeting a receptive population and selling to consumers wanting an HMO
- Well-organized and managed operation

Operational Success Factors
- Professional sales staff
- Excellent consumer relations
- Access to care assured
- Excellent information systems
- Excellent provider relations
- Top level management commitment to the product and a strong corporate culture
- Select receptive providers
- Strong provider reimbursement incentives
- Effective risk-sharing mechanisms
- Utilization controls and quality assurance that works
- Excellent provider communications and feedback channels

SOURCE: Adapted from Fox, P. D., and Heinen, L. (1987) *Determinants of HMO success.* Ann Arbor, MI: Health Administration Press.

of HMOs more than doubled from 1980 to 1990, with the greatest growth occurring in the individual practice association form. Health maintenance organization growth has been particularly dramatic in the western U.S., with nearly one-fourth of the entire western population now enrolled in these plans.

More than 33 million Americans now receive health care through a form of HMO. Some state Medicaid programs and the federal Medicare program are also using HMOs for their beneficiaries. The effort to enroll Medicare eligibles in federally qualified, prepaid, HMO-type provider systems is especially notable.

Organizational Evolution of Managed Care

The 1980s and the early 1990s saw further development and increased sophistication of managed care programs. While traditional health maintenance organizations continued to evolve and gain in popularity, other forms of managed care were also proliferating. Most of these newer forms of managed care consist of insurance products that use existing community-based resources, somewhat analogous to the concept of the IPAs.

Among the most popular and rapidly developing forms of managed care has been the preferred provider organization, or PPO. The PPO combines fee discounting on the part of participating providers with some IPA concepts.

In the PPO, a sponsor, which may be an insurance company, an employer, or another entity, contracts with participating hospitals, physicians, medical groups, and other providers to offer services to enrollees in the PPO. Generally, the providers are reimbursed on a contracted-fee basis using an established fee schedule for specific procedures or on a defined, preestablished discount from the provider's usual and customary fees. The PPO concept also incorporates requirements for use review and other quality controls.

Enrollees in the PPO must use contracted providers to obtain the maximum benefit under the plan. Care obtained outside of the contracted network of providers results in substantially reduced levels of coverage. Typically, PPOs require a standard deductible and a copayment of 10 percent of allowable charges for covered services rendered by providers who are participating in the plan. They also require a 30 or 40 percent copayment, based on allowable charges, for nonparticipating provider-source care. Obviously, consumers have a substantial financial incentive to obtain care from within the network.

Most health insurance companies now offer some kind of PPO. Many employers no longer even offer an indemnity option to their employees, thus forcing them to choose between PPOs and other forms of managed care.

A further variant on the PPO concept is the exclusive provider organization or EPO. In this form of managed care, consumers must use participating providers. Providers are assured a greater pen-

TABLE 13-4. Health Maintenance Organization Enrollment: United States, Selected Years

Plans and Enrollment	1980	1990
Plans	Number	
All plans	235	572
Model type:		
Individual practice association	97	360
Group	138	212
Geographic region:		
Northeast	55	115
Midwest	72	160
South	45	176
West	63	121
Enrollment	Persons in Thousands	
Total	9,078	33,028
Model type:		
Individual practice association	1,694	13,741
Group	7,384	19,287
Federal program:		
Medicaid	265	N/A*
Medicare	391	1,842
	Number per 1,000 Population	
Geographic region:		
Northeast	31.4	145.6
Midwest	28.1	126.2
South	8.3	70.5
West	121.8	232.1

*N/A = not available.

SOURCE: National Center for Health Statistics. (1991). *Health, United States, 1990* (DHHS Publication No. [PHS] 91-1232). Washington, D.C.: U.S. Government Printing Office.

etration of the marketplace by having enrollees in the plan channeled to them. The EPO is even more restrictive than the PPO and thus further reduces consumer choice.

There are, of course, other variations on the managed care concept, and other aspects of managed care are discussed elsewhere in this book. The remainder of this chapter discusses many of the unique aspects of managed care as they pertain to the organization, structure, and operation of health care systems and also as they affect the providers themselves. Both the positive and negative aspects of managed care are highlighted, particularly as they represent likely attributes of any further reorganization of the nation's health care system (14).

General Concepts of Managed Care Programs

A number of operational characteristics of managed care plans are unique. Many approaches to providing care under managed care programs are designed to affect the operation and structure of the health care system and, in particular, to affect the use of services by consumers. Therefore, many of these concepts have significant impact on quality, access, costs, and other key components of health services delivery. Some represent threats to such time-honored values as consumer choice, free access, avoidance of involvement of insurers in the patient–provider relationship, and other key principles that are now being called into question.

The Gatekeeper

Among the most important concepts underlying many managed care plans is the role of the primary care physician (PCP) as a gatekeeper. This approach has long been used in health maintenance organizations.

The gatekeeper concept is that one individual, usually a PCP in family practice, internal medicine, or, less often, pediatrics or obstetrics/gynecology, is responsible for all primary care for the patient. The PCP also determines when referral to specialists is needed and provides an oversight and coordinating role for the patient's health care needs. The gatekeeper concept is designed to manage the patient's use of resources, to reduce the self-initiated use of specialty services, and to ensure overall coordination, not duplication, of care.

The gatekeeper can function smoothly in patient care management, but can present a barrier to access to specialty services. The PCP may under- or overrefer to specialists, depending on practice patterns and financial incentives. While the conventional wisdom is that gatekeeper physicians are cost-effective and can improve the quality and coordination of care, limited empirical evidence for such a conclusion is currently available.

Utilization Oversight

Utilization review and its associated procedures is an integral part of managed care. The concepts of utilization review revolve around monitoring the use of services and determining the appropriateness of the care that is provided (15). Utilization review usually occurs at the level of the provider organization. The managed care contract from the insurance entity or other sponsor frequently stipulates the nature and extent to which managed care contractors must perform utilization review.

Most utilization review focuses on either the use of inpatient hospital services or referrals for expensive and complex secondary and tertiary care. To be effective, utilization review must include analysis of physician practice patterns and individual physician behaviors within contractor organizations. Utilization review may also examine the use of services on a patient-specific basis to detect inappropriate or abusive use of the system by consumers.

Networks

Managed care programs that follow the independent practice association or community-based model—as opposed to the closed panel, staff group practice model—develop networks of providers. Some networks are composed of group practices rather than solo practitioners. These networks are made up of participating providers who sign contracts with the managed care sponsor and agree to the specified terms and conditions of the plan, including such factors as fee schedules, discounts, and utilization review requirements.

Many managed care programs focus their network development on PCPs and hospitals. Less

common is the development of networks that include specialty care providers, although these providers increasingly are also being included in the networks to gain greater control over their use and costs. Networks allow the managed care sponsor to provide beneficiaries with some selection of PCPs, hospitals, and other providers and, more important, to provide direct control over the participating providers within the health care delivery system that the network creates.

Consumer Controls

Control over the behavior of consumers is achieved through a variety of mechanisms. Obviously the networks themselves, and the use of gatekeepers, serve to channel patients. In addition, managed care programs, and especially HMOs, may influence access to care by creating a variety of barriers such as the waiting times for appointments mentioned previously.

Patients with severe problems and expensive care needs are "controlled" through the use of various forms of case management. In case management, an experienced professional with knowledge of the health care resources available to the network monitors the care provided to the patient to determine whether the care is necessary and is being provided in the most cost-effective setting. Case management may involve bringing to bear specialized resources such as home health services to meet patient needs, perhaps in lieu of hospitalization.

Case management is a rapidly growing area of the health care industry, but the evidence thus far is not conclusive regarding the extent to which case management can reduce costs and at the same time improve efficiency and patient outcomes. Case managers can be supportive and of great assistance to patients and their families.

Consumer Issues Associated with Managed Care

Several important consumer issues arise in managed care programs, some of which have been touched upon already in this chapter. It is important to emphasize that the benefit package and administrative structure of managed care programs are generally advantageous to the consumer. Balancing the issues of access and use controls, managed care programs tend to offer a more comprehensive package of benefits than traditional indemnity plans.

Covered preventive services often include, at little or no cost to the patient, routine physical examinations, including vision and hearing screening, well-child care, and patient education services. Coverage for reproductive health needs, such as infertility diagnosis and treatment, may be more extensive in managed care programs. Reimbursement of services provided by contracting chiropractors, podiatrists, mental health professionals, and certain other service providers may also be more lenient.

Administrative operation of managed care programs, from the viewpoint of the consumer, may also offer advantages. In most managed care programs, paperwork is virtually eliminated for the consumer, with the burden of claims processing and copayment collection placed on the providers. This approach is helpful to the consumer, but it also reduces the administrative costs of the program for the sponsor. Consumer-initiated claims processing generally occurs only for care obtained outside of the provider network.

Finally, most managed care programs also include a number of other consumer activities. These include a membership department to cope with any administrative problems that arise, including such routine matters as changing primary care providers.

Consumer complaints are usually accommodated by the plan as well. But problem resolution may ultimately be the responsibility of the provider organization. Most managed care programs also use compulsory arbitration in the settlement of malpractice-related disputes, a potentially cost-effective approach.

Reimbursement and Pricing Considerations

Managed care programs pay providers using a number of mechanisms. In a staff model, group practice-type HMO, physicians are reimbursed on a salary basis with some incentive compensation, usually distributed at year end based on factors related to individual productivity and plan profitability. In IPAs and certain other managed care programs, participating community-based physicians may be reimbursed on a traditional, fee-for-service, discounted fee basis, or they may receive capitation payments with additional incentive compensation. PPOs and similar types of managed care programs generally reimburse on a discounted, fee-for-service basis.

Most managed care programs reimburse hospitals on a predetermined, negotiated, often per-diem, basis. Payment of specialty service providers and other services, if under contract with the plan, will be based on a preestablished, negotiated fee schedule, usually at a discount from usual and customary fees.

Risk Sharing

Of increasing importance and interest in managed care is the use of risk-sharing pools of various sorts. These vary widely, and no optimum form of risk sharing has yet been identified. In general, risk pools involve the establishment of a pool of money from which certain services are paid throughout the year. The funds remaining at year end are divided between the providers and the insurer. The risk pools are often separate for physician and hospital services, and generally do not include specialized referral providers, who are used on an as-needed basis.

The general concept of the risk pools is to provide an incentive to reduce use, and particularly hospitalization and specialty referrals. The extent to which risk pools are effective in doing so, and the question of whether they result in underuse of needed services, has not yet been fully determined.

There is, as reflected by the risk pool concept, a general belief that risk must be shared between providers and insurers to ensure containment of costs and use. Since patients are affected by this structuring of the system they are, in a sense, also involved in the risk-sharing concept, but more as silent partners.

Another aspect of sharing risk in managed care includes reinsurance for provider organizations, which may be built into the contract by the insurer in the form of stop-loss insurance. The insurer, while trying to obtain the best possible prices from providers, also has an important incentive to be sure that providers are solvent and reasonably happy with the contract. The insurer must ultimately also guarantee that patients are satisfied, at least to the extent that they don't leave the plan en masse. Thus insurers must monitor not only costs, but also patient satisfaction and use of services.

The Effect of Managed Care on Provider Organizations

A number of key considerations involve provider organizations that participate in managed care programs, particularly PPO- and IPA-type plans. One of the most important and practical issues, especially in regard to the medical staff, is the effect on physician practice patterns of having both fee-for-service and prepaid or managed care patients.

A hospital may enter into managed care contracts independently, through its medical staff, or by using owned resources such as a hospital-sponsored group practice. Managed care may require extensive reorganization of hospital services, especially in ambulatory care (16).

From a managerial perspective, a group practice (or hospital) participating in a managed care contract wants its physicians to "control" their use of services, especially hospital care, for enrolled patients. At the same time, these physicians would tend to increase fee-for-service revenue by enhancing use, including laboratory and radiological services, and referrals within the group to specialty providers.

This conflict in incentives places the group and its administrator in the position of sending diametrically opposed signals to physicians regarding utilization and revenue enhancement. In addition, utilization review, with a focus on use as opposed to quality, is likely to be more aggressive for managed care patients.

A related complication of managed care is physician reimbursement. In a staff model, group practice HMO, all physicians are reimbursed identically, and all patients are seen under a relatively uniform health plan. In a group practice or other physician setting where both fee-for-service and managed care patients are being seen, physician reimbursement becomes much more complex. The group must determine the extent to which incentives can be provided for physicians to enhance use by fee-for-service patients and reduce use by managed care patients.

Physicians may resent the apparent interference by the group, and the various insurance plans, in their practice of medicine. Physicians may also resent having large panels, or numbers, of patients assigned to them under managed care. These conflicts are not easily resolved (17). They also raise the issue of whether two standards of care are being provided based on a patient's payment source.

Another concern on the part of group practices, and even solo physicians participating in managed care plans, is the risk of adverse selection. Participating providers may be able to limit the total number of beneficiaries for which they assume responsibility, but they generally cannot screen such beneficiaries based on clinical criteria to protect against adverse selection. As a result, and especially in contracts that require a high degree of risk sharing, providers can be at substantial liability in the event of adverse selection. Some protection is offered if the provider contract includes provision for stop-loss coverage.

Managed care contracting insurers or employers will generally require some degree of reporting on the part of participating providers. For group practices with large numbers of covered beneficiaries,

TABLE 13-5. Key Principles of Managed Care

- Reduced consumer administrative requirements
- Reduced utilization, especially of inpatient services
- Broader benefit structure, especially for preventive services
- Enhanced provider risk sharing
- Greater management control over providers and consumers

---

data requirements might be more extensive than for solo practitioners in an IPA-type arrangement. IPAs also require billing arrangements that usually meet reporting needs themselves.

These reporting requirements mandate that the provider have an adequate management information system to collect data and generate required reports (18). In addition, pricing of contracts by participating providers requires management information systems that allow for the determination of true costs and analysis of use patterns (19). Since contracts are often bid competitively, a participating provider wants to be sure to submit a winning bid, but at the same time must protect against bidding too low (20).

The dollar amounts involved in these contracts, when substantial numbers of lives are covered, can be quite high, so miscalculations can result in very significant losses. Most contracts are negotiated for a one-year period and provide no opportunity for renegotiation during the contract performance period.

Risk management is also an essential component of these contracts. This includes, in addition to previously discussed binding arbitration, maintaining positive patient relations, enhancing patient-provider interaction so as to reduce the threat of patient complaints and malpractice litigation, and other legal and operational considerations. Risk management also involves fair and accurate bidding for contracts; monitoring of use as well as costs; utilization review; a variety of quality assurance mechanisms; adequate underwriting and stop-loss protection; and, of course, malpractice coverage and adequate reserves in the event of losses.

Finally, managed care requires positive relationships among participating physicians, physician groups, and hospitals (21,22). Hospitals and their medical staffs often need to cooperate in bidding for contracts, and managed care changes the relationships between physicians and hospitals (23). Hospital care must be carefully managed, and quality assurance, utilization review, stop-loss protection, and other aspects of risk management must be incorporated into the relationship with the hospital (24).

The hospital may have an independent relationship with the insurer or employer sponsoring the plan, or it may contract through the participating medical group. Relationships with participating specialty and other service providers must also be managed from administrative, pricing, quality, and utilization control perspectives.

Challenges and Opportunities for Managed Care

While there are many recent developments in managed care, the fundamental concepts of prepayment have existed for quite some time. In recent years, there has been a great deal of experimentation with different forms of prepayment. Systems of care have been developed to provide reasonable quality at controlled costs and to yield positive reactions from providers, patients, employers, and the federal government.

In all likelihood, experimentation with managed care is not yet over. Some of the key principles of managed care that appear to have been validated are presented in table 13-5. Many of these principles, such as prospective payment and utilization controls, are likely to be permanent fixtures of the U.S. health care system.

Further enhancements are likely in the evolution of managed care plans. Intervention in the health care system by the federal government, such as is exemplified by Medicare prospective payment and by resource-based relative-value scales (25), may substantially affect the evolution of managed care plans. Any national health care financing scheme is also likely to use various aspects of managed care.

Other Concerns and Pitfalls

Other issues in managed care that must be considered include antitrust, particularly as it relates to the formation of provider networks for purposes of contracting (26); consumer dissatisfaction with limitations on choice of providers; viability of plans in the face of the rapid proliferation of plan sponsors; viability of hospitals, groups, and other providers that are excluded from networks; physician and other professional provider satisfaction (or more likely dissatisfaction); contract limitations and requirements, such as utilization review; and other constraints on practice patterns.

Numerous other potential pitfalls exist in managed care, including financial failures of insurers; inadequate numbers of beneficiaries to provide a critical mass; the effect of the aging of the population on cost trends; the long-term effect of deep discounting on providers; conflicts among providers, insurers, and employers; assurance of quality of care (27,28); and, ultimately, the effect of managed care on the promotion of health, prevention of disease, and enhancement of client well-being.

While managed care has come a long way, many challenges and uncertainties remain (29). The role of managed care in the future of our nation's health care system, while likely to continue, remains somewhat uncertain.

References

1. Kongstvedt, P. R. (1989). *The managed care health handbook.* Rockville, MD: Aspen Publishers.
2. Freund, D. A., & Hurky, R. E. (1987). Managed care in Medicaid: Selected issues in program origin, design, and research. *Annual Review of Public Health. 8.* 137–163.
3. Fox, P. D., & Heinen, L. (1987). *Determinants of HMO success.* Ann Arbor, MI: Health Administration Press.
4. Pauly, M. V., Hillman, A. L., & Kerstein, J. (1990).

Managing physician incentives in managed care: The role of for-profit ownership. *Managed Care. 28.* 1013–1026.
5. Garnick, D. W., et al. (1990). Services and charges by PPO physicians for PPO and indemnity patients: An episode of care comparison. *Medical Care. 28.* 894–906.
6. Schroer, K. A., & Penn, D. A. (1987). *Hospital strategies for contracting with managed care.* Chicago: American Hospital Association.
7. Feldman, S. (Ed.). (1991). *Managed mental health services.* Springfield, IL: Charles B. Thomas.
8. Wells, K. B., Manning, W. G., Jr., & Valdez, R. B. (1990). The effects of a prepaid group practice on mental health outcomes. *Health Services Research. 25*(4). 615–625.
9. Wagner, E. H., & Bledsoe, T. (1990). The Rand health insurance experiment and HMOs. *Medical Care. 28*(3). 191–200.
10. Ellsbury, K. E.., & Montano, D. E. (1990). Attitudes of Washington State primary care physicians toward capitation-based insurance plans. *Journal of Family Practice. 30*(1). 89–94.
11. Hillman, A. L., Pauly, M. V., & Kerstein, J. J. (1989). How do financial incentives affect physicians' clinical decisions and the financial performance of health maintenance organizations? *New England Journal of Medicine. 321*(2). 86–92.
12. Manton, K. G., Tolley, H. D., & Vertrees, J. C. (1989). Controlling risk in capitation payment. Multivariate definitions of risk groups. *Medical Care. 27*(3). 259–272.
13. Murray, J. P. (1988). A follow-up comparison of patient satisfaction among prepaid and fee-for-service patients. *Journal of Family Practice. 26*(5). 576–581.
14. Prottas, J. M., & Handler, E. (1987). The complexities of managed care: Operating a voluntary system. *Journal of Health Politics, Policy and Law. 12*(2). 253–269.
15. Romeo, S. J. W. (1988). The economic effects of utilization review in prepaid care. *Medical Group Management. 35*(3). 54–86, 60.
16. Matson, T. A. (Ed.) (1990). *Restructuring for ambulatory care: A guide to reorganization.* Chicago: American Hospital Publishing.
17. Kahn, L. (1987). A physician's view of managed care. *Health Affairs. 6*(3). 90–95.

18. Huth, S. (1988). Claims data is key to managed care program. *Employee Benefit Plan Review. 42.* 56–60.

19. Traska, M. R. (1988). Managed care: Whoever has the data wins the game. *Hospitals. 62*(7). 50–53, 55.

20. Wrightson, W., Jr. (1990). *HMO rate setting & financial strategy.* Ann Arbor, MI: Health Administration Press.

21. Valentine, S. T. (Ed.). *Physician bonding: Developing a successful hospital program.* Gaithersburg, MD: Aspen Publishers.

22. Shortell, S. M. (1991). *Effective hospital–physician relationships.* Ann Arbor, MI: Health Administration Press.

23. Goldstein, D. E., & McKell, D. C. (1990). *Medical staff alliances: How to build successful partnerships with your physicians.* Chicago: American Hospital Publishing.

24. Bermans, N. F. (1985). Joint ventures in ambulatory care. *Journal of Ambulatory Care Management. 8*(4). 79–87.

25. Hsiao, W. C., Braun, P., Dunn, D., & Becker, E. R. (1988). Resource-based relative values: An overview. *Journal of the American Medical Association. 260*(16). 2347–2353.

26. Shouldice, R. G. (1988). Antitrust and managed care. *Medical Group Management. 35*(4). 12–13, 33.

27. Wolfson, J., Levin, P. J., & Campbell, J. D. (1988). Beyond the cost of health care: The new era of quality and liability in managed care. *Journal of the Florida Medical Association. 75*(3). 165–168.

28. Brook, R. H., & Kosecoff, J. B. (1988). Competition and quality. *Health Affairs. 7*(3). 150–161.

29. Boland, P. (1991). *Making managed healthcare work: A practical guide to strategies and solutions.* New York: McGraw Hill.

PART SIX

Assessing and Regulating System Performance

Chapter 14

Influencing, Regulating, and Monitoring the Health Care System

Stephen J. Williams
Paul R. Torrens

In recent years, and particularly with the enhancement of fiscal pressures in the health care environment, the processes of monitoring, evaluating, controlling, and influencing the functioning of the system have gained great importance. These mechanisms involve the monitoring of information related to pricing, costs, use, quality, and, in a broader sense, efficacy and effectiveness of services. These processes are a complex and multifaceted effort on the part of payors, providers, government, and consumers.

This chapter takes a comprehensive and integrated view of these mechanisms, their operation, and their purposes. The chapter examines how the operation of the health care system is changed, influenced, controlled, and monitored. Everyone involved in the health care system is affected by the mechanisms discussed in this chapter. A thorough understanding of these mechanisms is essential for all participants in the health care system and is also key to understanding the possible future evolution of the system itself, as discussed further in the last chapter of this book.

In summary, the evolution of voluntary and mandated efforts to control, monitor, and change the health care system is discussed in this chapter in detail, focusing especially on issues of use, access, and quality. The discussion begins with the development of voluntary health planning.

Voluntary Health Planning and Mandated Regulation

Encouragement of voluntary efforts to plan local health services and to provide incentives to hospitals and other organizations to cooperate in the effort to reduce duplicated services has a long history in the United States. Volunteerism stems from both the initiative of industry and the desire of government to promote cooperative ventures. From an external "regulatory" perspective, voluntary planning is designed to provide a mechanism for the industry to police itself with the objectives of reducing duplication and improving access to care. Unfortunately, the individual objectives of the industry and of government are not necessarily consistent with each other.

From an industry perspective, voluntary planning is primarily focused on reducing competition, gaining an edge in the marketplace, and protecting an institution's existing markets. The fundamental inconsistencies of voluntary planning have been well demonstrated. The conclusion is inevitable that government requests for voluntary planning yield advantages for individual institutions but not necessarily for the community.

Purposes of Planning

Voluntary planning, like regulation, price controls, and other forms of external intervention in the health care system, is designed to influence the operation of the system in such a way as to promote collective social objectives, rather than each institution's objectives. The increasing complexity of the health care system, and of our society in general, suggests a need for planning. From an individual institutional perspective, strategic planning is essential to the development of services, marketplaces, resources, and competitive advantages. In a centrally controlled health care system, such as a health maintenance organization (HMO) or internationally in a national health service, the planning function is critical to the allocation of resources and to the assurance that consumer needs are met (1). In a competitive marketplace, as exists generally in the United States, institutional planning is, as noted above, essential to the long-term viability of each hospital, group practice, or other provider. But under competition, the voluntary planning role is essentially absent, and substituted in its place is the influence of the market and the resulting evolution of services independent of any clear, external plan.

The extent to which planning is voluntary rather than mandated is a function of philosophy, economics, national political agendas, and many other complex, socially determined factors. As discussed later in this chapter, voluntary planning in the United States has failed to accomplish significant social objectives. However, a more aggressive, mandatory approach to planning, such as is evidenced in other types of centrally controlled health care systems, can lead to a highly rational allocation of resources and cost-effective decision making. Whether such an approach will ever occur in the United States is an issue of economics and politics.

Early History of Planning

Health planning in the United States had its origins in the 1930s and 1940s. Early forms of health planning were primarily the result of community-wide voluntary organizations established by hospitals in such areas as New York City. These agencies, often called hospital councils, cooperated on a narrow range of services and support functions that were mutually beneficial to member hospitals. For example, some early forms of shared services included management information systems and computers, centralized laundry services, fund raising, and limited services for the medically indigent. These agencies were effective only to the extent that all participating hospitals were able to gain an advantage through the cooperative planning function (2).

In other words, voluntary planning worked only on a limited basis and only in instances where every participating organization ended up a winner. Trade-offs that would have resulted in one participant's losing key services, revenue, or market presence were not likely to be the subject of the voluntary planning effort. As a result, voluntary planning in this early stage did not serve a key or central function in maximizing access to services or in reducing the cost of services on a communitywide basis.

To a limited extent, these voluntary planning agencies (which in some forms exist to this day) did serve some beneficial role for their participating institutions. Hence, it would not be appropriate to view voluntary planning as a total failure, but rather as a limited success and one oriented more toward institutions than communities (3).

The next stages of institutional and community-wide planning occurred concurrently with increased federal government involvement in the health care system. Increasing use of regulatory, as opposed to voluntary, approaches to affecting the operation of the health care system began to evidence themselves in the early development of the next stage of health planning. The financial support for these planning approaches also shifted somewhat from philanthropic donations, such as those supporting the hospital councils in their earlier years, to government support with implicit strings attached.

In a sense, the development of these government interventions in the planning process was also an outgrowth of earlier historical precedents. One of these was the report of the Committee on the Cost of Medical Care, mentioned in an earlier chapter, which suggested that the United States develop a more planned, regionalized health care system similar to the one subsequently developed in the United Kingdom as a result of the Dawson Report recommendations.

The increasing emphasis on planning also occurred concurrently with the development of hospital councils in such cities as New York, Rochester, and Pittsburgh. However, these early movements toward a more planned health care system were never successfully incorporated into national health care policy and a nationally managed system.

The Hill-Burton Program

World War II led to the diversion of national resources to the war effort. After the war, it was widely recognized that the nation's hospitals had suffered as a result of a shortage of resources. In addition, the increasing suburbanization of our nation led to the need for expansion of hospital resources into these suburban areas. The legacy of the Great Depression and World War II was a hospital system in the United States severely lacking in modern amenities, with existing hospitals requiring substantial modernization and expansion and, at the same time, a rapidly developing need for increasing the dispersion of hospital resources

into the new communities being built outside core urban areas.

Recognizing this national need, Congress passed the Hill-Burton program, officially titled "The Hospital Survey and Construction Act of 1946." This act also represented the first federally mandated health planning initiative in the United States. States were required to inventory existing hospitals and determine the need for construction of new hospitals and renovation of existing hospitals. Resources were provided from the federal government for construction and renovation of hospitals in response to a need for hospital beds as evidenced by the application of these mandated planning methodologies.

From a technical perspective, planning approaches required under the Hill-Burton Act were rather simplistic and based on bed-to-population ratios. More important, however, is the recognition that, for the first time, external intervention in the system to promote the planning of health-related resources was encouraged and financially supported by the federal government. In addition, from a social perspective, the Hill-Burton program was designed to reduce or eliminate shortages of hospital facilities in rural and relatively poor regions.

The Hill-Burton program was eminently successful in allocating construction funds for development of hospital resources. Indeed, in some locations the act may have led to the development of excess resources, particularly with subsequent changes in medical and surgical practice. In addition, as hospital bed deficiencies were eliminated, Congress changed the nature of the Hill-Burton Act to increasingly emphasize hospital renovation, and then to expand into ambulatory care services (4).

From a planning perspective, the Hill-Burton Act represented very limited success in encouraging significant planning activities, at least beyond those mandated for the allocation of federal support for hospital construction. Program administration was conducted at the state level by state agencies and with the advice of hospital planning councils made up of industry and government representatives.

Neither consistent and well-designed decision-making guidelines nor significantly advanced health planning methodologies were used in the planning process. In later years, federal involvement in planning at the local level built on this early experience, but, as will be evidenced below, with not much greater success.

The "Great Society" and Subsequent Planning Efforts

Various federal programs were designed to encourage planning activities at the local level. The Regional Medical Programs Act was a federal grant program implemented at the local level with a focus on funding planning and related projects for specific health care problems, such as heart disease and cancer (5). Allocation of federal financial support for medical school development and other related activities also was associated with some mandated planning requirements.

However, the next major, and more all-encompassing, effort to promote voluntary health planning occurred with the passage of comprehensive health planning legislation in the mid-1960s. Comprehensive health planning, or CHP, was the precursor to the most recent, and now defunct, effort to combine voluntary and mandatory planning and regulation under a federal initiative in the National Health Planning and Resources Development Act of 1974.

Comprehensive health planning was developed with the recognition that Medicare and Medicaid funding had to be tied to attempts to encourage more cost-effective provision of health services and reductions in duplication of resources. CHP was a voluntary program to promote significant health planning activities at the local level with state supervisory oversight. Under CHP, a statewide agency, the CHP(a) agency, supervised the overall planning effort in each state.

Local planning agencies, CHP(b) agencies, were created in designated regions throughout each state; the mandate of these agencies was to conduct the actual local planning effort. CHP was committed to consumer involvement through membership on various advisory councils. These agencies were funded primarily through federal and state grants with some supplementation from other local sources.

Limited empirical evidence suggests that the CHP voluntary planning effort was generally unsuccessful in achieving the social goals of enhancing access and quality and reducing cost and duplication of services. As with other voluntary efforts, these agencies could rely only on providers' goodwill. Successful change was possible where it was beneficial to organizations to participate in the planning process. As a result of the voluntary nature of the effort, and the tendency for any individual institution to look out for its own interests, communitywide goals and objectives were difficult to achieve.

Certificate of Need

Increasing recognition that voluntary efforts were likely to continue to be unsuccessful in achieving broad, communitywide objectives led various states to move from a voluntary planning effort to an enhanced regulatory approach. The regulatory mechanism used to implement these efforts was termed "certificate of need" (CON) (6). In essence, CON was a process by which hospitals or other health care providers seeking a substantial expansion of their scope of services or physical facilities would have to have prior approval from a government-endorsed entity (7). In the early days these were the CHP(a) and CHP(b) agencies; later they were the planning agencies created under the National Health Planning and Resources Development Act of 1974.

Organizations without CON approval were in violation of state law. The review of the request for authorization for additional resources or expansion of services was based on the voluntary planning agencies' assessment of health care resource needs in the community. Hence, a somewhat analytical and methodologically sound approach was used to assess the extent to which these requests met community needs and promoted social objectives.

Other Federal and State Programs

Many other federal and state initiatives aimed at changing the operation of the health care system were also enacted into law in the 1960s and 1970s. These programs included an experimental health services delivery system designed to develop new health care systems and numerous reorganizations of the federal bureaucracy and of individual agencies involved in health care. Increasing emphasis was also placed on conducting research related to access to health care, quality of care, and other aspects of the operation and functioning of the health care system.

The National Health Planning and Resources Development Act of 1974

From a health planning perspective, the most recent landmark legislation was PL 93-641, the National Health Planning and Resources Development Act of 1974. This law was the last major federal initiative designed to promote health planning on a communitywide basis. These efforts were subsequently abandoned by the Reagan administration in the early 1980s with a move toward a procompetitive, marketplace-driven health care system.

The National Health Planning and Resources Development Act of 1974 essentially folded all of the prior legislation and agencies into a new structure somewhat analogous to CHP. Statewide entities called State Health Planning and Development Agencies (SHPDAs) were established, and a state health-planning council, the State Health Coordinating Council (SHCC), served as an advisory mechanism at the state level in setting overall policy.

At the local level, new planning agencies, called Health Systems Agencies (HSAs), were established; they were analogous to the CHP(b) agencies and actually conducted local planning efforts in their own communities. Extensive political processes occurred in the establishment of these local agencies and in defining the geographic areas for which each agency was responsible. These agencies were also designed to provide opportunities for consumer involvement in policy making through advisory councils and the use of public hearings. At the federal level, overall policy was the responsibility of the Secretary of the Department of Health, Education, and Welfare (now the Department of Health and Human Services), assisted by a national health planning council representing various constituencies.

To provide greater impact, the HSAs in the states where CON existed were given authority to conduct CON reviews and make recommendations at the local level to the state planning agency. The state agencies had statutory authority to approve or disapprove applications submitted for services and facilities expansion under the CON laws.

At the federal level, to provide increased powers for the planning agencies, Section 1122 of the Social Security Act, as amended, provided that hospitals and other Medicare providers had to meet all planning mandates. Failure to comply resulted in a disallowance of Medicare reimbursement for that portion of new construction, or facilities expansion, that was denied planning approval. Thus, the local and state health planning agencies had authority to conduct voluntary assessments of health planning needs; inventory existing resources; determine deficiencies; and, on a mandatory basis, recommend and implement CON and Section 1122 regulations.

Numerous deficiencies were inherent in this voluntary, and limited mandatory, approach. First, the entire health care system of the nation was "grandfathered" in. Planning agencies had no authority to effect facility or service closures. Second, extensive political involvement was inherent in the process. Intervention by various state legislatures resulted in some circumvention of the process. The planning agencies' ability to conduct and implement analytical and apolitical assessments was limited. In addition, those hospitals and other providers with the greatest fiscal resources were able to develop the most sophisticated analytical planning documents and applications, as well as to

TABLE 14-1. Concepts of Regionalization

Population served	Defined geographically or by enrollment
	Health care needs identifiable
System requirements	Coordinated, systematic networks
	Integrated
	Primary care-based
Resource allocations	Dynamic needs-based planning
	Resource-based decision making
	Prospective budgeting
	Utilization controls
	Assured access
	Consumer involvement/feedback and provider accountability

exercise the greatest influence on the political process. Attempts to increase consumer involvement were also difficult to implement and led to increased bureaucratic activity and process without necessarily enhancing substance or outcomes.

Thus, PL 93-641, while well-intentioned, realistically resulted in complex and relatively ineffective planning processes. The lack of overall control over all health care resources, and the need to focus primarily on the encouragement of voluntary cooperation by providers, which had already proven to be ineffectual, effectively doomed this entire approach. Even the mandated aspects of the effort, CON and Section 1122 review, have been shown to have had minimal effect on the proliferation of health care resources and on the containment of costs (8). The lack of a comprehensive, mandated approach to the planning process and the reliance on consumer involvement, voluntary cooperation, limited methodological approaches, and other deficiencies all contributed to a process that came to be viewed by the incoming Reagan administration as a clear failure, and indeed a hindrance, in promoting effective marketplace decision making in a procompetitive environment.

Planning does work. Evidence from national health services, such as in the United Kingdom, as well as from United States self-contained and centrally managed health care systems, such as Kaiser, the military, and the Veterans Administration, clearly indicate that centrally controlled, aggressively managed planning does work on a mandatory basis. The process of regionalization, the characteristics of which are represented in table 14-1, requires that such planning be centrally controlled, conducted for a definable population, and be associated with the ability to control the distribution of both existing and new resources within the system (9).

Deregulation of Planning

The philosophical origins of reducing government intervention in the national economy, with the subsequent change in attitudes toward health services-related planning and regulation, occurred during the Carter administration as federal regulatory authority over a number of industries was changed to a more market-focused orientation. Government involvement in decision making was decreased, especially in the areas of strategic pricing and marketplace decisions on the part of industry. Among the industries where government intervention was decreased in this period were the airlines and telecommunications.

It is important to note that deregulation and reduced governmental involvement in market-related planning does not preclude intervention related to health and safety issues. In the airline industry, for example, the termination of Civil Aeronautics Board authority related to market entry and pricing did not reduce involvement of the Federal Aviation Administration in safety-related regulatory processes, such as aircraft and pilot certification; air traffic control; and aircraft design, assembly, and maintenance.

In the health care industry, mandatory government involvement related to health and safety factors has always existed and remains active to this day. These interventions include fire safety regulations, building codes, and food service regulation. Sanitation, fair labor practices activity, and other government involvement also continue to be prevalent in the health care industry. Antitrust policy, securities regulation, and a number of other market-related interventions have had a mixed experience in this industry.

The Reagan administration accelerated the deregulatory processes initiated by the Carter administration. Deregulation expanded in the scope of economic activity no longer covered. Deregulation and a reduced emphasis on communitywide planning as it relates to services, facilities, and marketplaces have been characteristic of the procompetitive stance of both the Reagan and Bush administrations.

Pricing regulation, however, has experienced a somewhat different philosophical approach, with a mixed philosophy related to government purchases of health care services, particularly under Medicare, as discussed elsewhere in this chapter and throughout this book. Health and safety interventions, as noted above, have been maintained at previous levels by federal, state, and local governments. Most of these interventions are not federally controlled, although a number are affected by Medicare certification and other federal programs. In recent years, there has also been increasing interest in the regulation of laboratories, drug companies, and other parts of the health care system.

Early action on the part of the Reagan administration led to Congressional repeal of most aspects of the National Health Planning and Resources Development Act of 1974. From a philosophical perspective, this deregulatory attitude was based on a belief that, first, the regulatory cost exceeded the regulatory benefits; and second, the economic marketplace would serve to meet social goals. It is interesting to note that a number of states have maintained CON authority, although the minimum size of projects requiring such approval has been substantially increased.

With the exception of those states with current CON authority, hospitals and other health care providers have generally been able to enter markets at will, to expand or contract physical facilities, and otherwise to determine their own strategic plans, subject to the health and safety constraints

mentioned previously and to certain pricing limitations. Some early indications, not yet fully determined, of the effect of this procompetitive environment on the industry can be observed.

Removing the yoke of regulatory process, and the implied threats of the voluntary planning agencies, has resulted in an increased proliferation of health care facilities and resources in many areas of the country. Increased competition has also led to consolidation and other changes in the operation of certain aspects of the system, particularly in the hospital sector. The for-profit industry has been particularly affected by pricing constraints and market competition leading to significant divestitures and reorganizations. Many proprietary companies are refocusing their efforts on more profitable product lines, such as drug and alcohol rehabilitation, rather than on traditional acute-care hospital services.

The consolidation and realignment of the airline industry following deregulation is particularly interesting in view of indications that the health care industry is also moving toward a more vertically and horizontally integrated and consolidated form. Hospitals have increasingly viewed competitive pressures as forcing greater integration of their services by either acquiring other product lines or arranging joint ventures or affiliation agreements to ensure adequate patient volumes, especially for inpatient and ancillary services. Hospitals and hospital systems are increasingly merging with each other, and with other parts of the health care system, to provide a more comprehensive set of services that can then be sold to employers through managed care entities and other arrangements.

It is too early to determine the extent to which consolidation will be the norm nationwide, but if present trends accelerate and a competitive market remains, it is possible that these consolidated systems will result in relatively fewer vertically integrated provider systems in each marketplace competing for insured patients including employer groups. Federal antitrust policy related to the health care industry is in too early a stage of evolution to anticipate how such policy will adapt to this new marketplace and whether antitrust policies will ensure that the fewer, more integrated, producers are still competing fairly.

Other Regulatory Interventions

Voluntary programs to achieve socially desirable goals through the types of planning activities discussed above would be as far as government would go if they were successful. The overwhelming evidence, of course, is that such voluntary and limited regulatory approaches do not achieve government and social objectives. As a result, other forms of more aggressive intervention in the health care system's operations have occurred, and will likely occur again, as government seeks to modify the health care marketplace further. Since each institution or provider system seeks to maximize its own market share, profits, and other objectives, regulatory intervention is aimed at forcing compliance with socially mandated government goals related to such issues as access, costs, and quality.

Regulatory intervention as attempted in the United States historically has been highly imperfect. At the extreme, regionalized systems, including national health systems, offer the most ideal environment for imposing regulatory mechanisms. The marketplace-driven environment typical of the United States offers the least receptive environment for regulatory intervention, since the goals of each participant in the marketplace differ both from each other and from society's overall goals. The absence of a clear national health policy, and changes over time in federal and local policy have also muddied the waters and inhibited the success of regulatory efforts. Failure to agree on outcome measures for health services and specific criteria by which to evaluate those services, particularly in the absence of a clear national agenda, make intervention that much more difficult.

Ultimately, regulation, particularly that carried out by governments, must be based on national consensus regarding the role of government and an acceptance of intervention in the marketplace.

Philosophically, regulation is most acceptable as it relates to health and safety concerns shared by society at large. Regulation in our environment is least acceptable with regard to specific operational decision making in freely operating markets. In health care, however, the conflict between individual welfare and freedom of market activity is much more complex and pronounced, since a failure of the market to provide adequate services to members of the society can lead to disastrous consequences for those individuals. All of these highly complex considerations must be weighed in determining the nature and role of intervention in the system, and in establishing national health policy.

Types of Market Interventions

Intervention in the marketplace has historically occurred along a number of specific lines. These are, in part, indicated in figure 14-1.

Subsidy interventions have two focuses. Supply-side subsidies provide financial or in-kind assistance to individuals lacking such resources for purposes of purchasing health care in the marketplace. Examples of these types of subsidies include Medicare and Medicaid, as well as other programs designed to assist the medically indigent. In a few instances, such as for end-stage renal disease, which is administered as a benefit under the Medicare program, and emergency response communications systems, subsidies are available to all members of the society. These subsidies can be in the form of vouchers, dollars, or income-tax deductions or credits. The nature of these subsidies, and individuals' ability to use such subsidies freely in the marketplace, can have a significant effect on the structure and response of the health care system.

A second group of subsidies focuses on increasing the supply of services available in a community. These supply-side subsidies include grants to providers for facilities expansion or construction, grants to medical schools and other health professions' schools to increase the supply of providers, direct grants to subsidize services, and other efforts to

Type of Regulation	Aimed at Individuals	Aimed at Institutions
Subsidies	Supply 　Training grants Demand 　Medicare/Medicaid 　Tax exemptions/credits 　Entitlement programs	Supply 　Construction grants, 　　loans, loan guarantees 　Tax exemptions Demand 　Tax exemptions to 　　employers
Entry Restrictions	Personnel licensure	Facilities lincensure Capital expenditure 　controls
Rate Controls	Fee schedules	Rate-setting commisssions Medicare prospective 　payment reimbursement
Quality Controls	Professional review 　organizations Utilization review Preadmission authorization Second-opinion surgery 　reviews	Certification for Medicare 　and Medicaid

Figure 14-1. Illustrative regulatory mechanisms.

increase the supply of health-related resources. The Hill-Burton program is an example of a supply-side subsidy.

The next category of intervention involves controls over entry into the marketplace. Entry controls, from an antitrust perspective, are of particular interest in their role in reducing competition. To some extent, entry controls in the health care system reduce competitive pressures when they reduce the number of providers or institutions offering services. However, in the health care industry, entry controls are also used (at least ostensibly) to control the quality of care. Entry controls include the licensing process for professional providers, such as physicians or nurses, as well as licensing and certification of institutional providers.

The extent to which government uses entry controls as a mechanism for reducing competition, either explicitly or implicitly, is somewhat unclear.

It could be argued, for example, that in areas such as nursing, the marketplace can determine the adequacy of an individual's professional training and experience. This would alleviate the need for licensure, except for the purpose of reducing the availability of such individuals in the marketplace. Another example in which entry controls may be of questionable quality control need is licensure of nursing home administrators.

A third category of government intervention involves controlling prices. Price controls can assume many forms. In a monopoly, such as natural gas retail distribution, government uses control of pricing to protect the consumer from price gouging by the provider, since alternative providers are not readily available. In the health care industry, price controls are used primarily as mechanisms for a forced reduction in the costs of services (10). For example, price controls have been imposed in the health care industry through hospital cost and rate-setting commissions, which have directed pricing of hospital services (11,12). Government has also controlled prices in this and other industries to contain "inflationary" price increases, such as during World War II and during the Nixon administration's efforts to moderate inflation through a nationwide price freeze.

Government price controls are also used in entitlement programs, such as Medicare, to control expenditures and provide incentives, particularly under prospective reimbursement, for cost containment (13,14). In a regionalized health care system, price controls are generally not relevant, since providers are reimbursed through prospectively budgeted dollar allocations rather than through fee-for-service or negotiated pricing mechanisms.

Intervention aimed at controlling or affecting the quality of services provided in the health care industry represents another significant area of regulation. Quality controls also include, and often are a major focus of, utilization controls, which in turn are also designed to affect costs of services (15). Control over the quality of care and related issues is discussed in more detail later in this chapter.

As noted earlier, other forms of intervention relate to health and safety requirements as well as to maintaining a competitive marketplace through the promotion of antitrust policy. Again, although antitrust policy has not been extensively enforced in the health care industry, the 1980s' and 1990s' philosophical approach of a competitive market suggests the need to ensure that price fixing, collusion, monopolistic behavior, and other anticompetitive activity does not occur (16). It is government's role to perform these tasks.

Regulatory Constraints

Both planning and regulation require the availability, development, and use of adequate methodologies to analytically determine what needs exist in a community and how to meet those needs. Our national legal system and the Constitution itself require that due process be followed in any activity involving government intervention in the market-place. Even voluntary planning, to be effective, requires a process that brings the key participants into the planning effort to gain their perspectives and their loyalty in the implementation of new policy. Thus, the methodological, political, and economic aspects of planning and regulation are complex and must be carefully weighed in the design of any interventions.

The long-term viability of any interventions and the assurance of ongoing public accountability on the part of government and providers mandate the development of a positive political environment for such efforts. Weighing the burdens of these interventions and their costs against the public's benefits, and convincing providers, consumers, and other constituencies of the value of such activity is essential (17).

Ultimately, providing quantitative, analytical evidence that such interventions, whether they be voluntary or mandatory, actually do achieve their objectives is critical. Creating a structure for promoting, measuring, and ensuring the quality of care, for example, provides no benefit if it cannot be analytically proven that such a structure in fact leads to better care for consumers and does not hamper the operation of the system on the part of providers.

The many unique characteristics of the health care marketplace also further complicate any attempt to determine which interventions make sense. The role of insurance in insulating consumers from health care costs, the lack of a normal economic market as a result of the provider's ability to generate demand, and other complex factors must be considered.

Monitoring and Regulating the Quality of Care

While this chapter thus far has focused on planning and regulating health care resources and their use, this section of the chapter discusses evaluation and regulation of the quality of care. It is first necessary to define what is meant by quality of care.

Measuring and ensuring the quality of care through external interventions in the health care system has value only if "quality" can be improved as a result of the effort. Extensive empirical evidence developed over the years suggests that quality of care varies considerably across physicians and hospitals. When specific quality standards are developed by experts and are applied to data from clinical practices, the evidence indicates that practice patterns frequently do not comply with such recognized standards.

Quality review processes are also a component of physician continuing education and institutional quality improvement efforts. Data assessment is useful in identifying areas in which physicians' skills and institutional operations are deficient. This evaluative or feedback mechanism is important in continuing quality improvement. Over the last few years, increasing recognition in U.S. industry of the need for enhancing the quality of products and services has gained great favor, the success of Japanese industries proving a motivating factor. The health care industry, sometimes a laggard in such efforts, is now moving more aggressively in quality enhancement.

From a payor's point of view, such as under federal entitlement programs or insurance plans, the quality of care provided is a measure of the value of the commodity purchased. Expenditure of dollars by employers, governments, insurers, or consumers purchases a product with measurable quality content. Purchasers want the best quality of product for their dollars. Payors are increasingly recognizing that they should expect certain quality standards to be met. Consumers, too, need to be more vigilant in assessing quality, although their evaluation is based on substantially different criteria from those used by payors or providers, as discussed further below.

What is Quality?

From a medical care perspective, quality is the degree of excellence or conformity to established standards and criteria (18). Defining quality is a difficult task, and instituting measurement and assurance of quality is a challenge. Even physicians

have difficulty in identifying and obtaining consistently high-quality care (19). From a societal point of view, the policy question has to be raised as to what level of quality of care we wish to ensure for all of our citizens. Is it feasible for all Americans to receive the "best" quality of care, or are we seeking to ensure that everyone receives at least a minimum standard of quality of care? The relationship between health care outcomes (and health itself) and the quality of care is not always clear-cut. Difficulties in relating health care services to quality of life and patient well-being further complicate definitions of quality and the determination of our society's objectives in enhancing, maintaining, and ensuring quality.

Consumer expectations of quality may differ substantially from professional observers' perspectives. Patient satisfaction may be more associated with provider attitudes, convenience, access, costs, and similar considerations, while professional assessments of quality may focus on technical indicators, thoroughness of the provider's efforts, and appropriate application of sophisticated technologies. Lacking generally agreed-upon quality objectives for the nation, performance is more difficult to evaluate.

Assessment of quality must also address difficult appropriateness of care issues. An emphasis on preventive services may be more important than worrying about what happens should prevention fail. There are even instances in which individuals were misdiagnosed as having diseases that, in fact, they did not have, leading to substantial personal dislocation in spite of the provision of good-quality care after the diagnosis (20,21). Thus, quality must be viewed from both broad societal perspectives as well as individual episodes of care.

Assessment versus Assurance

In examining the quality of health care, two key aspects of the quality issue are differentiated. Quality assessment is the process by which the quality of care is measured. Quality assessment involves a multitude of methodologies, some of which are applicable only to sophisticated special studies, while others can be applied on an ongoing basis. Quality assessment includes the processes of defining how quality is to be determined or measured, identification of specific measurement variables, collection of data, and analysis and interpretation of the results of the assessment (22).

Quality assurance is the process of institutionalizing, or conducting on an ongoing basis, quality measurement activities and combining these with feedback mechanisms aimed at continual quality improvement. Quality assurance primarily involves those activities conducted on an ongoing basis in institutional settings, such as hospitals and large group practices. Government mandates and certification requirements, such as those mentioned in the earlier discussion of regulation, generally focus on meeting minimum quality specifications.

Feedback mechanisms include physician education in various forms, and hospital and institutional operations reviews and enhancements. Quality assurance also includes licensure and certification review processes that may lead to suspension of privileges with continuing evidence of extremely poor quality.

Quality Assessment

An extensive body of literature has been accumulated on assessments of the quality of health care in this country and internationally; it is beyond the scope of this chapter to review this material. The measurement of quality is now based on three major criteria areas developed originally by Avedias Donabedian and others (23). These are structure, process, and outcome. While other formulations for approaching quality of care have been developed, this approach is the most widely recognized and understood.

Structure Measures

Structural measures of the quality of care focus on the context of the environment within which services are provided. Table 14-2 illustrates categories of structural measures of the quality of care. Struc-

TABLE 14-2. Illustrative Categories of Quality of Care Structure Measures

Institutional	Facilities licensure
	Compliance with health and safety codes
	Medical staff appointments and reviews requirements
Individual Professional	Licensure
	Board certification

tural measures include such indicators as board certification of physicians, licensure of facilities, and availability of various supplies and equipment.

The structure within which care is provided reflects the adequacy of providers and facilities, as opposed to what these individuals and organizations actually produce and how they produce it. These measures indicate the extent to which providers, facilities, and organizations have adequate capability to provide the services they offer. Structure also indicates the extent to which organizations and individuals meet certain generally accepted criteria for justifying valid participation in the health care marketplace. Structural inadequacies represent failures to meet these standards, especially with regard to minimum training requirements, health and safety codes, adequacy of facilities and equipment, and the like.

Structural measures generally do not offer adequate specificity to differentiate the capabilities of providers or organizations beyond meeting minimal standards. In addition, the relationship between structure and other measures of quality, such as outcomes, must be clarified to ensure that enforcing structural standards leads to better results (24).

Process of Care

The second major area of quality assessment is the process of care (25). Examples of process categories are listed in table 14-3. Process measures the specific way in which care is provided. Examples of process include which diagnostic procedures or laboratory tests are performed, and the specific content of physician/patient interactions. Process measures are often evaluated against national criteria and standards for specific diagnostic categories and procedures, particularly surgical procedures. For example, established criteria from national organizations, such as the American College of Surgeons or the American Academy of Pediatrics, exist for specific diseases, such as ear infections, to evaluate whether a physician performed the correct tests in assessing patient status, and particularly in determining the appropriateness of surgical procedures, such as myringotomy.

As with structure, it is important to relate process to patient care outcomes. Extensive research has been performed examining the process of care for numerous diagnostic procedures.

Clinical protocols which outline analytically, using a decision-mapping format, the specific procedures to be followed for suspected diagnoses or for patient principal complaints have also been developed. These algorithms are particularly useful in assessing clinical performance by physicians and other practitioners, as well as for guiding mid-level providers such as nurse practitioners. Finally, clinical protocols focusing on the process of care are increasingly being used as the basis for computerized teaching and are even being combined with multimedia computers to add visual images to instructional material.

Outcomes of Care

The last category of quality assessment measurement is the outcome of care. Outcome measures midpoint and end results of the clinical care process and includes infection rates, morbidity, and mortality (table 14-4). In many respects, outcome measures are the most important indicators of the quality of health care services in that they essentially combine all other indices by examining the end results of care (26,27). However, outcome measurement is often difficult to relate analytically to structure and process. Many factors influence outcomes, including patient compliance with med-

TABLE 14-3. Illustrative Process Categories to Measure Quality of Care

- Laboratory test performed
- Radiology tests performed
- Diagnostic approaches used
- Drugs prescribed
- Therapeutic procedures performed

TABLE 14-4. Illustrative Categories of Outcome Measures of the Quality of Care

- Morbidity
- Mortality
- Infection rates
- Complication rates
- Recovery rates
- Functional disability
- Days of work lost

ical regimens, the natural course of disease, other patient behaviors and physical and mental characteristics, and side effects and adverse consequences not directly attributable to the care process itself. It is also frequently difficult to separate out the contributions of each provider or organization to the overall care process. Special approaches, such as the Tracer Method, which follows the progression of care for a specific treatment, have attempted to do this. Ideally, outcome measurement should directly relate, in a quantitative, measurable manner, changes in patient health associated with specific medical care interventions. The reality is that this is extremely difficult to accomplish.

Outcome measurement can use individual indices of morbidity and mortality, such as death rates and infection rates. In addition, multifaceted scales have been developed which combine many indicators or subindicators of health into one measurement instrument. These indexes include various health risk appraisal and health status instruments, such as the Sickness Impact Profile (28). These more complex instruments are particularly useful in measuring progress for diseases, such as arthritis, where sensitive measurement of patient behavior or functional change is needed.

Data Sources

Data for quality assessment are drawn from numerous sources. These include patient medical records, which are abstracted for data analysis; patient questionnaires administered to determine satisfaction and other indicators of quality of care; hospital records of patient transactions; public records, such as birth and death certificates; insurance and entitlement program claim forms; and direct observation of patient and provider interactions.

Data collection is a complex and sophisticated topic in the context of quality care. Data must accurately reflect the actual care provided to ensure the validity of the information obtained. Data collected must relate to specific indicators of quality, and must fit an overall, logical protocol for assessment. Reliability is important in assuring that data elements are accurately and comparably measured for different providers and patients (29). Reliability is particularly important in ensuring that equal and fair evaluations of providers occur across patients and hospitals.

Evaluations that are more subjective in nature, such as those resulting from professional observation, must be accurately constructed to assure reliability. Data must be consistent in the sense of ensuring that for each measure, response categories are comparable across evaluation activities and that interpretation of data is consistent with the data collection criteria. Since quality assessments involve serious judgments regarding professional and institutional competency, fairness, accuracy, and consistency are particularly important.

Numerous data difficulties exist in the area of quality assessment. Frequently, medical records are poorly composed or lack key information. Particularly outside the hospital setting, medical records can be haphazard and a poor indicator, in themselves, of the care provided. Providers, under the pressure of time and patient demands, may hurriedly record information in the medical record.

Problems of accuracy and completeness are inherent in such a process.

Quality Assurance

A wide range of quality assurance activities exists; some activities are mandated, others are voluntary. Quality assurance consists of ongoing applications of quality assessment methodology. As a result, quality assurance requires that assessment methods—applicable on an ongoing, rather than one-time, basis—be used, except for special studies conducted in conjunction with either research or one-time investigations.

Patient Satisfaction

Ongoing quality assurance includes patient satisfaction measurement. Patient satisfaction is difficult to measure in a meaningful way, since most surveys of individual patients at specific institutions or providers generally indicate a high degree of patient satisfaction. Satisfaction measures are obtained through interviews or questionnaires and may be intimidating to the patient. Designing questions that differentiate elements of patient satisfaction is not easy. Patient answers are particularly difficult to discern with regard to the technical quality of care as opposed to the general environment within which services are offered. To be truly effective, patient satisfaction questionnaires must be provider-specific and must seek out negative or adverse perceptions.

Provider organizations are sometimes loathe to encourage expressions of negative sentiment on the part of patients for fear of creating an adversarial environment or raising difficult points that may not readily be answered by the provider organization. Patient satisfaction questionnaires typically elicit responses such as patient dissatisfaction with the cost of services, the amount of time that the physician spends with the patient, or the extent to which the physician explains the medical problem to the patient. As is the case for many quality-of-care assessment issues, the ability of the provider organization to respond to these indicators of dissatisfaction may be limited by physician attitudes, fiscal constraints, and other complex factors.

Statutory quality assurance often focuses on structure, process, and outcome requirements that are specified by law or are required for reimbursement purposes. Structural quality assurance requirements that stem from the legal constraints within which organizations operate in health care include, as mentioned previously, personnel and facility licensure and certification requirements. Physicians, nurses, and certain other personnel must be licensed, usually by state authorities, to practice. Physicians may be certified by various medical specialty boards as well. The extent of medical staff board certification in specialties for which services are offered is often used as an indicator of institutional quality. Facility licensure is a less sensitive indicator of quality, since an unlicensed facility cannot legally operate. Accreditation of hospitals and certain other facilities by the Joint Commission on Accreditation of Health Care Organizations (JCAHCO) is a voluntary process that focuses most directly on structure; recently JCAHCO has increased its weighing of outcome-related accreditation criteria. The broad licensure privileges associated with professional and facility licenses and certifications suggest that these indicators have limited value in differentiating quality. For example, physicians are generally licensed to practice medicine and surgery, broadly defined.

Utilization Review

A variety of mechanisms associated with monitoring and evaluation of the quality of care fall under the rubric of utilization review (UR) (table 14-5). In most institutional settings, quality assurance and utilization review are functionally combined. Many of the same data sources apply for application in utilization review and quality assurance.

Utilization review aims at assessing and affecting the use of services and serves as a mechanism for quality assessment in the context of inappropriate

TABLE 14-5. Illustrative Utilization Controls by Category

Type of Control	Control Mechanism
Supply of services	Unavailability of service
	Queues
Financial	Price
	Benefit limit
	Exclusions
	Deductibles
	Coinsurance
Service authorizations	Certification
	Prior authorization
	Preadmittance screening
	Recertification
Reviews	Claims review
	Professional standards review
	Institutional review
	Medical audit
	Service accounting
Legal	Malpractice litigation

utilization. Utilization review is also associated with a number of insurance mechanisms required for hospital use, and especially for surgical procedures.

The primary objective of utilization review is to monitor, and provide appropriate incentives to influence, the use of health care services. UR also serves to determine the extent to which such use meets established criteria and standards, particularly for hospital care. Many quality assessment studies that involve issues of utilization review have been conducted. Utilization review both augments quality assessment and assurance and contributes to reimbursement policy and control.

Utilization review includes examining hospitalization rates of use both in the aggregate and for specific patients, providers, and procedures. Utilization review involves determining the appropriateness of hospital admissions and lengths of stay, as well as the frequency of specific diagnostic and therapeutic procedures, especially surgical procedures. Also included in utilization review is comparative analysis within and across institutions for specific procedures and diagnostic categories to determine appropriateness of practice patterns at each institution.

There has been considerable interest in utilization review and its association with quality assessment, particularly as it pertains to hospital admissions and the performance of elective surgical procedures (30). Extensive quality assessment research has suggested that such elective procedures have often been performed inappropriately, possibly as a result of financial incentives under fee-for-service medical practice. Most notable are the now-classic research studies of small-area analyses comparing geographic subdivisions of various states to determine differences in rates of performance of such elective procedures as hysterectomy, appendectomy, myringotomy, tonsillectomy, and adenoidectomy (31). Other research has focused on the substantial regional and institutional differences in rates of cesarean section. Reductions in rates for these elective surgical procedures have occurred, possibly the result of these studies (32).

UR and Reimbursement

Utilization review also includes mechanisms to regulate reimbursement under various insurance and entitlement programs. In this context, utilization review is less directed at quality of care than at controlling the use of services to reduce costs. Under federal and state entitlement programs, utilization review has been used to manage patient care, particularly for hospital inpatient services. The insurance industry, particularly under managed care, relies heavily on utilization review mechanisms to monitor and control use of services as well.

Any movement toward increased rationing of health care, such as has been proposed in various states (most notably Oregon) and which occurs in some other countries' health care systems, will have to be based on rational resource decisions and careful controls over use of services (33,34,35). Both regional controls, such as those discussed in

the first part of this chapter, and quality and use of controls will have to force more rational use of resources to gain more care for more people at lower costs than would otherwise be the case.

Reimbursement-related utilization review mechanisms include prior authorization before hospitalization, or before performing certain surgical procedures. A second opinion prior to surgery is another review provision, optional under Medicare, that has been popular, but has had mixed results (36,37,38). These requirements are explained either in the enrollee's plan description or to providers, particularly under entitlement programs and some managed care plans and health maintenance organizations.

Prior utilization may be combined with concurrent review, and other forms of recertification following admission, to monitor patient length of stay and service use. Concurrent review is designed to pressure practitioners to discharge patients from the hospital more rapidly. Failure to comply with utilization review requirements may result in the patient's or institutional provider's losing coverage for all or a portion of the hospital stay.

PROs

Utilization review as mandated under the Medicare program is conducted by professional review organizations (PROs). PROs conduct admission reviews to determine medical necessity and the appropriateness of each setting. Readmissions are examined to determine whether an admission follows a recent discharge solely for purposes of increasing Medicare reimbursement; discharge and readmission would result in multiple payments. PROs are also charged with examining possible premature discharges of patients to increase hospital revenues.

Special rules apply to mental health admissions and a number of other situations. Random sampling of medical records is conducted for purposes of checking diagnosis-related group category assignment by the hospital to avert DRG creep and mislabeling. Special consideration is also given to outliers with regard to extended length of stay and additional reimbursement.

Thus, PROs use utilization review and other techniques primarily to guard against unnecessary admissions, expensive outliers, early or premature discharge (called "dumping"), medical record miscoding to enhance reimbursement, validation of DRG assignment, and to protect against "churning," or unnecessary discharge and readmissions. Since prospective payment incentives differ substantially from the retrospective reimbursement system that existed prior to October 1983, PRO functions now focus on protecting the government from different types of fraud and abuse as compared to the earlier professional standards review organizations under retrospective reimbursement (39).

Valuing Utilization Review

Utilization review and other processes, such as second-opinion surgical programs, must be examined critically from a cost/benefit perspective. Utilization review may discourage needed services and may question physician clinical decision making.

Physicians frequently complain that they are on the front line assessing the patient's needs and that utilization review personnel, including highly skilled nurses and physicians, use secondary data to form judgments. Physician judgments, given that medical practice is an art as well as a science, need to be accounted for in the general scheme of these mechanisms. Clinical decision making has to be left to the front-line providers, while at the same time some significant degree of oversight and review of the care process must exist to protect patients from poor-quality care and to maintain reasonable cost controls in the system (40).

Toward An Integrated Approach

This chapter has reviewed the many external and internal influences on the practice of medicine that affect the functioning of the health care system.

The primary purpose of most of these interventions is to modify the operation of the system and the participants in the system, both providers and consumers, in such a manner as to improve access, ensure quality, reduce costs, and provide oversight of the clinical decision-making process (41).

Total Quality Management

Total quality management (TQM), a concept drawn from the industrial sector, is starting to gain ground in the health care industry (42). This approach is typified in the Japanese automotive industry, and it creates an environment where all aspects of production are oriented toward consumer-related objectives and the production of a high-quality product with minimal defects. In health care, total quality management is seen as a mechanism and philosophy that incorporates risk management, quality assurance, and patient satisfaction objectives (43,44). Employee motivation, enhancement of technical quality, excellence in structural and process aspects of care, and reduction in mistakes related to both clinical and administrative treatment of patients are also key factors that are included in a total quality commitment. While the transfer of the TQM concept from the industrial to service sectors of the economy may encounter some difficulties, many of the principles inherent in TQM will be quite beneficial in health care and, if implemented successfully, may significantly enhance quality and patient satisfaction (45).

Risk Management

Risk management, consistent with TQM and oriented to self-regulation, has also gained greater attention in recent years in all settings, but especially in the hospital (46). Risk management, consisting of a variety of proactive efforts to prevent adverse events related to clinical care and facilities operations, is especially focused on avoiding medical malpractice (47). Malpractice serves as a deterrent to poor technical quality of care and provides redress for patients experiencing such care. However, malpractice concerns also result in the practice of defensive medicine, leading to additional tests and procedures and increased health care costs. Finally, patient satisfaction and physician–patient interactions are highly correlated with malpractice litigation, again emphasizing the need for an integrated, consumer orientation in health care (48).

Due Process

Determining what care is appropriate, allowing some leeway for the provider on the front lines, defining what is good and bad care, and offering incentives that promote all the positive aspects of this external review process are exceedingly difficult challenges. Government and insurers alike have historically been loathe to interfere in the practice of medicine. Only recently, for example, has the Medicare program determined that reimbursement for some procedures, such as coronary artery bypass surgery, would be limited to facilities meeting certain performance criteria, such as minimum quantities of procedures.

Our constitutional legal system, with its due process and burden of proof requirements, increases the difficulty of implementing government rules on medical practice. Insurance companies, not as subject to such constraints, still have concerns about imposing guidelines on practitioners, particularly because such guidelines could lead to adverse patient outcomes. Thus, regulating system performance with regard to clinical practice is very difficult to accomplish. Furthermore, the scientific epidemiological basis for many clinical judgments is still somewhat limited.

The nation's health care system is slowly moving toward greater integration of these regulatory and review mechanisms. The system isn't government run yet, although there are many forms of government involvement in the pricing, quality, and operations of the system. These interventions, like the system itself, need to be rationalized. Rather than following an ill-conceived, piecemeal approach, any such interventions must logically fit all

other aspects of the system's structure, incentives, financing, and social goals. Mechanisms aim at both interaction of providers and communities and providers and patients. Since most of these mechanisms are in one way or another related to each other, and to reimbursement policy, it is essential to move toward a logical integration of all approaches. These control mechanisms are integrally related to the structure of the overall system and have to be part of the design of the system's structure itself. And the structures of the provider and financing organizations themselves need to adapt to changes in modern management theory and practice, using the experiences of other industries and countries (49). These issues are discussed in more detail in the remaining chapters of this book.

References

1. Roemer, M. I. (1985). *National strategies for health care organization: A world overview.* Ann Arbor, MI: Health Administration Press.
2. Gottlieb, S. R. (1974). A brief history of health planning in the United States. In C. C. Havighurst (Ed.). *Regulating health facilities construction* (pp. 7–26). Washington, DC: American Enterprise Institute for Public Policy Research.
3. Klarman, H. E. (1978). Health Planning: Progress prospects and issues. *Milbank Memorial Fund Quarterly. 56.* 78–112.
4. Lave, J. R., & Lave L. B. (1974). *The Hospital Construction Act: An evaluation of the Hill-Burton program* (pp. 41–43). Washington, DC: American Enterprise Institute for Public Policy Research.
5. Bodenheimer, T. S. (1969). Regional medical programs: No road to regionalization. *Medical Care Review. 26.* 1125–1166.
6. Hyman, H. H. (Ed.). (1977). *Health regulations: Certificate of need and Section 1122.* Germantown, MD: Aspen Systems Corp.
7. Havighurst, C. C. (1973). Regulation of health facilities and services by "certificate of need." *Virginia Law Review. 59.* 1143–1232.
8. Salkever, D. S., & Bice, T. W. (1979). *Hospital certificate of need controls: Impact on investment,*

costs, and need. Washington, DC: American Enterprise Institute for Public Policy Research.

9. Pearson, D. A. (1976). The concept of regionalized personal health services in the United States, 1920–1975. In E. W. Saward (Ed.). *The regionalization of personal health services* (pp. 10–14). New York: Prodist.

10. Gabel, J., & Ermann, D. (1985). Preferred provider organizations: Performance, problems, and promise. *Health Affairs. 4.* 24–40.

11. Sloan, F. A. (1983). Rate regulation as a strategy for hospital cost control: Evidence for the last decade. *Milbank Memorial Fund Quarterly. 61.* 195–221.

12. Eby, C. L., & Cohodes, D. R. (1985). What do we know about rate setting? *Journal of Health Politics, Policy and Law. 10.* 299–323.

13. Coelen, C., & Sullivan, D. (1981). An analysis of the effects of prospective reimbursement on hospital expenditures. *Health Care Financing Review. 2.* 1–40.

14. Kidder, D., & Sullivan, D. (1982). Hospital payroll costs, productivity, and employment under prospective reimbursement. *Health Care Financing Review. 4.* 89–100.

15. Brook, R. H., Williams, K. N., & Rolph, J. E. (1978). *Controlling the use and cost of medical services: The New Mexico experimental medical care review organization.* Santa Monica, CA: The Rand Corporation.

16. Havighurst, C. C. (1980). Antitrust enforcement in the medical services industry: What does it all mean? *Milbank Memorial Fund Quarterly. 58.* 89–123.

17. Cromwell, J., & Kanak, J. R. (1982). The effects of prospective reimbursement programs on hospital adoption and service sharing. *Health Care Financing Review. 4.* 67–88.

18. Donabedian, A. (1981). *Exploration in quality assessment and monitoring* (vol. 2): *The criteria and standards of quality.* Ann Arbor, MI: Health Administration Press.

19. Bunker, J. P., & Brown, B. W., Jr. (1974). The physician-patient as an informed consumer of surgical services. *New England Journal of Medicine. 290*(19). 1051–1055.

20. Bergman, A. B., & Staemm, S. J. (1967). The morbidity of cardiac non-disease in school children. *New England Journal of Medicine. 276.* 1008–1013.

21. Sackett, D. L., Taylor, D. W., Haynes, R. B., et al. (1977). The short term disadvantage of being labeled hypertensive. *Clinical Research. 25.* 266.

22. Williams, K. N., & Brook, R. H. (1978). Quality measurement and assurance. *Health Medical Care Services Review. 1.* 3–15.

23. Donabedian, A. (1980). *Exploration in quality assessment and monitoring* (vol. 1): *The definition of quality and approaches to its assessment.* Ann Arbor, MI: Health Administration Press.

24. Shortell, S. M., & LoGerfo, J. P. (1981). Hospital medical staff organization and quality of care: Results from myocardial infarction and appendectomy. *Medical Care. 19.* 1041–1056.

25. Donabedian, A. (1968). Promoting quality through evaluating the process of patient care. *Medical Care. 6.* 181–202.

26. Schroeder, S. (1987). Outcome assessment 70 years later: Are we ready? *New England Journal of Medicine. 316.* 160–162.

27. Wennberg, J. E., Bunker, J. P., & Barnes, B. (1980). The need for assessing the outcome of common medical practices. *Annual Review of Public Health. 1.* 277–295.

28. Bergner, M., Bobbitt, R. A., Krenel, A., et al. (1976). The Sickness Impact Profile: Conceptual formulation and methodological development of a health status index. *International Journal of Health Services. 6.* 393–415.

29. Goldman, R. L. (1992). The reliability of peer assessments of quality of care. *Journal of the American Medical Association. 267*(7). 958–960.

30. Wickizer, T. M., Wheeler, J. R. C., and Feldstein, P. J. (1989). Does utilization review reduce unnecessary hospital care and contain costs? *Medical Care. 27.* 632–647.

31. Wennberg, J., & Gittelsohn, A. (1973). Small area variations in health care delivery. *Science, 182.* 1102–1108.

32. Dyck, F. J., Murphy, F. A., Murphy, J. K., et al. (1977). Effect of surveillance on the number of hysterectomies in the province of Saskatchewan. *New England Journal of Medicine. 296.* 1326–1328.

33. Grannemann, T. W. (1991, Fall). Priority setting: A sensible approach to Medicaid policy? *Inquiry. 28*(3). 300–305.

34. Klevit, H. D., Bates, A. C., Castanares, T., Kirk, E. P.,

et al. (1991). Prioritization of health care services: A progress report by the Oregon State Health Services Commission. *Archives of Internal Medicine. 151*(5). 912–916.

35. Hadorn, D. C. (1991). Setting health care priorities in Oregon: Cost-effectiveness meets the rule of rescue. *Journal of the American Medical Association. 265*(17). 2218–2225.

36. Ruchlin, H. S., Finkel, M. L., & McCarthy E. G. (1982). The efficacy of second-opinion consultation programs: A cost-benefit perspective. *Medical Care. 20.* 3–20.

37. Martin, S. G., Schwartz, M., Whalen, B. J., et al. (1982). Impact of a mandatory second-opinion program on Medicaid surgery rates. *Medical Care. 20.* 21–45.

38. Brook, R. H., & Lohr, K. N. (1982). Second-opinion programs: Beyond cost-benefit analysis. *Medical Care. 20.* 1–2.

39. Bellin, L. E. (1974). PSRO: Quality control? Or gimmickry? *Medical Care. 12.* 1012–1018.

40. Schwartz, W. B. (1987). The inevitable failure of current cost-containment strategies. *Journal of the American Medical Association. 257.* 220–224.

41. Donabedian, A., Wheeler, J. R., & Wyszewianski, L. (1982). Quality, cost, and health: An integrative model. *Medical Care. 20.* 975–992.

42. Casalou, R. F. (1991). Total quality management in health care. *HHSA. 36*(1). 134–146.

43. Berwick, D. M. (1989). Continuous improvement as an ideal in health care. *New England Journal of Medicine. 320*(1). 53–56.

44. McLaughlin, C. P., & Kaluzny, A. D. (1990). Total quality management in health: Making it work. *Health Care Management Review. 15*(3). 7–14.

45. Albrecht, K. G., & Bradford, L. J. (1990). *The service advantage: How to identify and fulfill customer needs.* Homewood, IL: Jones-Irwin.

46. Youngberg, B. J. (Ed.). (1990). *Essentials of hospital risk management.* Rockville, MD: Aspen Publishers.

47. Orlikoff, J. E. (1988). *Malpractice prevention and liability control for hospitals* (2nd ed.). Chicago: American Hospital Publishing.

48. Cunningham, L. (1991). *The quality connection in health care: Integrating patient satisfaction and risk management.* San Francisco: Jossey-Bass.

49. Eskildson, L., & Yeats, G. R. (1991). Lessons from industry: Revising organizational structure to improve health care quality assurance. *QRB Quality Review Bulletin. 17*(20). 38–41.

PART SEVEN

National

Health Policy

Chapter 15

Health Policy and the Politics of Health Care

Philip R. Lee
A. E. Benjamin

Political considerations have significantly affected nearly all of the developments discussed in this book. However, the importance and central role of health care policy analysis and politics can best be highlighted by directly discussing these issues. That is the purpose of this chapter. While many of the topics mentioned here have been discussed from a variety of perspectives in other chapters, the policy and politics of changes in health care in the nation are the focus here, and examples of developments in health care serve as illustrations of the central role of political forces in shaping our health care system. The philosophies and processes discussed in other chapters, especially in chapter 4 are further analyzed here.

Government plays a major role in planning, directing, and financing health services in the United States. The significance of the public sector is apparent as one considers the following: Public programs account for approximately 40 percent of the nation's personal health care expenditures, most physicians and other health care personnel are trained at public expense, almost 65 percent of all health research and development funds are provided by the government, and most nonprofit community and university hospitals have been built or modernized with government subsidies. The bulk of government expenditures are federal, with state and local governments contributing significant, but much smaller amounts.

Health policies and programs of the U.S. government have evolved piecemeal, usually in response to needs that were not being met by the private sector or by states and local governments. The result has been a proliferation of federal categorical programs administered by more than a dozen government departments. Over the years, new programs have been added, old ones redirected, and numerous efforts made to integrate and coordinate services. In the 1980s a major effort was made by the Reagan administration to significantly diminish the federal role in domestic social policy through the transfer of some programs to the states, reduced federal funding or elimination of federal support entirely. The effort has been only partially successful and has not changed the basic configuration of publicly supported health programs, although the burden of financing now falls more heavily on state and local governments. Functions of the public and private sectors have become increasingly interrelated, and roles are often poorly delineated. There can be little argument that the primary function of most government programs in health has been to support or strengthen the private sector (e.g., hospital construction, subsidy of medical student training, Medicare) rather than to develop a strong system of publicly provided health care.

Although U.S. government policies have evolved over a 200-year period, most of those affecting health services have developed since the enactment of the Social Security Act of 1935. Many federal health programs evolved because of failures in the private sector to provide necessary support—for example, biomedical research; others arose because results of the free market were grossly inequitable—for example, hospital construction; and some programs, such as Medicare and Medicaid, developed because healthcare was so costly that many could not afford to pay for necessary health services. Some federal health programs, such as biomedical research, potentially benefit everyone, while others, such as the Indian Health Service, reach only a small but needy segment of the population. Some programs, such as poliomyelitis immunization and health personnel development, have been effective in achieving their goals; others, such as health planning, have probably not realized even limited objectives; still others, such as Medicare, have reached some goals, although at a much higher cost than originally anticipated.

The process by which health policy is made in this country can be best understood by considering a fundamental paradox in American health care: government spends more and more money to support a wide range of health programs, services, and agencies, yet the role of government in the reform of our health care system remains limited and halting. Government is faced with a crisis in

health care, defined primarily in terms of rising costs to public treasuries, while proposed solutions are framed in terms that do not address in a comprehensive fashion the sources of demand on the public purse. Indeed, solutions to the cost crisis have combined withdrawing benefits from those very recipient populations whose health care needs justify government intervention with attempts to reduce costs by either stimulating competition or regulating (reducing) payment to hospitals, nursing homes, and physicians. While federal policies may move in one direction, state policies may move in another. To understand this paradox, it is necessary to consider several characteristics of public policy making and thus to explore the sources of the paradox and the nature of policy processes in health.

Dimensions of Policy Making in Health

Policy making in health care crosses several levels of government and hundreds of programs, is complex, and no single analytical scheme can do it sufficient justice. Still, public policy students have identified five dimensions of the policy process: 1) the relationship of government to the private sector, 2) the distribution of authority within a federal system of government, 3) pluralistic ideology as the basis of politics, 4) the relationship between policy formulation and administrative implementation, and 5) incrementalism as a strategy of reform. Each will be considered in detail.

Public and Private Sector Politics

Although the role of government in health care has grown considerably in recent years, that role remains relatively limited. The U.S. government is less involved in health care than are the governments of many other industrialized countries (1). This circumstance derives primarily from a persistent ideology that identifies the market system as the most appropriate setting for the exchange of health services and from a related belief that private sector support for public sector initiatives can be acquired only through accommodation to the interests of health care providers. The significance of the market ideology has been elaborated in analyses of the passage of Medicare and Medicaid in 1965 (2,3). The persistence of doubts about the appropriate role of government is certainly apparent in the renewed vitality of neoconservatism, in which it is argued that the market can better respond to the economic and social problems of our time if it is unfettered by government intervention (4).

Uncertainty about the role of government in health care has numerous consequences. The primary concern is the absence of any design or blueprint for governmental reform (5). Instead, the public sector (with its relatively immense capacity to raise revenues) is called on periodically to open and close its funding spigots to stimulate the health care market. Hospital construction and physician education are prominent examples of public activity. Not only is there no blueprint for public sector action, but governments in America harbor grave doubts about the appropriateness of regulation as a public-sector activity. Dependence at the federal level on "voluntary approaches," such as the reduction of hospital costs in the late 1970s, delayed serious consideration of more stringent measures even as the costs to government of hospital care continued to rise dramatically (6).

A Federal System

The concept of federalism has evolved dramatically in meaning and practice since the founding of the republic more than 200 years ago. Originally, federalism was a legal concept that defined the constitutional division of authority between the federal government and the states. Federalism initially stressed the independence of each level of government from the other, while incorporating the idea that some functions, such as foreign policy, were the exclusive province of the central government, while other functions, such as education, police protection, and health care, were the responsibility of regional units—state and local government.

Federalism represented a form of governance that differs both from a unitary state, where regional and local authority derive legally from the central government, and from a confederation, in which the national government has limited authority and does not reach individual citizens directly (7,8).

Shifts in responsibilities assigned to various levels of government do not pose a serious problem for health policy if at least two conditions are met: 1) administrative or regulatory responsibilities and financial accountability are consonant, and 2) the various levels of government possess the appropriate capacities to assume those responsibilities assigned to them. Important questions can be raised regarding whether either of these conditions has been met in the development of health policy during the last two decades.

Analysis of federal-state relationships in programs as divergent as Medicaid, provider licensure, and family planning under Title X of the Public Health Service Act have suggested that the structure of these relationships produces outcomes widely held to be dysfunctional (e.g., Medicaid cutbacks) because one level of government (e.g., the states) can do nothing else under the conditions established by another (e.g., the federal government). The disjunction between administrative responsibilities and financial accountability (i.e., the term of federalistic arrangements) in these cases has yielded results for which governments and the recipients of health care ultimately have paid a price. What seems to matter most in the structure of relationships within federalism is not so much the distribution of activities but the relationships among levels of government (9).

For allocations of authority among levels of government to work, it is important that governments possess those capacities appropriate to the responsibilities they confront. Governments must possess the capacity to generate revenue, the capability to plan and manage policies and programs, and the political will to plan and implement needed reform. State and local governments have been found wanting in each of these respects. Because state governments do not tax as heavily as the federal government (10), their capacity for generating new revenues is limited. Many states, moreover, are viewed as having inadequate administrative infrastructures, lacking sufficient sophisticated management techniques, and having limited capabilities in the conduct of policy analysis and planning.

Finally, there is evidence that state and local governments may have less political will to make decisions in the public interest than the federal government. Wide variations among states in program outputs (e.g., Medicaid) suggest significant inequities. The argument is not that every state, if freed from federal constraints, would establish standards for health programs that are certain to fall below former federal standards. Rather, it is that some states will surely exceed some federal standards and others will fall far below what is generally considered adequate. At the heart of this problem, many argue, is the reputedly greater susceptibility of state governments to interest group pressures and narrow conceptions of the public good.

Perhaps the most significant instance of the failure of the states to provide their citizens equal rights and equal protection has been in the area of civil rights. In education, housing, health care, and virtually every area of domestic social policy, it has been necessary for the federal government, particularly the federal courts, to require compliance with federal laws and regulations.

There is some countervailing evidence that the capacity and will to govern is becoming more widely diffused within the federal system. States (taken as a group) have spent a higher percentage of their budgets on health care than the federal government has, even though absolute federal expenditures for health have grown to more than double state and local health expenditures combined (11). A considerable increase at the state level in the conduct of policy analysis and its use in policy deliberations is one indication that state capacity to plan and manage is improving (12). Regarding inequities and political will, on the other hand, little counterevidence has emerged to challenge the argument that the states are more vulnerable to interest groups (e.g., provider groups in health) and that the result is a wide program variation among states in response to provider—not consumer—interests. The structure of federalism enables provider groups to maximize their power at the expense of consumer interests (9,13).

In a recent monograph on federalism and the national purpose, Brizius (14) groups the arguments favoring centralization into eight clusters of related principles: 1) national purpose, 2) national security, 3) equity, 4) guaranteeing rights, 5) efficiency, 6) competence, 7) uniformity, and 8) unity. In contrast to the principles tending toward centralization are those that support greater decentralization and the maintenance of a truly federal system. Brizius groups 12 arguments for decentralization into seven principles: 1) diversity, 2) political sovereignty, 3) guaranteeing rights, 4) limits on power, 5) accountability, 6) efficiency and competence, and 7) competition.

The argument regarding centralization and decentralization has not been settled, despite a vigorous debate in the past decade. No agreement has been reached on the vital question of the distribution of authority and responsibility among various levels of government. The federal government finances hospital and medical services for the elderly through Medicare; it contributes at least 50 percent of health care costs for Medicaid beneficiaries, is the major supporter of biomedical research, provides a limited amount of support for a variety of health services (e.g., mental health, family planning, crippled children's services, AIDS, substance abuse), is the sole regulator of the entry of new drugs into the market, and plays a critical role in the regulation of environment and occupational health.

States spend a large portion of their general fund budgets on health care for the poor (Medicaid), on mental health services, on the support of a range of public health programs, and on the education and training of health professionals.

Local governments remain an important provider of health care, particularly hospital, outpatient and emergency care for the poor, mental health and substance abuse services, and a variety of public health services. Both state and local governments are mandated by higher levels of government (by either regulation or court order) to provide services or implement various environmental health or occupational health and safety regulations.

Pluralistic Politics

"Pluralism" is a term used by political theorists to describe a set of values about the effective functioning of democratic governments. Pluralists argue that democratic societies are organized into many diverse interest groups, which pervade all socioeconomic strata, and that this network of pressure groups prevents any one elite group from overreaching its legitimate bounds. As a theoretical framework for explaining the political context of policy making, this perspective has been criticized relentlessly and appropriately (15,16). As an ideology that continues to influence the way elites and masses view government, pluralism becomes a basis for considering some essential elements of the process of public decision making in this country.

Interest groups play a powerful role in the health policy process. Most federal and state laws designed to address the health care needs of the population are shaped by the interaction among interest groups, key legislators, and agency representatives. Ginzberg (17) has identified four power centers in the health care industry that influence the nature of health care and the role of government: 1) physicians, 2) large insurance organizations, 3) hospitals, and 4) a highly diversified group of participants in profit-making activities within the health care arena.

The influence of these power centers is evident in policies at all levels of government. The development of Medicare and Medicaid policies reflects the powerful influence of physicians, hospitals, and nursing homes as well as their allies in the health insurance industry. For example, in enacting Med-

icare, Congress ensured that the law did not affect the physician–patient relationship, including the physician's method of billing the patient. The system of physician reimbursement adopted by Medicare was highly inflationary because it provided incentives to physicians to raise prices and to provide ancillary services, such as laboratory tests, electrocardiograms, and X-ray films. Hospital reimbursement historically has been based on costs incurred in providing care, creating strong incentives to provide more and more services. Despite the impact of steadily rising Medicare costs on the Social Security trust fund, on Social Security taxes (paid by employers and employees), and on the elderly, until recently, Congress has steadfastly refused to alter Medicare's methods of payment to physicians and hospitals. It was not until 1989 that the U.S. Congress adopted a set of policies to reform payments for physicians' services in the Medicare program. Also, many features of the program, patterned on principles developed by the medical industry, have had remarkable staying power.

The passage of a hospital prospective payment system (PPS) for Medicare by Congress in 1983 signaled a potential shift in the power of key interest groups in health. Recent history has made it clear that an apparent legislative defeat (e.g., the passage of Medicare) can subsequently become an important source of benefits and power for ostensibly losing interests (e.g., the medical lobby). The implementation of PPS has not been a fiscal disaster for hospitals, as some predicted, and it remains to be seen whether federal payment reforms will effect any fundamental alteration in the role of major power centers in health care.

As the case of Medicare suggests, health policy in the United States has been a product largely of medical politics (18). Marmor et al. (19) describe the political "market" in health (i.e., institutional arrangements among actors in the political system) as imbalanced. In an imbalanced market, participants have unequal power, and those with concentrated rather than diffuse interests have the greater stake in the effects of policy. At least until recently, provider interest groups have had a far greater stake in shaping health policy than have consumer interests. Recently, large employers have become increasingly important in the health policy debates at the federal and state levels, particularly on issues related to health care cost containment.

Some observers argue that the rising costs of health care may be changing the configuration of interest groups seeking to influence health policy. In recent years, steadily escalating costs have stimulated other interests, especially labor, business, and governments themselves into giving greater attention to health policy and its implications. Polls of public attitudes show a growing dissatisfaction with health care financing in the United States and a strong desire for major reforms (20,21). In other words, their interests may be shifting from diffuse to concentrated. The result may be that increased competition in the political marketplace from a more diverse set of participants will lessen the dominance of medical provider groups (22). The pluralist dream of effective interest groups that prevent any one group from overreaching its legitimate bounds continues to influence our thinking about health care.

Policy Implementation

The nature of the health process is determined not only by the balance between provider and consumer interests but also by the relationships of these interests to government actors. Public policy students have observed that policy making moves through at least three stages: 1) agenda setting, the continuous process by which issues come to public attention and are placed on the agenda for government action; 2) policy adoption, the legislative process through which elected officials decide the broad outlines of policy; and 3) policy implementation, the process by which administrators develop policy by addressing the numerous issues unaddressed by legislation (13,23). An important element of the health policy process involves the relative roles of elected officials and

professional administrators. As one moves from agenda setting to policy adoption and implementation, it can be argued that the role of elected officials becomes more remote and that of administrators more crucial.

No policy theorist has pressed this argument with more conviction than Lowi (24). A central theme in what he calls interest-group liberalism is the growing role of administrators in politics. According to Lowi, in a period of resource richness and government expansion, such as the 1960s, government responded to a range of major organized interests, underwrote programs sought by those interests, and assigned program responsibility to administrative agencies. Through this process the programs became captives of the interest groups because the administrative agencies themselves were captured. Interest groups dominate the policy process, he argues, not only through their influence on the legislative process (policy adoption) but also through control of administration (policy implementation). In effect, governments in the United States make policies without laws, and they leave the law making to administrators.

The study of policy implementation in health has received increased attention in recent years (25,26,27,28). Not surprisingly, the landmark legislation creating Medicare and Medicaid in 1965 has been the subject of much of this analysis. A study of Medicare by Feder is especially enlightening (29). She describes a number of crucial decisions related to the nature of the federal role that were not addressed by the legislation and discusses the process by which the Social Security Administration subsequently addressed these decisions. Feder argues that the agency could have pursued two fundamentally different strategies. Using a cost-effectiveness strategy, the agency could have assessed the impact of alternative approaches to a problem (e.g., hospital payment) on cost and quality and selected a course that would achieve maximum health care value per dollar spent. As an alternative, with a balancing strategy, the agency could have sought to identify relevant political actors (e.g., the American Hospital Association), weighed their capacity to aid or threaten program survival, and selected those policies that minimize political conflict (29).

Feder makes a persuasive argument that the Social Security Administration selected a balancing strategy. She traces the various consequences for the public interest of an approach that administratively transfers policy discretion to those provider groups with the greatest stake in the content of that policy. For those directly involved in the implementation of the Medicare program, the primary motivation was not only to minimize political conflict, but also to ensure access for elderly Social Security beneficiaries to hospital and physician services. At one point these were jeopardized because of the vigorous enforcement of the Civil Rights Act by the U.S. Public Health Service and the Social Security Administration on instructions of the Secretary of Health, Education, and Welfare. When compliance with the Civil Rights Act was assured in hospitals, particularly in the South and Southwest, access barriers disappeared. Reimbursement policies followed the intentions of Congress and achieved the initial objective of ensuring high levels of hospital and physician participation in Medicare.

Incremental Reform

The powerful role of administrators in the implementation of policy is derived in part from the broad and ambiguous nature of much federal and state health legislation. Despite dramatic improvements in the capacity of congressional staff to conduct policy analysis, the constraints of politics are such that ambiguity frequently is employed to ensure the passage of legislation.

The public policy process in American government can best be described in terms of an incremental model of decision making (30,31). Simply stated, this model posits that policy is made in small steps (increments) and that policy is rarely modified in dramatic ways. Major actors in the

political bargaining process, whether legislators, interest groups, or administrators, operate on the basis of certain rules, and these rules are founded in adherence to prior policy patterns. Because the consequences of policy change are difficult to predict and because unpredictability is risky in the political market, policy makers prefer reform in small steps to more radical change.

An example of incremental change was the gradual evolution of the National Institutes of Health from a small federal laboratory conducting biomedical research in the 1930s to a multibillion-dollar research enterprise. The addition of new institutes took place over a 50-year period. Budgets also grew gradually, beginning after World War II. Even when major health policy initiatives were adopted, such as Medicare and Medicaid, the change was in the source of funds to pay for medical care for the elderly and the poor, not in the organization or provision of medical care.

The incremental model was elaborated by decision theorists concerned with ways that policy makers managed a large information load and the uncertainty of their political environment. Quite a different view, but one that is compatible with this perspective, has been developed by Alford (32). Alford addresses the nature of reform in health care and its ideological basis. He identifies three approaches to reform, including market reformers, who call for an end to government interference in health care delivery and the restoration of market competition in health care institutions, and bureaucratic reformers, who blame market competition for defects in the system and call for increased administrative regulation of health care. What these perspectives share, notes Alford, is that each leads to incremental reform as well as the extent to which they challenge fundamental patterns of policy is limited. A third approach, the structural interest perspective, begins with an analysis of the ways in which the other two accept and benefit from current arrangements in health care. This perspective is formulated to challenge the effective, institutional control exercised by dominant structural interests that benefit from continuance of the system in its present form. As Alford makes clear, the market and bureaucratic approaches are descriptive of the limits of health care reform, and they underlie resistance to change in the health system.

Relatively little research in the United States has examined the institutional and class basis of public policy, including health policy (33). Those who hold that defects in health care are rooted deeply in the structure of a class society would radically alter the present health care system, creating a national health service, with decentralization of administration and community control over health care institutions and health professionals. Those who view defects in health care as having a class basis believe that tinkering with the health care system itself cannot achieve the desired outcomes but that these will follow major structural changes in society.

European countries that practice a parliamentary rather than representative democracy can effect larger changes more swiftly. In the parliamentary form of government, party policies are implemented speedily because the winning party practices bloc voting. Delay is caused only by the inability to achieve power. In representative governments, the parties cannot manage the discipline necessary to enforce party loyalty to programs or policies because elected representatives owe more, or at least as much, to their personal appeal as to party designation. The party discipline of parliamentary government is replaced by the quest for consensus in representative government, and consensus is most readily achieved when proposed reforms involve only modest change.

A Historical Framework: The Development of Health Policy from 1798 to 1988

Although the federal system in the United States has evolved continuously, at certain periods in our history the relationship among the federal, state, and local governments has undergone dramatic change. The major shifts in intergovernment rela-

tions were often the result of a crisis (the Civil War, the Great Depression, civil rights issues) rather than the result of a critical examination of the issues.

Public health and health care did not loom large in the policy debate about federalism until the late 1940s, when President Truman advocated a program of national health insurance, and again in the 1960s, when implementation of Medicare transformed the role of the federal government in health care. Over the years, however, health policy issues (e.g., federal regulation of food and drugs, federal support for biomedical research, hospital construction, and health professions education) have raised critical issues about the role of government in health care, intergovernmental relations, and the role of the private sector.

The private sector in the United States has always maintained a larger role in health care than it has in most other industrial nations. This has been true in both the financing and delivery of services. While it is not possible to do full justice to the rich history of health care policy here, an effort is made to present highlights in the development of health policy that reflect the manner in which much has changed and much has stayed the same.

The slow emergence of public policies and programs related to health and health care in the United States has generally followed the pattern of other industrial countries, particularly those in western Europe (34). At least three stages in the process have been identified:

1. Private charity, including contracts between users and providers, and public apathy or indifference
2. Public provision of necessary health services that are not provided by voluntary effort and private contract
3. Substitution of public services and financing for private, voluntary, and charitable efforts

Although these three stages have been identified within many nations, different patterns have been observed among industrial countries. Political parties in the United States have been more reluctant than those in European countries or Canada to challenge the medical profession, hospitals, and the health insurance industry to promote health care reform.

The role of government at the federal, state, and local levels in public health and health care evolved partly in response to changes occurring in the health care system (35). With the major changes in health care that have occurred over the past 200 years, particularly those in the past 50 years, has come a transformation in the role of government.

The Early Years of the Republic: A Limited Role for the Federal Government (1798–1862)

During the early years of the republic, the federal government played a limited role in both public health and health care, which were largely within the jurisdiction of the states and the private sector. Private charity shouldered the responsibility of care for the poor. The federal role in providing health care began in 1798, when Congress passed the Act for the Relief of Sick and Disabled Seamen, which imposed a 20-cent per month tax on seamen's wages for their medical care. The federal government later provided direct medical care for merchant seamen through clinics and hospitals in port cities, a policy that continues to this day. The federal government also played a limited role in imposing quarantines on ships entering U.S. ports in order to prevent epidemics (34). It did little or nothing, however, about the spread of communicable diseases within the nation, a problem that was thought to lie within the jurisdiction of the individual states.

Through the 18th, 19th, and early 20th centuries, the major diseases in the United States, as in Europe, were infectious diseases, as discussed in Chapter 1. Tuberculosis, pneumonia, bronchitis, and gastrointestinal infections were the major killers. As the sanitary revolution progressed in the 19th century, social and economic conditions advanced, nutrition improved, reproductive behavior was modified, the burden of acute infection de-clined, and the burden of chronic illness began to rise. National health policies during the 18th and 19th centuries were limited to the imposition of quarantines to prevent epidemics and the provision of medical care to merchant seamen and members of the armed forces. In laws beginning with the Act Relative to Quarantine of 1796, Congress preempted state and local authority and put an end to long-standing federal–state disagreements regarding the authority to prevent and control epidemics of yellow fever and chlorea, as well as recurring outbreaks of plague and smallpox (36).

States first exercised their public health authority through special committees or commissions. Most active concern with health matters was at the local level. Local boards of health or health departments were organized to tackle problems of sanitation, poor housing, and quarantine. Later, local health departments were set up in rural areas, particularly in the South, to counteract hookworm, malaria, and other infectious diseases that were widespread in the 19th and early 20th centuries.

The Evolution of Health Policy: The Emergence of Dual Federalism and the Transformation of American Medicine (1862–1935)

The Civil War brought about a dramatic change in the role of the federal government. Not only did the federal government engage in a war to preserve the union but it also began to expand its role in other ways that significantly altered the nature of federalism in the United States. This changing federal role was reflected in congressional passage of the first program of federal aid to the states, the Morrill Act of 1862, which granted federal lands to each state. Profits from the sale of these lands supported public institutions of higher education, known as *land-grant colleges* (37). Toward the end of the 19th century, the federal government began to provide cash grants to states for the establishment of agricultural experiment stations. While the federal role generally was expanding, the change had little impact on health care. An important exception occurred in the late 1870s when the Surgeon General of the Marine Hospital Service was given congressional authorization to impose quarantines within the United States.

While the first state health department was established in Louisiana in 1855, it was not until after the Civil War that the states began to assume a more significant role in public health. Massachusetts established the first permanent board of health in 1869. By 1909, public health agencies were established in all the states. During this period there also was rapid development of local health departments. State and local governments based their policy changes and management practices on the rapid advances in the biological sciences. Drawing on these advances, state and local health departments moved beyond sanitation and quarantine to the scientific control of communicable diseases (38).

The basic policies that created both state and local health departments derived from the police power of state governments (39). Thus the states, and not the federal government, were the key to translating the scientific advances of the late 19th century into public health policy and the dramatic improvements in public health that followed.

The most significant role played by state governments in personal health care during this period was in the establishment of state mental hospitals. These first developed as a result of a reform movement in the mid–19th century led by Dorothea Dix. Over the next century, state mental institutions evolved into isolated facilities for custodial care of the chronically mentally ill. The development of these asylums reinforced the stigma attached to mental illness and placed the care of the severely mentally ill outside the mainstream of medicine for more than a century (40).

Hospitals began to evolve in the 19th century from almshouses that provided shelter for the poor. Hospital sponsorship at the local level was either public (local government) or through a variety of religious, fraternal, or other community groups. Thus the nonprofit community hospital was born; this institution, rather than the local public hospital,

gradually became the primary locus of medical care. Physicians provided voluntary services to the sick poor in order to earn the privilege of caring for their paying patients in the hospital (41). Hospital appointments became important for physicians in order to conduct their practices. Hospitals increased in number in the late 19th century and began to incorporate new medical technologies, such as anesthesia, aseptic surgery, and later, radiology. Although charity was the major source of care for the poor, public services also began to grow in the 19th century. Gradually, local government assumed responsibility for indigent care. The development of the hospital is discussed further in Chapter 6.

After the Morrill Act the next major change in the role of the federal government came more than 40 years later in the regulation of food and drugs. After 20 years of debate and much public pressure, Congress enacted the Federal Food and Drug Act in 1906 to regulate the adulteration and misbranding of food and drugs, a responsibility previously exercised exclusively by the states. The law was designed primarily to protect the pocketbook of the consumer, not the consumer's health. While it provided some measure of control over impure foods, it had little impact on impure or unsafe drugs (42). The legislation not only represented a major change in the role of the federal government but also provided the constitutional basis for present-day regulation of testing, marketing, and promotion of prescription and over-the-counter drugs.

A number of other important developments in the early decades of the 20th century had a strong impact on health care and health policy. Among the most significant were reforms in medical education that transformed not only education but also professional licensing and, eventually, health care itself. The American Medical Association and the large private foundations (e.g., Carnegie and Rockefeller) played a major role in this process. Voluntary hospitals also grew in number, size, and importance. Medical research produced new treatments. Infant mortality declined as nutrition, sanitation, living conditions, and maternal and infant care improved. Health care changed in significant ways, but it was little affected by public policy.

The Evolution of Health Policy: From Dual Federalism to Cooperative Federalism (1935–1961)

The Great Depression brought action by the federal government to save banks, support small business, provide direct public employment, stimulate public works, regulate financial institutions and business, restore consumer confidence, and provide Social Security in old age. The role of the federal government was transformed in the span of a few years. Federalism evolved from a dual pattern, with a limited role in domestic affairs for the federal government, to a cooperative one, with a strong federal role.

The Social Security Act of 1935 was certainly the most significant domestic social legislation ever enacted by Congress. This marked the real beginning of what has been termed "cooperative federalism." The act established the principle of federal aid to the states for public health and welfare assistance. It provided federal grants to states for maternal and child health and crippled children's services (Title V) and for public health (Title VI). It also provided for cash assistance grants to the aged, the blind, and destitute families with dependent children. This cash assistance program provided the basis for the current federal–state program of medical care for the poor, initially as Medical Assistance for the Aged in 1960 and then as Medicaid (Title XIX of the Social Security Act) in 1965. Both later programs linked eligibility for medical care to eligibility for cash assistance. More important, however, the Social Security Act of 1935 established the Old Age, Survivors' and Disability Insurance (OASDI) programs that were to provide the philosophical and fiscal basis for Medicare, a program of federal health insurance for the aged, also enacted in 1965 (Title XVIII of the Social Security Act). Passage of the Social Security Act of 1935 was significant, for it provided the basis

for direct federal income assistance to retired persons and established the basis for federal aid to the states in health and welfare; however, this legislation did not include a program of national health insurance. This was due principally to the opposition of the medical profession to any form of health insurance, particularly publicly funded insurance.

In 1938, after the death of a number of children due to the use of Elixir of Sulfonamide, consumer protection became an important issue for policy makers. This disaster resulted in the enactment of the Food, Drug and Cosmetic Act of 1938, which required manufacturers to demonstrate the safety of drugs before marketing. This law was a further extension of the federal role and was consistent with other major changes in that role that occurred during the 1930s. After the passage of this act, little change was made in drug regulation law until the thalidomide disaster in the early 1960s.

Growing attention to maternal and child health, particularly for the poor, was reflected in grants to the states and in a temporary program instituted during World War II to pay for maternity care of wives of Army and Navy enlisted men. This means-tested program successfully demonstrated the capacity of the federal government to administer a national health insurance program. With rapid demobilization after the war and opposition by organized medicine, the program was terminated; but it was often cited by advocates of national health insurance, particularly those who accorded first priority to mothers and infants.

Introduction of the scientific method into medical research at the turn of the century and its gradual acceptance had a profound effect on national health policy and health care. The first clear organizational impact of the growing importance of research was the transformation of the U.S. Public Health Service Hygienic Laboratory, established in 1901 to conduct bacteriologic research and public health studies, into the National Institutes of Health (NIH) in 1930, with broad authority to conduct basic research. This was followed by enactment of the National Cancer Act of 1937 and the establishment of the National Cancer Institute within the framework of NIH. There followed multiple legislative enactments during and after World War II that created the present institutes, focused primarily on broad classes of disease, such as heart disease, cancer, arthritis, neurologic diseases, and blindness. In the 15 years immediately after World War II, NIH grew from a small government laboratory to the most significant biomedical research institute in the world. NIH became the principal supporter of biomedical research, quickly surpassing industry and private foundations. Indeed, in the period after World War II until the 1960s, federal support for biomedical research represented one of the few areas of health policy in which the federal government was active. The influence of organized medicine was a critical factor in limiting the federal role in other areas during this period.

In addition to federal support for biomedical research, largely through medical schools and universities, and a limited program of grants to states for public health and maternal and child health programs, federal policy related to hospital planning and construction became of primary importance. After World War II, it was evident that many of America's hospitals were woefully inadequate, and the Hill-Burton federal–state program of hospital planning and construction was launched in response in 1942. Its initial purpose was to provide funds to states to survey hospital bed supply and develop plans to overcome the hospital shortage, particularly in rural areas. The Hill-Burton Act was amended numerous times as its initial goals were met. This legislation provided the stimulus for a massive hospital construction program, with federal and state subsidies primarily for community, nonprofit, and voluntary hospitals. Public hospitals, supported largely by local tax funds to provide care for the poor, received little or no federal support until the needs of private institutions were met. The program became a model of federal–state–private sector cooperation in the distribution of substantial federal resources. It was a prime example of cooperative federalism and the major force—until enactment of Medicare and Medicaid—behind

modernization of the voluntary community hospital system.

After World War II, President Truman urged Congress to enact a program of national health insurance, funded through federal taxes. President Truman's efforts and those of his supporters in Congress and organized labor were thwarted, again largely as a result of opposition by the American Medical Association. No progress was made in extending the federal role in financing of medical care because the medical profession argued that voluntary health insurance, such as Blue Cross, and commercial insurance could do the job.

By 1953, when the Department of Health, Education, and Welfare (now the Department of Health and Human Services) was created, the federal government's role in the nation's health care system, although limited, was firmly established. This role was designed primarily to support programs and services in the private sector. Biomedical research, research training, and hospital construction were the major pathways for federal support. The Food and Drug Administration also became part of DHEW and was its primary regulatory agency. Traditional public health programs, such as those for venereal disease control, tuberculosis control, and maternal and child health, were supported at minimal levels through categorical grants to the states. Federal support for medical care was restricted to military personnel, veterans, merchant seamen, and native Americans until 1960, when enactment of the Kerr-Mills law authorized limited federal grants to states for medical assistance for the aged. This program proved short-lived, but it highlighted the need for a far broader federal effort in medical care for the poor and the aged.

The Transformation of Health Policies: The New Frontier, The Great Society, and Creative Federalism (1961–1969)

A number of major federal health policy developments took place between 1961 and 1969, during the presidencies of John F. Kennedy and Lyndon B. Johnson. Although federal support was extended directly to universities, hospitals, and nonprofit institutes conducting research, most federal aid in health was channeled through the states. The term "creative federalism" was applied to policies developed during the Johnson administration that extended the traditional federal–state relationship to include direct federal support for local governments (cities and counties), nonprofit organizations, and private businesses and corporations to carry out health, education, training, social services, and community development programs (7). The primary means used to forward the goals of creative federalism were grants-in-aid. More than 200 grant programs were enacted during the five years of the Johnson administration.

The first major health policy changes after the election of President Kennedy again was the result of a crisis. The thalidomide disaster in Europe had little direct impact in the United States because the Food and Drug Administration had not approved the drug for marketing here. The disaster nonetheless focused renewed attention on the problems of drug safety, efficacy, and promotion, and led to the most sweeping reforms of federal drug laws in 24 years. The 1962 amendments to the Food, Drug and Cosmetic Act specified that a drug must be demonstrated to be effective, as well as safe, before it could be marketed. Advertising also was strictly regulated, and more effective provisions for removal of unsafe drugs from the market were included (42).

The categorical programs that developed during the period of creative federalism were numerous and varied. Some programs were based on disease (heart disease, cancer, stroke, and mental illness); some, on public assistance eligibility (Medicaid); some, on age (Medicare, crippled children); some, on institutions (hospitals, nursing homes, neighborhood health centers); some, on political jurisdiction (state or local departments of public health); some, on geographic areas that did not follow traditional political boundaries (community men-

tal health centers, catchment areas, the Appalachian Regional Commission); and some, on activity (research, facility construction, health professionals training, and health care financing) (36).

Among the more important new laws enacted during the Johnson administration were the Health Professions Educational Assistance Act of 1963, which authorized direct federal aid to medical, dental, pharmacy, and other professional schools, as well as to students in these schools; the Maternal and Child Health and Mental Retardation Planning Amendments of 1963, which initiated comprehensive maternal and infant care projects and centers serving the mentally retarded; the Civil Rights Act of 1964, which prohibited racial discrimination, including segregated schools and hospitals; the Economic Opportunity Act of 1964, which provided authority and funds to establish neighborhood health centers serving low-income populations; the Social Security Amendments of 1965, particularly Medicare and Medicaid, which financed medical care for the aged and the poor receiving cash assistance; the Heart Disease, Cancer and Stroke Act of 1965, which launched a national attack on these major killers through regional medical programs; and the Comprehensive Health Planning and Public Health Service Amendments of 1966 and the Partnership for Health Act of 1967, which reestablished the principle of block grants for state public health services (reversing a 30-year trend of categorical federal grants in health). This legislation also created the first nationwide health planning system, which was dramatically changed in the 1970s to focus on regulation of health care as well as health planning (43). It should be noted that not until the Nixon and Reagan administrations was the block grant concept widely applied to federal grants-in-aid to the states. Of the many new health programs initiated during the Johnson presidency, only Medicare was administered directly by the federal government.

The programs of the Johnson presidency had a profound effect on intergovernmental relationships, the concept of federalism, and federal expenditures for domestic social programs. Grant-in-aid programs alone (excluding Social Security and Medicare) grew from $7 billion at the beginning of the Kennedy and Johnson administrations in 1961 to $24 billion in 1970, at the end of that era. In the next decade the impact was to be even more dramatic as federal grant-in-aid expenditures for these programs grew to $82.9 billion in 1980. "Grants-in-aid," note Reagan and Sanzone (7), "constitute a major social invention of our time and are the prototypical, although not statistically dominant [they now constitute over 20 percent of domestic federal outlays], form of federal domestic involvement."

The programs of the Johnson administration not only had a significant effect on the nature and scope of the federal role in domestic social programs but also had important consequences for health care. Federal funds for biomedical research and training, health personnel development, hospital construction, health care financing, and a variety of categorical programs were designed primarily to improve access to health care and secondarily to improve its quality. Increased attention during this period was given to the notion of health care as a right, a concept similar to the principle of the "earned right" that underlies the Social Security system (44,45).

Although there was a profound change in the role of the federal government, many policies adopted during this time reflected the interests of the medical profession, the hospitals, and the health insurance industry. Medicare and Medicaid hospital reimbursement policies were designed to ensure hospital participation. Adoption of the cost-based method of reimbursement proved a boon for hospitals but was very costly for the taxpayer. Policies designed to meet the physician shortage of the 1960s eventually developed full support from organized medicine. Designed to strengthen the capacity of the nation's medical schools to respond to a nationally perceived need, these policies also provided direct benefit to an interest group of growing power—medical schools.

Health Policy in an Era of Limited Resources: From Creative Federalism to New Federalism and a Return to Dependence on Competition and the Private Sector (1969–19??)

During the 1970s, President Nixon coined the term "New Federalism" to describe his efforts to move away from the categorical programs of the Johnson years toward general revenue sharing, through which federal revenues were transferred to state and local governments with as few federal strings as possible, and toward block grants, through which grants are allocated to state and local governments for broad general purposes. During the Nixon and Ford administrations (1969–1977), considerable conflict developed between the executive branch and the Congress with respect to domestic social policy, including the New Federalism strategy originally advocated by President Nixon. Congress strongly favored categorical grants, with their detailed provisions, and was opposed to both revenue sharing and block grants. This period also witnessed an erosion of trust between federal middle management and congressional committees and subcommittees (46).

President Nixon also differed sharply from President Johnson in his explicit support for private rather than public efforts to solve the nation's health problems. On this fundamental issue the Nixon administration made its position clear: "Preference for action in the private sector is based on the fundamentals of our political economy—capitalistic, pluralistic and competitive—as well as upon the desire to strengthen the capability of our private institutions in their effort to provide health services, to finance such services, and to produce the resources that will be needed in the years ahead" (47).

Although the Nixon administration attempted to implement its New Federalism policies across a broad front, progress was made primarily in the fields of community development, personnel training, and social services. Categorical grant programs in health continued to expand despite attempts by both the Nixon and Ford administrations to transfer program authority and responsibility to the states and to reduce the federal role in domestic social programs. During the period 1965–1975, more than 75 major pieces of health legislation were enacted by Congress, indicating continued support for the categorical approach by the federal government (43).

Although categorical health programs proliferated in the 1960s and 1970s, the expansion of two programs—Medicare and Medicaid—dwarfed the others. While these programs contributed to medical inflation, their growth was due largely to the rising costs of medical care in the 1970s. Federal and state governments became third parties that underwrote the costs of a system that had few cost-constraining elements, and the staggering expenditures had profound effects on health policy.

The federal government's response to skyrocketing health care costs (and thus governmental expenditures) assumed a variety of forms. Federal subsidies of hospitals and other health facility construction were ended and replaced by planning and regulatory mechanisms designed to limit their growth. In the mid–1970s health personnel policies focused on specialty and geographic maldistribution of physicians rather than physician shortage, and by the late 1970s, concern was expressed about an oversupply of physicians and other health professionals (48). Direct subsidies to expand enrollment in health professions schools were cut back and then eliminated. Funding for biomedical research began to decline in real dollar terms when an abortive "war on cancer" launched by President Nixon appeared to produce few concrete results and when Medicare and Medicaid preempted most federal health dollars.

More important than the constraints placed on resources allocated for health care were regulations instituted to slow the growth of health care costs. Two direct actions were taken by the federal government: 1) a limit on federal and state payments to hospitals and physicians under Medicare and Medicaid (included in the 1972 Social Security Amendments) and 2) a period of wage and price control applied to the general economy when the Economic Stabilization Program was introduced to dampen increasing inflation. Wage and price controls on hospitals and physicians were continued after the general restrictions were removed. When controls were lifted in 1974, health care costs again began to climb.

Another regulatory initiative was designed to control costs through limiting the use of hospital care by Medicare and Medicaid beneficiaries. Although the original Medicare and Medicaid legislation required hospital utilization review committees, these appeared to have little effect on hospital use or costs. In 1972 amendments to the Social Security Act (PL 92-103) required the establishment of professional standards review organizations (PSROs) to review the quality and appropriateness of hospital services provided to beneficiaries of Medicare, Medicaid, maternal and child health, and crippled children programs (paid for under authority of Title V of the Social Security Act). PSROs were composed of physicians who reviewed hospital records in order to determine whether length of stay and services provided were appropriate. Results of these efforts have been mixed. In only a few areas where PSROs have been in operation is there evidence that cost increases have been restrained, and in these areas it is not clear that the PSRO has been a critical factor.

An attempt also was made to control costs through major changes in the organization of medical care, as discussed throughout this book. Efforts were made to stimulate the growth of group practice prepayment plans, which provide comprehensive services for a fixed annual fee. These capitation-based prepayment organizations were defined in federal legislation enacted in 1973 as health maintenance organizations (HMOs). Studies have demonstrated that HMOs provide comprehensive care at significantly less cost than fee-for-service providers, primarily because of lower rates of hospitalization (49). Predictably, the federal stimulus for development of HMOs encountered strong resistance from organized medicine. Nevertheless, the program successfully enhanced professional and public awareness of HMOs and assisted in the development of a number of small prepaid group practices. The impact on costs at the national level, however, remained minimal.

An additional regulatory initiative enacted during President Nixon's second term was the National Health Planning and Resource Development Act of 1974 (PL 93-641). This law incorporated some of the planning principles from the Partnership for Health Act of 1967 and the Heart Disease, Cancer and Stroke Act of 1965, both of which were terminated with the enactment of PL 93-641. In addition to the health planning responsibility assigned to state health planning and development agencies (SHPDAs) and to local health systems agencies (HSAs), the law required that health care facilities obtain prior approval from the state for any expansion, in the form of a "certificate of need" (CON).

The National Health Planning and Development Act was enacted when decentralization of government authority and new federalism were primary strategies for achieving national objectives and when the role of special interests, such as organized medicine, was expanding at both federal and state levels. State and local health planning agencies created by the law resisted efforts to impose what they considered to be too much federal direction and regulation. With few exceptions, HSAs were not part of local government, but rather nonprofit private agencies strongly influenced by health care providers, particularly physicians and hospitals represented on their boards of directors. Although health planning agencies were concentrating their efforts on health care costs, particularly those generated by additional hospital beds and technology, these efforts appeared to have little effect in the face of inflationary pressures from the hospital reimbursement policies of Blue Cross, Medicare, Medicaid, and commercial health insurance carriers. The regulatory role that they were required to play, particularly the approval (or disapproval) of the certificate of need required for new hospital and nursing home construction, created growing resistance among providers. Although this regulatory role apparently has had little impact on total investments by hospitals (50), provider opposition

to it led to growing efforts to limit the authority of health planning agencies.

Although the New Federalism advocated by President Reagan was a dramatic departure from previous policies and trends because of the scope of his proposals, the roots of these policies were first evident in the comprehensive Health Planning and Public Health Service amendments enacted in 1966 during the presidency of Lyndon Johnson. They were increasingly evident in both the policy initiatives and the budgetary decisions of Presidents Nixon and Ford. The Nixon and Ford New Federalism policies were not only similar to those later advocated by President Reagan, but their fiscal and monetary policies also were designed to reduce the growth of federal spending and program responsibility.

During the presidency of Jimmy Carter (1977–1981), there were few new health policy initiatives. The Carter administration tried without success to get Congress to enact hospital cost-containment legislation. Special interests, particularly hospitals and physicians, again prevailed. They were able to convince Congress that a voluntary effort would be more effective. Escalating health care costs did moderate during the debate in Congress, but when mandatory controls were discontinued, costs rose at a record rate. The picture in the late 1970s was one of frustration with efforts to control costs. Concern about access to care became a secondary consideration.

In 1979, when legislative authority for health planning was renewed, two conflicting congressional attitudes emerged: 1) an antiregulatory, procompetitive sentiment that was to grow in the 1980s (51) and 2) a continuing movement toward decentralization of existing planning and regulatory programs, providing state and local authorities with increasing responsibility. Congress was not anxious to spend more money on medical care, and the procompetitive approach was promoted as a more effective means of cost containment than continued expansion of regulatory cost controls.

Since it is inherently difficult to make specific changes in health planning and regulatory processes that increase beneficial competition, these new provisions simply added impossible goals to the already lofty purposes identified for health planning—improving access and assuring quality of care while controlling costs. These procompetitive, antiregulatory, and prodecentralization forces found full expression two years later with the enactment of the Omnibus Budget Reconciliation Act of 1981 and in efforts in 1982 to eliminate federal support for local health planning efforts.

The Reagan administration accelerated the degree of pace of change in policy that had been developing since the early Nixon years. The most prominent shifts in federal policy advanced by the Reagan administration that directly affected health care were 1) a significant reduction in federal expenditures for domestic social programs, including the elimination of the revenue-sharing program initiated by President Nixon; 2) decentralization of program authority and responsibility to the states, particularly through block grants; 3) deregulation and greater emphasis on market forces and competition to stimulate health care reform and more effective control of health care costs; 4) tax reductions, despite significant increases in the national debt, with a resulting decline in the fiscal capacity of the federal government to fund domestic social programs; and 5) Medicare cost containment through the implementation of a prospective payment system for hospitals based on costs per case, using diagnosis-related groups (DRGs) as the basis for payment.

An important consequence of the block grants enacted by Congress at the urging of the Reagan administration is that the wide discretion that these grants provide to the individual states fosters inequities in programs among the states. This, in turn, makes it impossible to ensure uniform benefits for target populations, such as the poor and the aged, across jurisdictions or to maintain accountability with so many varying state approaches (13). Because the most disadvantaged individuals are heavily dependent on state-determined benefits, they are especially vulnerable in this period of economic flux. These policies also have increased

pressure on state and local governments to underwrite program costs at the same time that many states, cities, and counties are under mounting pressure to curb expenditures.

Although the Reagan administrations strongly favored deregulation and stimulation of procompetitive market forces, this had little impact on federal health care policies except in the health planning area. The federal health planning legislation was not renewed in the 1980s, but a number of states continued to operate certificate of need programs in an attempt to control the proliferation of expensive technologies.

In contrast to eliminating health planning as a means of regulation, the Reagan and Bush administrations have used regulations to limit hospital reimbursement and physician fees in the Medicare program.

At the state level, however, major changes are under way that respond to the growing influence of the free-market ideology. In California, major reforms were enacted in 1982 in an attempt to increase competition among hospitals and reduce the costs of Medicaid in that state. Private insurance companies were also authorized to contract directly with hospitals through preferred provider contracts in an attempt to stimulate price competition among hospitals.

Congress has considered a number of procompetition proposals related to Medicare, Medicaid, and private health insurance. Although the proposals differ in detail, several elements characterize the procompetitive approach: 1) changes in tax treatment for employers, employees, or both, regarding employer contributions to health insurance plans (not supported by Congress in the 1980s but may be enacted in the 1990s if costs continue to escalate; 2) establishment of incentives or requirements for employers to offer employees multiple choices of health insurance plans, subject to certain limitations with respect to coverage of services and cost sharing, including catastrophic illness benefits and preventive care; and 3) establishment of Medicare voucher systems under which elderly and disabled individuals would receive a fixed-value voucher that could be applied toward the purchase of a qualified health insurance plan (unlikely to be enacted).

Although recent federal procompetition–deregulation policies have attracted the greatest attention, it is the dramatic reduction in federal fiscal capacity due to tax cuts and the growing federal deficit that have had the most immediate effect on health services. While the federal government is debating cost-containment strategies, a number of states have moved to restrict expenditures for Medicaid beneficiaries because of the continued impact of high costs on Medicaid expenditures at the state and federal levels. Several states, including California, have enacted dramatic policy changes, restricting patients' freedom to choose providers, reducing levels of hospital and physician reimbursement, and shifting the burden of large numbers of poor patients back to local government.

The politics of limited resources began to dominate the U.S. political scene in the 1970s, and this continued into the 1980s, with little prospect of change. The prolonged period of postwar economic growth, based on productivity gains, came to a halt in the early 1970s, and the additional resources needed in domestic social programs and defense have been more and more constrained as a result. Controlling the costs of health care has become a critical need at the federal and state levels. In the 1970s, policy efforts focused more on limiting federal and state expenditures in Medicare and Medicaid than they did on dealing with the root causes of the problem—the growing supply of physicians; the rapid growth in biomedical technologies in health care; and reimbursement incentives in Medicare, Medicaid, and private insurance mediated through the fee-for-service health care system that have led to enormous inflation in health care costs. With the advent of the prospective payment system (PPS) for Medicare, enacted by Congress in 1983, federal policy makers began to attack these perverse reimbursement incentives. The comprehensive physician payment reforms in the Medicare program, including a Medicare fee schedule, volume performance standards, and a limit on balance billing by physi-

cians, enacted by Congress in 1989, suggests a growing interest in Congress to control cost increases through regulation rather than procompetitive strategies.

Whether these approaches to restraining hospital and physician expenditures are effective remains to be seen. Unless they are applied broadly to the private sector, it is likely that they will restrain the rate of increase in Medicare expenditures but increase those in the private sector due to cost shifting. Given a policy process characterized by limited government roles, federalism, pluralism, administrative bargaining, and incrementalism, prospects remain relatively dim for controlling expenditures in ways that protect vulnerable groups such as the poor and the elderly. It is increasingly evident that those groups whose needs originally inspired special programs are relinquishing the gains achieved in access to care.

The cost-containment strategies of the past decade, particularly those since 1981, combined with the effects of the recessions of 1981–1982 and 1990–1992 on unemployment and access to private health insurance; the growth of the undocumented alien, immigrant, and refugee populations; and the diminishing commitment to provide for the near poor and the working poor has led to a significant increase in the number of uninsured and underinsured. Census Bureau data for 1984 revealed that 17 percent of the population under age 65 years (35 million people) lacked any health insurance, an increase of more than 20 percent since 1979 (52). These figures dipped slightly in the late 1980s with the country's economic recovery but have been rising again with the recession of 1990–1992.

Federal policies related to Medicare and Medicaid, taxes, and refugees and undocumented aliens; state policies related to health care cost containment and Medicaid, ranging from California's procompetitive approach to New York's regulatory strategy; and the policies of private insurance companies and employers related to private health insurance, competition, and cost containment have all contributed to the rising number of uninsured and underinsured. Because the working poor, the disabled, refugees, new immigrants, undocumented aliens, and workers in small businesses do not have the influence of the large employers, the insurance industry, physicians, hospitals, and other influential participants in health policy, it is unlikely that their voices will be heard, unless the costs of their care impose such a burden on state and local governments and community hospitals (i.e., bad debt and charity care) that these groups will gain allies willing to advocate on their behalf. Because the interests of these groups remain diffuse in terms of potential for political action, it is unlikely that they can compete effectively in the policy process with the interest groups that have long influenced the shape of public policy in health.

The continued rise in health care costs has become the dominant health policy issue of the 1990s. Between 1970 and 1990, the share of gross national product spent on health care rose from 7.3 percent to 12.3 percent. National health spending in 1991 rose 11 percent over 1990, to $738 billion. This was the fifth consecutive year of double-digit annual increases (53). The U.S. Department of Commerce has projected increases in 1992 of $817 billion, a record 14 percent of GNP. The Commerce Department also projects that costs will continue to increase at 12–13 percent per year for the next five years. Estimates for the year 2000 imply that the percentage of GNP devoted to health care will likely exceed 16 percent and may even exceed 20 percent.

Families and businesses pay for health care directly through health insurance premiums and out of pocket (e.g. deductibles, copayments) and indirectly through payroll, income, and other taxes that pay for public programs. According to a 1991 report by Families USA Foundation, the United States spent $6,535 per family for health care in 1991; approximately two-thirds of health care costs are paid by families and one-third is paid by businesses (54).

For two decades health care spending in the United States has outpaced the growth of the rest of the economy, with consequences for workers (depressed wages), businesses (a growing share of profits to health care), families (rising out-of-

pocket costs and rising taxes to pay for public programs), and government (increasing share of government expenditures for health care).

Various attempts to control the continuing rise in costs, particularly the growing emphasis on competition in the 1980s, have failed. One result has been a growing interest on the part of U.S. policy makers in the success of other industrialized countries in controlling costs while providing universal health insurance (e.g., Canada, the United Kingdom, Germany, Japan) or a national health service (U.K.).

One significant question for the 1990s is whether the United States will continue its unique approach to health care cost containment, which emphasizes competition and limited use of regulation, particularly in the Medicare and Medicaid programs, or adopt more comprehensive strategies pursued successfully in France, Germany, and Japan—three countries with systems that resemble our own. These countries provide near universal access to health insurance through mandated employment-based insurance with government subsidies for the elderly and the poor. Health insurance is provided by multiple third-party private insurers, largely nonprofit, which must provide minimum coverage that includes a wide range of benefits. Health care services in these countries are provided by physicians in private, fee-for-service practice and by private and public hospitals.

The greatest difference between these three industrialized countries and the United States are the regulations imposed on payments to physicians and hospitals. Virtually all payers must abide by standardized rates which are not set unilaterally by the government but emerge as a result of negotiations among physicians, hospitals, and third-party payers, as well as the government in France and Japan. In addition to price controls, budget controls are used in France, Germany, and Japan to set overall limits on spending. When coupled with mechanisms to enforce these limits, the controls have been quite effective.

While two fundamentally different approaches to cost containment have been advocated and applied in the past 15 years—regulation and competition—it appears that a mixed system will emerge in the United States because of the strong role of the private sector, a federalist system of government, the dominance of pluralistic politics, and a penchant for incremental reform.

In his critical analysis of health planning in the United States, France, England, and Quebec Province in Canada, Rodwin calls for "regulated competition" (55). Enthoven (56), in his most recent contribution to the policy debate about the role of competition, calls for both "managed competition" and universal health insurance. Whether health policy makers decide on competition, regulation, "regulated competition," or "managed competition," there is no way to escape the need to link health planning and health care financing. It is critical that reimbursement systems—whether capitation or fee-for-service—encourage hospitals, physicians, nursing homes, pharmacists, and other providers to pursue society's interests as well as their own.

There are signs of an emerging consensus amid all the conflicts and tensions engendered by the need to constrain the growth in the health care sector. Various forces will affect future policies: some, such as the aging of the population, are beyond the control of policy makers; others, such as the rapid increase in physician supply and the use of an increasing number of new technologies in health care, are amenable to more direct policy interventions. One of the keys will be to reach agreement on the nature and scope of universal health insurance. Another will be to modify reimbursement policies to achieve appropriate policy goals. Still another will be to deal realistically with the failure of the "free market" and unregulated competition to assure equity.

The regulatory approach to cost containment began to gather support again in the 1980s with Medicare's prospective payment system in hospitals in 1983, and the adoption of a Medicare fee schedule by Congress in 1989. In addition to the Medicare fee schedule, Congress adopted an expenditure target, called a volume performance standard, to limit the rate of increase in expenditures for physicians' services. Both the Medicare fee schedule and the volume performance standard drew on the experience of other countries, particularly Canada and Germany. The fact that other major industrialized nations had managed to provide universal health insurance and control costs was a lesson that was gradually beginning to be appreciated by U.S. policy makers.

In addition to this evident failure of U.S. health care cost containment efforts and the apparent success of countries that have provided universal coverage with effective cost containment, there has been a substantial change in public attitudes favoring health care financing reform (20). This change in public attitude and the growing dissatisfaction of Americans with the present system of health care financing and the rising costs of care may overwhelm the special interests (insurance companies, physicians, hospitals) that have long thwarted comprehensive reforms in health care financing and cost containment.

Health care became a major political issue in 1991 and is likely to remain so until the problems of health care cost containment and universal access to health insurance are solved in the United States. The next major chapter in national health policy may well be written before the elections of 1996.

References

1. Jonas, S., & Banta, D. (1981). Government in the health care delivery system. In S. Jonas (Ed.). *Health care delivery in the United States*. New York: Springer.
2. Marmor, T. R. (1973). *The politics of Medicare*. Chicago: Aldine.
3. Vladeck, B. C. (1980). *Unloving care: The nursing home tragedy*. New York: Basic Books.
4. Wade, R. C. (1982, August 1). The suburban roots of new federalism. *The New York Times Magazine*. 20, 21, 39, 46.
5. Ginzberg, D. (1978). Health reform: The outlook for the 1980s. *Inquiry*. *15*. 311–326.
6. Pechman, J. A. (Ed.). (1979). *Setting national prior-*

ities: The 1980 budget. Washington, DC: The Brookings Institution.

7. Reagan, M. D., & Sanzone, J. G. (1981). *The new federalism* (2nd ed.). New York: Oxford University Press.

8. Hale, G. E., & Palley, M. L. (1981). *The politics of federal grants.* Washington, DC: Congressional Quarterly Press.

9. Vladeck, B. C. (1979). The design of failure: Health policy and the structure of federalism. *Journal of Health Politics, Policy and Law. 4.* 522–535.

10. Reagan, M. D. (1972). *The new federalism.* New York: Oxford University Press.

11. Clarke, G. J. (1981). The role of the states in the delivery of health services. In S. C. Jain (Ed.). *Role of state and local governments in relation to personal health services.* (Reprinted from *American Journal of Public Health.* [1981]. *71.* pp. 59–69.)

12. Lee, R. D., & Staffeldt, R. J. (1977). Executive and legislative use of policy analysis in the state budgetary process. *Policy Analysis. 3.* 395–405.

13. Estes, C. L. (1980). *The aging enterprise.* San Francisco: Jossey-Bass.

14. Brizius, J. A. *Federalism and national purpose* (pp. 72–98). Working paper 2, Project on the Federal Social Role, National Conference on Social Welfare, Washington, DC.

15. Schattschneider, E. E. (1960). *The semisovereign people.* New York: Holt, Rinehart & Winston.

16. Bachrach, P. (1967). *The theory of democratic elitism: A critique.* Boston: Little, Brown.

17. Ginzberg, E. (Ed.). (1977). *Regionalization and health policy.* Washington, DC: U.S. Government Printing Office.

18. Silver, G. A. (1976). Medical politics, health policy, party health platforms, promise and performance. *International Journal of Health Services. 6.* 331–343.

19. Marmor, T. R., Wittman, D. A., & Heagy, T. C. (1976). The politics of medical inflation. *Journal of Health Politics, Policy and Law. 1.* 69–84.

20. Blendon, R. J., & Taylor, H. (1989). Views on health care: Public opinion in three nations. *Health Affairs. 8.* 149–157.

21. Blendon, R. J., et al. (1990). Satisfaction with health systems in ten nations. *Health Affairs. 9.* 185–192.

22. Feldstein, P. J. (1981). The politics of health. In P. R. Lee, N. Brown, & I. V. S. W. Red (Eds.). *The nation's health: Article booklet* (pp. 40–42). San Francisco: Boyd & Fraser.

23. Sabatier, B., & Mazamania, D. (1979). Conditions of effective implantation. *Policy Analysis. 5.* 481–504.

24. Lowi, T. J. (1979). *The end of liberalism: The second republic of the United States.* New York: Norton.

25. Silver, G. A. (1978). *Preface: The uncertainties of federal child health policies.* Hyattsville, MD: National Center for Health Services Research.

26. Kingdon, J. W. (1984). *Agendas, alternatives, and public policies.* Boston: Little, Brown.

27. Sabatier, P. A. (1988). An advocacy coalition framework of policy change and the role of policy-oriented learning therein. *Policy Sciences. 21.* 129–168.

28. Oliver, T. R. (1991, July). *A conceptual guide to policy implementation.* Unpublished manuscript, University of California, Institute for Health Policy Studies, San Francisco.

29. Feder, J. M. (1977). *The politics of federal hospital insurance.* Lexington, MA: Lexington Books.

30. Lindblom, C. E. (1959). The science of "muddling through." *Public Administration Review. 10.* 79–88.

31. Wildavsky, A. (1964). *The politics of the budgetary process.* Boston: Little, Brown.

32. Alford, R. R. (1975). *Health care politics: Ideological and interest group barriers to reform.* Chicago: University of Chicago Press.

33. Estes, C. L. (1982). Austerity and aging in the United States: 1980 and beyond. *International Journal of Health Services. 12.* 573.

34. Lee, P. R., & Silver, G. A. (1972). Health planning— a view from the top with specific reference to the USA. In J. Fry & W. A. J. Farndale (Eds.). *International medical care.* Oxford, U.K.: Medical and Technical Publishing Co., Ltd.

35. Torrens, P. R. (1988). Overview of the health services system. In S. J. Williams & P. R. Torrens (Eds.). *Introduction to health services* (3rd ed.). New York: Wiley.

36. Lewis, I., & Sheps, C. (1983). *The sick citadel: The American academic medical center and the public interest.* Cambridge, UK: Oelgeschlager, Gunn and Hain.

37. Hale, G. E., & Palley, M. L. (1981). *The politics of federal grants.* Washington, DC: Congressional Quarterly Press.

38. Miller, C. A., Moos, M. K., Kotch, J. B., et al. (1981).

Role of local health departments in the delivery of ambulatory care. In S. C. Jain (Ed.). *Role of state and local governments in relation to personal health services.* Chapel Hill: University of North Carolina Press.

39. Miller, C. A., Gilbert B., Warren, D. G. (1977). Statutory authorizations for the work of local health departments. *American Journal of Public Health. 67.* 940–946.

40. Foley, H. A. (1975). *Community mental health legislation.* Lexington, MA: Lexington Books.

41. Silver, G. A. (1976). *A spy in the house of medicine.* Germantown, MD: Aspen Systems Corp.

42. Silverman, M., & P. Lee. (1974). *Pills, profits, and politics.* Berkeley: University of California Press.

43. U.S. Department of Health, Education and Welfare. (1976). *Health in America 1776–1976* (DHEW Publication No. [HRA] 76–616). Washington, DC: U.S. Government Printing Office.

44. Lee, P. R., & Jonsen, A. R. (1974). The right to health care. *American Review of Respiratory Diseases. 109.* 591–593.

45. Callahan, D. (1977). Health and society: Some ethical imperatives. *Daedalus. 106.* 1.

46. Walker, D. (1981). *Toward a functioning federalism.* Cambridge, MA: Winthrop.

47. Richardson, E. L. (1971). *Towards a comprehensive health policy in the 1970s.* Washington, DC: U.S. Department of Health, Education and Welfare.

48. Lee, P. R., LeRoy, L., & Stalcup, J. (1976): *Primary care in a specialized world.* Cambridge, MA: Ballinger.

49. Luft, H. S. (1980). *Health maintenance organizations: Dimensions of performance.* New York: Wiley-Interscience.

50. Salkever, D. S., & Bice, T. W. (1976). The impact of certificate-of-need controls on hospital investment. *Milbank Memorial Fund Quarterly. 54.* 185–214.

51. Budetti, P. (1981). Congressional perspectives on health planning and cost containment: Lessons from the 1979 debate and amendments. *Journal of Health and Human Resources Administration. 4.* 10–19.

52. Blendon, R. J., Aiken, L. H., Freeman, H. E., et al. (1986). Uncompensated care by hospitals or public insurance for the poor. *New England Journal of Medicine. 314.* 1160–1163.

53. U.S. General Accounting Office. (1991, November). *Health care spending control: The experience of France, Germany, and Japan* (GAO Publication No. [HRD]-92-9). Washington, DC: U.S. Government Printing Office.

54. Families USA Foundation. (1991, December). *Health spending: The growing threat to the family budget.* Washington, DC: Author.

55. Rodwin, V. G. (1984). *The health planning predicament* (p. 303). Berkeley: University of California Press.

56. Enthoven, A. C. (1986). Managed competition and health care and the unfinished agenda. *Health Care Financing Review* (Ann. suppl.). 120–150.

Chapter 16

Understanding the Present, Planning for the Future: The Dynamics of Health Care in the United States in the 1990s

Paul R. Torrens
Stephen J. Williams

After having read all of the separate chapters in this book about the various parts of the American health care system, the reader might well ask, "What does all this mean for the future? Where is health care in the United States going in the 1990s and what is the dynamic force that is driving the health care system of this country?" The purpose of this final chapter is to introduce a set of ideas that may possibly explain why there is so much "activity" in health care in the United States and at the same time, so little progress in solving our major problems. The purpose of this chapter is to provide an understanding of the basic dynamics that are driving the American health care system, so that the reader can better understand the central forces directing the future of health care in the United States.

Health Care in the United States: A Continuous Circular "Gaming" System

The model that best describes the current American health care system is that of a continuous, circular "gaming" system. In this model, the rapid rise in health care costs sets off a series of events that ultimately affect the entire U.S. health care system and eventually lead to even higher health care costs in the future. Briefly stated, the rise in health care costs has an impact on those organizations and agencies (employers and insurance programs, primarily) that pay the health care bills and forces them to take cost-containment actions. These efforts of the payors to contain health care costs (to contain health care *expenditures,* more accurately) have an impact on the providers of care, particularly hospitals and physicians. These providers find their sources of revenue being constrained as a result of the payors' health care cost-containment efforts, so they then take actions of their own in reaction to the efforts of the payors. These actions of the health care providers, in turn, often affect patients and communities which must then try to take whatever actions they can to lessen the impact.

The result of this chain of events is a circular

system that merely passes along the effects of one particular set of changes to another part of the system, which in turn takes actions of its own to pass the problem along further. The end result of this set of dynamic forces is a continuous, circular system that encourages (some would even say, forces) each individual part of the system to figure out how to play the "game." Each individual part of this circular "gaming" system expends a tremendous amount of effort to solve its particular limited problems and very often does so with an elaborate display of talent, energy, and sophistication. Unfortunately, this limited and somewhat self-interested set of individual solutions to limited problems does not really succeed in containing the rise in health care costs, and this inevitably leads to a new round of individualized efforts by payors to contain the new increases in health care costs. Tragically, the need for each individual part of the circular "gaming" system to deal with its limited problems, and to treat other parts of the system as adversaries, prevents all of the individual parts of the system from coming together to mutually and cooperatively solve systemwide problems that are not amenable to individual, limited solutions. The ultimate tragedy and irony of this circular "gaming" system of health care is that it not only does not solve the initiating problem (the rapid rise in health care costs), but it also prevents any broad, cooperative efforts that would be necessary to solve the problem.

The Reasons for the Rise in Health Care Costs

As a first step in understanding this model of American health care as a circular "gaming" system, it is important to identify the basic reasons for the rise in health care costs in the United States. It is also important to understand that these reasons are the result of significant *successes* and not failures of the individual parts of the American health care system. One of the most unfortunate views of the health care system in the United States today is that there is something "wrong" or "bad"

about the rise in health care costs, when the reasons for that rise are directly related to the American society's desire for better health care. Health care in the United States is not a "failure"; it is not providing a product that no one wants. We are not operating a "going-out-of-business" sale in health care. Quite the contrary, in fact. The reasons for the rise in health care costs are that the product (20th-century health care) is very effective and is actively desired by everyone in the United States.

Four particular "successes" have led to the rise in health care costs. The first of these has been the expansion of our supply of hospital facilities and beds, beginning shortly after World War II, largely as a result of the federal government's Hill-Burton program. Under Hill-Burton, federal funds were made widely available for construction of new hospitals throughout the country and for vigorous expansion of old ones. It was the stated goal of this program to improve access of the American people to modern hospital care no matter where they lived in the United States, and it was remarkably successful in meeting that objective.

The second reason for the rise in health care costs has been the increasing number of physicians available throughout the United States, again beginning in the 1950s. At that time, it was felt that there was a "shortage" of physicians in the U.S., particularly in rural areas and in such fields of medicine as general practice/family practice. The solution to this perceived shortage of physicians was to expand the country's capacity to produce them. This was done by greatly increasing the number of medical schools that were educating and training physicians in this country, as well as by expanding the capacity of already existing medical schools so that they could produce even larger graduating classes. This effort to expand the supply of physicians was done in direct response to the country's desire to have better access to physician care and the effort was extremely successful. However, this improved access to physician services, together with expanded access to hospital services, has greatly increased use of physician and hospital services, resulting in significant rises in health care costs.

The third major "success" leading to the rise in health care costs has been the phenomenal expansion of health insurance coverage to the American people, again a post–World War II occurrence. While it is true that the United States does not have universal insurance coverage of its population, it is estimated that more than 85 percent of the population do have access to health insurance of one kind or another. This expansion of insurance coverage from a relatively rudimentary coverage at the end of World War II to the expanded coverage of today has made it easier for the American public to use the expanded supply of physicians, hospitals, and hospital beds. More doctors, more hospitals, and more health insurance coverage have all contributed to increased use and ultimately to the rise in health care costs.

The fourth major "success" underlying the rise in health care costs has been the remarkable growth in medical science and health care technology since the end of World War II. American society has provided immense sums of money for the development of medical science and technology, primarily through funding the National Institutes of Health and related researchers throughout the country. The return on this investment in terms of an extraordinary array of new discoveries and technologies has been remarkable, but also very expensive to implement. The new technologies require significant capital investment, call for increasingly sophisticated and well-trained personnel for their implementation, and absorb a rapidly growing amount of operating revenue to maintain.

Our society has approved these developments and has provided financial support not only for the initial development of new technology but also for the capital and operating funds to make it widely accessible. It should not be a surprise to anyone that the combination of expanded physician supply, number of hospitals and hospital beds, and insurance coverage, together with an impressive new array of technology, should lead to an explosive rise in health care costs.

It is important to note that American society has actively supported each of these four separate "success" stories. These were not events that were forced on a reluctant or unwilling public, but rather were seen as important social advances. The "failure" of our society, however, has been its lack of willingness to develop a system that would integrate and, to some degree, supervise and control these individual developments. This lack of an overarching social structure that could integrate these four success stories has been likened to an airplane manufacturer that develops four extremely powerful jet engines and then mounts them on an airplane body with each engine pointing in a slightly different direction. Such an airplane would probably fly only in circles. In the same fashion, it should be obvious that without a broader system of social influence and control, the four major "successes" would never come together into a well-integrated system of health care that could also contain the rise in costs for that care.

It is important to understand that the rapid rise in health care costs in recent years and the attempts to control that rapid rise are the central, motivating dynamic in the organization and operation of U.S. health care today. The single most important factor influencing virtually all aspects of the health care system is the rise in health care costs and our various piecemeal attempts to contain it. The following sections of this chapter describe how these dynamics play out in practical terms.

Impact of Rising Health Care Costs on Payors/Actions Taken by Payors in Response to Rising Health Care Costs

The rise in health care costs has had a major impact on the payors of health care expenses, particularly the three major elements in the payor section of the American health care system: Medicare, Medicaid, and corporate employers. With the rise in health care costs, each of these payors has faced tremendous challenges and has had to initiate major efforts to contain their expenditures.

For some years, Part A of the federal Medicare program has been paying out more money each year than it has taken in in revenues. This has resulted in significant operating deficits in Part A of the Medicare program. Since that part is supposed to be self-sustaining (that is, maintained solely by contributions from future beneficiaries and not subsidized by general tax revenues), it has been forced to use accumulated reserves from previous years to meet this deficit. Unfortunately, those reserves from previous years have been dwindling and face exhaustion some time after the year 2000 unless something is done to reverse the flow. These predictions of future financial catastrophe for Part A have been a significant stimulus to the Health Care Financing Administration (HCFA) to control health care costs and to reduce (or cap) Part A expenditures.

HCFA has taken a number of steps to reduce its expenditures in both Part A and Part B. First among these efforts has been the implementation of the diagnosis-related groups (DRG) method for paying hospitals for their care of Medicare beneficiaries. As a result of this new method of payment, hospitals are no longer paid according to the number of individual services they provide or the number of days that Medicare beneficiaries remain in there. Instead, they now receive a fixed sum of money for each admission, that sum being determined by the admitting diagnosis, not by the volume of services provided. This form of payment provides a strong incentive to hospitals to become more efficient in their operations, but it also invokes a number of unintended reactions within hospital organizations, as we shall see later. The overall effect of this new system of payment for hospital care has been to significantly slow the rise of Medicare's outlays for its beneficiaries' hospital services.

A second major strategy employed by Medicare has been to encourage Medicare recipients to join health maintenance organizations and other forms of prepaid group practice plans. The purpose of this strategy is to move as many Medicare beneficiaries as possible into a form of health care delivery that is covered by a single *per capita* payment for care, regardless of the volume of services delivered. This allows the Medicare program to better predict and control its annual beneficiary expenses. At present, only a small percentage of Medicare recipients have chosen to leave fee-for-service medical care to join health maintenance organizations or prepaid group practices, but their percentage is growing and this managed-care approach remains a significant long-term cost-containment strategy for the Medicare program.

A third strategy of reimbursement reform that is being used by Medicare is the resource-based relative-value system (RBRVS) format for paying physicians. This system attempts to rationalize Medicare payments to physicians by reducing reimbursement to some physicians (who are currently thought to be overpaid) and to increase reimbursement to other types of physicians (who are thought to be underpaid). Although this system is supposed to be "budget neutral" for the present and is not avowedly intended to reduce total Medicare budgetary outlays for physician services, it does establish a long-range method for reviewing and resetting the level of reimbursement to physicians in a manner that is different from that used before. It is an attempt to rationalize physician payments, to shift certain financial incentives among physician groups, and to provide a long-term mechanism for more effectively controlling Medicare payments to physicians for their services.

Finally, the Medicare program is also initiating a wide variety of small reforms that influence various aspects of the reimbursement policy and, therefore, various parts of the American health care system. In some cases, for example, the contributions of Medicare beneficiaries for their participation in the Medicare program and for their receipt of health care at the time of service is being increased, thereby shifting more of the cost of medical care back to the beneficiaries themselves, even if only in small amounts. Attempts have also been made to review the Medicare reimbursement practices to teaching hospitals for postgraduate medical education and at the same time, to review reimbursement practices for hospitals that supposedly have a disproportionate share of poor and indigent patients. Other types of regulatory reform related to physician ownership of laboratory and other ancillary services to which physicians themselves might refer patients are also being put in place.

At the same time that Medicare is trying to protect itself from the effects of rising health care costs, individual state Medicaid programs are also battling to control their expenditures, which now represent a major percentage of each state's government outlays. A typical state Medicaid program reaction has been to reduce or restrict eligibility for services as much as possible. States have also attempted to hold down expenditures by limiting increases in payment rates to physicians and hospitals as much as possible. In some states such as California, the state Medicaid program has established a program for contracting directly with certain hospitals for in-patient care of Medicaid recipients; this has resulted in a more competitive approach toward hospitals' ability to care for Medicaid patients and has given the state Medicaid program more leverage with those hospitals that do contract for care. Finally, some state Medicaid programs, like the federal Medicare program, are attempting to move Medicaid recipients into health maintenance organizations and managed care programs, in order to control use and costs more effectively.

Some of the most active cost-containment methods are being put into place by employers and by the health insurance carriers they use to provide coverage for their employees. Many employers are trying to reduce benefit packages seen as overly generous in the past; this has been particularly true in the case of mental health benefits. In other instances, employers have attempted to increase the employee cost sharing for health insurance benefits and for health services, with varying degrees of success; in a number of instances, these efforts to shift some of the cost back to the employee have led to prolonged labor disputes.

Many employers, acting through their insurance intermediaries, have initiated stringent utilization review methods, often employing the new utilization review and control companies that have sprung up for this purpose. After a rather slow start, companies have been strongly encouraging their employees to move into health maintenance organizations and managed care programs of one kind or another; in the case of mental health benefits, some employers have virtually removed the individual fee-for-service aspects of mental health coverage and have substituted managed mental health programs for the entire mental health benefit. Finally, in geographic areas where particular employers exercise control over a significant share of the health care market by reason of the number of their employees, employers have become more active in seeking direct contracts with individual providers at competitive prices for selected high-cost (and usually high-technology) procedures.

Impact of Payors' Actions on Providers/Actions Taken by Providers to Adapt to Payor Efforts

All of these activities by the payors to reduce or control their expenditures have not gone unnoticed by health care providers, particularly physicians and hospitals. In each case, the providers have reacted exactly as one might expect: they have looked for ways to reduce their operating cost or to increase their revenues from other sources.

In the case of hospitals, the change to a DRG system of reimbursement by Medicare has been a strong incentive for improved operational efficiency. This has meant a general downsizing of hospitals and their staffs and has prompted a major attempt by most hospitals to manage their resources and activities more carefully. Hospitals have invested significant amounts of money in new information systems that allow them to identify their operating costs more accurately at the source and to monitor their cost variations more easily. These systems also allow hospital managers to make better, more informed judgments about allocations of resources to services that are more likely to generate increased revenues.

At the same time, hospitals have realized that they are participating in an increasingly competitive marketplace, one in which other hospitals are now seen as competitors. Hospitals have developed active marketing and advertising programs to seek new "business" and have worked diligently to develop new "product lines" (new types of services that can attract new patients and/or physicians).

In many instances, hospitals have begun to work more closely with their medical staffs to develop joint ventures; these are undertaken both to attract new business to the physician and the hospital and to strengthen the attachment of physicians to their hospitals. In many instances, hospitals and their medical staffs have developed new types of group-practice arrangements that will allow the hospitals to seek contracts from health maintenance organizations on behalf of physicians and the hospitals together. Indeed, the modern large hospital without some type of organized mechanism by which hospital and physician can seek outside contracts, is seen as a weak and noncompetitive institution that may eventually suffer badly in an aggressively marketed health care system.

At the same time as hospitals are being affected by payors' actions, individual physicians are being affected as well. As physicians see more and more of their fee-for-service patients being siphoned off to HMOs and other types of managed care programs, these physicians feel forced to sign contracts with such programs to accept their enrollees. Often the physicians feel that if they do not participate in these contracted programs, they may eventually find themselves with fewer patients or none at all.

In the same fashion, physicians may purchase and operate various types of ancillary services, such as clinical laboratories, diagnostic imaging centers, home health agencies, and the like; they may operate these as joint ventures with other physicians or perhaps even with hospitals. At the same time, other physicians are adding various types of laboratory or other testing services in their offices, performing those ancillary services themselves that previously had been sent out of the physicians' offices.

Just as hospitals are feeling the need to draw closer to their medical staffs, individual physicians are beginning to feel the need to draw closer to their hospitals. The medical staffs of many hospitals have taken the lead in developing parallel medical service organizations that are intended to allow hospitals and physicians to enter into business and contractual relations together with outside groups. Though these types of hospital–physician joint medical care organizations would have been unlikely 10 years ago, they are now a well-accepted part of the hospital landscape for physicians. In some instances, the financial strength and vigor of these organizations is serving as a means of actually attracting new physicians to the medical staffs of individual hospitals.

In addition to physicians and hospitals, other types of providers are scrambling energetically to maintain their level of economic return, as well as their share of the marketplace. Individual practitioners such as physical therapists and nurses, who previously might have only been employed by institutions, are now developing new outpatient and homecare service programs that they can own and operate themselves. These include home health agencies that provide nursing services, physical therapy, nutrition services, etc. as well as specialized types of programs to deal with problems or patient groups, such as work-related injuries in worker compensation programs. The fact that these particular health professionals are less well placed to develop new types of business enterprises and services than physicians has constrained these efforts somewhat but has not held them back entirely.

Impact of Provider and Payor Actions on Patients and Communities/Actions Taken by Patients and Communities to Adapt

As might be expected, as the payors and the providers move to adapt to changing environments, patients and communities have felt the impact of their actions and they have attempted to adapt too. Unfortunately, in our system of health care, individual patients and their communities are least able to protect themselves from the actions of payors and providers.

The rising costs of health care have had several effects on patients and communities, either directly or through the actions of payors and providers. The costs of health insurance have soared and individuals have felt that effect either in the cost of their insurance coverage (if they are paying for their own insurance) or in the cost of their share of the insurance premium (if their employer pays for most of it). The individual's share of medical and hospital payments (that portion not covered or only partially covered by insurance) has also increased as the total amount of the bill has increased.

Not only has the price of health insurance coverage gone up, the availability of insurance, at any price, has changed. Many individuals have found that they cannot purchase health insurance, either because of previous medical conditions or because of limited small group acceptance by many major health insurance carriers. Individuals are increasingly reluctant to change jobs if they are covered for medical care at one job but are uncertain about the range of coverage at another. As has been well documented by a number of researchers, the number of uninsured has increased significantly in recent years; what has not been as well documented has been the increase in under-insurance of those people whose policies are no longer as broad or as beneficial as in the past.

Communities have found themselves affected by the changes in health care as well. With many state Medicaid programs reducing eligibility for health insurance coverage, the burden of providing care to those who were previously covered now falls to the local government health care system. This has resulted in increased financial burdens for these communities as well as serious overcrowding and diminished efficiency at local government health facilities. In some communities,

the rising costs of health insurance coverage are said to have contributed to the loss of individual businesses or the decision of businesses to discontinue providing insurance. In other communities, there have been forced closings of important public services, such as trauma centers or mental health services, in both the public and private sectors, because of economic pressures on these services.

The rising cost of health care and decreased access for some people has also made these subjects important items in public debate and political campaigns. After the 1991 Pennsylvania senatorial election, it was said that the candidate's position on national health insurance was a positive force in his being elected. In the presidential campaigns of 1992, health care and health insurance "reform" received a great deal of attention (if not action) both by the candidates and by the public. In numerous labor union contract negotiations, changes in health insurance benefit packages were major items and caused difficulties and sometimes actual strike actions.

While it cannot be said that the American people are of one mind about what to do with regard to health care or health insurance reform, it is clear that the public is increasingly knowledgeable and concerned about the rise in health care costs. It is also increasingly obvious that various segments of the American public who can band together and protect themselves from the impact of payor and provider actions are doing so, further fragmenting the system and its participants. Just as with the rest of the U.S. health care system, the American public and its communities are learning that they have to protect themselves in whatever way they can.

Impact of All the Combined Changes on Health Care Costs in the U.S. Health Care System

As was mentioned at the beginning of the chapter, the great irony of all these changes and activities is that they have not resulted in any more significant control of health care costs than previously. It is clear that individual efforts and realignments have had at least some effect on keeping the rise of health care costs from being even worse than it is at present, but it must be admitted that none of the cost-control efforts that have been made, either individually or collectively, has resulted in an orderly, effective system for containing future costs. It is quite clear that costs will continue to rise rapidly and that the "gaming" nature of the individual parts of the health care system will continue, as these individual parts struggle to ensure their survival. Indeed, it seems likely that the dynamics of U.S. health care will continue to be determined by efforts to either contain health care costs or protect and maximize reimbursement.

The dilemma facing future health care in the United States is that there seems to be no relief in sight from the present system, while at the same time there is no agreement on the establishment of a new and better system. Workers in the health care system in the future will continue to be forced to adopt survival tactics until some new type of structure comes along that allows all parties to participate in broader, systemwide solutions. It seems clear that the energies of many capable, well-trained, well-intentioned health care professionals will be focused on fixing leaks in the lifeboats rather than on launching new ships.

This vision of the American health care system is admittedly a pessimistic one, just at a time when the public should be optimistic about the things that can be accomplished in health care today. At the very moment when the scientific and technological side of health and medical care stands poised to develop and deliver major new breakthroughs in treatment and prevention, the financing and delivery side of the system is facing its worst strains. Unfortunately, until the financing and service delivery aspects of health care can be improved, much of the potential of the marvelous new science and technology may remain unfulfilled.

There is simply no way that this society can begin to unleash the potential of these new tech-

nologies; there is simply no way that this society can address the need for newer types of services such as long-term care, mental health services, gene therapy, and other molecular biology advances, unless a way of controlling the rising cost of care is found for the services that we have now. The rise in the cost of the present array of services will soak up so much added revenue that there will be none left to permit movement into new services of any kind. At the same time, individual participants in the system are becoming increasingly frightened about moving away from protecting their part of the system, since they see no better alternative on the horizon and have no desire to commit professional suicide for themselves and their institutions.

It must be stated very directly and firmly that the health care system is bogged down in problems that it did not create by itself and that it cannot solve by itself either. It is clear that the larger society must understand that the system has followed a series of mixed messages from the public in its desire for the best in health care and has found itself caught in a continuous, circular, self-repeating situation that it cannot break. Indeed, the *only* way in which solutions can probably be obtained is for society to come to grips with some important questions, such as the limits of its ability to provide care and its willingness to assume a more supervisory and even regulatory control of a system that can no longer handle its own problems. The ideal circumstance would be for the various parts of the American health care system to come together voluntarily to solve those broad systematic problems that no one can solve separately, but that seems highly unlikely.

The future challenge to health care professionals is to understand the dynamics driving the health care system (the rapidly rising costs of care) and to work at several levels to improve the situation. On one level, *every* health care professional must understand that control of rising health care costs is his or her *primary* responsibility. On a broader level, each health care professional must work in his or her individual practices, institutions, and programs to contain health care costs in an organizational manner. Finally, on the broadest (and possibly most important) level, each health care professional must work actively to make society at large understand its responsibility to create new social forms of organization, supervision, and per- haps even control of the health care system itself. The people of the United States and their various representatives can no longer expect the system to solve its own problems; they must provide a new means and a new format for approaching these problems and creating new solutions.

Index